I dedicate this book to the thousands of practical nursing students who shared their lives with me over several decades, teaching me resilience, as they overcame amazing obstacles to become LPNs. They have left an indelible mark on my life. I am humbled by their accomplishments, despite the struggles they have faced, and thank them for the many lessons learned.

In addition, I dedicate this book to my parents for instilling in me an "open mind," a desire always to do more, a zest for life, and a love of family and friends. My accomplishments would be small if not for the support and love of my husband, Duane; our boys, CJ and David; our girls who joined our family, Hilary and Stephanie; and the special girl who has stolen my heart, our granddaughter, Kamy. I only hope she has the opportunity to be influenced by people who will expand her thinking, as my nursing students and colleagues have done for me over the years.

Patty Knecht

Acknowledgments

- Nancy O'Brien, Executive Content Strategist, Nursing, who convinced me that I could find the time and would enjoy the challenge. Early on, Nancy's encouragement was invaluable.
- Heather Rippetoe and Heather Bays, Senior Content Development Specialists, and Lisa Bushey, Project Manager, were lifelines, providing wisdom and direction regarding format, editorial issues, and organization hints. Their words were encouraging and provided timely feedback to countless queries.
- Signe Hill and Helen Howlett, the original authors, whose work provided a strong foundation for countless students and provided a solid foundation for myself as a new author. I am grateful for their dedication and continual improvement of this textbook over the years.
- Reviewers provided critical feedback, suggesting additions and deletions to this edition. This has enhanced the applicability of the textbook to meet students' learning needs in an evolving health care system. I thank them for their candor and consider them partners in this project.
- The faculty, staff, students, and graduates of the Chester County Intermediate Unit Practical Nursing Program, who provided continual support and challenged my thinking, resulting in continual pursuit of knowledge.
- Mentors at Penn State University, National League for Nursing, and many others who listened, supported, and facilitated my growth in writing skills. Although painful, without all of you, this opportunity would have never occurred. Many thanks!
- Michael S. Hill for his earlier contributions to Chapter 22: *Finding a Job: What Works, What Doesn't*. Many of his concepts continue to be relevant and are contained in this new edition.
- A special thanks to my husband, Duane. His positive attitude empowers me to accept new challenges and reach high. As he emerged as a great cook, he ensured I was nourished to continue this important work. Without his support, I might have quit on several occasions.
- To our children: "You are the wind beneath my wings." I marvel at the obstacles you overcame and who you have become and hope that your lives will be filled with love and happiness rooted in family, a rewarding career, and a passion for what is good and just.

Reviewers

Teresa J. Brooks, RN, BSN, MSN
Assistant Professor
Academic/Clinical Instructor
Iowa Lakes Community College
Spirit Lake, Iowa

Shelley Eckvahl, MSN, RN
Professor
Nursing
Chaffey College
Rancho Cucamonga, California

Beverly S. Ferguson, MSN, BSN, RN
Practical Nursing Instructor
Traviss Career Center
Lakeland, Florida

Louise S. Frantz, MHA, Ed, BSN, RN
Practical Nursing Program Coordinator
Pennsylvania State University—Berks Campus
Reading, Pennsylvania

Sharon Ivy Gordon, MSN, RN, CNOR(E)
Practical Nursing Program Director
Health Education Center
Penn State Lehigh Valley
Allentown, Pennsylvania

Kimberley Kelly, RN, BSN, MSN
President/School Director
The Vocational Nursing Institute
Houston, Texas

Lauralee S. Krabill, MBA, RN-BC, CNOR
Director of Allied Health and School of Practical Nursing
Sandusky Career Center
Sandusky, Ohio

Donald A. Laurino, MSN, CCRN, CMSRN, PHN, RN-BC
Lead Instructor
American Career College at St. Francis
Lynwood, California

Kyra McCoy, RN
Nursing Program Director
Edmonds Community College
Lynnwood, Washington

Betty Jo Mitchell, RN
Child Health Consultant
Dryades YMCA
New Orleans, Louisiana

Sandra A. Rank, MSN, RN
Program Administrator
Auburn Practical Nursing Program
Auburn Career Center
Concord Township, Ohio

Christine Sproles, RN, MSN
Nursing Instructor
Fortis Institute Nursing
Pensacola, Florida

Sarah E. Whitaker, DNS, RN
Consultant
Real Nurses Agency
Memphis, Tennessee

Elizabeth Woodward RN, BSN
Nursing Program Coordinator
State Fair Community College
Eldon, Missouri

Nancy York, RN-BC
Director
District 1199c Training and Upgrading Fund PN
  Program
Philadelphia, Pennsylvania

ELSEVIER

3251 Riverport Lane
St. Louis, Missouri 63043

SUCCESS IN PRACTICAL/VOCATIONAL NURSING:
FROM STUDENT TO LEADER, EIGHTH EDITION

ISBN: 978-0-323-35631-2

Nursing Diagnoses. From Herdman, T.H., Kamitsura, S. (Eds.) (2014) NANDA International, Inc. Nursing diagnoses: definitions & classifications 2015-2017, (ed. 10). Kaukauna, WI: NANDA International, Inc. Published by John Wiley & Sons, Ltd. Companion website: www.wiley.com/go/nursingdiagnoses.

In order to make safe and effective judgments using NANDA-I diagnoses, it is essential that nurses refer to the definitions and defining characteristics of the diagnoses listed in this work.

NCLEX®, NCLEX-RN®, and NCLEX-PN® are registered trademarks and service marks of the National Council of State Boards of Nursing, Inc.

Previous editions copyrighted 2013, 2009, 2005, 2001, 1997, 1993, 1988.

Library of Congress Cataloging-in-Publication Data

Names: Knecht, Patricia (Patricia A.), author. | Preceded by (work): Hill, Signe S. Success in practical/vocational nursing.
Title: Success in practical/vocational nursing : from student to leader / Patricia (Patty) Knecht.
Description: 8th edition. | St. Louis, Missouri : Elsevier, [2017] | Preceded by Success in practical/vocational nursing : from student to leader / Signe S. Hill, Helen Stephens Howlett. 7th ed. c2013. | Includes bibliographical references and index.
Identifiers: LCCN 2016016044 | ISBN 9780323356312
Subjects: | MESH: Nursing, Practical | Nurse's Role | Nursing Theory | Vocational Guidance
Classification: LCC RT62 | NLM WY 195 | DDC 610.73/0693—dc23 LC record available at https://lccn.loc.gov/2016016044

Content Strategist: Nancy O'Brien
Content Development Manager: Laurie Gower
Content Development Specialist: Heather Bays
Publishing Services Manager: Jeff Patterson
Project Manager: Lisa A. P. Bushey
Designer: Renee Duenow

Printed in the U.S.A.

Last digit is the print number: 9 8 7 6 5 4

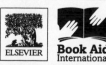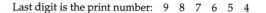

8 EDITION

Success in Practical/ Vocational Nursing

From Student to Leader

Patricia (Patty) Knecht, PhD, RN, ANEF
Chair, Division of Nursing
Immaculata University
Immaculata, Pennsylvania;
Formerly, Director of Practical Nursing
Chester County Intermediate Unit,
    Practical Nursing Program
Downingtown, Pennsylvania

ELSEVIER

LPN Threads

Standard LPN Threads series features incorporated into *Success in Practical/Vocational Nursing: From Student to Leader*, 8th edition make it easy for students to move from one book to the next in the fast-paced and demanding LPN/LVN curriculum. The following features are included in the LPN Threads:

- A **reading-level evaluation** is performed on all LPN texts to increase the consistency among chapters and ensure that the text is easy to understand.
- **Full-color design, cover, photos,** and **illustrations** are visually appealing and pedagogically useful.
- **Objectives** (numbered) begin each chapter, provide a framework for content, and are important in providing the structure for the TEACH Lesson Plans for the textbook.
- **Key Terms** with phonetic pronunciations and page number references are listed at the beginning of each chapter. Key terms appear in color in the chapter and are defined briefly, with full definitions in the **Glossary.** The goal is to help the student reader with limited proficiency in English to develop a greater command of the pronunciation of scientific and nonscientific English terminology.
- A wide variety of **special features** relate to critical thinking, leadership and management, and more. Refer to the "To the Student and Instructor" section of this introduction on page ix for descriptions and examples of features from the pages of this textbook.
- **NCLEX Review Questions** and **Critical Thinking Scenarios** presented at the end of chapters give students opportunities to practice critical thinking and clinical decision-making skills with realistic student/patient scenarios.
- **Key Points** at the end of each chapter correlate to the objectives and serve as a useful chapter review.
- A full suite of **Instructor Resources,** including TEACH Lesson Plans, Lecture Outlines, and Power-Point Slides, Test Bank, Image Collection, and Open-Book Quizzes, is included on the Evolve site.
- In addition to consistent content, design, and support resources, these textbooks benefit from the advice and input of the **Elsevier LPN/LVN Advisory Board**.

LPN Advisory Board

To the Student and Instructor

I am excited to introduce you to the 8th edition of *Success in Practical/Vocational Nursing: From Student to Leader.* The changes and additions to this edition are based on formal and informal instructor and student feedback of the 7th edition. Their suggestions, emerging workforce and nursing education trends, and the evolving health care market have been carefully evaluated and formed the basis for the updates and new chapters included in this edition.

Following in Hill and Howlett's footsteps, information provided is focused on realistic information and presented in a concise format. Bullets, charts, and figures are used to facilitate the ability to scan the information when pressed for time. Scenarios and interactive exercises are used to engage students and provide opportunities for peer-to-peer and peer-to-faculty dialogue, both in and out of the classroom. NCLEX-style questions were developed to provide the student with quick feedback regarding comprehension of content knowledge, followed by critical thinking scenarios designed to facilitate application of knowledge and to foster robust discussion. The introductory scenarios included in some chapters are purposely placed to provide context for the upcoming reading and, it is hoped, trigger the student's sense of inquiry.

Updated and new content is woven throughout all of the chapters. However, three chapters—Chapter 3: Community Resource; Chapter 18: Work Force Trends: How to Find a First Job You Will Love; and Chapter 19: Licensure and Regulation: Know Your State Practice Act—are infused with new concepts, providing to the students and faculty content that sparks realistic, straightforward conversation regarding the value of the LPN, workforce trends, state regulations governing the LPN practice, and key information critical to safe practice and NCLEX PN® success. In addition, Chapter 3 provides an in-depth discussion to assist the student in identifying community resources. The resources discussed can be a current lifeline for the practical nursing students and also provide the required LPN knowledge to assist patients and families in the near future.

Most importantly, this textbook has been designed as a journey. The journey begins as a student and never ends. As nurses we are continually learning and striving to exceed our personal and professional expectations.

Leadership exists from the bedside to the boardroom. The realistic material presented in this textbook will assist you in becoming and growing as a leader. Best of luck as you study to become an LPN/LVN, a trusted, respected profession.

TEACHING AND LEARNING PACKAGE

We provide a rich, abundant collection of supplemental resources for both instructors and students.

FOR THE INSTRUCTOR

The comprehensive Evolve Resources provide a wealth of material to meet your teaching needs. Instructors will have access to all of the student resources, as well as the following:

- An ExamView Test Bank contains NCLEX-PN® Examination–style questions that include multiple-choice and alternate format item questions.
- TEACH PowerPoint Presentations (including Audience Response Questions) include approximately 1100 slides with annotations.
- TEACH Lesson Plans in the new updated TEACH format are based on textbook chapter objectives. These lesson plans provide a roadmap to link and integrate all parts of the educational package and can be modified or combined to meet your scheduling and teaching needs.
- An Open-Book Quiz is provided for each chapter in the textbook.

FOR THE STUDENT

- Evolve Student Learning Resources include NCLEX-PN® Examination–style interactive review questions that test your knowledge and help you prepare for licensure.
- Helpful Phrases for Communicating in English and Spanish are also provided.
- Additional ancillary material is included to supplement the content of the chapters.

I welcome your comments and suggestions. You can contact me in care of the customer service department at Elsevier (support.elsevier.com). I wish you well in your school year.

Patty Knecht

Reading and Review Tools

Objectives introduce the chapter topics.

Key Terms are listed with page number references, and difficult medical, nursing, or scientific terms are accompanied by simple phonetic pronunciations. Key terms are considered essential to understanding chapter content and are defined within the chapter. Key terms are in color the first time they appear in the narrative and are briefly defined in the text, with complete definitions in the Glossary.

Each chapter ends with a *Get Ready for the NCLEX-PN®Examination!* section that includes (1) **Key Points** that reiterate the chapter objectives and serve as a useful review of concepts, (2) a list of **Additional Resources**, (3) a set of **Review Questions for the NCLEX-PN®** **Examination** with answers located in the back of the book, and (4) **Scenarios** with answers located on the Evolve site.

References and Suggested Readings in the back of the book provide resources for enhancing knowledge.

CHAPTER FEATURES

Keep in Mind Boxes—introduce the reader to the underlying theme of the chapter.

Critical Thinking Boxes—encourage problem-solving for both academic and personal situations.

Coordinated Care Boxes—are presented in four ways to introduce the reader to leadership and management in nursing:
- Management Tools—provide practical instructions and resources and have the reader apply learned concepts to specific situations.
- Management Hints—provide tips for handling management situations.
- Leadership Activities—provide students with exercises to practice their leadership skills. Instructions and needed resources are provided.
- Leadership Hints—give helpful hints to follow and remember when in a leadership situation.

Professional Pointers—give readers advice on nursing best practices in the professional arena.

Try This Boxes—challenge students to imagine, visualize, and think outside the box.

Contents

Personal Resources of an Adult Learner

Objectives

On completing this chapter, you will be able to do the following:

1. Identify yourself as a traditional or nontraditional adult learner.
2. Identify personal resources that will facilitate your success in a practical/vocational nursing program.
3. Using your birth date, identify your generation and characteristics of this generation viewed as a resource for success in a practical/vocational nursing program.
4. Identify factors and issues that could interfere with your use of resources in the practical/vocational nursing program and strategies to address these factors and issues.
5. Discuss personal responsibility for learning and active participation in the learning process.
6. Discuss your rights as an adult learner.
7. Identify various types of evaluation used in a practical/vocational nursing program.
8. Create a personal plan, inclusive of your unique resources, aimed at successfully completing a practical/vocational nursing program within the designated time frame.

Key Terms

active learning (ĂK-tĭv LĔRN-eng)
constructive evaluation (kŏn-STRŬ K-tĭvē ē-VĂL-ū-ā-shŭn)
facilitator (fă-SĬL-ĭ-TĂ-tŏr)
First Amendment (ă-MĔND-mĕnt)
formal education (FŎR-măl)
generalization (GĔN-ĕ r-ă-lĭ-ZĂ- shŭn)
generational personality (GĔN-ĕr-Ā- shŭn ăl)
informal education (ĭn-FŎR-măl)
learner (LĔR-nĕr)

paradigm (PĂR-ă-DĪM)
performance evaluation (pĕr-FŎR-măntz ĭ-văl-ū-Ā-shŭn)
positive mental attitude (PŎS-ĭ-tĭv MĔN-tăl ĂT-ĭ-tood)
referral (rĭ-FŬR-ăl)
returning adult learner (rē-TŬRN-ĭng ă-DŬLT LĔRN-ĕr)
self-directed learner (SĔLF-dĭ-RĔCT-ĕd LĔRN-ĕr)
self-evaluation (SĔLF-ē-VĂL-yoo-ā-shŭn)
teaching (TĔCH-ĭng)
traditional adult learner

CJ, Stephanie, Katie, and Hilary have just finished their orientation for the Success Practical Nursing Program. As they exit the building, they overhear two other students, David and Olivia, who appear to be recent high school graduates, talking about the age, cultural, and educational differences of the class. David states, "Those older students asked way too many questions and could barely fill out the information online. I just wanted to get out of there." Stephanie approaches David and states, "Hi, David, I am one of those older people. I will try to be careful with my many questions but I love how diverse the class is—I was afraid I was going to be the only older student. It will be interesting to see how we all learn together. I look forward to learning with you." Shrugging his shoulders, David walks to his car. "Well," CJ states, "being a realist, let's hope for the best. It seems like understanding yourself and each other is critical to your personal and the program's success. All of us being different can be a strength, if we understand each other and keep communication open. Let's hope for low drama and keep it positive."

As you read the chapter, think about these students' comments. What knowledge will you develop to help you better understand yourself and others? Learning as a team is powerful. Remember, nursing is a team sport. Your educational journey with your team is beginning . . .

THE ADULT LEARNER AND RESOURCE MANAGEMENT

As an adult learner, resource management is a key to success. A successful person/student knows their key resources, where to find them, and when and how to use them effectively. Unfortunately, we often neglect to engage our resources in a timely fashion. We have all heard the expression "too little, too late." The chapters in Unit 1 are designed to assist you in creating a strong plan to engage your resources "just in time," ensuring success. Understanding your role as an adult learner, including your unique personal attributes, is one of your most valued resources. Self-discovery as an adult learner is a key first step to success. Let's start by understanding the different types of adult learners.

The adult learner (one who acquires knowledge and skills) comes in all ages, and it is possible to have **learners** from five generations in your nursing class. Depending on birth year, generational groups can be characterized. Time frames and names for the five generations vary among authors, but each generation is separated by approximately 20 years (Box 1-1).

Box 1-1   The Five Generations

- Matures (The Silent Generation) born 1925 and 1945
- Baby Boomers (Boomers) born between 1946 and 1964
- Generation X (Gen X) born between 1965 and 1980
- Generation Y (Millennials/Net Generation) born between 1981 and 1994
- Generation Z born after 1994

Data from Halfer D, Saver C: Bridging the generation gaps. Nursing Spectrum/Nurse Week, 2008; Riggs CJ: Multiple generations in the nursing workplace: part I. *J Contin Educ Nurs, 44*(3), 105-6, 2013.

Try This

The Five Generations

Using Box 1-1, identify your generation.

People born around the same time generally develop a **generational personality** of how they think and what they value. This personality is shaped by a common history of cultural events, images, and experiences. Income, religion, education, and geography also influence your generational personality. Understanding your generational perspective and the views of different generations will improve your communication and collaboration with your classmates, faculty, mentors, and colleagues.

Your goal is to be aware of each generation's shared experiences. Avoid stereotyping individuals of a specific generation. A stereotype is a false assumption. It is an expectation that all individuals within a specific group will act exactly the same because they are members of that group. Stereotypes ignore the individual differences that occur within a specific group, for example, a generational group. See Box 1-2 for characteristics of each generation.

Box 1-2   Characteristics of the Five Generations

TRADITIONALIST (THE SILENT GENERATION)
- Depending on birth year, generational personalities may be shaped by the Great Depression, World War II, and/or the Korean War.
- Are more conservative, prefer formal titles, are more formal with intrapersonal interactions, seek conformity.
- Consider work an obligation. Prefer one-to-one meetings and formal memos. Do not like ambiguity or change, prefer to learn in formal, structured ways, oriented to the past but are adaptable.
- Digital immigrants. May be reluctant to use advanced technology; and need more time and hands-on to learn modern technology devices and protocols.

BABY BOOMERS
- Depending on birth year, generational personalities may be shaped by Watergate, the Vietnam War, the space race, civil rights, women's liberation, and the assassinations of John and Robert Kennedy and Martin Luther King.
- Dedicated, highly motivated and hard-working, idealistic.
- Prefer learning in a relaxed, organized, and respectful atmosphere; like group discussions.
- Digital immigrants and have varying technology skills.

GENERATION X (GEN X)
- Depending on birth year, generational personality may be shaped by the Challenger explosion, the end of the Cold War, MTV, AIDS, Google, Amazon, and dual career households.

- Accept diversity, less judgmental, pragmatic (practical), flexible, self-reliant (had Boomer parents), multitask well, used to change, informal.
- View work as a challenge and opportunity to make changes in the world. Intolerant of "busywork," like small chunks of information, prefer self-study.
- Digital immigrants and are technically literate.

GENERATION Y (MILLENNIALS)
- Depending on birth year, generational personality may be shaped by Columbine, 9/11, the Clinton scandal, and the Afghanistan and Iraq wars.
- Dynamic, confident, straightforward, opinionated, optimistic, sociable, embrace change, multitask, like group discussion.
- View work as a means to an end and have a sense of entrepreneurialism.
- More tolerant of people different from them; for example, race and sexual orientation.
- Digital natives (Net Generation); grew up using cell phones and computers.

GENERATION Z
- Generational personality is influenced using technology and always being highly connected.
- Prefer using smart phones and would rather text than talk.
- Desire collaboration, are creative and want to impact the world.
- Digital natives.

Data from Halfer D, Saver C: Bridging the generation gaps. *Nursing Spectrum/Nurse Week*, 2008; Hartner K: Generational diversity. *ADVANCE Newsmagazines for LPNs*, February 20, 2007. http://lpn.advanceweb.com/Common/Editorial/PrintFriendly.aspx; Olson M: The millennials: first year in practice. *Nursing Outlook* 57:10-7, 2009; Billings D, Halstead J: Teaching in nursing: a guide for faculty, St. Louis, 2009, Elsevier/Saunders; Mehallow C: Generational conflict in nursing: how to relate to colleagues across generations. http://career-advice.monster.com/in-the-office/workplace-issues/generational-conflict-in-nursing/article.aspx; Riggs CJ: Multiple generations in the nursing workplace: part I. *J Contin Educ Nurs, 44*(3), 105-6, 2013.

Try This

Your Generational Personality

Using Box 1-2, Characteristics of the Five Generations, identify the characteristics of your generation that do/do not apply to you. Discuss with a classmate or family member generational characteristics that cause you to be judgmental. Seek to understand why this characteristic is viewed as important to the respective generational group.

The **traditional adult learner** comes to an educational program directly from high school or as a transfer student (i.e., from another program of study). They are in transition from late adolescence to young adulthood. In addition to their own developmental tasks, these students are being propelled into situations of responsibility for others. Traditional adult learners grew up in a digital, wireless world and are known as the "Net Generation/Millennials."

The **returning adult learner** has been out of school for several years. Many of these learners have not taken any courses since high school. Returning adult learners include Generation Xers, Baby Boomers, and Matures. Returning adult students are experiencing many different life transitions and have diverse reasons for enrolling in nursing school. Perhaps an employer shut down a business, or a layoff occurred resulting in a need for job training. In addition, a change in marital status, children leaving the household, change in the health of a spouse, or an impending retirement might have created a need for a stable income source, including health insurance benefits. Lastly, recent retirement may also have provided the time to pursue personal passions. Despite these diverse reasons, a common theme prevails across generations, simply stated as, "I always wanted to be a nurse." Because of valued life and work experiences, returning adult learners have built a strong foundation for the personal commitment and transitions needed in nursing school and practical/vocational nursing. Complex lives, inclusive of competing demands from grown children and aging parents, can contribute to the stress of nursing school.

A subset of the returning adult learner are those adult learners with prior education beyond high school. This learner shares some of the characteristics of both traditional and returning adult learners. However, this adult learner might have technical school or college experience or an undergraduate or graduate degree in a discipline other than nursing. Depending on the level of academic success and degree of program completion, this learner may have a strong academic skill set. However, in some cases, this adult learner has had limited success in the academic world and often questions their abilities. It is common that adult learners who have been unsuccessful in many other types of postsecondary programs can excel in a practical/vocational nursing program when academic and social support services are readily available and easily accessible. Reasons for choosing to enroll in the practical/vocational nursing program include the following:

- Desire to change careers
- Attraction to nursing
- Desire to acquire new job skills
- Lack of financially sustainable employment in the area for which the person has a degree
- Strong projected job demand in practical/vocational nursing

Regardless of the reason for enrolling in the 9-month to 1-year practical/vocational nursing program, most learners find this program meets their needs in both time and cost. The diversity of the learners is a benefit to practical/vocational nursing programs. Nursing in general and practical/vocational nursing in particular are challenged to build a diverse nursing workforce to meet the needs of our changing demographics in the United States. Learning together with students from diverse backgrounds contributes positively to building a culturally competent skill set.

Critical Thinking

Which Type of Adult Learner Am I?

Which type of adult learner are you? Survey your classmates. Determine which ones consider themselves to be traditional or nontraditional. Identify different strengths that you can share with each other.

FORMAL AND INFORMAL EDUCATIONAL EXPERIENCES

Generalizations can be made about each type of learner. Keep in mind that generalizations are broad, sweeping statements. The characteristics of each type of adult learner are not found in every individual.

- Traditional adult learners are accustomed to **formal education**. The practical/vocational nursing program in a vocational-technical school, junior college, or private school is an example of a program of formal education.
- Nontraditional adult learners might not have been in a classroom for some time or may have recently graduated from college. In either case, they have been learning. However, most often their education has been informal. Examples of their informal educational experiences include learning new technology for personal and business use, developing time management and organizational skills while managing an office or household and leading a community volunteer event. These experiences will be invaluable when learning new material.

◎ Try This

Informal Educational Experiences

List at least five informal educational experiences you have had since high school.

1.
2.
3.
4.
5.

How will these informal educational experiences positively impact your success in nursing school?

GEARED FOR SUCCESS

All adult learners have strengths that assist them in succeeding in the practical/vocational nursing program.

Traditional adult learners:

- Are at their prime physically, are filled with energy and stamina, and often have fewer out-of-school responsibilities to distract them from their studies.
- Are experts at educational routine and have been given the opportunity to develop reading, writing, studying, and test-taking skills.
- Are digital natives who have always had cell phones and computers in their lives. They know how to register for classes and take tests online. When they need information, they "Google," and when they want to contact a friend, they send a text or instant message. They live by social media. Facebook, Instagram, LinkedIn, and gaming are everyday communication tools.

Nontraditional adult learners:

- May feel they have energy drain caused by their varying family responsibilities.
- Have had responsibilities and life experiences that help them relate well to new learning, make sense out of it, and get the point quickly. These serious learners are focused on classroom/clinical work.
- Are digital immigrants who have had to learn to live in a digital world. Some find it easy to adapt, but others may find it more difficult to do so. When these learners need information, they consider going to the library, seek out paper resources, and enlist children and younger friends to use technology. Communication with friends and family can vary greatly from using their landline, cell phone, or email. They are novices at social media and are learning daily how to improve communication via social media.
- Most are mature, motivated, and **self-directed learners** who have set goals for themselves. Many have made economic, personal, and family sacrifices to go back to school.

Depending on their level of academic success, they may have developed a strong academic skill set or have struggled and never really achieved academic success.

? Critical Thinking

Reasons I Can Succeed

Identify and list three attributes you possess that will help you succeed in the practical/vocational nursing program.

1.
2.
3.

LIABILITIES AND HIDDEN DANGERS

All adult learners are geared for success, and each group has its own strong points. However, each group also has some liabilities, things that could stand in the way of success. Identifying these liabilities is a key strategy required to develop a successful plan for success.

HIDDEN DANGER SHARED BY ALL ADULT LEARNERS

One of the greatest liabilities shared by all adult learners is the fear of failure. Fear of anything is a very strong motivator, but in a negative sense. Fear of failure in school is a feeling that usually develops as a result of past negative experiences with learning situations. Perhaps you did not do well in some high school or college classes. Maybe you did not study, studied the wrong way, or allowed yourself to be put down by teachers or professors in the past. Maybe you allowed yourself to underachieve because of peer pressure. Regardless of the cause, you may look at school in a negative, threatening way.

Your past is history. You have a clean slate ahead of you! Many adult learners with the same history and fears as you have succeeded in their educational programs. You are an adult in an adult educational experience. Begin to picture in your mind the rewards of succeeding in the practical/vocational nursing program. Forget the failures and setbacks you may have suffered in high school and other educational experiences. Replace your fear of failure with the desire for success. Keep your thoughts positive, and practice these positive thoughts continuously. Watch the content and tone of your thoughts and words. Negative thoughts and words can play like a song in your head. As surely as you learned this negative script, you can learn a positive script. However, it does take time. Replace your "I cannot" and "I never could" with "I want to," "I can," "I will," and "I am going to." Avoid dwelling on the past and look to the future. Go all the way with PMA: **positive mental attitude**. If you consistently expect to succeed, and combine this expectation with hard work in your studies, you *will* succeed. Did you know that your brain believes anything you tell it? If it learned to believe you could fail, it can also learn to believe you can succeed. Start today to engage in positive self-talk. Positive music lyrics can also help. Listen to lyrics such as "Fight Song" from Rachel Platten when you feel discouraged.

Surround yourself with positive peers. Sometimes students who may not have succeeded in other nursing programs or a previous nursing course may be your classmates. Active listening to this group of peers can be positive and assist you in avoiding common student pitfalls. However, remember that reasons for lack of academic success are varied, personal, and confidential. If negativism prevails, politely avoid these conversations. New beginnings are good for all!

DANGERS FOR THE TRADITIONAL ADULT LEARNER

The following examples of dangers for traditional adult learners are examples of generalizations. They may or may not apply to the traditional adult learners you know.

Grade Expectations

A grade of C on a test or for a nursing course surprises some traditional adult students because, despite the effort put into studying in high school, they always received A grades. The same studying routine will not lead to success in your nursing program.

Traditional adult learners often have fewer outside responsibilities to distract them from their studies. Some traditional adult students lack time-management skills or motivation when it comes to studying. Some may still be in the same habits they became comfortable with in high school. Study time required to master content in a practical/vocational nursing program is personal to each student. However, if you are accustomed to receiving an A in high school for minimal effort, you will typically not experience this reward in the practical/vocational nursing program.

Social Activities

Some traditional adult learners may allow social activities and recreation to compete with school and study time. In a 24/7/365 wired/wireless world, they are accessible at all times to friends and family through social media. They need to learn to "turn it off." Set limits by sharing your class and clinical schedules with family and friends, and restrict being contacted to emergencies only during those times. Develop awareness of the chance to get distracted when online and for valuable time to slip away. Be cognizant of the need for some down time daily, even if it is only 15 minutes. The need to clear your mind and reenergize is critical to your success.

Employment

The amount of time occupied by employment outside of school hours may be another interference for some traditional adult learners. Ask yourself, "How much of the time that I am employed outside of school is necessary for food, shelter, and other realistic expenses?" Many explanations can be given for the liabilities listed here for traditional adult learners. Some traditional adult learners may still be working at developing an awareness of who they are and what life is all about for them. Some may lack a sense of direction and have no clear goal or idea of what they really want to do in life. Some may lack inner motivation to be a practical/vocational nurse. These learners can succeed by taking responsibility for making decisions about priorities and personal use of time that will help them meet the goals they have established for themselves.

DANGERS FOR THE NONTRADITIONAL LEARNER

Physical

Nontraditional adult learners may recognize that they do not have a strong academic skill set. Their reading, writing, test-taking, and study skills may be rusty. Technology skills may pose even more of a challenge. Physical changes occur as adults age and can affect learning. The senses of vision and hearing are at their peak in the adolescent years and decline very gradually through the adult years. Energy level has also been reported to have decreased and impacted study time. As the decades go by, these adults may notice the need for more illumination when they read or perform skills in the clinical lab. Experiencing eye strain can contribute negatively to energy level. In addition, hearing in the classroom and when performing certain nursing skills may be a challenge. Learn to seek out solutions early. Assistive devices are available to address these issues.

Social and Family Responsibilities

Diverse and competing family, employee, and student roles need to be juggled effectively. These demands can come from husbands, wives, significant others, mothers, fathers, daughters, sons, grandparents, employees, and/or volunteers. Returning to school may result in feelings of guilt because they know it will affect their relationships and routines outside of school.

Because of their many roles, returning adult learners have more demands placed on them. Some families may not support the student's choice to continue their formal education. Spouses/significant others may object to the extra demands placed on them. Care of children and aging parents may provide a continual feeling of inadequacy. Common comments include: "I feel like I am not doing anything well" and "No one is happy, particularly me." Recognize and acknowledge this inherent struggle. Identify resources to assist and do not hesitate to reach out to confirm your feelings of frustration, guilt, and inadequacies before the stress level mounts.

Managing time will assist. Realistic goal setting is essential. Four hours of sleep nightly will not be a viable long-term plan for success.

All humans when faced with obstacles have thoughts of giving up at some point. The strategies in this book will assist you in recognizing that your feelings are normal, help you to learn to anticipate some of the usual roadblocks, and identify and implement quick solutions to keep you on the road to success. A solid realistic plan is the key.

Personal Needs for Improvement

Identify and list three things that could stand in your way of success in the practical/vocational nursing program.

1.
2.
3.

SPECIAL CHALLENGES FOR PRACTICAL/VOCATIONAL NURSING STUDENTS

No matter what type of adult learner you are, some learners have special challenges to success in practical/vocational nursing. Learners with a spouse/significant other at home may be extremely busy with school and family affairs. Learners with aging parents may be involved with their needs for assistance. Single parents may feel overwhelmed when the learner role is assumed in addition to all their other roles. It may be good for learners with spouses/significant others to imagine what it would be like to be a learner without these individuals to offer support.

Practical/vocational nursing students who speak English as their first language sometimes indicate the difficulty of course work and the amount of time it takes to complete assignments. It may be insightful for these learners to imagine being responsible for the same amount of course work when English is their second language. Learners who speak English as a second or additional language need to strive continually to understand content presented in a language that is different from their native tongue. Reading assignments need to be translated by these students to their native language to be understood. Taking a test requires extra effort, as these students may need to translate test directions and items to their native language for understanding before answering an item. This is comparable with presenting English-speaking learners with textbooks and tests written in Spanish or Russian with the need to translate both to English.

These learners described are typical of the demographic of a practical/vocational nursing student. It is important to remember there are approximately 700,000 licensed practical nurses (LPNs) in the United States (Health Resources and Services Administration [HRSA], 2014). Thus facing the preceding challenges is common, and many graduates have achieved success despite the great odds that needed to be overcome. They are a testimonial that success is within your reach, even if you are faced with these special challenges.

STRENGTHS OF ALL ADULT LEARNERS

All adult learners possess unique strengths. These strengths often are the opposite of the dangers

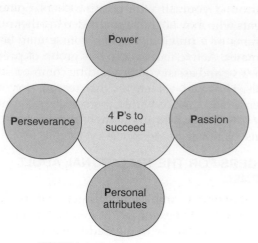

FIGURE 1-1 The four "*P*"s of success.

discussed above. Most importantly, each adult learner needs to recognize that you would not be accepted into a practical/vocational nursing program unless you were able to demonstrate the essential academic skills necessary for success. Couple this with passion, self-confidence, perseverance, physical health, and a good plan (inclusive of identified academic and social supports), and you are ready to soar to success. Focus on the four "*P*"s to create your personal plan for success (Figure 1-1). The four "*P*"s are Power, Passion, Perseverance, and Personal Attributes. Power is essential; belief in yourself and your ability to be successful is inherent to success. Passion fuels your inner drive when the barriers seem insurmountable, and perseverance ensures that you stay on track when exhaustion hits and all seems astray. Lastly, self-reflection to identify your personal attributes is essential to a realistic and successful plan. Personal attributes include finances, time, social supports, and academic skill set. An unrealistic evaluation of personal attributes, despite power, passion, and perseverance, can lead to an unsuccessful outcome resulting in course or program failure.

LEARNERS HAVE RIGHTS

As an American citizen, you need to start thinking about some fundamental rights that you have been granted through the U.S. Constitution that will affect you as a learner. The **First Amendment** gives you freedom of expression as long as what you want to express does not disrupt class or infringe on the rights of your peers. So when your instructor asks you to join in a discussion, do not be afraid to do so. Instructors want your input in a class session. They have no intention of holding your comments against you. The Fourteenth Amendment assures you due process. Due process means that if you are charged with a violation of policies or rules, you will be presented with evidence of your misconduct and will be entitled to state your position. So relax. The institution in which you are enrolled cannot terminate you at a whim, nor does it want to. It exists to help you succeed. A more detailed account of these two rights can probably be found in your school's student handbook. If you do not have a copy of the student handbook, download an online copy or obtain one from the student services department. An important learner's right is the right to have an organized curriculum and a responsible instructor who is prepared to teach it. You have the right to know the requirements of each course and how you will be graded for each course. Although your tuition and fees do not pay for all the services you receive through your school, you are the most important person in the educational system. You are the customer! You do not interfere with the instructor's or any staff's work; you are the focus of it.

RESPONSIBILITIES OF LEARNERS

The first responsibility of learners is to learn. The author of this book wants you to test your knowledge regarding the process of learning before you read any further. Read the following four statements and decide whether they are true or false. As the chapter continues, these statements will be discussed. You will be expected to check the accuracy of your responses. Remember, your answers are for your eyes only.

[?] Critical Thinking

Responsibilities of Learners

Read the following four statements, and indicate whether each is true or false.
1. The instructor has the responsibility for my learning.
2. If I fail, it is the responsibility of the instructor.
3. If I succeed, the credit for my success should go to the instructor.
4. My instructor has the responsibility to pass on to me all the information I will need to know in my career as a practical/vocational nurse.

TEACHING VERSUS LEARNING

Years ago, a wonderful thing happened in the area of adult education. Teachers were exposed to the difference between **teaching** and learning. Great emphasis was placed on the role of the learner. Changing emphasis from teaching to learning is called a **paradigm** (a way of thinking) shift. Learners need to be aware of the exciting world of learning and the roles of teaching and learning in that process. In doing so you will know what is expected of you as an adult learner.

Passive Learners

Many of us have had educational experiences in the past that encouraged dependency and passivity on the part of the learner. Think back to the educational experiences you have had. Did they involve sitting in classes in which the teacher did most of the talking and you just took notes? Did you view the teacher as someone who possessed knowledge and somehow was going to pass it on to you? And, if you did not pass, did you say, "The teacher flunked me"? When you think about it, these situations are characterized by the adjectives *dependent* and *passive*.

The last time you were dependent from necessity was when you were an infant. Even then you were far from passive. When you observe a 6-month-old infant, the spirit of inquiry is evident as they gaze to look up and watch a fan, reflect in the mirror and see their reflection, and listen intently as the sounds change on the television. We all inherently have a spirit of inquiry that resides within us. When you became a toddler, you became very independent and began to learn about the world in earnest. You very actively pursued your learning; that is, the acquiring of new knowledge and skills. And you did it with gusto! Now you are an adult learner. How unfair of an instructor to expect you to become dependent and passive in your learning. This is especially true because studies have proven that people learn best when they are actively involved in their own learning and have an interdependent relationship with the instructor.

Instructors—Facilitators of Learning

You have already learned that it is the instructor's responsibility to set up a curriculum. Your state's board of nursing dictates the core content of the curriculum in a school of nursing. It is then up to the faculty of your school to decide how that content will be included in the nursing program. Some practical/vocational programs might use the general structure of the National Council Licensure Examination for Licensed Practical Nurses (NCLEX-PN®) examination in developing a curriculum. Instructors act as **facilitators** of your learning. They are responsible for creating an environment in which learning can take place. They do this by arranging for a variety of activities and experiences, which trigger your spirit of inquiry. In addition, they provide access to academic resources to seek knowledge, discuss, debate, and make conclusions. A critical part of facilitation involves being available to you when you encounter questions and problems you cannot solve. Instructors also have the responsibility to evaluate learning. They do so by testing and observing learners.

As a student, you have not only the right but also the responsibility to talk to an instructor when you have a concern about your relationship with him or her. Under rules of assertiveness, always go to the source. Follow the chain of command to resolve your concerns. The same rule applies if you have a problem with a classmate. Approach the classmate, not another student.

Active Learning

To *learn* is to acquire knowledge and skills. The verb *acquire* means to obtain or gain by your own effort. As a learner in a practical/vocational nursing program, you need to be your own agent of knowledge and skill acquisition. You have the personal responsibility to acquire the knowledge and skills needed to be a practical/vocational nurse. **Active learning** is not a passive activity. As a learner, you must open yourself up, reach out, and stretch to gain knowledge and skills. To be successful, you must be personally involved in your learning. It is impossible for instructors to pour knowledge and skills into your head. You need to become self-directed and curious in your learning. You need to use critical-thinking skills to help you comprehend what you read in texts and journals, what you see on PowerPoint presentations, DVDs, online resources, and what you hear in class discussions. Instructors will not hover over you and guide your every step. Instructors are there to facilitate your learning and be a mentor and coach.

Do not expect the instructor to assume your skill for you, be your medical dictionary, or reteach Chapter 2 in *Anatomy and Physiology* because you did not have time to study. Instead, expect your instructor to observe you while you are trying to work through a difficult skill. The instructor will make suggestions and demonstrate a point here and there to help you along. If you are having trouble, expect your instructor to help you put a definition of a medical term in your own words. Expect the instructor to answer specific questions you may have about Chapter 2 in *Anatomy and Physiology*. These are the roles of teacher and learner and examples of their interdependency. If you are to learn and succeed in practical/vocational nursing, you need to become actively involved in your own learning. You say you are too old to learn? You say you cannot teach an old dog new tricks? Much study has been done in this area. To date, studies of adult learning clearly indicate that the basic ability to learn remains essentially unimpaired throughout the life span. Now review the answers to your true/false questions from the Critical Thinking exercise earlier in the chapter. Are there any answers you want to change before looking at the key?

1. *False.* You have the responsibility for your own learning. You must become actively involved in the learning process.
2. *False.* If you fail, it is your own fault. Adult educational programs are geared for success. You are geared for success. Although you could list many reasons why you might not succeed, the teacher failing you is not one of them. Learners sometimes allow themselves to fail.
3. *False.* When you succeed (and you are perfectly capable of doing so), only you can take credit for the success. You were the person who assumed responsibility for your own learning. You became actively involved in the learning process.
4. *False.* Instructors have had much experience in nursing. They do not know all the experiences you will have in your career as a practical/vocational nurse. Even if they did, there would be no time or way to transfer this knowledge to you. Instructors help learners learn how to learn. This is important in an ever-changing field such as nursing. Your instructors will encourage you to develop critical-thinking and problem-solving skills, which will enable you to handle new situations as they arise in your nursing career.

If you had no wrong answers, you should be an expert on learning. Now put your expertise to work for you. If you had one or more wrong answers, the author suggests you reread the "Teaching versus Learning" section in this chapter. Chapters 2, 5, and 19 will help you to become an active learner and a critical thinker and be successful in the practical/vocational nursing program, on NCLEX-PN®, and as a candidate for an LPN/Licensed Vocational Nurse (LVN) nursing position.

ROLE OF EVALUATION

The second responsibility of learners is to receive and participate in evaluation. Evaluation plays an important role in your education in the practical/vocational nursing program and throughout your career. You have set a goal to become a practical/vocational nurse. As the year goes on, your instructors will evaluate you in several different ways to determine whether or not you are progressing in the achievement of that goal. When you graduate, you will be evaluated periodically while on the job, sometimes as a means of determining whether or not you are to receive a salary increase. At other times you will be evaluated to see if you are functioning well enough to keep your job. Evaluation in the practical/vocational nursing program occurs in several areas: written tests, presentations, and evidenced-based papers and projects that measure your knowledge of theory and understanding of that knowledge, and **performance evaluations** that measure your ability to apply your knowledge in the clinical area. Performance evaluations occur in the clinical simulation lab and a diverse array of clinical settings. Evaluation in these areas is a learning experience in itself. Following evaluations, students should assess their strengths and weaknesses and create a plan to improve their knowledge and performance accordingly.

Theory Tests

Learners and instructors look at test results very differently. Learners focus on the number of items they answered correctly. They need to identify what they did right on a test so they can apply the process of getting the right answer to future tests and apply this information in the clinical area. In addition, learners are often only focused on the grade. In a nursing program, identifying knowledge that you have not conquered is essential to your eventual success on the NCLEX-PN exam. Thus instructors often focus on the specific items the learner(s) got wrong. Wrong items indicate critical knowledge the learner does not have. Understanding why each answer choice was incorrect is also a great learning experience. Do not just ask for your grades. Try to arrange time with your instructors to review your tests. It is inaccurate to say that grades do not count. You must earn the minimum grade established by your nursing program. But consider this: If you got 80% on a test, it means you did not answer 20% of the questions correctly. Now place yourself in the patient's slippers. What about the 20% of the test questions your nurse got wrong? Was it something the nurse should have known to care for you safely? Also, this 20% of information not learned may impact your ability to successfully pass the NCLEX-PN on the first attempt. For this reason, try to look at tests as learning experiences. Be as interested in your wrong answers as you are in your correct answers. Take time to look at your tests with the goal of understanding why the correct answers are correct and why the wrong answers you gave are wrong.

Clinical Performance Evaluations

The most meaningful evaluations you will receive during the year will be the performance evaluations given while you are in the clinical simulation lab and diverse clinical areas. Because these evaluations give you an opportunity for career and personal growth, understanding this form of evaluation and the responsibilities you have with regard to it is important. Clinical performance evaluations also provide an example of how to evaluate others in your expanded role.

In the clinical area, instructors will be observing you as you care for patients. They are observing you to discover the positive things you are doing to reach your goal of becoming a practical/vocational nurse. These behaviors are to be encouraged. They indicate that learning has taken place, you are applying your knowledge, and you are growing and progressing toward your goal. Instructors are also observing you to discover behaviors that stand in the way of reaching your goal. These behaviors are to be discouraged. Your instructor will update you daily on your progress in a verbal or written manner. At the end of a clinical rotation, you will receive a written performance evaluation during a conference with your clinical instructor.

From the start you need to look at performance evaluations as a two-sided coin. The instructor is on one side, and you are on the other. As part of their job, instructors have the responsibility of evaluating your performance. As a learner, you have the responsibility of being aware of your clinical behaviors. You are responsible for **self-evaluation**. Practical/vocational nursing students, at the time of graduation, should be able to look at their nursing actions and be aware of their strong behaviors and behaviors that need improvement. Developing the ability to be aware of one's behaviors begins with day one in the practical/vocational nursing program, including the simulation laboratory. A learner does not automatically have this skill. Learners must consistently work at viewing themselves objectively. Instructors will help in this area. For example, when learning how to make a bed, ask yourself, "Is the finished product as good as I had intended it to be when I started?" Do not wait for the instructor to identify areas of success or areas that need improvement. Peer learning and continual evaluation is a great strategy to implement in both the simulation lab and the clinical area. Each one of your peers will bring unique strengths and resources to the learning experience. View this as a resource and use it on a daily basis. For example, have a peer critique your lab procedure before the clinical skills evaluation by the instructor. Filming (if available) can be a powerful tool in the simulation lab. Direct observation of our skill performance encourages immediate focus to improve in identified weak areas and correct errors accordingly.

Professional Pointer

Objective awareness of one's own behaviors is an important skill to have as an employee.

Think back to when you received comments from your teachers and parents about your behavior in grade school and high school. How did you feel when you received these comments? Many people grow up with negative feelings about these episodes of criticism and even about the word itself. Criticism means evaluation. Some people attach a negative meaning to criticism and view it as a put-down.

The phrase "constructive criticism" may evoke negative feelings. The phrase "**constructive evaluation**" is frequently used instead. This choice of words may help you look at evaluation of your behaviors in a positive way. Distinguish what is being evaluated. You must separate your behaviors or actions from yourself, the person.

Constructive evaluation directed toward your behaviors has no bearing on your value as a person. Look at your behaviors either as being positive and helping you to reach your goal, or as needing improvement. Behaviors that need improvement should be modified so you can reach your goal of being a practical/vocational nurse.

As you progress in the nursing program, you will learn about a systematic way of conducting patient care called the "nursing process" (see Chapter 12). An important part of the nursing process is evaluation of patient goals while giving patient care. If your actions are not helping patients reach their goals, they need to be modified. Knowledge of the nursing process will help you develop your ability to look at your actions and evaluate them. Comments from instructors will help your self-awareness.

A good way to start learning self-evaluation is to look at yourself in everyday life. Ask yourself how you look through the eyes of others:

- How would you like to be your own spouse?
- How would you like to have yourself as a learner?
- How would you like to be your own mother or father?
- How would you like to be your own nurse?

If you would not like to be any of these people, identify the reasons why.

Another good exercise is to make two lists: a list of your assets or strong points and a list of your liabilities or areas that need improvement. When asked to evaluate themselves, learners traditionally rate themselves more negatively. They tend to neglect their strong points. Identifying strong points is not proud or vain behavior. It is dealing with yourself honestly and openly. After you have identified assets and liabilities, review your assets periodically. Make an effort to grow these strong points while modifying your liabilities. Work on one liability at a time. If you do so, your assets list will grow and your liabilities list will shrink.

A good place to start self-evaluation in nursing is in the skills lab of your basic nursing course. Observe the results of your actions. Are you using a drape during procedures to avoid chilling and invading the patient's privacy? Are you aware of the effect of the tone of your voice on your instructors and peers?

Evaluation is an ever-present reality in any career. Getting into the practice of self-evaluation early in your program of study will help you to develop a skill you will use daily in your career and personal life.

? Critical Thinking

Self-Evaluation

List one of your strong areas you identified as a new practical/vocational nursing learner. (Review your answers to **Critical Thinking: Reasons I Can Succeed** earlier in the chapter.)

List one area needing improvement that you have identified as a practical/vocational nursing student. (Review your answers to **Critical Thinking: Personal Liabilities** earlier in the chapter.)

? Critical Thinking

Plan to Eliminate My Areas That Need Improvement

Discuss with an instructor, peer, or significant other the areas you identified as needing improvement. Request verification and identification of any other areas you have not identified. Avoid the temptation to become defensive and list why these areas exist. Instead, focus on developing a plan to eliminate at least one of your areas that need improvement. How can you convert this area into a strength?

DEALING WITH REFERRALS

If you are evaluated by your instructor as having areas that need improvement, the instructor might refer you to a counselor at school. Examples of areas that require a referral are a grade below passing in a major test and frequent absences from class. Counselors at technical colleges and junior colleges are academic counselors who have expertise in helping students identify reasons for academic problem areas. A referral to a counselor is an attempt to help you succeed. These counselors can help students set up a plan of action to remedy the problem. We have seen some students resist going to the counselor because they think it is a waste of time. An external counseling system may also exist. Be proactive. In most schools, you can initiate the need for assistance before the instructor referral. If you are struggling with academic or clinical performance, seek out help early and often. In addition, remember that counselors can also assist with a variety of personal crises. These could be extreme situations such as death of a loved one or an abusive situation, or they could be less urgent but still important, such as struggling with time management or communication skills.

? Critical Thinking

Referral to Counselor

Identify how you access counselors at your school.

What could be one reason for thinking that an appointment with the counselor is a waste of time?

Consider one potential area that you may need to access a counselor while enrolled in school.

OTHER RESPONSIBILITIES OF LEARNERS

In addition to assuming responsibility for your own learning, becoming actively involved in the learning process, and receiving and participating in evaluation, it is necessary to be aware of some other responsibilities you have as a learner:

1. Be aware of the rules and policies of your school and the practical/vocational nursing program. Abide by them.

2. When problems do develop, follow the recognized channels of communication both at school and in the clinical area. The rule is: Go to the source. Avoid "saving up" gripes. Instead, pursue them as they come up. Deal with them in an assertive manner (see Chapter 9).

3. Be prepared in advance for classes and clinical experiences. You expect teachers to be prepared, and they expect the same of you. When you are unprepared for classes, you waste the time of the instructor, your peers, and yourself. When you are unprepared for clinical experiences, you are violating an important safety factor in patient care. When you are scheduled for the clinical area, your state board of nursing expects you to function as a licensed practical/vocational nurse would function under your state's Nurse Practice Act.

4. Seek out learning experiences at school and in the clinical area. Set your goals higher than the minimum. In postconference, use your peers and the experiences and knowledge they have and learn from one another.

5. Seek out resources beyond the required readings. Examples of these resources can be the learning resource center, information from past classes, electronic resources at the clinical sites, and the Internet.

6. Assume responsibility for your own thoughts, communication, and behavior. Avoid giving in to pressure from your peers. BYOB: be your own boss.

7. Be present and on time for classes and clinical experiences. Follow school and program policies for reporting absences. Frequent absences and late arrivals, despite a passing grade average, could result in disciplinary action up to and including dismissal from the program. In addition, developing a strong commitment to be dependable and accountable will contribute to job success and advancement in the future.

8. Be an active, self-directed learner. Know what you know, what you do not know, and where to find the evidence needed.

9. Treat those with whom you come into daily contact with respect. Be mindful of their rights as individuals.

10. Remember, the clinical area can be very stressful for the student, instructor, staff member, and patient. You must remain professional at all times. Learn the fine line between assertive and aggressive. Observe others for their response to challenging situations and self-evaluate often.

11. Seek out your instructor when you are having difficulties in class or the clinical area. Often instructors can tell when students are having problems. More important are the times when they cannot tell, and only the student knows a problem exists. Do not be afraid to approach your instructors. They are there to help you.

12. Keep a record of your grades as a course proceeds. At the beginning of a course the instructor and/or your course syllabus will explain the method of calculating your final grade. You are responsible for knowing your average grade at all times.

Get Ready for the NCLEX-PN® Examination!

Key Points

- Adult learners develop diversity in age, resulting in differing ways of thinking and valuing.
- The adults in your class could be Matures (The Silent Generation), Baby Boomers, Generation Xers, Generation Ys (Millennials), and Generation Z.
- Adult learners can be classified as traditional adult learners and nontraditional learners.
- Each category of adult learner possesses characteristics that can help the learner succeed in the practical/vocational nursing program.
- Each group of adult learners also possesses characteristics that can prevent success.
- Liabilities occur in areas in which learners have control over their solutions. Implement the solutions early. Seek assistance when the solutions are not evident.
- Although learners have rights, they also have responsibilities. Important responsibilities include taking an active part in the learning process and participating in the evaluation of their learning and growth.

Additional Learning Resources

evolve Go to your Evolve website (http://evolve.elsevier.com/Knecht/success) for the following FREE learning resources:
- Answers to Critical Thinking Scenarios
- Additional learning activities
- Additional Review Questions for the NCLEX-PN® exam
- Helpful phrases for communicating in Spanish and more!

Review Questions for the NCLEX-PN® Examination

1. Select the appropriate behavior for the student practical nurse/vocational nurse (PN/VN).
   1. To accept responsibility for personal success, including grades, in the nursing program.
   2. To be as passive a learner as you can possibly be both in classes and in the clinical area.
   3. To learn everything from the nursing instructors that is needed to function as a PN/VN.
   4. To blame the nursing instructor for any failures that occurs in class or the clinical area.

2. A practical/vocational nursing learner has been referred to the counselor because of a failing grade on the last test in Nursing Fundamentals. Which of the following learner responses indicates the student understands the purpose of the referral?
   1. "The instructor does not like me and wants me to quit the program."
   2. "This is a warning that I will be asked to withdraw from the program."
   3. "The purpose of a referral is to help me identify problems to avoid failure."
   4. "A psychologist will evaluate me for psychological problems that may be interfering with success."

3. A student practical nurse/vocational nurse (PN/VN) has just received the end-of-course clinical evaluation. Which of the following attitudes is most appropriate regarding the role of evaluation of students in the clinical area?
   1. Instructors and PN/VN students have the responsibility to identify positive behaviors and those that need improvement.
   2. It is the job of the instructor only to identify positive clinical behaviors and behaviors that need improvement.
   3. When PN/VN students identify positive behaviors, it indicates that they are proud and overly confident individuals.
   4. When behaviors that need improvement are identified, clinical evaluation may destroy self-esteem in the PN/VN student.

4. Four practical nurse/vocational nurse (PN/VN) students were absent the day tests were returned and reviewed in a pediatric course. Which of the following students has a plan that will benefit the student in future testing and clinical situations?
   1. The student who on the next class day will ask the instructor for the grade on the test for personal records.
   2. The student who on the next clinical day asks the instructor to schedule time to go over test items that were correct.
   3. The student who thinks that because the test is over, it is unnecessary to review test items because the grade is final.
   4. The student who asks when there is time to go over all the test items so the reasons for wrong answers can be identified.

Alternate Format Item

1. Which of the following students is *not* demonstrating behavior for success in the practical/vocational nursing program? *(Select all that apply.)*
   1. A recent high school graduate who expects the instructor to teach her everything she needs to know.
   2. A student who is a mother of four and spends time in the library each afternoon reviewing class notes.
   3. A student who has not been in school for 20 years and seeks out the instructor when content is not understood.
   4. A student with college experience who works part-time and joins a group that crams before each examination.
   5. A student who speaks English as a second language and studies every night in preparation for class and clinical.

2. Olivia, 37, just started the practical nursing program at the local technical college. Her class is composed of students in their late teens, twenties, thirties, fifties, and one retired man. From the following list of generalized characteristics, select those that describe Olivia's generational age. *(Select all that apply.)*
   1. Accepts diversity in the members of her class.
   2. Is more formal when approaching classmates.
   3. Works long hours to get the job done.
   4. Does not readily use the computer lab.
   5. Is self-reliant when learning nursing skills.

Critical Thinking Scenario

Amy, 36, has been accepted to the practical nursing program. Initial excitement is followed by concern. Amy begins to think: "Can I really do this? I have three kids, am a single parent, and haven't had any classes since high school! And high school was a bad dream for me. I never got along with my teachers. And how am I going to be able to afford school both in time and money? I work full-time now and have a hard time making ends meet in time and money. And I heard you have evaluations of what you do when taking care of patients. I don't like people being critical of me." Identify at least three different areas Amy should evaluate before enrollment. What can you suggest to Amy to include in a success plan to help her with her concerns?

Academic Resources (Study Skills and Test Strategies)

Objectives

On completing this chapter, you will be able to do the following:

1. Use techniques in learning situations that will increase your degree of concentration, improve your listening skills, enhance your comprehension (understanding) of information needed for critical thinking as licensed practical nurse/licensed vocational nurse (LPN/LVN), and develop your ability to store information in long-term memory.
2. Use hints for successful test taking when taking tests in the LPN/LVN program.
3. Identify your knowledge of your school's learning resource center (LRC).
4. Discuss the value of reading assignments in periodicals.
5. Use a digital database, and locate an article related to nursing.
6. Discuss six hints used to gain full value from mini lectures and PowerPoint presentations.
7. Discuss the use of the resources such as labs, study groups, the Learning Management System (LMS), electronic devices, and mannequins in your personal learning.
8. Describe how digital databases, nursing organizations, guest speakers, and mobile devices help you stay current in practical/vocational nursing.
9. Identify academic resources, in your local community, based on your unique personal qualities that will assist you to SUCCEED.

Key Terms

active listener (ĂK-tĭv LIS-ĕn-ĕr)
app (ăpp)
blended course (BLEN-dĕd)
bucket theory (BŬK-ĭt)
call number (kăl)
case scenario (kas sĕn-ĂR-ē-ō)
comprehension (KŎM-prē-HĔN-shŭn)
computer-aided instruction
computer simulation (SIM-ū-LĀ-shŭn)
cooperative learning (kō-WŎP-ĕr-ă-TIV)
copyright laws (KŎP-ē-rīt)
course outlines (kŏrs ŌWT-līn)
discussion buddy (dĭs-KŬ-shŭn)
distance learning (DIS-tăns)
distracters (dĭ-STRĂK-tĕrz)
electronic devices (Ē-lĕk-trŏn-ĭc)
electronic simulation
external distractions (ĕks-TŬRN-ăl dĭ-STRĂK-shŭns)
interlibrary loan services (ĭn-TĕR-Lī- brĕr-ē)
internal distractions (ĭn-TŬRN-ăl dĭ-STRĂK-shŭns)
Internet
key
key concepts (kē kŏn-sĕpts)
Learning Management System (LMS)

learning resource center (LRC)
lecture-discussion strategy
mnemonic devices (nĭ-MŎN-ĭc)
mobile devices
nursing skills lab (NŬR-sĭng skĭlz)
online catalog
options (ŎP-shŭns)
passive listener (PĂ-sĭv LIS-ĕn-ĕr)
peer-reviewed
periodical index (PIR-ē-ŏd-ĭ-kăl ĭn-DEKS)
periodicals (PIR-ē-ŏd-ĭ-kălz)
podcast (PŎD-căst)
reference materials (REF-rĕnts mă-TER-rē-ăls)
simulation (SIM-ū-LĀ-shŭn)
stacks
static simulation
passive listener (PĂ-sĭv LIS-ĕn-ĕr)
stem (stĕm)
study group (STŬ-dē groop)
study skills lab (STŬ-dē skĭlz)
syllabus
tutoring (TOO-tŏr-ēng)
virtual clinical excursions (VER-choo-ăl)
understanding (ŬN-dĕr-stăn-dĭng)

13

Success is dependent on a strong self-analysis. Knowing who you are, what your academic strengths are, and how to find/use available academic resources will help you to SUCCEED!

During lunch, five students, Olivia, Katie, Alessandra, Lisa, and Jonathon sit together and discuss the morning's class about academic success. Olivia states, "I am kind of scared. That pile of books and list of assignments due next week is overwhelming. There were times the instructor was going so fast that I could hardly keep up." Lisa continues, "I agree. I was grateful when she outlined on the whiteboard a chart with the schedule of our clinical, class, and lab days, although I could tell some people were bored with this detail. It was very confusing until I saw it on the board. It helped me to organize my week." Katie chimes in, "I felt the same way and realized that I need to see things in writing. Just hearing the information is often confusing to me." Alessandra states, "I can see how everyone learns differently. There are many resources. I think we will need to carefully identify what works best for each of us and not assume a peer's successful study strategies will definitely be our best option. They may work, but not if we are a different type of learner. For example, I want to join a study group but know that I am a solitary learner. So I will need to choose carefully and balance the study group with solo study. I am excited but a bit nervous. Oh, it's 11:56. Let's go. I don't want to be late for class."

A solid academic self-analysis is essential. This analysis already began when you completed the required nurse entrance test. Although several types of tests are used for nursing school entrance, most measure key areas of academic aptitude. They are a good starting point to a self-analysis. Examining test results can assist you in determining how to focus your efforts. For example, in your test, were you strong in reading comprehension, mathematic calculations, or making deductions? If your overall math grade was below average (below the fifty percentile), what specific math concepts do you need to review? If you did not take a nurse entrance test, examine your performance on prerequisite courses (if required) for areas needing further development.

In addition to this analysis, you will also want to ask yourself several other questions:
- What is your learning style?
- Do you have solid study skills?
- What are academic resources? Are they available to you, and how do you use them?

Let's start by identifying your learning style.

Identify your learning style(s): Discuss how your learning style can impact your learning, comprehending, retaining, and applying information in the care of patients. Remember: Everyone's learning style is unique.

Everyone learns differently. Some student practical nurses/student vocational nurses (SPNs/SVNs) take voluminous notes. Some just listen. Others learn best by hands-on activities and group instruction. In contrast, some are solitary learners and prefer to learn independently on the computer. Listen to student conversations about studying to get clues on different styles of learning. Examples include, "I like absolute silence;" or "I like my music blaring;" or "I study best in the wee hours of the morning;" or "I like to munch when I study;" or "I make up rhymes to help me remember;" or "I read on a treadmill;" and so on. All students can be equally successful. There are many theories about what affects learning style.

Take a few minutes to list your "favorites" when studying.

Brain dominance impacts the way you think. Your thinking style impacts the way you learn. Your learning style is the way you receive information most efficiently and effectively.

BRAIN DOMINANCE

The battle of biology (hardwiring) versus socialization (how you are raised) in brain development is finally backed by scientific evidence. Originally, biology alone was credited for male/female differences in areas such as learning and behavior. For a number of years, until the late 1980s, the importance of socialization became the focus. It was thought that men and women became what they are based on their specific socialization. Looking back, it has not worked out this way, and both boys and girls have suffered because of this singular emphasis.

RIGHT AND LEFT SIDES OF THE CEREBRUM

We often hear people talk about being "right brained" or "left brained." In reality no one is completely "right or left brained." We achieve our best when both sides of our brain work together, as partners. For example, the left side of the brain is verbal and fluent, and without the help of the right side to add tone and inflection, it would make our speech robotlike. In school, the left side of the brain helps break down information so we can master it. The right side gives a total picture of our learning (Figure 2-1). However, specific parts of the brain impact different attributes.

RIGHT-BRAIN-DOMINANT INDIVIDUALS

Primarily **right-brain-dominant** individuals tend to be intuitive, imaginative, and impulsive. They prefer to start out with a broad idea and then pursue supporting information. They learn best by:
- Seeing and doing in an informal, busy, somewhat unstructured environment
- Simulations, group discussions, panels, and activity-based learning. This group will embrace the "flipped classroom"

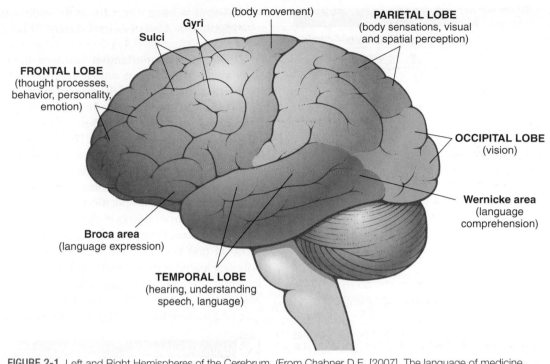

FIGURE 2-1 Left and Right Hemispheres of the Cerebrum. (From Chabner D.E. [2007]. The language of medicine [ed 11]. St. Louis: Elsevier.)

LEFT-BRAIN-DOMINANT INDIVIDUALS

Left-brain-dominant learners tend to be analytical, rational, and objective. They learn best by:
- Putting together many facts to arrive at an understanding
- Having traditional lectures, demonstrations, and assigned readings

THINKING STYLE

Usually one side of the brain is dominant and affects the way you process information. The two most common styles are linear and global. **Linear thinkers** (also known as left-brain dominant):
- Prefer a very structured approach to learning. They are most comfortable doing things in order. For example, when going to their first day of the nursing program, linear thinkers will have checked ahead of time the route they will take, which door to go in, where the room is located, the time they are expected to arrive, and what supplies they are expected to bring.
- They will review the information carefully *before* leaving home.

Global thinkers (also known as right-brain-dominant):
- Are more comfortable going to the nursing program their first day by accessing information and relating it to their overall goals. They will just get into their vehicle and drive, without any preplanning, on that first day.

LEARNING STYLES

Learning takes place in different ways. It is important not to pigeonhole anyone, including yourself. Everyone is capable of learning with any learning style and will use another style to reinforce learning.

PERCEPTUAL LEARNING STYLES

Perceptual learning style refers to our three main sensory receivers:
- Visual (learn primarily with their eyes)
- Auditory (learn primarily by listening)
- Kinesthetic/tactual (learn primarily by hands-on tasks)

The majority of individuals in Western countries prefer the visual learning style. The next most natural is auditory, and the least common is the movement (kinesthetic) and tactile (touch) style. Many practical nursing programs, particularly hour-based programs, have more "hands-on" training than a traditional prelicensure registered nurse (RN) program. This can attract students who have a visual or kinesthetic learning style.

◎ Try This

Self-Evaluation of Sensory Learning Style Directions

Underline the symbol that is most accurate for each statement.

	YES	SOMETIMES	NO
Prefers to talk rather than read.	•	△	□
Likes to touch, hug, and shake hands.	△	□	•
Likes to brainstorm in groups.	•	△	□
Uses finger spelling as a way to learn words.	△	□	•
Prefers written directions.	□	•	△
Sings or talks to self.	•	△	□
Likes to take notes for studying.	□	•	△
Remembers best by doing.	△	□	•

Continued

Try This

Self-Evaluation of Sensory Learning Style Directions—cont'd

	YES	SOMETIMES	NO
Likes or makes charts and graphs.	□	•	△
Learns from listening to lectures and tapes.	•	△	□
Likes to work with hands.	△	□	•
Might say, "I don't see what you mean."	□	•	△
Good at jigsaw puzzles and mazes.	□	•	△
Has a good listening skill.	•	△	□
Presses pencil down hard when writing.	△	□	•
Learns words by repeating out loud.	□	•	△
When traveling, prefers to have oral directions.	•	△	□
Plays with objects during the learning period.	△	□	•

Count all of the symbols. The highest number indicates the sensory reading preference.

Key
□ = visual • = auditory △ = kinesthetic/tactile
Adapted from the Barsch Learning Style Inventory, Penn State Learning Style Inventory, and the University of Georgia Education Technology Center Learning Style Inventory.

Critical Thinking

Summarizing Your Learning Styles

After you have completed the Self-Evaluation of Sensory Learning Styles exercise, make two columns on a piece of paper. Label the columns "A" and "B." Write the statements you answered as "Yes" or "No" in column "A," and write the statements you answered as "Sometimes" in column "B." You have identified your sensory learning style. The "Perceptual Learning Style Preference" section tells you how the information can be helpful to studying.

PERCEPTUAL LEARNING STYLE PREFERENCE

People think differently. They think in the system corresponding to the sense of vision, hearing, or kinesthetic/tactile.

- **Observers: Visual learners** have two subchannels: visual linguistic and visual spatial. **Visual-linguistic** learners learn best through reading and writing. They tend to remember what they read. They like to write down directions and pay better attention to traditional lectures if they watch them on a DVD, YouTube, or PowerPoint presentation. **Visual-spatial** learners do less well with reading generally, and they learn best through charts, demonstrations, videos, and other visual materials. They can easily visualize faces and places and seldom get lost in new surroundings. Observers tend to say, "I see what you mean" or "I think you mean. . . ."
- **Listeners: Auditory learners** think in terms of hearing, talk to themselves, or hear sounds. They may move their lips and read out loud. They learn best by hearing

and tend to have difficulty with reading and writing assignments. Listeners tend to say, "I hear what you are saying."

- **Doers: Kinesthetic/tactual learners** have two subchannels: movement and touch. They tend to lose interest during class if there is no movement or external stimulation. Kinesthetic learners experience feelings in regard to what is being thought about. They learn best by moving, doing, touching, experiencing, or experimenting. Sometimes learners with this style are categorized as slow learners because the information is not presented in their learning style.

Being identified as a specific type of learner does not mean that a learner thinks exclusively in any one of these overall systems. What it means is that most people think more in one system than another. There are ways to enhance learning by supporting the overall system. No learning preference is better than another. It is usually easier to feel connected to someone who shares a similar learning preference: "We think in the same language."

Critical Thinking

Think about instructors you have had from the lower grades to the present. Which instructor was your favorite? What was their teaching style? Did it match your favorite style of learning?

Professional Pointer

A learning preference is just that. Think about resources available to reinforce information using your preferred learning style.

Visual Learner

If you are a visual learner, you learn best by watching a demonstration first. Make this preference work for you by using the following techniques:
- Sit in the front seat of a face-to-face class.
- Stay focused on the teacher's facial expression and body language.
- Take notes in class, and highlight, color code, and use mind maps to process and learn content.
- Rewrite notes in your own words as a form of studying (e.g., write notes or draw pictures in the margin of your book or as a note on the screen).
- Use index cards for review or memorization.
- Review YouTube clips or videos, DVDs, podcasts, and so on.
- Look for reference books that contain pictures, graphs, or charts, or draw your own.
- Request demonstrations and observational experiences before practicing a new skill.
- Try to "picture" a procedure rather than just memorizing steps.

Auditory Learner

If you are an auditory learner, you learn best by hearing. Make this preference work for you by using the following techniques:
- Listen carefully if the instructor summarizes what you will be learning, points out what is important to

remember, and summarizes what has been covered during class.

- Read aloud or mouth the words. Concentrate on hearing the words, especially when reading test questions.
- When attending a lecture, listen to the words instead of taking notes during class. Audio-tape the presentation and discussion if the instructor and students grant permission. Play the tapes back several times. Playing the tape in the car, while doing routine tasks, or just before sleeping can be beneficial to learning.
- Find a "study buddy" or group with whom to discuss class content. Compare notes and verbalize the information to aid in learning the material.
- Request permission to make audiotapes or oral reports (instead of written reports) for credit.
- Make up silly rhymes or songs (mnemonic clues) to remember key points.
- Request a verbal explanation of illustrations, graphs, and diagrams.

Kinesthetic/Tactual Learner

If you are a kinesthetic learner, you learn best by touching, moving, or hands-on tasks. Traditional lectures, in which one is required to sit, read, or listen for long periods of time, may be difficult for you. It is a problem to process both visual and auditory input.

Using your muscles by gesturing can help improve memory of information by matching a gesture to information that needs to be remembered. When the gestures and word are associated in your mind, performing this gesture can retrieve the word. Physical motion can jog memory and promote recall. You should see the motions students go through during an examination. Make this preference work for you by using the following techniques:

- Handle the equipment before you practice a nursing procedure.
- Move while reading or reciting facts (e.g., rocking, pacing, or using a Stairmaster or stationary bike).
- Change study positions often. During traditional lectures, you may want to sit in back so you can stand up and take notes without being too obvious.
- Use background music of your choice when studying away from school.
- Take short breaks and do something active during that time.
- Offer to do a project as a way of enhancing a required classroom presentation. For example, if you have been asked to explain how oxygen gets out of a capillary and carbon dioxide gets in, develop a project to use as the basis for your explanation.
- Use arrows to show relationships when taking notes. Use flash cards, games, mnemonic clues, and other gamelike activities to reinforce content of long reading assignments.
- Highlight key concepts; make diagrams and doodles.

CATEGORIES OF MULTIPLE INTELLIGENCES

Gardner (1999) described what he termed "multiple intelligences" as being more accurate than the single measure of the intelligence quotient (IQ) that most people are familiar with. The seven identified intelligences include the following:

1. Linguistic
2. Logical/mathematical
3. Spatial
4. Musical
5. Bodily/kinesthetic
6. Interpersonal
7. Intrapersonal

This knowledge provides additional information that will further enhance your learning.

IDENTIFYING AND USING THE INTELLIGENCES

LINGUISTIC LEARNER (THE WORD PLAYER)

If you are a **linguistic learner**, you learn best by saying, hearing, and seeing words. You like to read, write, and tell stories. You are good at memorizing names, places, dates, and trivia. Make this preference work for you by using the following techniques:

- Take notes when you read this text and reduce the number of words you have included in the notes. Your love of words and vocabulary may cause you to become distracted from the key points. Use these notes as your study source.
- Review all written work before handing in the assignment. Delete extra words and phrases that are not directly related to the topic.

LOGICAL/MATHEMATICAL LEARNER (THE QUESTIONER)

If you are a **logical learner** as well, you learn best by using an organized method that involves categorizing, classifying, and working with abstract patterns and relationships. You are good at reasoning, math, and problem solving. Make this preference work for you by using the following techniques:

- Take the time to organize a method of study that fits you personally.
- Redo your notes to fit your study method, categorizing the material under titles and themes.

SPATIAL LEARNER (THE VISUALIZER)

If you are a **spatial learner**, you learn best by visualizing, dreaming, working with colors and pictures, and studying diagrams, boxes, and special lists in the textbook/e-text. You are good at imagining things, sensing changes, puzzles, and charts. Make this learning preference work for you by using the following techniques:

- Make your own diagrams, boxes, or lists when they are not available in the text/e-text.
- Redo your notes using key concepts only.
- Box key information in the text. Highlight in your e-text.

MUSICAL LEARNER (THE MUSIC LOVER)

If you are a **musical learner**, you learn best by humming, singing, or playing an instrument. You are good at remembering melodies, rhythms, and keeping time. Make this preference work for you by using the following techniques:

- Play your favorite music, or hum while studying. Remind yourself which music relates to the content you are studying.
- Play an instrument while reviewing information in your head.

BODILY/KINESTHETIC LEARNER (THE MOVER)

If you are a **bodily/kinesthetic learner**, you learn best by touching, moving, and processing knowledge through bodily sensations. You are good at physical activities and crafts. Make this preference work for you by using the following techniques:

- Move around when studying. If you work out on a treadmill, stationary bike, or Stairmaster, it becomes a good time to read or review notes. You can also listen to podcasts or YouTube clips.
- Dance or act out concepts you are studying to experience the sensations involved.

INTERPERSONAL LEARNER (THE SOCIALIZER)

If you are an **interpersonal learner**, you learn best by sharing, comparing, cooperating, and interviewing. You are good at understanding people, leading others, organizing, communicating, and mediating. Make this preference work for you by using the following techniques:

- Organize and/or participate in a study group.
- Compare your understanding of material with that of other students.
- Practice mock simulations in the lab with a peer.

INTRAPERSONAL LEARNER (THE INDIVIDUAL)

If you are an **intrapersonal learner**, you learn best by working alone, self-paced instruction, and having your own space. You are good at pursuing interests and goals, following instincts, understanding yourself, and being original. Make this learning preference work for you by using the following techniques:

- Work on individualized projects.
- Contribute to team projects as needed. Align team projects with individualized projects.
- Trust your instincts in regard to study needs. (Gardner & Hatch, 1990)

Be aware of the type of learner you are, but do not limit yourself to those styles. Try out suggestions listed under other preferences. Some of them will further enhance your learning.

? Critical Thinking
Implementing Suggestions

Make a realistic plan involving learning styles that you think will work for you. Include observable, desired outcomes; a plan of action; and dates by which you will accomplish this plan. Remember that the dates are just educated guesses based on intimate knowledge of how you function. Be sure you note how you will determine progress toward a behavioral change. Use a format that works for you: columns, clustering, doodling, pictures, and so on.

👉 Professional Pointer

Identify your patient's learning style and use it as a basis to support teaching started by the RN or physician.

HOW WE LEARN

Scientists are not exactly sure how the brain can rewire itself with each new stimulation, experience, or behavior and cause learning. One idea is that a stimulus occurs and is processed in the brain at several different areas. Neural pathways (traces) become more and more efficient when a learning exercise, such as reviewing notes, is repeated. This is done through myelination (coating) of the neurons. Stimulation occurs when you learn something new. The mental or motor stimulation lights up the brain in several areas, producing even greater beneficial energy; for example, you receive a new assignment or have a new clinical experience.

The brain gets its energy for learning primarily from blood, about 8 gallons per hour. Remember to stay hydrated; drinking water is essential. According to Jensen (1998), "Dehydration is a common problem in school classrooms, leading to lethargy and impaired learning." Other factors that impede long-term memory include lack of sleep, multitasking, distraction, and lack of focus during class.

MAPPING (CONCEPT MAP)

Brain researchers have suggested an alternative to the linear method of note making. It encourages using the *right side* of the brain, with its emphasis on images. Color and drawings are processed by the right side of the brain and are important components of **mapping**. Information presented in a linear manner, as in traditional note taking, is not as easily understood as information presented by key concepts. The use of key concepts is the primary way in which the brain processes information. The brain takes these key concepts and integrates them in relationships. So if the brain does not work in lines or lists, the method of note making called mapping can enhance your ability to understand, review, and recall this information. Mapping is a method in which information is organized graphically so it is seen in a visual pattern of relationships. Mapping is most meaningful to the person who draws the map. Box 2-1 gives hints for note making, using the mapping method. Figure 2-2 is an example of

Box 2-1	Hints for Note Making: Mapping Method

Start with your note paper in a horizontal position.
- Start with a small circle in the middle of the paper.
- Put the main topic of activity in the circle.
- Add branches off the circle for important ideas and subtopics. Arrange these branches like the spokes of a wheel. Use a different-colored pen for each of the branches. Draw more branches off branches as needed for each topic. Draw a picture to go with each key topic or idea. Artistic ability does not count here. What is important is that the picture gives meaning to you!
- Visit the website www.lucidchart.com to create a concept map on your computer.

a summary using **clustering**, a basic form of mapping that helps simplify topics. Clustering is especially helpful for *visual* learners.

Some nursing programs have found mapping helpful in developing critical-thinking skills by having learners use this format to develop nursing care plans as concept maps, instead of the traditional column format. There are many web-based sites that will support creation of a concept map on your computer. Lucidchart is one example that is free (www.lucidchart.com)

VISUAL STRATEGIES TO ENHANCE UNDERSTANDING

Your scholastic world is bombarded with words, sentences, and paragraphs. One of the most beneficial

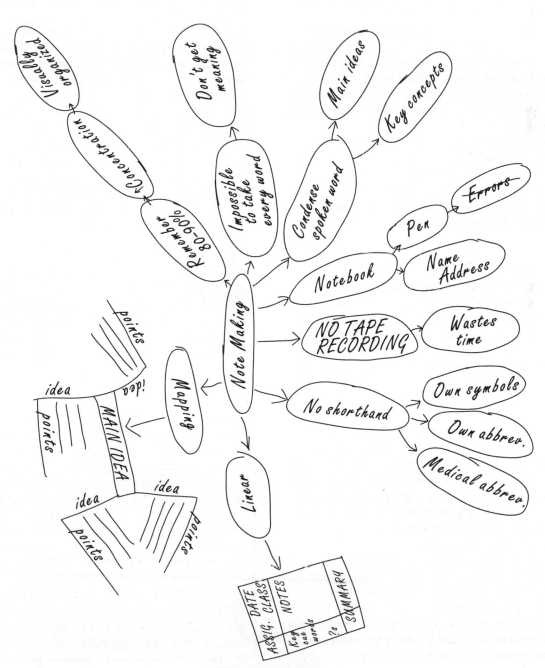

FIGURE 2-2 Clustering.

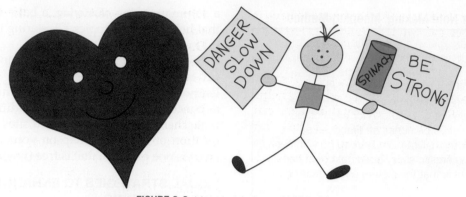

FIGURE 2-3 Idea sketch: Lanoxin (digoxin).

techniques to comprehend (understand) and remember all new information is to balance this verbal mixture with visual strategies. Each of the following visual strategies will help you understand and ultimately remember information better. They deal with the right side of the brain. You will be tapping a resource that possibly you have not used often if your left brain is dominant. These strategies include creating pictures and drawings that capture the key information.

Draw Idea Sketches

These drawings will probably be comprehensible only to you. The emphasis of **idea sketches** is not on the quality of the drawing but on the process you must go through to take a verbal concept and represent it graphically, without words. To go through this process, you must understand the verbal concept. You can even set it up as a cartoon. Use stick figures and describe the concept verbally. Figure 2-3 is an idea sketch illustrating the function of the drug Lanoxin (digoxin), which is used to slow and strengthen the heartbeat.

Use Color and Font Characteristics in Taking Notes

Use different color print, highlighters, crayons, or colored pencils in addition to underlining or highlighting sentences. If using a computer, changing the font characteristics is also a great tool. For example: use bold, underline, and italics features coupled with font color and highlight options to assist in categorizing information, thus enhancing your understanding and retention. These strategies help your brain organize and retrieve information more effectively.

Make Your Own Diagram as You Read

If you commit to memory by using words only, you are using only half of your brain's resources, those of the left side. If you also produce a sketch of that idea or view a sketch on a web site, you will have brought the right side of your brain into use. Using both sides of the brain enhances your success.

Engage in Mental Imagery

Engaging in **mental imagery** will help you remember material because it demands that you understand the information. When you use mental imagery, you become the idea that you are having difficulty understanding. The right side of your brain generates pictures of the idea, and the left side supplies the script to explain what is going on in the pictures (and always in your own words). Box 2-2 provides a mental image developed by a practical nursing student to give herself a simple understanding of the function of insulin, a hypoglycemic agent that increases glucose transport across muscles and fat cell membranes. Notice how she uses the senses of hearing and feeling and also body movement to help achieve understanding. She also uses a metaphor to tie it into something she is

---

Box 2-2 **Mental Images Depicting the Function of Insulin: I Am Insulin—A Job Description**

I am Insulin, and I am shaped like a canoe. In fact, I am a green canoe. My job is to make sugar or glucose in the blood available to most of the cells of the body for energy. I like my job. I like things that are sweet, but not too sweet, so normal blood sugar is just my thing. Sometimes after the person who owns the pancreas where I am stored in my canoe rack eats a meal, a whistle blows, and I know this is a signal to launch myself into the bloodstream. As I ride the currents of blood, I rock gently back and forth, and the sugar in my bloodstream jumps right in to be a passenger in the canoe. Blood sugar likes me. I think it is because I am green, but I might be wrong. When I am pretty full, but not full enough to swamp, I pass through the blood vessels, paddle through the sea of tissue fluid (boy, it smells salty) around the cells, and pass through the cell membrane. Then I deposit the sugar by making these molecules jump out of the green canoe and into the fluid inside the cell. I feel pretty important in my job. Without me, the blood sugar molecules would be unable to pass through the cell membranes. Because of this, I am given the official job title of hypoglycemic agent. I lower the level of sugar in the blood.

Excuse me! There goes the whistle.

trying to learn. The student recites the image to herself while she closes her eyes and visualizes it. First she had her roommate read the story while she visualized the scenario.

Perhaps a physiologist would wince at this description. However, it is nothing to be ashamed of if it helps you understand a concept. Plus, mental imagery can be fun. If you are a social learner, this could be a fun activity with peers, at the end of a long week. A difficult concept such as tonicity of fluids can become easy to remember.

? Critical Thinking

Increasing Understanding of Concepts

Choose a concept you are having trouble understanding in one of your nursing classes or text/e-book readings (i.e., trace a drop of blood), and try to increase understanding by using the following:
1. Draw an idea sketch.
2. Use mental imagery.
3. Locate an on-line resource.
Which strategy was most useful for the concept you chose?

UNDEPENDABLE MEMORY AND LEARNING SYSTEM

All students can experience barriers to learning. The discussion that follows is focused on strategies to assist students who are diagnosed or are possibly undiagnosed with attention deficit hyperactivity disorder (ADHD). Although the strategies discussed focus on this diagnosis, they can be helpful to all students, particularly when students experience high levels of stress (e.g., a new nursing student).

Average and above-average individuals with potential talent may embrace failure messages, low self-esteem, and loss of hope. Some of these people are part of a population that continues to live with untreated **adult attention deficit hyperactivity disorder (ADHD)**. Among the characteristics are an undependable memory and learning system and problems with self-regulation and self-motivation. The individual may have problems with procrastination, distractibility, organization, prioritization, and impulsive decision-making. Because of previous poor performance at school or work, they may have been labeled as "lazy," "stupid," or "crazy." Students diagnosed and treated with ADHD often become high achievers, experiencing academic success for the first time in their life.

POSSIBLE BEHAVIORS

- Procrastination
- Indecision, difficulty recalling and organizing details required for a task
- Poor time management, losing track of time
- Avoiding tasks or jobs that required sustained effort
- Difficulty initiating tasks

- Difficulty completing and following through on tasks
- Difficulty multitasking
- Easily bored
- Impatient
- Easily irritated
- Impulsive
- Endless energy

Adults with ADHD have experienced a lot of pain caused by repeated failure resulting in embarrassment, self-blame, and a loss of hope. Intelligence is not affected in ADHD. Excellent information is available at the National Resource Center (NRC) on ADHD, funded by the Centers for Disease Control and Prevention (CDC) (http://help4adhd.org). This is the nation's clearinghouse for the latest evidence-based information on ADHD. As a nursing student you will gain a deep understanding of the importance of reputable evidence. The CDC is a trusted government resource providing evidence and latest news regarding many health issues. Chapter 3 will address in detail community resources available to enhance your success.

SOME SUGGESTIONS FOR THE STUDENT WITH ATTENTION DEFICIT HYPERACTIVITY DISORDER (although they can help all learners!)

- Educate yourself about ADHD. Understanding the disorder is a useful tool in learning to manage symptoms.
- Get a coach; both a classmate and a friend/family member are ideal. A coach assists you in staying organized, encourages you, and reminds you to get back to work while supporting you. Humor can be helpful.
- Create a list of tasks to be accomplished, organizing tasks into manageable sections with deadlines. Prioritize your lists so the most important assignments are accomplished first.
- Procrastination is a major issue. Be alert to the possibility, and discipline yourself to avoid procrastination. Do not deviate from deadlines unless a crisis occurs.
- Color coding: The adult with ADHD is often visually oriented. Color helps to focus attention and also makes what you are looking at memorable. Use color in your text/e-book as you read to bring out important points. Highlight as you read and take notes on your computer.
- Pay attention to the different learning styles you read about in this chapter and try out the styles that appeal to you. The student with ADHD may need to multitask to study successfully (for example, listening to a study tape while jogging). Because physical activity is generally a part of ADHD, you may discover that reading or reviewing notes works best for you when you are on a Stairmaster, stationary bike, or other apparatus that moves. Having music may help drown out distracting noises when studying.

- Be alert to what time of day works best for you for studying. Decorate your personal study environment to inspire you. Invent your own way of studying. Do what works for you even if other students study differently.
- Note what is important and jot down ideas that invariably show up. Daydreaming is an important part of ADHD, and noting ideas may be a way of staying on task while studying and in class.
- When studying, give yourself a mini-time-out before you switch to a different subject. Transition is often difficult for the student with ADHD, and a little break will help in the transition.
- Find ways to recharge your batteries without guilt.

◎ Try This

Most students can benefit from some of the strategies noted above. List two that you will implement.

1.
2.

MORE BARRIERS TO LEARNING

Barriers may or may not be of your own making. Regardless of the reason for their existence, they belong to you now. It is up to you to identify if barriers exist and if they affect your learning. It is also up to you to seek help in dealing with the barriers, if needed. Your level of reading and math academic readiness, despite entrance test screening, can be a barrier. See Chapter 3 for specific details.

◎ Try This

Personal learning style related to academic readiness

Review your individual entrance test scores in comparison with the national average (50 percentile point on the test).

❓ Critical Thinking

Personal learning style related to academic readiness

Identify strategies discussed that can assist you in improving your reading, writing, or other related skills. Be specific. Based on your weak areas, list two implementations related to your learning style to improve in these areas.

1.
2.

INABILITY TO UNDERSTAND (COMPREHEND) CONTENT

Almost everyone in the United States can read and recognize words, but not everyone understands the meaning of the words they read. Years ago, a renowned reading researcher, Dr. Jeanne Chall, identified predictable stages of reading development, which are still valid today. They are as follows:

- Before a child starts grade school, the foundation for reading and learning has been established. By being read to, a child learns what books are for and how they are used. In addition, the alphabet is introduced.
- In grades 1 and 2, a child learns to translate written letters and symbols into sounds and words.
- In grades 3 and 4, the school-age child develops speed and accuracy in reading (fluency). The child has not yet learned to comprehend what is being read.
- In grades 4-8, the school-age child masters vocabulary and learns how to pick out the main parts when reading. This is the beginning of reading for content.
- In high school, students learn to weigh evidence in messages they are reading and evaluate and make judgments about what they read. These behaviors demonstrate the ability to read for content and understand what is being read.
- By the end of high school, adolescents have reached a stage in which they are able to manage their own learning process, choosing what to read, and knowing how to use what they have learned in areas of interest.

Many people in the United States have not reached the level of comprehending what they read. Memorization is not comprehension. Although some memorization is necessary, SPNs/SVNs must be able to analyze information critically and, in clinical, make deductions and conclusions about patient care. This is a role of a licensed person. Reading skills are important to your success.

PUTTING IT ALL TOGETHER

Quality education encourages you to explore and apply alternative thinking, multiple answers, and creative thoughts. You can become a self-directed learner using the following techniques:

- Practice thinking critically (see Chapter 5).
- Identify your major and specific learning styles. Studying becomes easier.
- Understand basic right- and left-brain functions and how they work together. It helps you appreciate your capacity for learning.
- Do your part to prevent dehydration when studying and participating in classes. Water is a major ingredient of blood, which motivates the brain. Nutrition and sleep are also important.
- Maintain a positive attitude as you continue to learn and apply what you are learning.
- Set realistic goals and evaluate the results to see whether or not these goals were met.

It is an obstacle to learning to believe learning can take place without effort.

- Remember that established preferences of learning may not be working for you. Learning styles can be changed or modified as needed. It is also worth it to try suggestions from other styles to see if the suggestions enhance your learning.

- Tie in new learning to previous lessons and experiences. This gives the material meaning and makes it easier to remember.
- Seek help when it is needed. See Chapter 3 for additional community resources. Do not hesitate to contact these sources and get help early! Once you have failed a test, it becomes difficult to meet the minimum grade to pass the course.
- Identify your reading level and make sure you reach your potential.
- Seek to understand the clinical task versus simply performing the steps. Practice with a partner while they are quizzing you, modeling the instructor's expected behavior.
- Question what you do not understand and question the source of information when you have reason to believe it is incorrect. Always be professional in your approach. Cite evidence when questioning the source.
- Remember that whatever your learning style is, the best memory is to write it down.

According to a Chinese proverb, "the weakest link lasts longer than the strongest memory."

Keep in Mind

Study Skills are critical to success in an LP/LV nursing program. They are learned skills and become habit once practiced well. It is never too late to improve your study skills!

Many educational institutions offer courses in how to study before learners enter a program, and have departments that offer study skills services after a learner has enrolled. There are millions of Internet sites that provide information about study skills. Visit Google "Pageburst," take a guided tour, check out the text and study skills, and see what can help you the most. Despite these resources, lack of study skills, including test-taking skills, is a major factor for failure or withdrawing from a nursing program. Learners who need these services are not always aware that they need them or try to develop them "too late." Often students do not focus on improving study skills until they have received several failing grades.

Learners cannot assume they have the study skills necessary to succeed in the LP/LV nursing program because they have attended high school or college. It is possible for students to have been successful in college in a different area of study (i.e., fine arts, music, history). It takes time and effort to comprehend, store, and recall the knowledge and skills needed for critical thinking in your chosen career.

GENERAL HINTS FOR LEARNERS

CONCENTRATION

Concentration is the ability to keep your mind completely on the task at hand. The major enemy of concentration is distraction. Many distractions in a learner's life compete with the need to focus on school assignments. These distractions can be summarized as two types: **external distractions**, which are those that come from outside you, and **internal distractions**, which are those that come from inside you. Remember your learning style preference and strive for a study environment that meets your unique needs.

External Distractions

External distractions occur in your physical and social environments. An obvious distraction is hunger and thirst. Be sure you have met your hunger needs before settling in to study. Nutritious snacks and water can provide a reason for needed breaks.

Personal study area. Your physical environment can be a potential enemy of concentration. Here are some tips to avoid distractions:

- Identify the type of environment that allows you to get the most out of your study time. Your grades will be the criteria by which you can judge whether your environment is helping or hurting. Everyone's environment is unique. Some students like total quiet, whereas others need music to drown out other distractors.
- Locate realistic indoor and outdoor areas for studying that are associated with learning. There is evidence that establishing specific study areas is beneficial. Your mind knows it is time to study and so does your family!
- Alternating areas where one studies can improve retention of information. The learning resource center can be used between classes and after school. At some schools, study rooms can be reserved.
- Have on hand the tools you will need, including course outline (syllabus), computer, Internet access, highlighter, print or e-book, and notes or reference materials.

Lighting. Eyestrain can occur if lighting allows glare, shadows, or flicker to exist in your study area.
- e-Readers may require additional external lighting.
- Reading lamps are available that advertise natural white light and a light grid to reduce eye-tiring glare.
- If a ceiling light is available, turn this on in addition to your table lamp to reduce shadows.
- A table lamp with a properly seated bulb needs to be shaded to reduce flicker.
- Your writing surface needs to be a light color to reflect light and reduce glare.
- If you experience symptoms of eyestrain, such as headaches, dizziness, tiredness, or blurred vision, when reading after you have tried to eliminate glare, shadows, and flicker, it may be time to have an eye examination to rule out the need for corrective lenses.
- Some learners discover they need glasses only after they enroll in an educational program that

demands much reading, such as the LP/LV nursing program.

- If you wear contacts, limit the amount of time that you read before switching to your glasses. You may experience dry eyes from significant reading especially on a computer screen. Seek medical guidance early to avoid any eye complications.

Background noise

- Television, iPods, and so forth can be distracting background noise to some learners, but others find that they study best with these devices.
- If these habits are interfering with your concentration and test grades, establish new habits.
- Be sure your family understands why you need to implement these changes.

Internet and social networking. Being online offers a vast amount of resources for all your classes.

- It is easy to get distracted by the information available on the Internet and social media sites.
- If you use search engines, e-book, and Twitter for personal and recreational purposes, you now need to learn how to use the Internet and social media professionally (see Chapter 18).
- Watch your time when you are online for educational, personal, or professional reasons because hours can slip by before you know it.
- Finding evidence and using websites to enhance understanding is a great strategy. However, time can slip away. For example, you may realize three hours has passed, and you have only completed 25% of the assignment, and the assignment is due in one hour. Be careful of this trap!

Your peers. Peers could be a possible external distraction. The energy devoted to any of the following behaviors can seriously deplete the energy needed to achieve success in the practical/vocational nursing program and can create unneeded stress and frustration. Answer "Yes" or "No" to the following questions about your peers in the LP/LV nursing program.

1. Are the people you associate with at school encouraging your progress in the practical/vocational nursing program?
2. Do you and your peers support and encourage one another?
3. Do you seek out other students who have negative attitudes? If so, what are the conversations you engage in during a supposedly relaxing coffee break?
4. Do the people you associate with love to belittle, complain, and tear down the instructor, the course, and various students in your group?
5. Does your anxiety level increase when you carpool with certain students on test days?
6. Can you identify a peer who is motivating to you?
7. Do your peers who are not enrolled in school pressure you to join them until late in the evening?

◉ Try This

Personal Distractions

List any external physical distractions that are affecting your concentration.

What can you do to eliminate these distractions?

Internal Distractions

You can have the study space, lighting, noise level, equipment, and peers for studying but still not be able to keep your mind on the task at hand. The culprit may be distractions arising from inside you. Common examples of internal distractions and suggestions for overcoming them follow.

Complaints of mental fatigue. Some learners confuse boredom with fatigue.

- Avoid studying one subject so long that you get bored with it.
- Keep your physical self-energized with proper nutrition, sleep, and exercise.
- At the first sign of getting tired, take a short break and come back to new material so that you can get your mental second wind.
- Intermix concepts you like to study versus areas you dread.
- Intermix reading, writing, and interactive assignments.

Daydreaming. Daydreaming can be a creative adventure or wasted time.

- Every time you find your mind wandering from the topic at hand, try putting a checkmark on a piece of paper that you keep at your side. This may remind you that you are drifting off and need to get back to work.
- Students who use this technique find that the number of checkmarks decreases dramatically with time.

LISTENING/VIEWING

The Active and Passive Listener/Viewer

Whether you are involved in a minilecture or a group discussion, viewing DVDs or YouTube clips, or watching a PowerPoint presentation as part of your course assignments, you are going to miss a lot if your mind wanders. Listening/viewing is much more than the mechanical process of hearing or seeing. There are two kinds of listeners/viewers. Which type are you?

- The **passive listener/viewer** receives sounds or sees words with little recognition or personal involvement.
- Passive listeners/viewers may be doodling, staring out the window, staring at the instructor, aimlessly trying to copy everything; all the while thinking about their children or significant others' needs.
- The **active listener/viewer** is always thinking, not just hearing or seeing words.

- Active listeners/viewers listen and look with full attention, are open-minded and curious, and are always asking themselves questions about content.
- The active listener/viewer, who really listens to hear and thoughtfully looks to see, is searching for relevant information, strives to understand it, and is always trying to figure out how content fits into the big picture, as you will also do in the clinical area.
- Active listeners/viewers realize that listening and seeing are important means of gathering information, and they work at developing these skills.
- Active listeners/viewers will identify words that are unfamiliar and seek out other resources to increase their understanding of the content while reading.
- The active listener/viewer searches for ways in which the words can be put to practical use regardless of the student's level of interest in, or degree of, fondness for the instructor or the instructor's dress or mannerisms. Box 2-3 gives you hints on how to become an active listener/viewer.

Try This

Active Versus Passive Listener/Viewer

Identify and list behaviors that indicate you are an active or passive listener/viewer.
My active listening/viewing behaviors:

My passive listening/viewing behaviors:
Discuss your comments with a peer. How can you increase your active listener/viewer skills?

Note *Making* Versus Note *Taking*

An important part of listening/viewing is remembering what you have heard or seen. Some students say that taking notes interferes with their listening/viewing skills. They are correct if they are in the business of taking notes. Research has shown that a student remembers only 50% of a 10-minute lecture when tested immediately afterward and only 25% of that lecture when tested 2 days later. You can improve those percentages to as much as 80% to 90%. Whether using your tablet or paper and pen, the secret is to engage in note *making* whenever you are listening/viewing. Because instructors derive

---

Box 2-3 Hints for Active Listening/Viewing in Classes

- Be well rested for class or activity.
- Complete assignments, extra readings, and exercises before class or activity.
- Focus on what is happening with the lesson. Listen and/or look for key information, central ideas, examples, and study hints.
- Capture key points of the PowerPoint presentations.
- Ask questions before, during, and after class.
- Make eye contact with the speaker.
- Listen when other students are speaking.
- Seek help when a difficult concept is not understood.

Box 2-4 Hints for Note Making

- When using a tablet or pen and paper, include the date and general topic of class/activity at the top of the page and any assignments that are given.
- Place specific topics of the class to the left of the page.
- Indent points as they are presented to explain/discuss the topic.
- Leave spaces between topics to add information to clarify the topic as needed.
- After class, in the left margin of a paper page, record any questions to clarify your understanding of the content.
- At the bottom of the page, summarize the content of the notes on that page, *in your own words*. This summary forces you to think about the ideas in your notes. You are critically thinking about the information, not passively copying it to be memorized later.

---

test questions from minilectures, discussions, activities, DVDs, PowerPoint presentations, and texts, that 80% to 90% of a specific learning activity could translate into a comparable test score. Note *making* will help you to pay attention, concentrate, and organize your ideas.

Note making hints

- Never try to capture every spoken or written word. This is note *taking*, and it is impossible.
- Actively listen/look for the main ideas. Capture them in a way that reflects your personal learning style or styles. You are recording ideas or **key concepts** that you will later add to, correct, and study. Your goal is to understand the information, *not* memorize it.
- Engage in note *making*, formulating condensations of what is said or seen in a textlike manner.
- Develop your own personal symbols, abbreviations, and/or shorthand of sorts to help you capture the main ideas, yet retain readability without having to completely transcribe the notes.
- With practice, notes will improve. Your goal is a set of notes you can use as part of test preparation.
- Outlining is a structured form of note making that starts with major points and indents supporting points. Numbers or letters can be used to outline but are not necessary. Indentations will do. Box 2-4 contains hints for note making.

Some students think that making notes alone will help them to retain the material. Active and frequent review of your notes is an important step in retention of material so that you can recall it at a later time.

HOW TO UNDERSTAND (COMPREHEND) INFORMATION

READING ASSIGNMENTS

"I read the material four times and got a D. My friend read the material once and got an A. It isn't fair." The learner who is speaking is correct. It takes a lot of time to read material four times for a test. The missing ingredient is the lack of **understanding (comprehension)** of information that is read.

- To think critically in nursing, you must have information.
- To acquire information, you must be able to read with understanding.
- Reading with understanding makes possible retention of the information.
- Retention ensures recall.

Earning only a D by merely reading words is a poor return on your time investment. Did you ever drive somewhere without remembering how you got there? That is the same as reading the text four times or getting to the end of a page and not knowing what you read. These readers have zoned out and have mindless reading. As they read, their minds will be somewhere else. They may be hungry, thirsty, tired, need to go to the restroom, or thinking about other things. Their comprehension of the information is low to absent, and test scores will suffer.

Because you are responsible for large amounts of reading in the practical/vocational nursing program, the ability to read with understanding is a necessary skill. Most of us are able to read printed words on a page. However, the reading demanded of a learner and future employee requires understanding of the meaning of the words read. Reading to learn and understand involves a rate of speed and degree of understanding that are effective.

You probably had to take a reading test as part of your preentrance tests for the LP/LV nursing program. Generally these tests are brief. If you scored low, you were referred for help with this skill. Perhaps you were one of those who achieved an acceptable score on these short-reading tests but could use some hints on how to increase your reading efficiency. Evaluate your reading habits by answering "Yes" or "No" to the questions in the following Try This exercise.

◎ Try This

Reading Habit Evaluation

Circle the reading habits that apply to you.

1. Do you ever reread a sentence before you come to the end?
2. Do you ever have trouble figuring out the main point of an author?
3. Do you stop reading every time you come across a word you cannot define and look up the word immediately?
4. Do you read novels, popular magazines, newspapers, and textbooks at the same speed?
5. Do you ever have trouble remembering what you read?
6. Do you have trouble understanding what you read?
7. Do you ever think of other things while you read?
8. Do you read every word of a sentence individually?
9. Do you focus on details when you read?
10. Do you tire quickly when reading?
11. Do you skip uncommon words when you read?

If you answered yes to any of the previous questions, you could benefit from help with your reading. A trip to your school's study skill center, or a consultation with your instructor for assistance with reading can help improve your skill in reading more efficiently and effectively.

Reading Effectively

- Read in phrases, a few words at a time, rather than word by word. Although the brain can view only one word at a time, it understands only when words are in phrases. For better understanding, you should read as you speak (i.e., in phrases).
- Put expression into your reading. You do not speak in a monotone, so why read that way? Musical learners can benefit by singing what they read.
- Be aware of your reading assignments that are technical or scientific in nature and vary your reading speed accordingly. The more recreational your reading material (e.g., novel or magazine), the faster you can read. For more technical or scientific material you must slow down. Regardless of your learning style, when the going gets tough in a paragraph of assigned reading, reading the difficult material aloud may help clear up more challenging information.
- Highlight unfamiliar words as you read. When you are finished reading, copy the words on an index card and look them up in the appropriate dictionary. Most of the unfamiliar words you come across will be medical terms, which can be found in a medical dictionary. At first you will think these words are Greek, and you are right. Quite a few of them are derived from the Greek language. The rest are derived from Latin. You may need to look the unknown words up immediately while you are reading. If so, be sure to reread the content.
- Write the definition on the other side of the card. Break down the word with vertical slashes into its prefix (the word beginning), root (core word), and suffix (word ending) so you can begin making associations with other words that have the same prefix, root, or suffix. If your medical dictionary does not include this information with each word, the information can be found in medical terminology texts or as part of a computer program of medical terminology. Be sure to listen to the word, particularly if you are an auditory learner or if English is not your first language.
- Nursing involves learning a new language. Regardless of learning style, include your own drawing to represent the definitions of these words with the verbal definition. This may help you recall the meaning of the word. Creating a song to remember difficult information can assist many learners. Using index cards allows your language development to progress because you can take the cards wherever you go. You can create flash cards on your computer,

use cards shared by others (i.e., cram.com), and retrieve these cards on your smart phone or tablet. Learning can occur whenever you have a few minutes to spare.

- Highlight key phrases in your text/computer resources/class notes and write notes in the margins. Highlighting will keep you active and result in the identification of key concepts for study and review.
- Audiotape words that you needed to define and also consider audiotaping your notes. Listen to this information when you are commuting, performing household chores, or walking between classes.
- Be sure to use resources provided by your instructor on the Learning Management System (i.e., Moodle, Blackboard, Angel). Determine mandatory versus optional assignments and resources. It is easy to become overwhelmed with all the resources available in today's digital learning environment.

Remember, an important part of any textbook is the index at the back of the book. This index will help you locate information quickly. The glossary (alphabetical listing of boldfaced terms in this text) at the back of the book will provide the definition of these words. Glossaries also usually exist in the textbook's web-based support materials or in e-books. In addition, pay close attention to charts, figures and tables, and recommended web sites. They are included to enhance your learning.

[?] Critical Thinking

Improving Reading Habits

Write your plan to increase your reading comprehension. Note how you will determine progress.

   Include in your plan, school and community resources.

REMEMBERING AND FORGETTING

We all can recall things from the past, indicating that our brains have the ability to store information. But how many times have you said, "I forgot" or "I cannot remember"? Possible causes of forgetting include a negative attitude toward the subject, which interferes with the motivation to remember. Valid as this cause of forgetting may be, perhaps the most common reason why students cannot remember is that they never understood, stored, and comprehended the information in the first place. Perhaps they did not listen/view actively, or they just read words and created a mental blur. Do not fool yourself when studying. Always close your book and describe "the top five" critical concepts regarding the area studied. Explaining health-related concepts to a peer or significant other who does not work in health care can be very helpful in determining if you understand the concept. Their questions and confusion will prompt you to seek additional knowledge.

FROM TEMPORARY TO PERMANENT MEMORY BY WAY OF A NEURAL TRACE

Once you understand information, you need to store that information so that you can recall it when needed on the clinical area (and on tests!). To store information in your long-term memory, a neural trace or record of the information must be created. It takes 4 to 5 seconds for information to move from the temporary (or short-term) memory to the permanent (or long-term) memory. To form a long-term memory of information, you must strive to understand that information. In doing so, you will give your brain the chance to lay down a neural trace. Presto! You have created a memory of that information. Short but frequent study periods with concentration will help you understand information and store it in your long-term memory. Then it is ready for recall. In addition, teaching a peer can be helpful as this helps you in improving your memory recall.

Remember that a positive mental attitude is a factor in learning, allowing you to understand and remember. Remind yourself that all the basic courses in your nursing program and college prerequisites are essential. They are the building blocks for all the remaining courses you will take in the practical/vocational nursing program. The following techniques help increase understanding of your studies by allowing neural traces to be recorded in your brain.

- Scan the reading material first, noting headings, bold words, charts, and tables.
- Next, read the entire selection. Continue to seek out key concepts, basic principles, and key ideas. Be selective and learn to sift out and reject unnecessary details. The activity of being selective helps you lay down neural traces. Emphasize accuracy, not speed. You want correct information to make a clear neural trace. It is difficult to unlearn wrong information and replace it with correct information. You cannot memorize everything. If you could, you would not have an understanding of anything. The student who focuses on memorization has difficulty in applying course information and solving problems in the clinical area.
- Short study periods followed by short rest periods are better than long study marathons. This type of study will reenergize you and allow neural learning to continue during rest periods. It seems that cramming for examinations is treated like a rite of passage among some students. Brain research has shown that short but frequent study periods help you store information in long-term memory. This will make the information available for testing and for application in the clinical area.
- Regardless of your learning style, use as many body senses and as much body movement as possible when trying to learn new information. Recite the information aloud as you read, using your own words. If you can explain it, you must understand it and will know it. Hearing you say the information

aloud is an additional channel that allows neural traces to be recorded.

- Write down the information in your own words. This muscle action will help you clarify ideas and improve thinking. *Do not copy word by word from a book*. Evidence does exist confirming that writing notes can be more beneficial than typing notes for some learners. Assess what works best for you and stick to it!

The techniques of using body senses and body movement are all elements of tactual learning and help lay down a neural trace. Try them, and see if they work for you. Adopt the suggestions that help you understand the material in your classes. They will increase your long-term memory of that information.

MEMORY AIDS

Mnemonic devices are examples of memory aids. Some examples include the following:

- *Rhymes*
  Thirty days hath September . . .
  I before *e* except after *c* . . .
  In fourteen hundred and ninety-two . . .
- *Acronyms*
  Every good boy does fine (to remember the line notes of the treble clef in music)

There are also devices in nursing that can help you remember information. For example:

- *CMTSP* (for assessment of the nerve and blood supply to an extremity)
  C = color
  M = motion
  T = temperature
  S = sensation
  P = pulse
- *PERRLA* (for assessment of the pupils)
  P = pupils
  E = equal in size
  R = round
  R = regular in shape
  L = react to light
  A = accommodation (pupils constrict)

Memorizing these acronyms can help the practical/vocational nurse remember groups of information. They do not take the place of or help you to understand the information. The Internet, including YouTube, has many examples created by other students.

SUCCESSFUL TEST TAKING

The majority of items on the National Council Licensure Examination for Practical/Vocational Nurses (NCLEX-PN®) are written at the application or higher levels of cognitive ability (NCLEX-PN® Examination, 2014). You can anticipate application-level or higher types of questions as part of theory tests in the practical/vocational nursing program. Application-level questions require you to know the information and then apply it to a clinical scenario.

Test-taking skills are divided into three general areas: preparing for the test, actually taking the test, and reviewing the test. The following sections address these areas.

PREPARING FOR THE TEST

- Preparation for test taking begins the first day of class with striving to understand information to do well on the test and meet clinical objectives.
- Clarify content to be covered on the test and the form of the test. The instructor will be measuring your understanding of all the objectives included on the test.
- Clarify the types of questions that will be asked on the tests. For example, will the test be multiple choice and/or short answer? Specific hints for taking multiple-choice, fill-in-the-blank, multiple-response, and prioritizing questions are included in this chapter.
- To store information in your long-term memory, review class information often.
- In study groups, write practice questions and share them to formulate complete accurate answers. Also, discuss the rationale (why) the other three answers are incorrect. Understanding why answers are wrong enhances deeper understanding of the topics.
- Cramming (last-minute studying of material for a test) sometimes results in short-term memory of material that might help you pass a test. However, because you did not engage in repetitions spaced over days, storage in long-term memory will not occur and application of the material to the clinical area will be difficult. In addition, you may score poorly on the final comprehensive exam, NCLEX-PN preparation examinations, and ultimately the NCLEX-PN.
- Do not reread the textbook. You have already completed your reading with understanding. Because you have studied the material periodically since the last test and used study skill techniques, all you need to do at this point is focus on your highlights, margin writings/onscreen notes, and index cards to check your understanding and retention of the information.
- The night before the test, go to bed at your usual time. Eat, hydrate well, and use relaxation techniques before the test.
- Be sure you have thoroughly completed any assignments that will be reviewed by the instructor as a "ticket to test."

TAKING THE NCLEX PN 2016

- If it is a group scheduled test, arrive at the classroom with plenty of time to get your favorite seat.
- Beware of peers who try to make you nervous by saying things like "You didn't study *that*, did you?" or "You mean you *didn't* study that?"
- If an online test, follow the rules for testing. Be sure to have any necessary ID/log in numbers.
- Be sure to complete accurately any information specific to the test, such as a test form (i.e., A or B).

- You organized your time and systematically reviewed for the test. Keep a positive mental attitude. Take slow, deep breaths to reduce tension.
- Avoid spending large amounts of time on difficult questions and avoid getting upset about them. Both of these activities waste time and do not earn points. Go on to the next question and return to the skipped item later. However, be aware that on the NCLEX-PN®, you will not be able to skip items and then go back to them. For the NCLEX-PN®, you need to answer each item as it comes up on the test.
- Take the full time for the test. If you finish early, try to answer the questions you skipped. Review your answers. Retake the question without looking at your previous answer selected. Compare your answers if more than one answer was chosen and decide which is the best possible answer. If a math exam, recalculate questions that caused you difficulty. Compare your steps and confirm that your final answers are the same. Do not look at your previous answer or work until you have recalculated and arrived at a final answer.
- Make sure you have not missed an item or group of items.
- If it is a paper multiple-choice examination with an answer sheet, make sure your answers match up with the proper slot on the answer sheet.
- If you are using a separate answer sheet that will be machine corrected, be sure you erase your first answer completely if you change answers.
- Should you change an answer? Although research has shown that test scores are generally improved by changing answers, we have seen some learners decrease their test scores by the same action. If you have given the item further thought and feel it should be changed, change it. Test by test, keep tabs on your test scores to see whether changing answers is helping your final score and modify your behavior accordingly.

REVIEWING YOUR TESTS

Remember, tests are a learning tool. When the examination is corrected and returned to you, do the following:

- Read the items you missed. Why are they wrong? Did you make a careless mistake? Did you know the material? Can you correct the item without looking in your textbook or notes? If not, look up the answer.
- Read the items you answered correctly. What did you do right to get credit for these items? Do you understand why the other answers were wrong or did you "luck out"?
- Decide which of your study skills and test-taking techniques are and are not working to your benefit. Modify your test-taking strategies accordingly.
- After reviewing their tests, some students realize that they need to study more, study differently, and/or read the test questions more analytically to succeed.
- Discussing content you did not know immediately after a test can assist in providing a deeper understanding and increase long-term retention

needed for the final exam, clinical practice, and NCLEX-PN.

Some students who have organized their notes and their time, and who systematically reviewed and understood the material, have nevertheless done poorly on tests. A reason for this could be that they did not follow the directions on the test. How well do you follow directions? Take out a blank sheet of paper and do the How Well Do You Follow Directions exercise in the Try This box.

How did you do? If you did not follow the directions, do you feel tricked? You were not. The directions were clear, and you simply did not follow them. Listen meticulously to oral directions and read the written directions completely before each test. To those of you who did follow the directions for this exercise, keep up the good work! If directions are ever unclear, ask the instructor before proceeding. Clarify the time limit of the examination. Now you are ready to begin. The hints in the following sections will come in handy for test taking.

◉ Try This

How Well Do You Follow Directions?

Directions: Read the following directions carefully. You will have 1 minute to do the exercise after reading the directions. Be sure to write legibly. When you have finished, check your answers against the directions before handing in the paper. Be sure to read the entire exercise before beginning.

1. On a sheet of paper, print your name in the upper left-hand corner, last name first.
2. Under your name, write the last four digits of your Social Security number.
3. In the upper right-hand corner, write the name and number of the course for which you are taking this exercise.
4. In the lower left-hand corner of the paper, write today's date.
5. In the lower right-hand corner, write your instructor's name, last name first.
6. Fold your paper in half lengthwise.
7. Number the left half of your paper 1 to 6, skipping three lines between each number.
8. Number the right half of your paper 7 to 12, skipping three lines between each number.
9. Now that you have read all the steps in this exercise, do only number 1 of the exercise and hand your paper to the instructor.

REDUCING ANXIETY BEFORE TESTING

Research shows that if a person does not do well on tests, odds are that he or she is less intelligent than the average student, has poor study habits, has weak test-taking skills, or is distracted by personal issues. Less intelligence does not apply or you would not have been admitted into the nursing program. Poor study habits do not apply if you established good study habits, organized your study time as suggested in this chapter, and made use of your personal learning style to comprehend course content. If poor study habits are an issue, you would notice it by poor test grades and should seek help.

Normal anxiety is your friend. This type of anxiety actually makes you sharper and more alert during a test. Only when anxiety overwhelms you does it become your enemy. Accept the energy resulting from normal anxiety as your partner. Total personal comfort is not the key. Normal anxiety leaves you somewhere between too much relaxation and too much tension, perfect for testing.

Make the days before testing work for you through your positive thinking. Think about what you think about. Are you in the habit of seeing yourself failing or just squeaking by? Because everyone daydreams and sets the stage for their reality, daydreaming is a natural way to practice being confident and successful. Visualization may be helpful. For additional ways to relieve anxiety, see the suggestions in Chapter 1.

Spend the evening before the test studying as needed but also focusing on one activity that normally relaxes/refreshes you. Get a good night's sleep by going to bed at your usual time. It is believed that sleep restores memories that were lost during a hectic day. Going to bed extra early and not falling asleep may result in a new worry. Follow through with your usual morning habits. Avoid forcing your system to adjust to a demand that is not a usual part of your routine.

⊚ Try This

Relax!

Make a *tentative* plan for what you will do the evening before any test examination.

HINTS FOR SPECIFIC QUESTIONS

The types of tests you will be taking in the practical/vocational nursing program, including the NCLEX-PN® examination, are achievement tests. They measure how much you have learned. Following are four types of questions found on the NCLEX-PN®. The same types will be used during testing in the practical/vocational nursing program.

Multiple-Choice Questions

- Multiple-choice questions are called items. Each multiple-choice question includes a **stem**, three **distracters**, and a correct answer, referred to as the **key**.
- The stem is the first line of a multiple-choice question.
- It defines the situation for which the learner must pick out the correct answer. The stem is presented as a statement or a question.
- Four statements, called **options**, follow the stem. Three of the options are incorrect answers and are called distracters. One of the options is the correct answer and is called the **key**.
- Distracters are presented to test whether you really have learned the material and can apply it.
- The format of the NCLEX-PN® examination is multiple-choice questions, most of which measure application or higher levels of nursing knowledge. Box 2-5 gives general hints for taking multiple-choice tests.

| Box 2-5 | Multiple-Choice Test Hints |

- Read over all the options given before making any decision.
- Eliminate the options you know are definitely wrong.
- Remember the course subject matter for which you are being tested.
- Eliminate options that are not related to the subject.

⊚ Try This

MULTIPLE-CHOICE QUESTIONS

Choose the appropriate option (the key) for the following multiple-choice statements. There is only one answer to each multiple-choice statement.

1. Multiple-choice questions are examples of:
   a. Sentences for which one-word answers are required.
   b. Questions or sentences with four options for answers.
   c. Two vertical columns that must be matched item by item.
   d. Statements that require a sentence on the answer sheet.
2. When answering multiple-choice questions, it is *not* appropriate to:
   a. Read all of the directions.
   b. Eliminate wrong options.
   c. Read each of the options.
   d. Ignore any negative words.

ANSWER TO MULTIPLE-CHOICE QUESTIONS

1. Key = b. A question or sentence is given with four options. Only one option, the key, is correct. The rest of the options are distracters; that is, options that are there to test whether you really have learned the material and can apply it. Option 1 describes fill-in-the-blank items, option 3 describes matching tests, and option 4 describes short-answer items.
2. Key = d. This multiple-choice item contains a negative word in the stem that can complicate things. Read the stem without the negative word to get some meaning out of it, and then read the options. One option should not fit in with the others. Now reread the original stem with the negative word and see whether or not the option you have already isolated fits in. Items with negative words in the stem are sometimes accused of being more of a reading test than a test of understanding of content. Although the test begins with directions, there may be additional directions before individual multiple-choice questions. These directions may ask you to select one best answer or select what is most important of four correct answers. *Do not stop reading when you think you have the correct answer.* There may be a better option yet to come. Options a, b, and c are true.

Multiple-choice questions are not "multiple-guess" questions. Think through each response thoroughly before choosing your answer. Should you ever guess? To be able to make a decision about guessing, you must know whether you will be penalized for wrong answers. Even if you are penalized, figure out the odds. If you can eliminate one distracter for certain, you have a better chance of answering correctly. Can you eliminate two out of four distracters? Your chances are now even better. You make the decision. Remember, on the NCLEX-PN® you will have to answer every item as it appears on the computer screen.

Fill-in-the-blank. These questions require you to calculate an item; for example, a medication dosage or intake and output. You may be asked to round the answer to the nearest whole number or the nearest tenth. Be sure to read directions carefully.

◎ Try This

Fill-in-the-Blank Questions

The LVN needs to chart intake for a patient. The patient drinks 8 ounces of coffee, a slice of toast, and 8 ounces of water. Record the intake in milliliters. (Fill-in-the-blank questions will be used in your courses with a clinical component.)

ANSWER

Intake is 480 mL. Thirty milliliters equals one ounce.

Multiple-response. A question is presented and you need to select all the options that relate to the information in the question. No partial credit is given. If there are five correct options and you select only four, you do not receive credit.

◎ Try This

Multiple-Response Questions

1. Indicate the strategies to improve reading comprehension. *(Select all that apply.)*
   a. Read text word by word.
   b. Highlight key information.
   c. Read quickly to complete the assignment.
   d. Avoid writing in book margins.
   e. Draw pictures to explain concepts.

ANSWER

b, e

Prioritizing. A nursing situation is presented and you need to prioritize (choose what you would do first, second, third, etc.) from a list of given steps or interventions. You would order the answer options from the first to the last step or priority. This is also called an ordered-response question.

◎ Try This

Prioritizing Question

Michael has decided he wants to be a practical nurse and work in long-term care. Prioritize the actions Michael must take to reach his goal.
   a. Pass all nursing courses.
   b. Obtain a job as a practical nurse.
   c. Pass the NCLEX-PN®.
   d. Investigate practical nursing.
   e. Be admitted to the nursing program.
   f. Graduate from the nursing program.

ANSWER

d, e, a, f, c, b

BEYOND THE BASICS OF STUDY SKILLS

Beyond the study skill methods reviewed thus far, many other academic resources are available to assist you. Identifying and using these academic resources will increase your likelihood of success. These Academic Resources are a critical component of your personal plan for success. As we discussed in Chapter 1, prioritization is important in time management. How you prioritize your use of academic resources will be important to your ability to SUCCEED!

💡 Keep in Mind

Knowing where and how to access nursing information makes keeping up-to-date for patient care and passing the NCLEX-PN® less stressful. In addition, it will protect your nursing license.

YOUR SCHOOL'S LEARNING RESOURCE CENTER

If you are a returning adult student, you know the **learning resource center (LRC)** as the library. Today, many students may never physically access the library but instead they use a virtual library. Whether you visit the library in person or virtually you will find today's library consists of books and countless electronic evidence-based resources. These diverse resources can support various academic levels and types of learning styles.

DIFFERENT STUDENT SKILL LEVELS AND DIFFERENT RESOURCES OF THE LEARNING RESOURCE CENTER

All LRCs have *similar* print and digital resources or access to these resources. However, not all LRCs are *equal* in technology. As a result, some small schools may use their affiliating clinical site libraries and electronic medical resources to supplement their school resources. The students' ability to use the LRC and related resources is very varied (Box 2-6). If you are skilled in this area, be aware that some of your peers may not be as skilled in using the LRC and its general resources and technology. Given differences in LRCs across schools and differences in the student's skill level, the discussion that follows focuses on what tasks are needed to obtain nursing information for class and clinical (Box 2-7).

- Box 2-6 includes a checklist of tasks you need to carry out to fully use the general print and digital resources and technology of your LRC for your student year and as a graduate.
- Box 2-7 includes a checklist of tasks you need to carry out to fully use the nursing resources and technology of your LRC for your student year and as a graduate.

Despite prior LRC experience, you need to identify and correct any deficiencies in regard to using nursing resources and technology in your school's and clinical site's LRC. Knowing how to carry through the tasks will save you energy, time, and frustration.

Box 2-6	Checklist of Tasks Needed to Fully Use Learning Resource Center General Resources and Technology

Identify which of the following tasks you are able to carry out in your LRC by writing "Yes" next to them. Write "No" next to the tasks you are unable to carry out.

- Does the LRC staff provide tours and/or orientation to services in person or online?
- Are library staff available to provide support by phone, e-mail, and/or real-time online?
- How does my LRC classify all of its print and digital holdings (books, videotapes, periodicals, CD-ROMs, DVDs, etc.)?
- How can I find the call number of a specific item?
- Once I have the call number, how can I locate a specific item?
- Where do I check out a specific item for home use?
- Can I access resources in my LRC from my home computer?
- How do I check out AV equipment for home use?
- How can I access needed resources that are not in my LRC?
- How can I access reference materials? (These would include an English dictionary, medical and nursing dictionaries, encyclopedias, almanacs, yearbooks, atlases, handbooks, and other similar categories of books.)
- Can I access learning resources in other schools' LRCs?
- Where is the circulation desk?
- Where are the copying machines? Do I need a code?
- Are there computers for personal use? Do they have Internet access?
- Where can I study in the LRC?
- How can I reserve a room for group study?
- Where are pamphlets located?
- Is there a Wi-Fi hot spot for a personal laptop, smart-phone, iPod Touch, or iPad (or other tablet)?

Box 2-7	Checklist of Tasks Needed to Fully Use Learning Resource Center Nursing Resources and Technology

Identify which of the following tasks you are able to carry out in your LRC and write "Yes" next to them. Write "No" next to the tasks you are unable to carry out.

- How do I access current print and digital nursing journals and periodicals?
- How do I access back issues of print and digital nursing journals and periodicals?
- How can I obtain a copy of articles in back issues of nursing journals and periodicals?
- How can I obtain a print or digital copy of an article in a nursing journal or periodical if my LRC does not subscribe to the publication?
- Does my LRC have online databases for nursing and general information?
- Where are the nursing texts located in the stacks?
- What is the procedure for accessing nursing materials that have been put on reserve for nursing classes?
- Are mobile devices available for use in the clinical area? If so, what nursing information is available for use with these devices? Are there any free or low-cost apps recommended?
- Are handheld computers available for class/clinical use?
- Can I use a tablet to meet my computer needs at school?
- Are earphones supplied?

◎ Try This

Checklist: General and Nursing Resources and Technology

On index cards or an electronic device, list the general and nursing LRC tasks from Boxes 2-6 and 2-7 with which you are *not* familiar. Indicate on your personal timeline when you will accomplish these skills.

WHERE TO START

Investigate your learning resource center. You need to know the physical layout of the LRC and general hours of operation. Is a tour available in person or online? Touring the LRC can save you many wasted hours and much frustration later in the school year. Ask the librarian the best way for you to find the answers to items on your checklists with which you are unfamiliar. LRC staff are available to answer questions. The LRC staff are experts in their field and can help you immensely.

General Information About Resources of the Library

Librarian. The librarian is a college-educated specialist who knows what the library has to offer in the area of information and where that information can be found. Look at the librarian as a professional educator about information for learning and as a person who is always ready to assist you. They are experts in identifying evidenced-based resources.

Circulation desk. The circulation desk is the area where library materials that can be checked out are processed. If materials that can be checked out are reserved by your instructor, they will probably be found here. Today, students often access materials electronically.

Online catalog. You can obtain a lot of information about your LRC by yourself once you understand the cataloging system. Most LRCs' card catalogs are online (computerized) catalogs. All print and digital materials found in your LRC are indexed in this computerized system. In addition to books, cataloged materials also include audiovisual materials (audio recordings, videos, CD-ROMs, DVDs, etc.). You can search for desired materials by subject, title, or author. The LRC may also have access to free or purchased access to digital databases. If the LRC does not have the material you are searching for, but another LRC on the online system does, this information might also be included.

In many systems students are able to access the **online catalog** and digital resources from home via computer, user name, and password. This system of cataloging saves students valuable time and energy. Keep your user name and password easily accessible to decrease frustration.

LOCATING IN-HOUSE RESOURCES

Libraries may choose to use either of two systems to classify in-house materials so they are easy to locate: the Dewey Decimal system and the Library of Congress classification system. Regardless of the system your library uses, the **call number** shown on the author, title, or subject screens is the same number as that on the material itself. Copy, in order, all the letters and numbers in the call number.

The Stacks

Armed with the call number, you can proceed to the **stacks**, the place where the majority of materials that can be checked out are located. The books are placed in call number order according to academic disciplines. When you do find the material you are looking for, note that materials covering the same subject are shelved in the same area. You might find additional useful material on the same shelf.

Reference Materials

Reference materials include dictionaries and other similar categories of books, including medical and nursing dictionaries, almanacs, yearbooks, atlases, encyclopedias, and handbooks. Some of these resources can be found online. You will find up-to-date information on any subject in this area. Print reference books generally do not circulate. Information from print reference materials may be copied on a copy machine if the book cannot be checked out. Online information can be printed. Be cautious to print only what is necessary. It is likely that you are allocated a certain number of copies per semester or program.

Interlibrary Loan Services

Interlibrary loan services allow your LRC to borrow materials you need that are not in your library's holdings. Print books and audiovisual materials are available through this service. A link for a digital full-text version of an article may be provided. If your LRC does not have the periodical in which an article you need is located, or an electronic subscription to the source, a photocopy of the article or a link, free of charge, might be obtained from a library that does have some form of the periodical.

Professional Journals/Periodicals

Practical/vocational nurses need to be aware of sources that will provide up-to-date, relevant, and accurate information on nursing topics. Professional journal/periodicals consist of articles containing news or material of current interest to a particular discipline. These are important, timely resources for a learner in a field that is changing as quickly as nursing and health care Because professional journals are published weekly, monthly, and quarterly (i.e., periodically), they are also called **periodicals**. Because of the frequent publication dates, they complement a comprehensive textbook that is published every several years. Given the quantity of articles, the titles and authors of various articles cannot possibly be included in the online catalog of the LRC. Instead, articles can be located using bound books called print periodical indexes and/or digital databases. Today, the digital database is the common source and often can be accessed from home via the Internet. Once the article is located it can be downloaded immediately to your computer or sent by e-mail via interlibrary loan. A unique digital object identifier (DOI) also exists today to assist in locating electronic documents. The DOI can identify a specific professional journal, article, or even a table within an article. The DOI is found in reference lists. You can click on the DOI and link directly to the journal/article (i.e., doi:10.1000/182), eliminating the need to use a digital database. This saves time! Professional journals of interest to practical/vocational nurses include, but are not limited to, *The Journal of Practical Nursing; Nursing Made Incredibly Easy; Nursing2016 (the year in the title changes as the year changes); Advance for Nurses;* and *The American Journal of Nursing.*

Try This

Professional Journals

Identify the location of the aforementioned nursing journals in your LRC. Determine which of them will help you keep up to date in nursing. Identify the location of other nursing periodicals.

Digital Periodical Databases/Print Periodical Indexes

Entries in **digital periodical databases/print periodical indexes** are listed by author, title, and subject. Read/view the help sections to ease your use of these resources. The following are two digital periodical databases/print periodical indexes that are of special value to practical/vocational nursing students. Your instructor may suggest others.

1. *Cumulative Index to Nursing and Allied Health Literature* (CINAHL®). This comprehensive and authoritative periodical index contains current listings for nursing and allied health fields and for others interested in health care issues, including biomedicine, consumer health, and alternative medicine. Nursing, allied health, and related journals are reviewed and indexed for over 11,000 topics. There are online

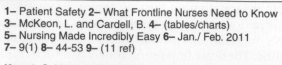

1– Patient Safety 2– What Frontline Nurses Need to Know
3– McKeon, L. and Cardell, B. 4– (tables/charts)
5– Nursing Made Incredibly Easy 6– Jan./ Feb. 2011
7– 9(1) 8– 44-53 9– (11 ref)

Key: 1. Subject. 2. Title of the article. 3. Authors of the article. 4. Additional information found in article. 5. Periodical in which the article appears. If the periodical is abbreviated, the periodical index in the front of the book will have a list of periodical abbreviations and the full name of the journal for which those abbreviations stand. 6. Date of publication. 7. Volume and number of periodical. 8. Page numbers of article. 9. Number of references used.

FIGURE 2-4 Cumulative Index to Nursing and Allied Health Literature.

tutorials to assist in understanding how to use the index. Figure 2-4 illustrates the information found in a typical entry in the CINAHL® print edition. Most schools have purchased access to online CINAHL® databases or have access via a clinical site. CINAHL® will be your primary source for current, accurate, and relevant articles used for evidence-based patient care.

2. *ProQuest.* This digital database collection covers all disciplines, providing access to dissertations and theses; three centuries of newspapers; more than 450,000 academic e-books; and a diverse collection of important scholarly professional journals and other content.

Your LRC will have a periodical listing that includes professional journals and magazines and the dates of the issues that are found in your library.

Remember, if the article you need is in a journal or magazine that is not held in your library in some form, see the librarian. The librarian can locate the article online in another library and arrange for you to receive a link or photocopy by interlibrary loan. Understanding how to use a digital database is a necessary skill.

◉ Try This

Locate the following article using the digital database CINAHL Search using the author and title of the article then search using the doi. Which was quicker?

Greenwood, D. (2015). Better Type 2 Diabetes Self-Management Using Paired Testing and Remote Monitoring. *American Journal of Nursing*, 115(2), 58-65. doi:10.1097/01. NAJ.0000460698.78499.33

Copyright laws prohibit the instructor from copying an article for each of you. For this reason, the required reading articles may be available on a reserve basis in the LRC by photocopy or digitally by a link within a Learning Management System (LMS). Copyright laws generally allow you to have one copy of an article (i.e., photocopy, print the reserve article, or download the article from the LMS). Because of copyright laws, use caution in redistributing the article electronically. This action may be prohibited.

Magazines and Newspapers

Include newspapers and popular magazines as sources of information on health-related topics. Magazine articles never replace professional journal reading, but they do provide information that your patients read. As one practical nursing student said, "I had better be up to date and understand what my patients are reading." Be aware of the author's expertise. Examine the author's demographic information and any funding received. This will help you identify possible author bias and evaluate the accuracy of the information on the topic.

RESPONSIBLE USE OF LEARNING STRATEGIES

Face-to-Face Class

Lectures/minilectures. Some of your teachers may have been taught using the "bucket theory" of education. The **bucket theory** suggests that merely by lecturing, a teacher can transfer knowledge from the teacher's mind to the mind of the student. This teaching method evolved from Aristotle's day. The teacher was considered the source and the vehicle of transmission of information, similar to a sage on the stage. Of course, the printing press, computers, and the Internet had yet to be invented!

Research has shown that students learn best from methods other than traditional lectures. Although traditional lecturing is an outmoded form of instruction, *brief lectures* (minilectures) can be valuable as a means of enhancing your assigned readings and clarifying information. A minilecture situation is a brief episode, taking only a portion of class time. Minilectures are intended to enhance your reading assignment, not replace it. A minilecture reflects the fact that the teacher spent time searching, reading, selecting, and organizing information for your benefit. The instructor has done all the work and has become smarter in the process. However, minilectures are passive learning experiences that do not actively involve you in the learning process. You need to remain especially alert and actively involved. The instructor may introduce various techniques (for example, Clickers) to keep you actively involved during minilectures as well as class in general.

Lecture-discussion. In the **lecture-discussion strategy**, the instructor shares several ideas with the class and then stops to let the class discuss the ideas. Sometimes the instructor may say that the next class will be nothing but discussion of the assignment. The instructor then acts as a discussion leader; or ideally a student may lead the discussion. An example of a learning strategy to help keep the discussion focused on course objectives includes the following:

- Box 2-8: an example of a learning strategy used in minilectures called **discussion buddy**
- Box 2-9: hints for participating in discussions and related activities

Box 2-8	Learning Strategy: Discussion Buddy

- You may be assigned to a discussion buddy before class.
- The two of you will be given a discussion task.
- Focus carefully on the minilecture and other resources on the Course Management System so you will be able to formulate an answer to the discussion task.
- After the minilecture, discussion buddies share their answers with one another. A new answer is formulated from both your responses.
- The instructor will choose students at random to share their newly composed answers with the class.

Box 2-9	Hints for a Discussion Class

- Be prepared to participate in the discussion by completing your assignment before class. This will allow you to be an active participant.
- Be sure you have made a list of questions about the assignment. Discussions are the perfect time to clear up questions.
- While other learners are speaking, listen to what they have to say. Some learners make the mistake of using other learners' speaking time to formulate their own comments.
- You may disagree with others during a discussion. Do so assertively and firmly. Provide evidence. Avoid yelling matches. It enriches your world to listen to another's point of view before responding.

Cooperative learning. **Cooperative learning** is a technique that emphasizes individual accountability for learning a specific academic task while working in small groups. The teacher is a facilitator. Cooperative learning encourages you to:

- be actively involved in your learning
- develop critical-thinking skills
- develop positive relationships with your peers
- develop the ability to work in a team situation, a skill an employer is looking for in an employee

What goes on in the classroom is just as important as what goes on in a reading assignment. There is, however, one great difference between the two: *You can repeat a reading assignment, but you can never repeat a missed face-to-face or synchronous online class.* Here are some hints to help you learn from any face-to-face *or synchronous online* class situation:

- Before taping a class activity, clarify if taping is allowed.
- Never skip a face-to-face *or synchronous online* class unless an emergency arises. Some students skip class to get another hour's sleep, use the time to prepare for another class or an examination, or get in their allowable number of absences. When an emergency does make it necessary for you to miss class, photocopying notes is not the answer to catch

Box 2-10	Verbal Cues for Key Ideas in Minilectures, Discussions, and Online Activities

"The most important difference is . . ."
"The major principle in this situation is . . ."
"To sum up . . ."
"The main point is . . ."
"Finally, . . ."
"In conclusion, . . ."
"Moreover, . . ."
"To repeat . . ."

up on what you missed. Ask a peer to go over his or her notes and tell you about the class. Recall what you learned about personal learning styles.
- Come to class prepared. By having the reading assignment completed before class, key terms and concepts will be familiar to you. You will be ready to participate in learning activities.
- Listen for verbal cues that will inform you of key points during minilectures (Box 2-10). Keep vigilant for nonverbal cues given by the instructor that will also inform you of key ideas. Examples are raising the hands; a long, dramatic pause; raising or lowering the voice; and leaning toward the class or into the computer screen. Be sure to copy everything that is written on the whiteboard/smartboard. If any review materials are provided, be sure to focus on these.
- The instructor speaks at a much slower rate than you are capable of thinking. The fact that you can think faster than the instructor can speak allows you to relate this new information to information you have learned in the past and to formulate questions that need clarification or for content you do not understand. Ask these questions in class and/or write down your questions during lecture to discuss with the instructor after class. It is *your* responsibility to question what you do not understand.
- Review your notes as soon after class as possible. This will improve your long-term memory of the information.
- Stay actively engaged while in class. Avoid using class time to work on other projects, such as care plans. Be an active listener.

Distance learning. Some of the courses in your practical/vocational nursing program or parts of courses may be available through **distance learning**. In this learning strategy, the student and teacher are separated by physical distance. The course may be synchronous (real time) or asynchronous (accessed at different times). In a synchronous class all of the students in the course and the instructor participate simultaneously by means of interactive website. This is similar to a face-to-face class. However, most common is an asynchronous format in which the students choose when they will attend class. In an asynchronous format, it is critical to adhere to due dates for posts and online discussions. A **blended course** (hybrid course) combines face-to-face instruction with online learning and is more common in an LP/LV nursing program.

Have the equipment needed, or access to equipment needed, to complete course assignments. You are in charge of your schedule. As with any class, self-discipline and motivation are important tools for success. The time management information in Chapter 1 will help you establish a weekly class and study schedule. The nature of the course requires you to have access to social media (i.e., LMS, e-mail, e-book, Google account and/or Twitter). Check these sites daily for messages from instructors and fellow students.

Study skills are a must. Distance-learning courses require much reading and self-discipline. The ability to understand information by means of the written word is important. Individual learning styles can impact your perception of distance learning.

Distance learning has proven to be at least as effective as traditional methods of instruction. Positive features include the fact that students become more active in personal learning and have more involvement in and control over the learning process. Some students report feeling less of a social connection. It is possible to plan a meeting with peers on campus or at a cafe to fulfill this need.

TECHNOLOGY USE DURING LEARNING ACTIVITIES

Class time requires active listening and participation in learning activities. Avoid using class time for snoozing, talking to friends, or any of the activities listed in Box 2-11. Your time in the LP/LV nursing program gives you the opportunity to sharpen (bring to an excellent level) professional behavior that is appropriate for your job as a practical/vocational nurse.

Box 2-11 Technology Courtesy for Learning Activities

- Check school policy for the use of cell phones, smartphones, iPod Touch, iPad, laptops, and so on.
- If cell phones are allowed, turn off the ringer and put it on vibrate.
- If it is necessary to return a call, leave the immediate area, quietly make your call, and quickly complete it.
- Avoid e-mailing, texting, tweeting, instant messaging, and playing games during class activities.
- Avoid surfing the Internet during class activities.
- Avoid listening to music on your iPod during class activities.

OTHER LEARNING RESOURCES

SYLLABUS AND COURSE OUTLINES

A **syllabus** is an up-to-date course document available by handout or online as part of a **Learning Management System (LMS)** at the beginning of a course. At a minimum, the syllabus includes a course description, course objectives, course requirements for a passing grade, required textbooks, grading scale, instructor information (office location, how to contact the instructor, office hours, response times for e-mails, etc.), course policies, and testing policies. A course outline may refer to policies in a student handbook. Be sure to review this material.

Your school may have **course outlines** for each course. These outlines are a great help to an adult learner. They contain unit-by-unit course objectives/student learning outcomes and content areas, which indicate what the learner must know to pass the course. Each objective/student learning outcome begins with a verb. Watch the verb carefully because it tells you the level of understanding you must achieve to meet the objective. If an objective states you must *list* something, that task is quite different from having to *compare* and *contrast* the same information. Instructors develop their test questions from the course objectives and course content. The course outline will include a list of resources indicating where the information to answer the objectives is found. Supplementary material in the form of worksheets, charts, activities, and additional reading may be included to round out your learning. An LMS contains complete online course content and includes, for example, a syllabus, library links, learning modules, a calendar for quizzes, tests, and assignments, chat rooms, and other features. If the amount of material is overwhelming, schedule a meeting with your instructor to prioritize the resource materials. This task could be dependent on your learning style. A tutor can also assist you.

STUDY GROUPS

Do you have a desire to achieve better grades? Do you need to study more effectively? Do you need a little support? Joining a **study group** is a great strategy! Students usually form their own study groups out of need. Studies have shown that despite each person's preferred learning style, *actively* participating in a study group can improve academic performance. *Actively* participating is the key! Sometimes students join a study group thinking that the group will help them pass, and they avoid active participation; these students are similar to freeloaders. Study groups work when students use them to become actively involved in their own learning. The group provides an outlet for discussion of material, which promotes retention. A diverse study group is generally most effective as each person's unique background stimulates the discussion.

Active study group members usually develop questioning and reasoning skills on a higher level.

TUTORING

Tutoring is a very select study group. Tutoring can be provided one on one or in small groups. For best results, the student arranges tutoring through a special department by means of instructor referral or self-referral. This referral can be electronic. The purpose of tutoring is to help a student understand the material better and pass the course. You must actively identify your learning needs. Specifically defining the content you do not understand will maximize your tutoring experience. Students who need tutoring *sometimes* have learning disabilities. In these situations, because of an excellent attitude on the part of these students and their active participation in the tutoring process, tutoring can be very beneficial.

NURSING SKILLS/SIMULATION LAB

The **nursing skills/simulation lab** is a resource that will allow you to practice and develop your physical nursing skills and clinical decision-making skills. This lab contains the physical items needed to make the practice area as similar to the workplace as possible. *Skills must be practiced.* In addition, the rationale for skills must also be verbalized. Reading about skills, watching a DVD or YouTube clip, and watching other students practice are only the first steps in developing a physical skill. *Practice until you are proficient in each skill so you feel competent performing these tasks in the clinical area.* Remember that you recall 10% of what you hear, 20% of what you see, 50% of what you read, and 90% of what you do. The Teton Lakota Indians have a proverb that summarizes how SPNs/SVNs need to approach the skills component of their nursing program: "Tell me and I'll listen. Show me and I'll understand. Involve me and I'll learn."

You will be required to make appointments to give a return demonstration of skills. Practice with a peer before this return demonstration. When you make an appointment with the skills lab, you are entering into an agreement with the lab personnel. Your responsibility is to practice the skill until you can perform it in the time frame of your appointment. If you are unable to keep your appointment, inform the lab personnel. This will allow them to schedule other students into lab time for skills testing.

Simulation is a learning activity that uses imaginary patient situations that mimic the reality of the clinical environment. The learner has the opportunity to think like a nurse and gather data, set priorities, plan, implement, and evaluate care in a virtual (reproduced/replicated by a computer) patient situation without risk to the patient. Simulation encourages decision making and critical thinking. Working as a team is often integrated into a simulation. It is ideal if students from different health programs can work collaboratively during a simulation.

Simulation can take many forms:

- **Case scenarios** can be delivered in a printed format or by computer. In each type, an imaginary patient story will bring reality to theory in the form of a clinical situation. Both forms may be used when the patient census is inadequate for patient assignments, when a desired patient situation is unavailable, or when enhanced learning of specific concepts is desirable. There are many web-based scenarios available (i.e., www.nln.org/professional-development-programs).
- **Computer simulation** can be a learning situation on CD inserted into a computer. The computer-patient simulation changes, as it would in the clinical area. This requires the student to evaluate the situation and plan new assessments (data collection) and interventions.
- **Static simulation** uses mannequins that are full-size body models or models of specific parts of the body made to be realistic. These mannequins are used for practicing skills before reaching the clinical area and returning demonstrations of procedures; for example, urinary catheterization, insertion of intravenous lines, and application of colostomy bags.
- **Electronic simulation** uses mannequins that are high-tech, more costly simulation models that can be programmed to set up different patient situations and allow practice of nursing procedures and data collection (assessment). Simchart for nursing can be used in alignment with a patient simulation. Simchart is modeled on an actual Electronic Health Record (EHR) used in a health care institution.
- **Virtual clinical excursions** are computer programs that electronically (controlled by a computer) provide a virtual hospital floor and patients whose conditions are constantly changing. This allows the student to practice in a safe environment. The data available mimic the data accessed if in a real clinical setting, thereby facilitating clinical decision-making as appropriate for the LPN/LVN role.

STUDY SKILLS LAB

If your school has a **study skills lab**, it is available to help you with academic problem areas. Examples of areas in which help is available are study skills, time management, reading (including vocabulary and comprehension), listening skills, math skills, test-taking skills (especially situation tests), note making, writing, and any other academic problem you may have. You can go to the skills lab on your own or by referral from your instructor or counselor.

No Time for Tutoring or the Skills Center

Some students who need tutoring or the study skills center state they do not have time to go for help. Be sure to create a plan that allows some accessibility during available tutor hours. At some time in the program, most students need to access the tutoring or the study skills center.

AUDIOVISUAL MATERIALS

In addition to minilectures, discussions/activities, textbooks, and articles, the instructor may have included videos, CDs, DVDs, PowerPoint presentations, **podcasts**, and other electronic resources as part of your assignment. Audiovisual (AV) materials are not considered extra or additional assignments. They are a significant part of all areas of learning. These learning resources give faith to the saying "A picture is worth a thousand words." AV materials provide an additional sensory channel for learning, compared with reading. In some nursing courses, especially autotutorial skills courses, the AV medium is the course. The student progresses independently, attending periodic lecture-discussion classes and seeking out the instructor when questions arise. Approach the AV material as you do a class. Realize that you have the option of repeating all or part of the material when you do not understand it.

INTERNET

The Internet offers unlimited resources on many subjects. The Internet is the physical infrastructure that allows the electronic circulation of billions of sites of information to Internet-ready computer users. An Internet provider charges a monthly fee and is a computer user's link to the Internet. Provider services can be dial-up modems, dedicated service lines (DSL), or broadband (high-speed Internet), meaning that you have instant access when your computer is turned on. Providers such as Comcast and Verizon provide broadband services. Broadband service is critical to effectively retrieve information from the Internet in a timely manner. In addition to computers, many types of electronic devices exist today to support students (i.e., iPads, tablets, smart phones).

The World Wide Web (www) is the most effective means of providing access to the vast amount of information available on the Internet. Everything on the Internet has an address (called a URL) that helps in locating a specific site. Most addresses begin with www, followed by a dot. The next letters in the address are specific to the site you wish to access; for example, www.ncsbn indicates the site that provides information about the national council of state boards of nursing (NCSBN). This is followed by three letters, called a domain name, which denote the site's source.

For example, the complete address for the site for information about NCSBN is www.ncsbn.org. The following are common domain names and their meanings:
- com: for-profit sites
- gov: government sites
- edu: colleges and universities that grant 4-year degrees
- org: usually reserved for nonprofit organizations
- net: network organizations
- mil: military

Search engines are programs that can help students zero in on the exact information for which they are searching. Search engines periodically scan the web and index it. Therefore, search engines are like the telephone book. Popular search engines include Google, Bing, Yahoo, Ask, and AOL. On Evolve are more suggestions of Internet sites that can be used by SPNs/SVNs as learning resources and for patient teaching resources.

It is necessary for the LPN/LVN to develop information literacy in finding health information for your patients and yourself. Although the Internet provides the means of obtaining that information, it is up to you to evaluate if that information is recent, accurate, and relevant. Wikipedia, known as a free online encyclopedia, is an example of a source that nursing students should *not* use to obtain information for class or clinical. Wikipedia is written by volunteers, and the articles can be edited by anyone with site access. The quality, accuracy, and appropriateness of Wikipedia articles are not checked by scholars in the related field of study (**peer-reviewed**).

Box 2-12 contains guidelines for gathering Internet information for your use or to share with patients. Let the user beware: Students can spend a lot of time on the Internet. To save time, take a few minutes to read the section that gives hints for using a specific site. Stay focused on your purpose. Avoid getting sidetracked.

Peer Assistance with Computer/Internet

If you do not have computer/Internet experience, ask students in your class who are familiar with using computers for hints on using this technology and information resource. Consider taking a short instructional course offered by your school or local library. In addition, you can ask the Internet a question when you are unsure of how to do or find something. Many refer to this action as "Google it."

MOBILE DEVICES

Because of Wi-Fi, your educational institution and/or clinical site may provide wireless access to the Internet. **Mobile devices** with **Internet** capabilities are useful for obtaining information for class and the

Box 2-12   Guidelines for Gathering Internet Information

- The Internet is not regulated in any way. Anyone can publish anything they want on the Internet. When searching the Internet, you can find the most recent and accurate information, as well as the most inaccurate and out-of-date information.
- Let the user beware: People can spend a lot of time on the Internet. To save time, take a few minutes to read the section that gives hints for using a specific site. Stay focused on your purpose. Avoid getting sidetracked.
- Check the professional credentials and qualifications of the author of the information.
- Determine the organization, group, agency and company that created the site. This will help you evaluate the credibility of the information. The domain name is helpful in evaluating credibility. For example, a site that has a ".gov" domain name may be more credible than a ".com" site that may be promoting a product.
- Check the date the information was created and last modified. This will ensure up-to-date material.
- What are the objectives of the author of the material? Does the author express opinions? Does the author have a personal bias?
- Seek the assistance of the librarian to effectively search key words.
- When conducting searches, supply key words to help the search tool narrow the document results to just the ones you want to see.
- When using key words for a search engine, use phrases or single words that are pertinent to your topic and describe it objectively.
- Use nouns only, and put the most important words that describe your topic first.
- When searching with a phrase (e.g., "study skills"), surround the phrase with quotation marks. This forces the database to search for words that are next to each other.
- Plus signs (+) or the word "AND" identify words that must appear in the search (e.g., nursing+practical).
- Minus signs (–) or the word "NOT" exclude words from the search (e.g., NCLEX-PN®, NOT NCLEX®-RN).

clinical area. Before utilizing the following information, clarify the policy of your school and clinical area for using computers and mobile devices while on the clinical area.

- **You must separate your private and professional uses of mobile devices.** If your device is capable of taking photos or videos, do not use these functions with patients. Health Insurance Portability and Accountability Act (HIPAA) requirements (see Chapter 7) prohibit the use of **electronic devices** for these purposes. If you are a student, you could be suspended or dismissed from the program. If you are licensed, you could receive a sanction regarding your license if you take photos or videos of patients in the clinical area.
- Nursing-based software that contains drug information, laboratory values, disease processes, and a medical dictionary is available as a subscription to be downloaded on your mobile device.
- Reference e-books for downloading on your mobile device can be purchased.
- **Apps** can provide instant clinical reference materials at the point of care for drugs, lab studies, and medical/surgical conditions. Some apps are free, but others charge a fee. Check the app store of your device.
- Check the appropriateness of selected software/apps with your instructor.
- Sites that provide information for mobile devices can be found on Evolve.

COMPUTER-AIDED INSTRUCTION

Computer-aided instruction (CAI) has the following benefits:
- Allows learners to be actively involved in their learning
- Encourages problem solving, a skill that employers expect of practical/vocational nurses
- Provides immediate feedback by quickly evaluating answers and decision-making strategies
- Provides an opportunity to develop the ability to follow directions

CAI simplifies concepts and reinforces skills that have been presented previously. If you do not have computer skills and CAI is used in your practical/vocational nursing program, you will be taught the skills necessary to use this type of teaching strategy. The process is simple even if you do not have any computer experience. The computer is essential in the clinical area to store and retrieve patient information via the Electronic Medical Record (EMR).

GUEST SPEAKERS

Nurses and other health professionals are sometimes invited to visit nursing classes as **guest speakers** or to make presentations via distance modalities (i.e., Skype, FaceTime, AdobeConnect, GotoMeeting, Podcast). These speakers donate their time to present current information on their areas of expertise and updates on specific nursing topics. Often their employers have released them to visit nursing classes.

Get Ready for the NCLEX-PN® Examination

Key Points

- Brain dominance impacts thinking style, which in turn impacts the way you learn.
- Each side of the brain processes things differently. It is accepted that the left hemisphere is more verbal and processes in parts and sequences. The right hemisphere is nonverbal and sees a total picture. A connection between the right brain and music has been established.
- The two most common thinking styles are linear (left-brain dominant) and global (right-brain dominant).
- Some people think in pictures (visual learners). Some hear sounds (auditory learners). Some experience a feeling in regard to what they are thinking about and learn best by doing (kinesthetic/tactile learners). Each learning style can be enhanced, and it is possible to use more than one learning style to reinforce learning.
- Multiple intelligences translate into learning styles. Identifying whether you are a linguistic learner (likes words and new vocabulary), a logical learner (organized and consistent), a spatial learner (prefers boxes and diagrams to words), a musical learner (likes to hum, sing, or play a musical instrument), a bodily/kinesthetic learner (likes touching and moving), an interpersonal learner (likes sharing, comparing, and cooperating), or an intrapersonal learner (likes working alone, self-paced instruction) further enhances your learning ability.
- Your personal attitude toward learning also influences the learning process. Attitude is closely related to whether you are a reactive learner who expects to be taught or an active learner who takes charge of his or her own education.
- Clustering, a form of mapping, is a method of note making. Concept mapping is a common strategy in nursing education programs.
- Visual strategies such as drawing idea sketches, using color in whatever form of note-making works for you, maximizing font characteristics when using a computer for note taking, diagramming information so it makes sense to you, and using mental imagery are all additional ways of study to assist in developing long-term memory of what you are studying.
- Most people in the United States can recognize words and read with fluency and accuracy. Because of being able to read with fluency and accuracy, there is an assumption that the person understands what they are reading. Studies show that many people in the United States have not progressed past the fourth-grade level in reading. In fact, newspapers and magazines are generally written at the fourth- to sixth-grade level.
- ADHD does not affect intelligence. There are numerous effective techniques to help the person diagnosed with ADHD succeed.
- Learning how to learn is important because study skills enable the SPN/SVN to understand (comprehend) and store in long-term memory the theory and skills required to be a practical/vocational nurse.
- When theory and skills are stored in long-term memory, they can be retrieved or recalled as the basis for critical thinking.
- Perhaps your most important skill for success in the LP/LV nursing program is your reading skill.
- There is no fast and easy way to learn information.
- Techniques that have been proven effective in increasing your level of concentration are creating personal study areas, evaluating the influence of peers, and decreasing daydreaming.
- Improving your listening/viewing skills requires you to be an active, rather than a passive, listener/viewer.
- Effective note *making* may enhance your ability to understand information.
- The LRC is your most valuable resource for learning as a student and for keeping up-to-date as a graduate.
- In addition to textbooks, minilectures, lecture-discussions, and cooperative learning are specific course-learning strategies that are used by the SPN/SVN.
- Methods of delivering instruction, such as distance learning, make learning more student-oriented.
- Additional learning resources include articles from periodicals, the syllabus, course outlines, LMSs, study groups, tutoring, audiovisual materials, the Internet, computer-aided instruction, web-based classes, and simulation.
- Staying current in practical/vocational nursing is made possible by using print or digital periodical indexes, CD-ROM databases, the Internet, skills labs, nursing organizations, community resources, and guest speakers.
- It is necessary for practical/vocational nurses to distinguish between personal and professional use of social media.
- After learning the information you need to be an LPN/LVN, you must demonstrate that learning has taken place by your performance in the clinical area and on tests.
- Determining your learning style and aligning key learning strategies and academic resources found in this chapter will help you obtain the information you need to SUCCEED in a practical/vocational nursing program and, ultimately, be a successful licensed practical/vocational nurse.

Additional Learning Resources

evolve Go to your Evolve website (http://evolve.elsevier.com/Knecht/success) for the following FREE learning resources:
- Answers to Critical Thinking Scenarios
- Additional learning activities
- Additional Review Questions for the NCLEX-PN® exam
- Helpful phrases for communicating in Spanish and more!

Review Questions for the NCLEX-PN® Examination

1. Which statement best describes how a *kinesthetic* learner will prefer to learn a lab skill?
   a. Watch a demonstration video and then practice the lab skill.
   b. Listen to a demonstration pod cast and then practice the lab skill.
   c. Draw a visual image of the lab skill and then practice the lab skill.
   d. Watch a demonstration interactive video while practicing the skill simultaneously.

2. Which statement best describes a student who primarily uses the left side of their brain?
   a. When learning a new procedure, you pay more attention to what the total information is rather than focusing on the steps.
   b. You break down information into smaller units and work to understand each step before proceeding to the next step.
   c. You have a tendency to give up on reading because it feels like too much of an overload.
   d. You would rather participate in a group demonstration to learn a concept.

3. Your instructor is involving all of the students in the teaching/learning process. You will work in groups of four. Your group decides to divide the responsibility based on each student's major learning preference. Which student(s) should be responsible for developing a concept map that aligns with the information being studied?
   a. Darius is a visual learner.
   b. Carlos is an auditory learner.
   c. Tom is a tactual learner.
   d. Jill is a logical/mathematical learner.

4. Which of the following statements describes the "S" step of the PQRST method of textbook study?
   a. Repeat, in your own words, the main points.
   b. Survey all of the material in the assignment.
   c. Periodically check to see what you remember.
   d. Carefully read charts, tables, figures, and boxes.

5. A nursing instructor suggests that an SPN/SVN receive help with study skills at the school's Skills Center. Which student response most accurately indicates that the student understands the purpose of the Skills Center?
   a. "I cannot afford the fee to attend study programs in the Skills Center at my school."
   b. "In high school, only students with learning disabilities attended the Skills Center."
   c. "It will take too much time out of my limited study time to go for help with studying."
   d. "Even a few visits to the Skills Center can help me get more out of my study sessions."

6. Classes in an LP/LV nursing program may be conducted in a lecture-discussion format. Select the student behavior that is *most* effective for this learning strategy.
   a. When time is needed to study for a test in a different class, arrange for a peer to take notes for you in your absence.
   b. Complete all assignments before going to class and prepare questions you have about parts of readings that are unclear.
   c. If you disagree with a student during a class discussion, interrupt the student and clarify the information, preventing other students from becoming confused.
   d. While the instructor is answering a student's question, review the notes and document any questions you need answered.

Alternate Format Item

1. Understanding information that is read in the LP/LV nursing program is necessary to save that information in long-term memory so it can be retrieved when needed for critical thinking. Which of the following students are using strategies that help in accomplishing this task? *(Select all that apply.)*
   a. Cole, while previewing a reading assignment, formulates questions from chapter titles that he can answer while reading the assignment.
   b. Juan takes a concept that he is having difficulty understanding and creates a story in his own words while visualizing the story.
   c. Cheyenne repeats what she reads in her own words after completing the assignment and again several times after the initial reading.
   d. Levi takes a verbal concept that he is having difficulty understanding and, without using words, draws a picture to explain the concept.
   e. Joan teaches a difficult concept to her significant other, assessing his understanding and answering his questions about the concept.

2. Which of the following are behaviors of active listeners during a class discussion in a medical/surgical class? *(Select all that apply.)*
   a. Daisy listens with full attention to whoever is speaking.
   b. Pao questions the content of the discussion.
   c. Sage thinks about the speaker's hairstyle.
   d. Isabella tries to relate this discussion to her last clinical assignment.
   e. Clay is working on the related care plan that is due later in the day.

3. A variety of learning resources and strategies are used in an LP/LV nursing program. Which of the following students are using these resources and strategies to their advantage? *(Select all that apply.)*
   a. Alberto joined a study group that meets every day after school to review and discuss class notes.
   b. Marta frequently skips lectures to study for a test in another class and finish care plans to submit by deadline.
   c. To help with time management, Julia borrows notes of the materials from friends who reviewed AV materials instead of watching them.
   d. Because of a long commute, Thai signed up for a distance learning class to save more study time.
   e. Mary's primary preparation for scheduled tests includes completing 50 NCLEX style questions.

Critical Thinking Scenario

Scenario 1

Amy has just completed her fourth week of the practical nursing program. She is frustrated with her low grades. She shares that she carefully examined how a few successful students/graduates studied and implemented similar strategies. Similar to them, Amy has been recopying her class notes nightly and using flash cards to study. She has discovered that recopying notes word for word is time consuming, and it is not helping her to understand and recall the information. As you chat with Amy you determine that Amy is an auditory learner. Provide some advice to assist Amy. Describe some alternative methods of studying to assist her.

Scenario 2

A new student who has been diagnosed with ADHD insisted on being in the back of the classroom and would walk around during class. A couple of the other students would periodically make a sarcastic comment directed at him. The instructor decided to change the order of chapters to be discussed in class, and today's discussion was about different learning styles and how to identify your personal style(s). When the instructor started talking about undependable learning styles, Joe began to listen. There were parts of what she said that sounded like him. The instructor also talked about impulsive behaviors, and Joe recalled his dad telling him many times that he keeps jumping into things without first thinking it through. Now it was this nursing program, and Joe already doubts his decision. Maybe there was finally information he could use. How would you suggest he get started and where he can get some support?

Scenario 3

Amy visited the counselor at school and discussed some time management strategies. Her situation at home has improved. While on a class break, Amy tells you she has improved how she manages her time but Amy earned a C in the first Fundamentals quiz and flunked the second quiz. She says she can't make sense of her notes and the night before the test is too late to clarify with peers what went on in class a week ago. What advice can you give Amy regarding study habits and reading assignments?

Scenario 4

Amy is present daily for class. Her grades have shown slow but steady improvement. While changing classes, Amy tells you she does not have time to go to the LRC because of child care responsibilities. Give Amy some suggestions for using the LRC.

Community Resources

Objectives

On completing this chapter, you will be able to do the following:

1. Identify community resources that can contribute to your success in the practical nursing program in regard to food, utilities, housing, finances, legal and medical needs, and transportation. Evaluate the ability of the community resource identified to effectively meet your needs.
2. Discuss why meeting your basic needs as described by Maslow's theory is critical to achieving success in the practical nursing program.
3. Discuss how the professional use of social media/social networking is a community resource.
4. Discuss how the various community resources can also support patients' needs.

Key Terms

community resources (kă-MŪ-nĭ-tē RĒ-sŏr-sĕs)
Maslow's human needs theory
nursing organizations (NŬR-sĭng ŏr-gă-nĭ-ZĀ-shŭns)

social media (SŌ-shŭl ME-dē-ăh)
social networking (SŌ-shŭl NET-wŏrk-ēng)

💡 Keep in Mind

It is essential to meet your and your immediate family's basic needs, such as food, shelter, and safety, to achieve success in a practical/vocational nursing program.

CJ and David are sitting waiting for the bus after school. CJ shares that his mom recently lost her job. With his three younger siblings living at home, he has increased his work hours to 32 hours per week to help out. He also shares that his grades are slipping and states, "I overheard my mom telling her friend about her fear of the cold weather and inability to pay the oil bill. Maybe I should withdraw from school and help her out. I am already working 32 hours per week, and I am not sure I can work many more hours and still be able to pass the course. My mom has always had a job. We really don't know what to do." David listens and responds, "I have been in tough spots with my family over the last several years. There are great community resources available. Mrs. Jones in the practical nursing office can help you and your Mom find help. This is my second time enrolled; last time I did just as you described. Increased my hours and ended up failing. It was not the right decision. I waited too long to ask for help — my ego would not let me. This time round, I am reaching out early if anything happens. I suggest you do the same. Let me know if I can help."

As you read this chapter, think of the resources that can assist CJ in this scenario. Do you need similar resources or different options? Most important, diverse community

resources can support you. It is important to keep an open mind.

Feeling true hunger, lacking sleep, feeling unsafe, or sensing a lack of belonging can impact your ability to learn. A famous psychology theorist, Abraham Maslow, in the late 1940s identified a hierarchy of needs known to be common to all people. (See Chapter 13 for more details.) **Maslow's human needs theory**, portrayed as a pyramid, has five steps, with the most basic needs existing at the bottom of the pyramid. The five steps include physiological needs, safety, love/belonging, esteem, and self-actualization. The first step, basic physiological needs (i.e., air, water, food, clothing, and shelter), is essential for human survival. Once these needs are met, the person will next focus on their safety needs, then love and belonging, esteem (i.e., respect), and self-actualization. To maximize your ability and success in a practical/vocational nursing program, it is important to feel respected and have self-confidence. These attributes are part of the fourth step of the pyramid, esteem. Thus difficulty meeting your physiological needs or safety needs can impact your ability to feel respected, be confident, and learn effectively. If you are hungry, thirsty, fear for your safety, fear for lack of food for yourself or your family, or feel unsafe, you need to address and resolve these issues the best you can. This will help you succeed as a student. This chapter is designed to provide examples of **community resources** that may assist you in your local area. Your school's counseling center is a great resource in identifying where these agencies exist and how you can contact them directly. The information in this chapter is provided to assist you in understanding what resources may be available and encourage you to seek assistance early and not to wait until the situation is very serious, possibly dangerous, negatively impacting your health and grades. In addition, this broad knowledge will provide information you can use to teach your patients about resources in the community. Community resources are a significant focus in health care reform. Our patients' hospital stays are very short and often nonexistent. Most care occurs in a community setting. Knowing community resources will be integral to your role as a student and an LPN/LVN, as you assist not only the patient but treat the family unit as a whole entity.

WHAT TYPES OF COMMUNITY RESOURCES EXIST?

Diverse types of community resources exist. School resources and your city, county, and state resources are available to assist you. Most communities have private resources as well. Frequently, religious organizations offer assistance and/or resources to individuals and families. Depending on the size of your school, your school community resources can include academic (i.e., writing center, mathematics center, office of career development, academic accommodations), financial aid, health services, housing, and social resources.

Keep in Mind

An orientation to your school resources is generally completed when you enter school. It is easy to forget what is available. Take a moment to visit your school's website. List some resources you think may be helpful in the near future. Bookmark the appropriate links for easy access when needed.

Community resources can be different across cities, counties, states, and the nation. However, common types of assistance are available in most areas of the country. The following major categories of community resources exist:
- Information and referral agencies
- Housing and shelter programs
- Financial and legal assistance programs
- Health and medical services
  - Drug & alcohol and mental health treatment centers
- Food programs
- Transportation programs
- Employment/educational/training programs

INFORMATION AND REFERRAL AGENCIES

Information and referral agencies can serve as your first stop if you are unfamiliar with services in your county. Often this may be where your school's counseling center refers you to determine the best resources to address your unique needs. These referral agencies provide free assistance in finding where to get help. They also may be able to guide you to resources based on income eligibility guidelines. Because many of the services available have income restrictions, knowing what is your best fit is important to save time in this process. As a student, your time is precious. For example, many resources using state and federal dollars have very rigid income eligibility limits. However, there can be some faith-based or philanthropy-funded resources that will evaluate your immediate situation, when qualifying you for a service. This can be helpful when you are a student, as your income has likely decreased dramatically. Despite your best-laid plans, the perfect storm may have hit (i.e., car died, child became very sick, and water pipes burst). Finding the right resource is key.

HOUSING AND SHELTER PROGRAMS

Adequate housing is an essential element of survival for you and your family. In addition, adequate housing will support you in your study habits as discussed in Chapter 2. There are a variety of shelters including homeless, women's, family, and youth shelters. Rehab centers also may provide short-term housing. Examples include the YWCA, YMCA, Salvation Army, and various other faith-related missions. Many counties and states will also have a homeless hotline that can be easily "Googled" if needed.

Housing programs can assist with rent, temporary housing, or even permanent housing. Many times, you may not even realize that you qualify for housing assistance because of a recent lay-off, divorce, or other life event. Rental housing assistance programs generally consist of affordable rental housing, housing counseling, rapid rehousing assistance, foreclosure/eviction assistance, home buying assistance, home repair programs, and weatherization services. Habitat for Humanity has a unique approach engaging the family with the community as they build the house. Contact your local housing authority to seek assistance.

FINANCIAL AND LEGAL ASSISTANCE PROGRAMS

Worry regarding finances and legal issues can be a reason that some students do not successfully complete a practical/vocational nursing program. There are community services available to help. Many of you are probably aware of the county assistance office also referred to as the *welfare office*. The type and amount of aid varies from state to state. The services provided through welfare include financial assistance for food (food stamps), child-care, unemployment, and housing. Lesser known services include assistance with your utility bill, credit counseling, tax preparation, and legal services. There are usually multiple legal aid services available in your community. Given that you are on a course to achieve a new financially sustaining career pathway, consider using financial planning and budgeting services. These services will assist you while you are in school on how to manage your bills and tuition needs; however, they will also assist you in future planning, including goal setting, debt reduction, credit repair, and savings/retirement programs. This truly is a great time to transform your life and create financial stability for the future. Tapping these resources during or close to completion of the program will empower you and your family for the future.

Civil legal service clinics and legal related workshops are conducted regularly and are free of charge. Topics can include: "How to have a criminal record (i.e., DUI) expunged?" and "Child Custody Laws – What you need to know." Citizenship educational classes and support are also available to assist in this complicated process. These services may be funded by governmental entities or faith-based centers. Immediately contacting any of these services, when needed, is a great first step in decreasing your stress level.

HEALTH AND MEDICAL SERVICES

Various types of health and medical services are available in your community. The cost of these services is usually on a sliding scale depending on your household income. These services may help you complete your physical and immunization requirements to attend clinical. Multiple clinics are available providing medical services. Maternal and child health consortiums, Planned Parenthood, and other women's services often exist independently to meet the unique needs of this population. Your local health care institutions, along with your public health department, offer a wealth of health and wellness classes and services to meet the community's needs, including your and your family's needs. Be sure to access them when needed.

Rehabilitation is available through drug and alcohol treatment centers and 12-step programs (i.e., Alcoholics Anonymous). Mental health crisis centers, and residential and day treatment centers, also exist to support community needs. Counseling services are often available through your Family Service county outreach office.

Maintaining dental hygiene is cost prohibitive because many people are uninsured or underinsured in this area of health care. Fortunately, dental services may be available for adults and children through local clinics and dental or dental hygiene schools.

Health insurance is available through your specific state's Affordable Care Act Health Insurance Exchange, and specific state-related children's insurance programs. Lastly, prescription expense assistance can be available through state, pharmaceutical funded programs, and local clinics.

⊚ Try This
Access Health Services

Visit the web site of your local hospital/health care system. Make a list of any services that they offer that may be helpful to you or your family. Determine if there is a charge and plan accordingly.

FOOD PROGRAMS

Countless food programs exist in our nation. They can be government, community, or faith-based funded. In recent years, there has been an increase in farm-raised produce that is harvested by volunteers and donated to food banks. This has assisted in improving the nutritional value offered by food banks and their ability to serve a nutritionally balanced meal. In addition to food banks, soup kitchens and other subsidized food events may exist in your local area. Hot meal programs may also be provided. Seniors and disabled individuals can have special programs that deliver meals to their doors (i.e., Meals on Wheels).

⊚ Try This

Identify a minimum of two food cupboards in your city/county. Determine the following:
- When are they open?
- Who is eligible?
- What foods are available?
- Is it client choice or prepackaged foods?
- Is there any assistance for individuals with dietary restrictions?

TRANSPORTATION PROGRAMS

Transportation can be a challenge for all students, particularly nursing students because of the travel required to attend diverse clinical sites. Given the complexity of scheduling clinical sites, it is unlikely that your school will be able to adapt to your unique transportation barriers when scheduling your clinical rotation. Most nursing schools, unless it is in a completely urban area, will counsel students about the necessity of a car while enrolled. Knowledge of public bus and train service may assist you in some situations; however, having a car in good condition is often essential. Car repairs are costly and can often be the "straw that broke the camel's back" when a student is missing clinical because of lack of transportation. Although these programs are limited, students should inquire regarding technical schools or auto shops that provide free repairs for people in financial need. An example of this type of program, Repair Angel, exists in the Philadelphia area. The auto shop owner covers the cost of the parts and some of their technicians donate their time to fix the car. Local practical nursing students have benefited from this amazing outreach service. Other examples include Cars4Causes, 1-800-Charity Cars, and access through Salvation Army or Habitat for Humanity.

Unique transportation programs exist for seniors and/or disabled people. In addition, some communities have volunteer transportation programs, often focused on a particular disease process, such as cancer. Although the hours that these services function may be limited, they may be instrumental to meet your family's needs while in school.

> **? Critical Thinking**
>
> - A student's car breaks down. It is going to cost $500 to repair. You find them crying in the parking lot and deciding not to return to school. What should you do?
> - You are discharging a patient from a rehabilitation center. They live alone and have limited family support in the area. How will they access outpatient therapy three days per week?

EMPLOYMENT/EDUCATIONAL/TRAINING PROGRAMS

Employment and educational training opportunities are available through your city/county. Some of you may have used these services to attain your GED® or prepare for the student nurse entrance test. Remember that if you need assistance with basic math, reading, or literacy skills, free programs exist in most areas of the country. If you need assistance, seek out the Adult Basic Education (ABE) or the adult literacy program in your county. You will receive free individual or small group training. Improving these basic skills will be integral to your academic success. See Chapter 2 for additional academic resources.

In your city/county there will be an employment center (i.e., Career Link). Many states have created a central resource center, where many of the resources noted above are available and combined with access to employment and educational/training opportunities. Most importantly, there may be a possibility that training dollars through the Workforce Investment Act are available to you to assist in paying your nursing tuition. If you are a dislocated worker or underemployed, you may be eligible for several thousand dollars in funding. When seeking access to these funds, inquire about the Workforce Investment Act funding and training grants. Use these as key words to narrow your search. Your school's financial aid office should also be able to assist you.

The Office of Vocational Rehabilitation (OVR) is available to assist people with disabilities to achieve employment and independence. This office may be able to assist with adaptive equipment or low-interest loans to assist a student. An example of a student who may seek out this service would be someone with a hearing disability who is in need of an expensive amplified stethoscope. OVR may be able to provide the evaluation and funding for this service.

There are many different types of employment services available. Although job-seeking skills are generally available through your school, additional services are available through these employment sites. Assistance with interview preparation, résumé creation, and possibly even clothing for an interview are a few of the services that can benefit you. Lastly, job locator/placement services will be a great resource upon successful completion of your practical/vocational nursing program or when you are looking for a suitable part time job while enrolled in the program.

> **◎ Try This**
>
> **Find a Community Agency**
>
> Identify an actual or potential need for a community resource as described above. Locate this community resource on the Internet and determine if you are eligible for their assistance.

> **? Critical Thinking**
>
> You see a peer who is crying in the parking lot as you exit school. You recognize the person from class and offer assistance. The person explains that their husband locked her out of the house and she stayed in their car last night. Tonight it is going to be cold. What advice will you share with this peer of yours?

BEYOND COMMUNITY RESOURCES

The Internet provides an opportunity for you to identify resources well beyond your school or local community to contribute to your success. Various nursing organizations, social media sites, scholarship opportunities, and academic and clinical resources are available on the Internet.

NURSING ORGANIZATIONS

Nursing organizations identify or offer speakers, seminars, and workshops on up-to-the-minute nursing topics and related health care topics. These programs are frequently made available to students, thereby enhancing their content knowledge and creating for them a new network of colleagues.

There are two long established practical/vocational nursing membership organizations in the United States: the National Association for Practical Nurse Education and Service, Inc. (NAPNES) **www.napnes. org** and the National Federation of Licensed Practical Nurses Association (NFLPN) **www.nflpn.org**. Both of these organizations are dedicated to promoting competence and advancing the profession of LPNs/LVNs. They provide continuing education, networking opportunities, and information regarding topics important to practical/vocational nurses. Visit the respective website for specific information.

SOCIAL MEDIA (ELECTRONIC MEDIA) AND SOCIAL NETWORKING

LinkedIn is a preferred professional network. In addition, nurses are using Facebook and Twitter, the most commonly used **social media** networks for communicating with family and friends, to communicate and collaborate with nursing organizations and keep up to date with colleagues. Professional organizations also use these networks to allow nonattendees to follow conventions, seminars, and so on. The interactivity of these sites allows one to consume as well as contribute information. It is critical to realize that social media and networking must be used with caution so as to develop an awareness of the professional versus personal use of these sites. The 2011 National Council of State Board Examiners (NCSBN) White Paper, "A Nurse's Guide to the Use of Social Media," states that 46 Boards of Nursing (BON) were surveyed by the National Council, and 33 boards reported receiving complaints about nurses who violated patient confidentiality/privacy by posting patient information on **social networking** sites. Sanctions ranged from a letter of concern, mandatory continuing education, to suspension of license.

- Violation of patient privacy is a violation of the Health Insurance Portability and Accountability Act (HIPAA) and can result in a fine for your employer and sanctions for you from your State Board of Nursing.
- Violation of patient confidentiality is also a violation of your professional code of ethics (see Chapter 6).
- Whether or not you engage in social media is a personal choice. If you choose to participate, carefully check the privacy policy of the site. Thoughtfully develop a profile and carefully set your privacy settings. Remember that caution is needed even when using privacy settings.
- Avoid putting on the Internet *anything* you would not put on television or the front page of a newspaper. Prospective employers may "Google" you. Be especially scrutinizing of pictures posted by you and your friends.
- LinkedIn is the biggest professional site, and interactions are more formal. This is a site for posting résumés, education, work history, accomplishments, and professional memberships. The goal is to connect with or remain connected with colleagues (Duffy, 2011). If you list your employer, remember that you are then a representative of that agency. The power of LinkedIn lies in making a second connection when job seeking. You leverage someone you know (your LinkedIn connection) to introduce you via email to their supervisor/administrator (their LinkedIn connection). This is especially helpful when job seeking.
- The NCSBN (2011) White Paper, "A Nurse's Guide to the Use of Social Media," and video are references to guide you. They are available at NCSBN.org.
- The American Nurses Association (ANA) has compiled a resource guide that nursing students can use to learn about professional use of social networking (http://www.nursingworld.org/socialnetworking toolkit.aspx).

Connecting with groups on social media provides an opportunity to chat with students throughout the country and in various levels of nursing education and experience. Facebook provides various opportunities for nursing students including:

- NurseGroups.com
- Nurses Notes by Johnson and Johnson

AllNurses.com represents a social media community exceeding 647,000 members and provides an opportunity for nursing students to connect with other students and nurses. A specific "student" site allows students the opportunity to discuss, debate, share best practices, and find camaraderie amid the perils of nursing school. Lastly, the Google site provides a Nursing and Allied Health Resource, consisting of a wide range of resources. Many resources are free; however, some do require a fee for access. This site is frequently updated and continually growing. Watch your time management while on these sites, and not just because of the fees. It is easy for several precious hours to slip away, leaving minimal time to study and prepare for the next day's class/clinical. Balance occurs when there is a great plan in place. Remember this author's four "P"s needed to create a plan to SUCCEED: Power, Passion, Perseverance, and Personal attributes. These Internet sites can fuel all four "P"s but also can limit your power, built through knowledge, if they conflict with study time. Use your social media savvy wisely. Create a plan and stick to it, changing it only when absolutely necessary!

Professional Pointer

Presentation of self on social media requires professional behavior. Try to "Google" yourself and critically evaluate all sources.

Try This

Social Media Policies

Investigate social media policies developed by your school, clinical areas, State Board of Nursing, and the National Council of State Boards of Nursing.

INTERNET ACADEMIC RESOURCES

Although many of the Internet-based academic/clinical resources are geared towards registered nurse (RN) students, practical/vocational nursing students can also benefit. For example, Practical Clinical Skills (www.practicalclinicalskills.com) is a website that provides free clinical simulation aids that help you in tasks such as assessing blood pressure, and simulating heart, lung and bowel sounds. This resource, although focused on RN students, provides an excellent resource that helps practical/vocational students to develop skills for real-life application. Sites, such as Off The Charts (http://ajnoffthecharts.com), sponsored by the American Journal of Nursing, also provide additional reference sources for students.

Get Ready for the NCLEX-PN® Examination!

Key Points

- Maslow's human needs theory, portrayed as a pyramid, has five steps, with the most basic needs existing at the bottom of the pyramid. The five steps include physiological needs, safety, love/belonging, esteem, and self-actualization.
- According to Maslow, if you are hungry, thirsty, fear for your safety, fear for lack of food for your children, or feel unsafe, you need to address and resolve these issues the best you can. If not, your learning can be affected.
- Community resources are a significant focus in health care reform. Our patients' hospital stays are very short and often nonexistent. Most care occurs in a community setting. Community resources will be integral to your role as a student and as an LPN, assisting not only the patient but also treating the family unit as a whole entity.
- Diverse community resources exist in your school community and community at large (i.e., city, county, state, nation).
- The following major categories of community resources exist: Information and Referral Agencies; the Housing and Shelter Program; Financial and Legal Assistance Programs; Health and Medical Services; Drug & Alcohol and Mental Health Treatment Centers; Food Programs; Transportation Programs; and Employment/Educational/Training Programs.
- All students may benefit by accessing a community resource while enrolled in a practical/vocational nursing program. Securing assistance before a crisis occurs is the goal.
- The Office of Vocational Rehabilitation (OVR) is available to assist people with disabilities to achieve employment and independence.
- There are two long established practical/vocational nursing membership organizations in the United States: National Association for Practical Nurse Education and Service, Inc. (NAPNES) and National Federation of Licensed Practical Nurses Association (NFLPN).
- Professional social media networks consist of varied groups including LinkedIn, Facebook, and Twitter. These sites are commonly used social media networks to communicate and collaborate with nursing organizations and keep up to date with colleagues.
- Social media and networking must be used with caution. Develop an awareness of the professional versus personal use of these sites.

Additional Learning Resources

evolve Go to your Evolve website (http://evolve.elsevier.com/Knecht/success) for the following FREE learning resources:
- Answers to Critical Thinking Scenarios
- Additional learning activities
- Additional Review Questions for the NCLEX-PN® exam

Review Questions for the NCLEX-PN® Examination

1. Maslow's human needs theory stresses the importance of humans meeting basic physiological needs and safety needs. If these basic needs are not met, the student may be unable to:
   a. Feel respected and have self confidence
   b. Sleep at night
   c. Access the digital database
   d. Identify a community resource
2. A student is struggling with basic math concepts in their pharmacology class. Which of the following may be a good community resource to access?
   a. Office of Vocational Rehabilitation
   b. Adult Basic Education (ABE) Program
   c. NFLPN
   d. Repair Angel
3. A practical/vocational nursing student is very active on social media. She is excited about being a nursing student. Today she took pictures during a clinical lab simulation and posted them on her Facebook page. The pictures included other students engaged in a catheterization simulation. Did this create a social media issue related to professionalism?
   a. Yes, she will probably be counseled or even suspended from nursing school.
   b. No, it is not really a big deal because it was not a real patient.
   c. No, it is in the spirit of team building that she posted the pictures.
   d. No, because it is a private site. However, it would be best in the future to ask her classmates before posting the pictures.

Alternate Format Item

1. Which of the following practical/vocational nursing students would benefit from seeking out a student assistance program or community resource? (Select all that apply.)
   a. Matt, whose wife just lost her job.
   b. Sophia, whose husband came home drunk the last three evenings.
   c. Elizabeth, who has a long history of credit card debt accumulation and now has poor credit.
   d. Dominic, who failed the first pharmacology test.
   e. Susan, who just won a $1000 scholarship.
2. Community agencies may be able to assist with the following: (Select all that apply.)
   a. Short-term rental housing
   b. Tax preparation
   c. Time management
   d. Anger management
   e. Citizenship

Critical Thinking Scenarios

Amy, continued . . .

Amy is now in her third month of the practical nursing program. She has been late for class four times and absent four days since school started. She is fearful she is going to be dismissed. She is thinking it is best to stop going to classes and just disappear. She is currently passing all the courses but her car broke for the third time this week. She does not have any money to get it fixed. In addition, her babysitter just gave her two weeks' notice that she is having surgery and will be unavailable for 3 months. Amy feels like the odds are impossible. This was her chance but now she feels defeated. She wants to run and hide. What suggestions would you give Amy?

4

How Practical/Vocational Nursing Evolved: 1836 to the Present

Objectives

On completing this chapter, you will be able to do the following:

1. Identify the year and place the first school of practical nursing was founded.
2. Name the school's most famous pupil.
3. Discuss the contributions of this most famous nurse.
4. Discuss how the evolution of practical nursing has influenced LPN/LVN practice today.
5. Present the rationale for your personal stand on entry into nursing practice.
6. Discuss the contribution of war nurses and early pioneers in nursing to overall nursing professional development.

Key Terms

Clara Barton
Cadet Nurse Corps
Mildred I. Clark
Jane Delano
Dorothea Lynde Dix
Glenna Goodacres
Anna Goodrich
Lystra Gretter

Anna Mae Hays
Lenah S. Higbee
Lillian Kinkela-Keil
Florence Nightingale
Notes on Nursing
M. Adelaide Nutting
Mary Seacole
Lillian Wald

Keep in Mind

The first nurses were practical nurses, and you are part of that proud heritage.

Today, formal educational programs are the norm for all nurses, including practical/vocational nurses. The length of the full-time program for the modern practical (or vocational) nurse is approximately 9 months to 1 year in most states. Part-time programs can last as long as 2 years.

MODERN PRACTICAL NURSES

Nursing has experienced many changes throughout its history (Table 4-1), and the changes continue. Two major changes that have occurred in practical nursing are a gradual increase in the required formal knowledge base and a requirement for licensing to practice practical nursing. Unlike the historically untrained or poorly trained practical nurse, who had unlimited and unsupervised freedom to practice, the present practical nurse is now trained in an educational program, consisting of theory, clinical simulation, and clinical hours. The practical/vocational nursing program prepares the student to successfully pass the National Council Licensure Examination for Licensed Practical Nurses (NCLEX-PN®) examination and meet minimum standards to practice safely as a graduate practical/vocational nurse. After licensing, the Licensed Practical Nurse/Licensed Vocational Nurse (LPN/LVN) is permitted to perform the job role of the LPN/LVN as aligned with the respective state regulations. Most state regulations stipulate that LPNs/LVNs work under the supervision of the Registered Nurse, physician, or physician extender (i.e., Nurse Practitioner).

FIRST SCHOOL OF NURSING (1836)

The first real school of nursing was founded by the Lutheran Order of Deaconesses under the supervision of a German pastor, Theodor Fleidner, in Kaiserswerth, Germany in 1836. The purpose of the program was to teach principles of nursing care to the Lutheran Order of Deaconesses. Many of the graduates of Kaiserswerth Deaconess Institute settled in other parts of the world and established similar programs. The school's most famous pupil was the Englishwoman, Florence Nightingale, the

Table **4-1**   **Nursing Milestones**

PERIOD IN HISTORY	EVENT
1836	First real school of nursing, in Kaiserswerth, Germany. Florence Nightingale attended for 3 months.
	Eighteen years later, after start of Crimean War, Nightingale nursed wounded with 38 self-identified (untrained) nurses.
1860	Nightingale established a school of nursing in England. She wrote several books. The most famous was *Notes on Nursing.*
Civil War (1861-1865)	In the South: Most nursing done by infantrymen assigned to the task. Southern women volunteered services. In the North: Dorothea Lynde Dix, a teacher, was appointed Superintendent of Nurses and organized a corps of female nurses (untrained).
1864	Clara Barton, a teacher, collected supplies for soldiers. This led to her appointment as Superintendent of the Department of Nurses for the Army.
1881	Clara Barton established the first chapter of the American Red Cross in Danville, New York.
1892	First class for formal training of practical nursing: YWCA, Brooklyn, New York.
1893	Nightingale Pledge written by Canadian-born Lystra Gretter, principal of Farrand Training School in Detroit.
	Henry Street Settlement founded by Lillian Wald, a social worker who graduated from a nursing program. Practical nurses pioneered in this new public health movement. They went into homes and taught the basics of cleanliness and control of communicable diseases to families in New York slums.
1893	Ballard School for Practical Nursing opened in New York.
1907	Thompson School for Practical Nursing opened in Brattleboro, Vermont.
1914	Mississippi is the first state to pass a law to license practical nurses.
1917	Standardization of nursing requirements for practical nursing by National League of Nursing Education (now the National League for Nursing [NLN]).
World War I (1914-1918)	Shortage of practical nurses. Army School of Nursing established. Highlighted the need for more and better prepared nurses. Smith Hughes Act of 1917 provided money for developing additional schools of practical nursing.
1920s	Acute shortage of practical nurses. Many did not return to nursing after the war.
1920-1940	Most practical nursing limited to public health agencies and visiting nurse associations.
1938	New York only state to have mandatory licensure.
World War II (1939-1945)	Shortage of RNs created need for LPNs. At home, practical nurses worked in clinics, health departments, industries, and hospitals. In the war, they ventured into hardship tours in Europe, North Africa, and the Pacific.
1940	The number of practical nurses peaked in 1940 at 159,009.
1941	NAPNES (National Association of Practical Nurse Education and Service), a nation's professional organization dedicated exclusively to practical nursing, was founded.
1943	Cadet Nurse Corps was founded; two-and-a-half-year courses to become nurses.
1944	Comprehensive study of practical nursing by U.S. Department of Vocational Education. This was the first time that tasks of practical nursing were agreed upon.
End of World War II	Nursing shortage saw movement of practical nurses into hospitals and gradually increasing responsibilities.
1949	NFLPN (National Federation of Licensed Practical Nurses) was founded to provide structure nationwide through which LPNs could promote better patient care and act on behalf of LPNs. The NFLPN-organized Joint Committee on Practical Nurses and Auxiliary Workers in Nursing Services recommended use of the title "licensed practical nurse" and differentiated between tasks of registered nurses and LPNs.
Korean Conflict (1950-1953)	Nurses finally became part of the military.
1951	*Journal of Practical Nursing* published by NAPNES (now *Practical Nursing Today*).
1952	Approximately 60% of the nurse workforce was made up of practical nurses.
1955	All states had licensure laws for practical/vocational nurses.
1957	NLN established a Council of Practical Nursing Programs.

Continued

Table 4-1   Nursing Milestones—cont'd

PERIOD IN HISTORY	EVENT
1960	By 1960, every state had a nurse licensure law.
1961	NLN began offering accrediting services for practical nursing programs
Vietnam War (1961-1973)	Military nurses were assigned to Vietnamese hospitals, MASH units, as flight nurses, and hospital ships.
1965	ANA (American Nurses Association) first moves toward two distinct levels in nursing: professional and technical.
1971	NBNA (National Black Nurse's Association) is established.
1975	1315 state-approved PN programs. More than 45,000 PN graduates. After 1975, number of PN programs and graduates declined.
1979	NLN published first list of competencies for practical/vocational nursing programs.
1980s	Resurgence of ANA moves toward two distinct levels of nursing. This resulted in some states adopting two levels of nursing and then rescinding their decision because of the nursing shortage.
1984	Creation of ALPNA (American Licensed Practical Nurses Association).
1989	The American Medical Association (AMA) initiated and subsequently dropped the registered care technician (RCT) proposal.
1990s	Unlicensed personnel are used for patient care. The number of hospital nursing jobs has decreased. The primary employment site has moved into the community.
1994	First computerized adaptive test (NCLEX-PN®) available to practical/vocational nursing graduates.
1995	Full-time nursing positions in hospitals decreased. Patient/nurse ratios increased. Primary employment in community continues.
1996	Long-term care certification examinations for LPNs/LVNs by National Council of State Boards of Nursing with the National Association for Licensed Practical Nurse Education and Service.
2000	Increased demand for LPNs/LVNs in nursing homes and extended care; demand down in hospitals.
Afghanistan War 2001–2014	Military nurses help set up surgical teams, MASH units, air evacuation, combat support units in Afghan and Iraqi hospitals.
Iraq War 2003–2011	Military nurses provide care and leadership to maintain the health and support units in Iraq.
2007	Nursing programs are turning students away because of the shortage of instructors.
2010	Institute of Medicine (IOM) Releases the Future of Nursing: Leading Chance, Advancing Health report.
2013	Health Resources and Services Administration (HRSA) report, *The US Nursing Service Report Trends in Supply and Education* released indicate a shift from acute care to long-term and community-based care.
2014	National League for Nurses (NLN) Releases Vision statement titled, *Recognizing the Role of the Licensed Practical/Vocational Nurses in Advancing the Nation's Health.*

LPN, Licensed practical nurse; *MASH*, mobile army surgical hospital; *NCLEX-PN*, National Council Licensure Examination for Licensed Practical Nurses; *RN*, registered nurse.

founder of modern nursing. She attended the school for 3 months and studied under Caroline Fliedner.

FLORENCE NIGHTINGALE (1820–1910)

Florence Nightingale was born in Florence, Italy. Her parents named her after the city and called her Flo. Nightingale's parents were wealthy, influential, and accepted in society. Florence was presented at court and was expected to follow the social pattern of other women of her day. Women were considered intellectually inferior to men. Education for middle-class and upper-class women often consisted of lessons in etiquette, dancing, music, manners, embroidery, painting, and modern languages. Instead of being tutored by governesses or in a private school, Nightingale's father tutored her in modern and ancient languages, history, composition, philosophy, and mathematics, including statistics. He was a strict disciplinarian, but she was an eager student (LeVasseur, 1998).

Nightingale turned down a proposal of marriage from a man her sister later married. Early on, Nightingale knew she had a purpose in life to fulfill. She begged her parents to permit her to go into the nurses' training program in Kaiserswerth, Germany. Her parents were not pleased, because nursing was seen as a job suitable only for lower-class women. As we know, Nightingale got her way. Upon graduation, she became superintendent for the Institution for the Care of Sick Gentlewomen in Distressed Circumstances, now the Harley Street Nursing Home in London (Romanoff, 2006). She began to take steps to make the work of nurses who served the gentlewomen easier. Dumbwaiters were installed so the nurses did not have to carry heavy trays up and down stairs. Nightingale also developed a system of call bells that could be seen in hallways to identify which person was summoning. Because the institution discriminated against Catholics and Jews, she dropped religion as a requirement for admission. Some of the governing board members were not happy with her changes.

The following year, as Nightingale was planning to become superintendent of King's College Hospital in London, the Crimean War broke out. She sent a letter to the Secretary of War offering her services. She did not know that he had also sent a letter to her requesting her assistance.

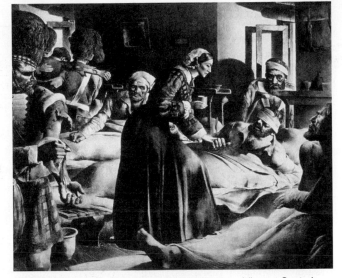

FIGURE 4-1 Florence Nightingale ministering to soldiers at Scutari (lithograph). (Courtesy National Library of Medicine.)

CRIMEAN WAR 1853 TO 1865

Shortly after the start of the Crimean War in 1853 (in which Britain, France, Turkey, and Sardinia fought Russia for control of access to the Mediterranean from the Black Sea), information about the neglect and poor care of casualties began to reach England. A correspondent for the *London Times* newspaper wrote vivid accounts of the deplorable conditions and lack of medical and nursing care for the British troops. The Sisters of Mercy tended Russian troops, the Sisters of Charity tended the French, and the wounded of England were almost completely neglected. The correspondent's charges were so persistent that a commission was sent to investigate. As a result, the Secretary of War decided that England, too, should have a group of women nurses to tend the war casualties.

The Secretary of War contacted Florence Nightingale and explained the situation to her. Because she had both nursing and administrative experience, the secretary perceived her as the one nurse in England capable of organizing and supervising care in a foreign land.

Being appointed to the task of organizing and supervising nurses during the Crimean War gave Nightingale an unexpected opportunity for achievement. She left for Crimea, taking with her 38 self-proclaimed nurses of limited experience, 24 of whom were nuns. On arrival, they found overcrowded, filthy hospitals with no beds, no furniture, no eating utensils, no medical supplies, no blankets, no soap, no linens, and no lamps. Wounded soldiers lay on the filthy floor in their battle uniforms (Figure 4-1). Soldiers were more likely to die from infected wounds than the wound itself. Nightingale took charge. Using the supplies she brought, and raising funds, she purchased supplies that doctors could not obtain for the army. Nightingale hired people to clean up the "hospitals" and established laundries to wash linens and uniforms and prepare nutritious meals. She expected a great deal of herself and those who worked with her. It was not an easy task. A major prejudice that had to

be overcome was that of medical officers, who considered the nurses intruders. The hours were long and difficult for Nightingale and her nurses. Many soldiers had family following them, and recreation rooms were set up for their use. She believed that the best nurses were those who had good character, who experienced a sense of calling, and who were well trained to meet the physical needs of patients. The barracks, a 4-mile labyrinth of cots meant for 1700 patients, packed in 3000 to 4000 patients. She did not want her nurses on the wards after dark and could often be seen after hours making additional rounds with her lamp to check on patients. The soldiers fondly referred to her as "Birdie." These extra efforts earned her the title, "The Lady with the Lamp," as immortalized in Longfellow's poem *Santa Filomena* (Box 4-1).

MARY SEACOLE; HONORED FOR HER WORK

Nightingale had help during many of those nights. **Mary Seacole**, a nurse from Jamaica, also played an important role in the history of nursing. She used her own money to build a lodging house in Crimea where she provided care for the soldiers. Seacole was especially knowledgeable about tropical medicine and used herbs and natural plant medicines to treat patients with cholera, yellow fever, malaria, and diarrhea. Both Seacole's government and the British Commonwealth honored her for the lives she saved (Cherry and Jacob, 2011).

DEATH RATE DROPS; NIGHTINGALE DECORATED

After 6 months, it was obvious that the efforts of Nightingale and her nurses were paying off. The death rate among the wounded dropped from 420 deaths per 1000 casualties to 22 per 1000. She stayed throughout the war and was the last to leave. Many of her nurses had become ill during the war and were sent home to recover. Nightingale became ill with Crimean fever,

Box 4-1   Santa Filomena

Whene'er a noble deed is wrought,
Whene'er is spoken a noble thought,
Our hearts, in glad surprise,
To higher levels rise.
The tidal wave of deeper souls
Into our inmost being rolls,
And lifts us unawares
Out of all meaner cares.
Honor to those whose words or deeds
Thus help us in our daily needs,
And by their overflow
Raise us from what is low!
Thus thought I, as by night I read
Of the great army of the dead.
The trenches cold and damp,
The starved and frozen camp—
The wounded from the frozen plain,
In dreary hospitals of pain—
The cheerless corridors,
The cold and stony floors,
Lo! in the house of misery,
A lady with a lamp I see
Pass through the glimmering gloom,

And flit from room to room.
And slow, as in a dream of bliss,
The speechless sufferer turns to kiss
Her shadow, as it falls
Upon the darkening walls.
As if a door in heaven should be,
Opened, and then closed suddenly,
The vision came and went—
The light shone and was spent.
On England's annals, through the long
Hereafter of her speech and song.
That light its rays shall cast
From portals of the past.
A lady with a lamp shall stand
In the great history of the land,
A noble type of good,
Heroic womanhood.
Not even shall be wanting here
The palm, the lily, and the spear.
The symbols that of yore
Saint Filomena bore.

—*Henry Wadsworth Longfellow*

probably typhus, and almost died. When she returned home, Queen Victoria decorated her for her efforts in the war.

? Critical Thinking

Medical Asepsis

Look up the word medical asepsis. Discuss with a peer how Florence Nightingale implemented many of the key aspects of medical asepsis to save the soldiers during the Crimean War. Does poor medical asepsis contribute to patient's deaths today? If so, discuss where and how.

NIGHTINGALE ESTABLISHES FIRST SCHOOL OF NURSING IN ENGLAND

One of Nightingale's major goals was to establish a school of nursing in England. An overwhelming number of physicians opposed such a school. Their opposition was that "because nurses occupied much the same positions as housemaids, they needed little instruction beyond poultice making, the enforcement of cleanliness, and attention to their patients' personal needs" (Kalish and Kalish, 1995). In 1860, Nightingale established the Nightingale Training School at St. Thomas Hospital in England. It was a 1-year program. She chose this site because of the hospital's reputation for progressive medical care. The school was independent from the hospital and financially independent as well. She believed nurses should work only in hospitals, not in private duty. Nightingale had strict admission standards that emphasized high moral character

and intelligence. She was strict with her nursing students. They were locked up at night as a way to assure the middle-class parents that their daughters were safe from harassment. Upon graduation, she gave the nurses gifts of books and invited them to tea. When her graduates went to work in far-off places, she sent flowers to welcome them to their new home (Romanoff, 2006).

Nightingale's personal and nursing decisions reflected the influence of works by Plato and Hippocrates. Examples include her decision to remain single, her sense of mission, her concern with patient environment, her focus on the whole patient, and her belief in the need for keen observation and assisting nature to heal the patient (LeVasseur, 1998). Nightingale wrote over 200 publications, the most famous of which is *Notes on Nursing*. Although she was reclusive, she was influential in matters of military and public health policy because she kept such precise notes, which included statistics. Nightingale's statistics, similar to evidence-based practice today, confirm her role as a visionary for the nursing profession.

💡 Keep in Mind

Like Florence Nightingale, the director of your nursing program will need to attest to your moral character when he or she notifies the respective state board of nursing that you have met all the practical/vocational nursing program requirements. Moral character is an essential component of a licensed nurse. Self-reflect on this fact often, ensuring your moral character is and remains strong.

NIGHTINGALE'S CORE BELIEF ABOUT NURSING

The core of Nightingale's spirituality was a belief in perfection. To her, nursing was a sacred calling, a commitment to work for mankind, not a business. Other Victorian women like her shared the sense of the sacredness of time and belief that wasting time was a sin. Nursing became a way for Florence Nightingale to work toward the perfection of mankind and her personal salvation. She was against licensure. To her it was too much like nurses being in a union. She eliminated prejudice against a better class of women entering nursing and created a push toward the development of nursing as a respectable vocation.

Nightingale was intelligent, well educated, and skeptical. This combination made her the foremost critic of the meaning of nursing and the nursing role. She continued to be involved in health policy well into her eighties. She was the first woman to receive the Order of Merit from the King of England. In 1910, she died in her sleep of heart failure at age 90. The government offered to bury her at Westminster Abbey, but according to her wishes, she was buried in the family plot at East Wellow, Hampshire. The marker reads, "F.N. Born 12 May 1820. Died 13 August 1910."

In 1893, **Lystra Gretter**, the principal of Farrand Training School in Detroit, and a committee modified the Hippocratic Oath. They named it the *Nightingale Pledge* as a token of esteem for the founder of modern nursing. It continues to be recited in many schools during graduation, primarily because of the mistaken belief that Nightingale wrote it. It reads as follows:

> *I solemnly pledge myself before God and in the presence of this assembly, to pass my life in purity and to practice my profession faithfully. I will abstain from whatever is deleterious and mischievous, and will do all in my power to maintain and elevate the standard of my profession, and will hold in confidence all personal matters committed to my keeping and all family affairs coming to my knowledge in the practice of my calling. With loyalty will I endeavor to aid the physician in his work, and devote myself to the welfare of those committed to my care.*

[?] Critical Thinking

Nightingale Pledge and Nursing

Review the Nightingale Pledge. Does it apply to the practical/vocational nurse in the twenty-first century? If you were to make changes, what would they be?

NIGHTINGALE MUSEUM ON THE SITE OF HER SCHOOL OF NURSING

In the spring of 1989, the Florence Nightingale Museum opened in London on the grounds of St. Thomas Hospital, the site of the Nightingale School of Nursing. The museum is a tribute to this nursing leader, despite the fact that she wrote in her journal, "I do not wish to be remembered when I am gone." Despite her great and courageous contributions to nursing, Florence Nightingale saw only her own faults and her failures.

EARLY TRAINING SCHOOLS IN AMERICA

Nurses in America were scarce and poorly trained. In 1849, Pastor Fliedner of Germany, who helped establish the first hospital and nursing school in Europe, came to America with four of his highly trained deaconesses. Although Pastor Fliedner was involved with establishing the first Protestant hospital in America, the deaconesses started the first formal training program for nurses in the United States. The hospital, known as the Pittsburgh Infirmary, still exists in Pennsylvania as the Passavant Hospital. The training program was separate from the hospital with the intent being to educate nurses.

As the nursing shortage continued, hospital-based schools of nursing emerged as a cost-effective (i.e., free) labor force for the hospitals. The living conditions and the long hours required a great deal of physical and emotional endurance of the students.

CIVIL WAR (1861–1865)

In the 1800s, women who worked in hospitals, particularly in the South, were victims of deep prejudice from men in general and especially from the medical profession. As one southern woman put it, "It seems strange that what the aristocratic women of Great Britain have done with honor is a disgrace for their sisters on this side of the Atlantic to do" (Kalish and Kalish, 1995).

Casualties were high on both sides during the Civil War. Many soldiers died right on the field, and others died because of a poorly trained medical corps. Southern women offered their services as volunteers, but most of the nursing was done by infantrymen assigned to do a task they did not want to do. It was many months before the Confederate government recognized southern women for their contributions.

In the North during the Civil War, women offered their services as nurses to the government. One hundred women were selected to take a short training course from doctors in New York. **Dorothea Lynde Dix**, a teacher by profession, was appointed Superintendent of Nurses. Her task was to organize a corps of female nurses. She would recruit only women who were younger than age 30 and plain looking; they wore simple brown or black dresses and were forbidden to wear hoop skirts or jewelry. Women who did not meet these criteria nursed anyway but without official recognition or pay from the government. In addition, as a longtime advocate for better conditions for those who suffered from mental illness, Dix went on to establish the first hospital for the mentally ill.

Clara Barton

Clara Barton, a teacher by profession, was one of the first civilians in the Civil War to round up army supplies. She rented a warehouse, filled market baskets, and encouraged friends to send food, blankets, and other supplies for the soldiers. Her efforts resulted in her being appointed Superintendent of the Department of Nurses for the Army in 1864. Clara Barton's efforts frequently found her on the front lines, and she nearly lost her life on two occasions. After the war, President Andrew Johnson commissioned her to do what she wanted to do: find missing prisoners of war. Later, while visiting in Europe for health reasons, she met J. Henri Dunant, founder of the International Red Cross. He asked for her help in introducing the Red Cross to America. Through Barton's efforts, the first chapter of the American Red Cross was established in Danville, New York, in 1881.

? Critical Thinking

What is the relationship between the American Red Cross and nursing?

FORMAL TRAINING: PRACTICAL NURSING

In 1893, the Ballard School under the auspices of the YWCA opened the first formal practical nurse program in Brooklyn, New York. The course lasted 3 months and focused on home health care for the chronically ill, invalids, children, and the elderly. It included cooking, nutrition, basic sciences, and basic nursing procedures. The graduates were referred to as attendant nurses. Other similar schools include the Thompson School for Practical Nursing, which opened in Brattleboro, Vermont, in 1907 and the Household Nursing Association School of Attendant Nursing, which opened in Boston in 1918. The Household School later changed its name to the Shepard-Gill School of Practical Nursing. The focus continued to be home nursing and light housekeeping duties. Hospital experience was not a part of the early programs. Before 1940, there were few controls, little education, practically no planning, and minimal supervision.

? Critical Thinking

As discussed above, the first formal practical nursing training focused on home health care of the chronically ill, invalids, children, and the elderly. Discuss with a peer how this aligns with practical/vocational nursing jobs found today.

NURSING IN THE HOME

Before World War I, most nursing done by practical nurses was home nursing, primarily because most people were cared for in the home. Even operations were performed in the home. There is some truth to how old Western movies portrayed surgery on the kitchen table. The nurse's 24-hour schedule included such procedures as cupping and applying leeches; preparing stupes for relief of abdominal distention, mustard plasters for relief of

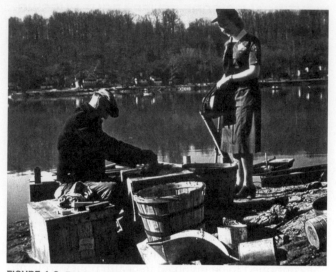

FIGURE 4-2 Public health nursing follow-up visits. (Courtesy National Library of Medicine.)

congestion, and poultices for drawing out pus from infections; and administering enemas, which were often nutritive enemas that contained eggnog with brandy or chicken broth. Intravenous infusions did not exist. Some practical nurses also assumed the then-accepted role of midwife. They taught new mothers the basics of cleanliness, diet, and child care (Figure 4-2). Approximately 1700 midwives attended 30% of all births in New York in 1919.

FROM HOME TO PUBLIC HEALTH NURSING

By the end of the nineteenth century, there was renewed interest in charitable work and concern for the sick. Practical nursing began to expand from home nursing to public health nursing, care of patients in the slums, school nursing, industrial nursing, and well-baby care. Once again, practical nurses pioneered in this new public health movement.

One of the best-known centers in 1893 was the Henry Street Settlement in New York. **Lillian Wald**, a social worker, graduated from nursing school and intended to become a doctor. Wald taught home nursing to immigrants and was so impressed by their need for medical care that she left medical school to begin a nursing service, the Henry Street Settlement. Practical nurses who were members of the Henry Street Settlement taught families in New York slums the basics of cleanliness and control of communicable diseases. There was a decrease in school absenteeism because the spread of childhood illness was reduced. School nurses visited schools and new mothers and their babies. They taught mothers the basics of preventing the summertime killer of infants: cholera infantum. It was estimated that their efforts resulted in the survival of 1200 more babies than usual during the hot summer months. Another original contribution of the nurses was the development of Little Mother Leagues in the slums, in which all girls older than age 8 were taught how to take care of their younger siblings, including the infants.

What programs exist in your local communities today aimed at decreasing the spread of communicable diseases?

TWENTIETH CENTURY

The nursing profession evolved to meet the nursing shortage and to make better use of nursing personnel. By 1903, states began to take steps that ultimately led to monitoring of practical nursing. During this period, nursing organizations were developed. The National League of Nursing Education (now the NLN) took the most influential step. In 1917, the league developed a nationwide system of standardization of nursing requirements for practical nursing.

MISSISSIPPI: FIRST TO LICENSE PRACTICAL NURSES

In 1914, Mississippi was the first state to pass a law licensing practical nurses. This was an important event because the public had no way of knowing who was providing nursing care. For centuries, self-proclaimed nurses were responsible for the majority of the nursing that was done. Licensing, however, was not mandatory, and by 1938, New York was the only state to have mandatory licensure. Today, all states require mandatory licensure for nurses, including practical nurses.

WORLD WAR I NURSES 1914 TO 1918

The history of nursing is also the history of war and hard-fought women's rights. Women were considered fragile and delicate and kept at home to raise their babies and keep house. World War I made it necessary for women to work outside the home so men could go to war. Poster campaigns depicted the glamour of war to persuade young women to sign up as doctors and nurses to help with the war effort. Women were encouraged to be tough, but they still struggled with those who did not want women working outside of the home. Nurses had been part of wars in the past but never as part of the military. World War I was the first war where nurses had professional training to serve. America declared war on Germany in 1917, and it was evident that there were not enough nurses to serve. **Jane Delano** of the American Red Cross began to recruit nurses and train and equip them for overseas duty. About 20,000 nurses were assigned to go overseas, and many of them stayed overseas after the war to help with the postwar relief programs.

The U.S. government insisted that only trained nurses could be sent to France with the Army. The reality was there were not enough nurses to meet both war and domestic needs. National nursing leaders **M. Adelaide Nutting, Anna Goodrich**, and Lillian Wald met and formed the National Emergency Committee on Nursing. As a result, the Vassar Training Camp was created to train college graduates in an intensive 3-month program to enter schools of nursing. Soon other universities began to offer similar nursing programs. In 1918, the Army School of Nursing was established at Walter Reed hospital in Washington, D.C. It extended similar programs to other military hospitals throughout the United States.

World War I nurses were not allowed to serve at the advanced dressing stations on the front lines, although some nurses showed up there. They served primarily in hospitals organized for treating the wounded: field hospitals, which were sometimes just behind the front; clearing hospitals (known as evacuation hospitals) that were 10 miles back from the front; and base hospitals, where all the wounded were eventually sent. They dealt primarily with communicable diseases, wounds, infections, shock, hemorrhage, and poison gas inhalation, and they even performed minor surgeries. The work was long and exhausting, with deplorable conditions and few supplies. Young nurses were exposed to horrors, not the glamour that had been advertised on the posters.

At the peak of the war, 23,000 (some sources say 30,000) nurses were in service, and none held a military rank. Although governed by military discipline, they were neither officers nor enlisted personnel. Because of this, they had no authority to direct corpsmen or orderlies or to take on administrative duties. After the war, through an amendment to the National Defense Act, the Army Nurse Corps was given officer status. This did not increase their pay or allowance to that of their male counterparts.

There is no record of a nurse dying because of combat, but about 260 nurses died because of the influenza epidemic of 1918. Many women were recognized for their service with awards. Three nurses received the Distinguished Service Award, and four Navy nurses were awarded the Navy Cross. In her book *Nursing, the Finest Art*, Donahue (1985) states, "One of the four, **Lenah S. Higbee**, the second Superintendent of the Corps, from 1911 to 1923, had a destroyer named in her honor on January 1945. This was the first time a fighting ship was named after a woman in the military service."

World War I emphasized what nurses of that time were capable of accomplishing. It also highlighted the need for more and better-prepared nurses. Moving nursing into colleges and universities was a major step for nursing education. Admission standards for nursing schools were raised, and the expectations of graduates were increased.

It was the service of women in the military that positively impacted women's rights: the Nineteenth Amendment, which was ratified in 1920. President Woodrow Wilson made a passionate plea to the Senate to pass the amendment. He pointed out how women were expected to work hard and make sacrifices without the privileges and rights men enjoyed.

Canadian Nurses in World War I

Unlike American nurses in the military, the Canadian nurses were given the designation of lieutenants in the army and were stationed at nursing care wards. Canadian nurses worked around the clock to treat the wounded, who were brought in on stretchers or just dragged in because no stretchers were available. They had thousands of wounded to care for and try to prevent the onset of infections. Many lives were saved because of the nurses' diligence.

The shortage of beds in the military hospitals often made it necessary to put the wounded on the floor. These wounded men were the victims of the many hungry rats that overran the hospitals and were fearless and not afraid to bite the wounded soldiers. A Hall of Honor was built in Ottawa, Canada, to remember and honor the Canadian nurses who stood so strong in times of such difficulty.

SMITH HUGHES ACT OF 1917

The home front was facing a battle of its own in 1917 and 1918, with a major epidemic of pneumonia in 1917 and a worldwide epidemic of Spanish influenza in 1918. The mortality rate was high, especially in 1918. The Smith Hughes Act of 1917 provided money for developing additional schools of practical nursing. The first high school vocational/practical nursing program opened at the Minneapolis Girls Vocational High School in 1919. However, the new schools could not supply nurses quickly enough to meet the severe shortage in the United States.

NURSES RETURN HOME: ACUTE NURSING SHORTAGE FOLLOWS WORLD WAR I

After the war, many nurses did not continue nursing. Some stayed overseas to help with relief efforts. This led to an acute shortage of nurses in the 1920s. Many more hospitals opened schools of nursing. Their real purpose was to provide staffing. Hospitals without schools were staffed heavily with untrained help.

From 1920 to 1940, six states made laws licensing practical nurses, but only a small number of practical nursing schools existed in the United States. Much of the nurse's work continued to be in public health agencies and visiting nurse associations.

DEPRESSION OF THE 1930S

During the Great Depression in the 1930s, many nurses lost their jobs or worked in hospitals for room and board rather than a salary. When it became fairly obvious that America was becoming involved in World War II, nursing leaders began to prepare for the need for nurses at all levels. They did not want to face the nursing shortage experienced during World War I. This was a monumental task because nursing had decreased in popularity as a vocation.

WORLD WAR II 1939 TO 1945

Although World War II began in 1939, the United States was unofficially involved by offering Lend Lease, which gave war materials to Allied countries in exchange for being allowed to use Allied bases. Initially noncombatants, American aircraft and warships escorted merchant ships and protected them against U-boat attacks. When Pearl Harbor was attacked, the United States declared war the following day. World War II involved about 50 countries and resulted in major changes throughout the world.

When Pearl Harbor was bombed on December 7, 1941, there were fewer than 12,000 nurses on duty in the Army Nurse Corps. Few of them had military experience and knowledge of Army protocol. Fifteen 4-week training programs were developed for new nurses. The programs stressed Army protocol; military customs and courtesies; field sanitation; defenses against air, chemical, and mechanized attacks; personnel administration; requisitions and correspondence; and property responsibility. More than 27,330 newly inducted nurses graduated from the 15 programs.

It became quickly obvious that there were not enough trained personnel to administer anesthesia. More than 200 nurses enrolled in the 6-month course on how to administer inhalant anesthesia, blood and blood derivatives, and oxygen therapy and how to recognize and treat shock. Nurses specializing in psychiatric care were in great need. One out of 12 patients in Army hospitals was admitted for psychiatric care. A 12-week course was developed by the surgeon general to teach nurses how to care for and medicate combatants with psychiatric disorders.

Approximately 59,000 American nurses served in the war. Army and Navy nurses served in both the European and Pacific theaters. They were closer to the front than in past wars. Nurses were assigned to field hospitals, evacuation hospitals, hospital ships, and as flight nurses on medical transport planes. Because of the care combatants received in field hospitals or during evacuation, fewer than 4% died from wounds or disease. The demand for nurses in the Army and Navy Nurse Corps helped create a nursing shortage at home. In 1943, Congress passed the Bolton Act, which became the basis for the **Cadet Nurse Corps**. The government subsidized schools that were willing to teach primary nursing skills in 2½ years. More than 150,000 nurses graduated from these programs. The Cadet Nurse programs were discontinued in 1948, but the public considered these programs a great success.

When the war ended, the Army was still segregated and still had a quota system for black nurses. Only 479 nurses of the 50,000 serving in the Army Nurse Corps were black nurses, and they were limited to taking care of black troops in black hospitals. The Army dropped its quota system in 1944 because of the negative public reaction. By the end of the war, black nurses had served in Africa, England, Burma, and the Southwest Pacific. Federal funding for the Cadet Nurse Corps made it possible for 2000 black students to enroll in the Cadet Nurse program.

Practical nurses played a significant role both at home and in World War II. At home, practical nurses worked in clinics, health departments, industries, and hospitals. At the battlefields, practical nurses and registered nurses could be found in both the European and Pacific theaters. Some officers were initially reluctant to have nurses assigned at combat zones. The dedication, organization, and professionalism proved their worth and won the respect of doctors, corpsmen, patients, and military command. Nurses adjusted to long hours with little rest, loss of electricity, bombings, kamikaze attacks, frequent moves and setting up of field hospitals, internment in concentration camps, deaths of patients and other nurses, wounds and diseases, and dealing with members of numerous cultures. It was noted that nurses adjusted to difficult and dangerous situations with a minimum of complaints.

Nurses received 1619 medals, citations, and commendations during the war, 16 of them posthumously to nurses who died as a result of enemy fire. After the war, nurses were eligible for the G.I. Bill of Rights, which entitled them to continue their education paid for by the government.

PRACTICAL NURSING RESPONSIBILITIES INCREASE AFTER WORLD WAR II

The end of World War II saw a continuing shortage of nurses. This shortage helped practical nurses play an important part in hospital nursing. Most hospitals gradually increased the responsibilities designated for the practical nurse. By the 1940s, there were nearly 50 approved practical nursing programs in the United States. The number of practical nurses in America peaked at 159,009 in 1940. By 1944, practical nursing was already experiencing a decline.

> **?** Critical Thinking
>
> How many practical nursing programs exist in your state today? How many LPNs/LVNs exist in the nation?

PRACTICAL NURSING DUTIES OUTLINED

In 1944, the U.S. Department of Vocational Education made a comprehensive study of practical nursing. This marked the first time that tasks of practical nursing were agreed on. Extensive specific duties were outlined, with an emphasis on maintaining aseptic technique. The phrases "to judge," "to appraise," "to recognize," and "to determine" were often used to describe the scope of the practical nurse's job.

> **?** Critical Thinking
>
> Discuss with a peer whether the phrases used in 1944 "to judge," "to appraise," "to recognize," and "to determine" describe the scope of the practical nurse's job today. What phrases would you suggest adding?

REGISTERED NURSE AND LICENSED PRACTICAL NURSE TASKS DIFFERENTIATED

Other important changes followed. In 1949, the Joint Committee on Practical Nurses and Auxiliary Workers in Nursing Services recommended use of the title "licensed practical nurse." Furthermore, the committee differentiated between the tasks of the registered nurse (RN) and the LPN. They saw the LPN as being under the supervision of the RN. The committee also suggested that practical nurses organize to make decisions on their salary, working conditions, and employment standards.

Because of the work of the Joint Committee, many practical nursing programs were strengthened with regard to content. They focused for the first time on the preparation of practical nursing instructors. Up to this point, any graduate nurse was eligible to teach practical nursing. During the 1950s, the number of programs continued to increase, and programs were extended to 9-, 12-, and 18-month programs.

THE KOREAN CONFLICT (ALSO KNOWN AS UNITED NATIONS POLICE ACTION OR THE SECOND INDOCHINA WAR) 1950 TO 1953

Many in the military believed that women had no place in the armed forces. The term used was *demilitarization*, and it took place rapidly after WWII. Many women lost their jobs in industry. Multiple reasons were given for sending women back to the kitchen, but one reason not discussed openly was that men would have difficulty reporting to women officers. It took 3 years for the government to determine that women were an integral part of the military. General Eisenhower finally clarified the issue by strongly recommending that women become a part of the U.S. military. Several senior officers who had worked with women during WWII had great praise for military women. This led to President Truman signing the Women's Armed Forces Act in 1948. By the time North Korea invaded South Korea, the number of women in the military was at an all-time low.

The United States entered the United Nations Police Action to support their ally South Korea when North Korea crossed the thirty-ninth parallel and invaded the Republic of South Korea. Because of the shortage of nurses in the military, nurses were recruited from civilian hospitals. According to records, 540 Army nurses served in Korea, and none died as a result of enemy action. Of the 3081 active-duty Navy nurses and 1702 reserve Navy nurses, according to records, none were killed or wounded because of enemy

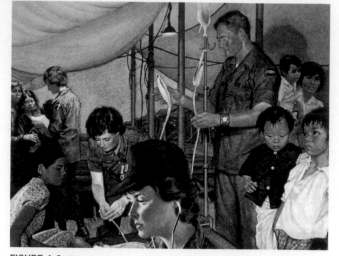

FIGURE 4-3 The American Soldier, 1975. In the foreground, as concerned relatives look on, an Army nurse checks an injured Vietnamese citizen. The scene is typical of many long evenings in tents set up as emergency medical stations on Guam, the first stop for the refugees. (Courtesy U.S. Army Center of Military History.)

action. The Navy nurses served on three troop ships in both U.S. and overseas hospitals. Army nurses cared for wounded in mobile army surgical hospital (MASH) units, prisoner of war camps, makeshift shelters, and hospital trains. Nurses were known for serving in MASH units where their responsibility was beyond that of the usual nurse. The shortage of medical personnel pushed them into doing work past their scope of nursing and into advanced practice. One such task was that of first assistant in surgery, which has now become an accepted part of RN advanced practice (RNFA) nursing (Figure 4-3).

Nurses also worked as flight nurses on evacuation aircraft. One of the women who served was **Lillian Kinkela-Keil**, a member of the Air Force Nurse Corps and one of the most decorated women in the U.S. military. Captain Kinkela-Keil flew over 200 air evacuation missions during WWII, as well as 25 trans-Atlantic crossings and she flew several hundred more missions as a flight nurse in Korea.

"Captain Kinkela-Keil was the inspiration for the 1953 movie *Flight Nurse* and served as technical advisor to the film. Her decorations include the European Theater of Operations with Four Battle Stars, the Air Medal with Three Oak Leaf Clusters, the Presidential Unit Citation with One Oak Leaf Cluster, the Korean Service Medal with Seven Battle Stars, the American Campaign Medal, the United Defense Medal, and the Presidential Citation, Republic of Korea. Captain Kinkel-Keil died in 2005 at age 88" (Wilson, 2011).

The Korean War is called *the forgotten war.* The men and women who served were forgotten, as was the war itself. Finding records and information about the war is also difficult to uncover. Little factual information is available to the public.

REGISTERED NURSES REACT

By 1952, nearly 60% of the nursing workforce was made up of practical nurses. In many instances, RNs expressed bitterness because hospitals, clinics, and other agencies were hiring practical nurses for less money and assigning tasks to them beyond their educational level. RNs also expressed concern that the public was unable to differentiate between the levels of nurses. Both wore the same type of white uniforms, caps, and pins. Many practical nurses quickly stopped wearing the practical nursing insignia, which was meant to identify the practical nurse. LPNs/LVNs performed tasks belonging to the RN one day and those belonging to nursing aides the next day. Many practical nurses felt trapped in such situations because of their need for employment.

PUBLIC LAW 911

In 1956, Public Law 911 provided for millions of dollars to expand and improve practical nursing programs. By 1975, there were 1337 programs, which graduated a total of 46,080 practical nurses. Approximately two-thirds of the practical nurses were employed in hospitals, 17.3% in nursing homes, 7.5% in private duty, and 6.5% in doctors' offices, clinics, and dental offices. Admission standards in most schools increased, as did the difficulty of the curriculum.

THE VIETNAM WAR 1961 TO 1973

The Vietnam War (1961–1973) was the longest war involving U.S. military forces. Numbers vary, but it is thought that about 7484 (79% female, 21% male) nurses served in the war (Martinez, 2010). Nurses enlisted for various reason including tuition forgiveness, free medical and dental care, opportunity to travel, and love for their country. All of the nurses volunteered and underwent a 6-week basic training course before being assigned to a 1-year stint in Vietnam. Assignments were primarily in Vietnamese hospitals, MASH units, as flight nurses, and on board the hospital ships USS *Repose* and *Sanctuary*. Most of the nurses were in their early twenties and recent graduates with less than 6 months of clinical experience.

Living conditions varied from bug-infested tents to air-conditioned trailers to small, single-occupant rooms. Nurses in field hospitals wore white duty uniforms, and the rest of the medical personnel wore lightweight olive drab made of cotton poplin. It was difficult to keep uniforms clean, and nurses preferred to wear fatigues when available.

Nurses performed duties beyond what they had learned in nursing school. The 6-month basic training did not adequately prepare the nurses, physically or emotionally. Nurses worked 12-hour shifts, 6 days a week. Days off were often canceled out of necessity when massive casualties arrived. Combat injuries were different in this war. Artillery was specifically designed to inflict massive, multiple injuries. Napalm, white phosphorous, and "antipersonnel" bombs were used as well. Napalm and white phosphorous burned tissue right down to the bone. Nurses described their orientation as being thrown into a "bloody hell" (Carlson, 2010). Nurses treated wounds they had never seen, did tasks beyond their nursing scope of practice, and dealt with illnesses such as typhoid, malaria, dengue fever, and bubonic plague. As in other wars, approximately 69% of admissions were for disease. In this war, it was malaria, viral hepatitis, skin diseases, venereal diseases, diarrheal diseases, and diseases of unknown origin. The rest were combat casualties. Assault rifles, rocket-propelled grenades, and booby traps were the major causes of wounds. Infection resulting from animal and human excreta in the paddy fields and waterways created additional problems in treatment.

As the war continued, service personnel were also being treated for drug addiction, especially heroin. Nurses had to deal with soldiers under the influence of illicit drugs. Nurses were told to control their emotions when dealing with severely wounded and dying soldiers. According to the Vietnam Veteran's Memorial Foundation, the hospital mortality rate was 2.6% per thousand in the Vietnam War compared with 4.5% during World War II.

In addition to practicing all the specialties, nurses also voluntarily gave medical assistance to Vietnamese civilians. This included basic care, immunizations, courses in child-care, and sick calls at orphanages.

Mildred I. Clark, chief of the Army Nurse Corps from 1963 to 1967, and **Anna Mae Hays**, chief of the Army Nurse Corps from 1967 to 1971, led the Army Nurse Corps during the Vietnam War. On June 11, 1970, Colonel Hays also became a brigadier general, the first woman and the first nurse in American military to attain general officer rank (West, Army Nurse Corps Historian).

Women were treated as second-class citizens both in the military and when they came home. Nurses suffered from posttraumatic stress disorder (PTSD), experiencing feelings of isolation and anger. They had difficulty finding employment and suffered bouts of crying and depression. Vietnam veterans found it difficult to receive treatment, and both men and women were treated badly by many in the public.

The Vietnam Women's Memorial, designed and sculpted by **Glenna Goodacres**, is on the National Mall in Washington, D.C. It is located at the south end of the Vietnam Veteran's Memorial and in the vicinity of the Three Servicemen memorial. The Goodacres monument shows three nurses in battle dress. One comforts a wounded or perhaps dying soldier, one is kneeling, and one is looking up in expectation.

? **Critical Thinking**

Preventing Posttraumatic Stress Disorder

If you were to join the military as a nurse and had to go into a war area, how would you prepare yourself to deal emotionally with the challenges you will face as a military nurse? What are work settings in the United States where you may experience PTSD?

NATIONAL BLACK NURSES ASSOCIATION

The National Black Nurses Association (NBNA) is a nonprofit entity, established in 1971. NBNA's mission is "to represent and provide a forum for Black nurses to advocate and implement strategies to ensure access to the highest quality of health care for persons of color" (NBNA, 2015). Multiple black nurses have contributed to the NBNA's legacy, establishing and growing this entity, beginning with the founder, Dr. Lauranne Sams, former Dean and Professor of Nursing, School of Nursing, Tuskegee University, Tuskegee, Alabama. NBNA represents 150,000 African American Nurses representing a diverse group of nurses (RNs, LPNs/LVNs, nursing students, and retired nurses) focused on providing culturally competent health care to African Americans.

IRAQ WAR 2003 TO 2011 AND THE AFGHAN WAR 2001 TO 2014

The U.S. involvement in the Afghanistan war (2001) was a result of the attacks on the Twin Towers in New York City on September 11, 2001. The war in Iraq (2003) began as a result of a belief that Iraq had weapons of mass destruction, which it did not. Very little has been written about nurses' experiences in Afghanistan and Iraq.

The Air Force sent 4060 nurses to Afghanistan and Iraq. Since 2003, the U.S. Navy deployed 1193 nurses to Iraq and 403 nurses to Afghanistan. In addition, since 2007, over 100 nurses were deployed as part of the International Security Assistance Force in Afghanistan (Bolvin, 2010). They quickly helped set up surgical teams and mobile hospitals to receive casualties. Issues arose regarding the lack of critical care nursing experience and the lack of experience using some equipment before deployment. Nurses were also assigned to air evacuation units, combat support units in Afghan and Iraqi hospitals, and hospitals for detainees. Living quarters varied from tents to primitive plywood shacks to container housing, depending on where they were sent. A layer of fine sand covered everything, showers were scarce, and feeling dirty all the time was common. Sanitation and sewer systems were minimal, and with the high temperatures, the smell of sewage was often in the air.

Some nurses described Afghanistan and Iraq as noisy, smelly places. It is not unusual to burn excreta and surgical waste. At the beginning of the war, little food was available, and most meals consisted of ready-to-eat fare, with water stored in containers that tasted like chlorine and was always warm because of the heat. This is a reason soldiers and medical people requested Kool-Aid and Crystal Light packets to add to the water (Desch and Doherty, 2010).

For nurses working in countries beyond our borders, being culturally sensitive when providing care to patients is an even greater issue. Patients' cultural preferences must be integrated into the plan of care. Nursing and medical care extends to America's wounded troops, civilians, National Army soldiers, and other coalition soldiers from around the world.

Although it is acceptable in Afghanistan for a male to be a nurse, male nurses cared for males only, and female nurses cared for female patients only. Families, when available, were involved in the care of hospitalized patients. Equipment and medicines were needed. Diarrheal illness was an issue in the civilian community, as was malaria, parasites, polio, and a protozoan illness caused by sand flies (especially in children playing in the sand).

Troops experienced severe injuries from mortar fire and roadside explosive devices, as well as gunfire. Approximately 2% to 4% of the troops experienced gastrointestinal illness with nausea, vomiting, and diarrhea.

Although many nurses were not directly in harm's way, they are at risk for PTSD because of constant fear, exposure to trauma and loss, ethical dilemmas, and fatigue (Bolvin, 2010). Each individual undergoes an assessment when he or she returns to this country. Sometimes symptoms do not appear until later, or the individuals' answers during an exit assessment may trigger concern and follow up. They may be concerned about how they will be viewed when they are back home. It is not unusual for a nurse to grieve the person he or she was before going to Afghanistan or Iraq. Others appreciate professional growth and all that they learned to do and deal with, building their courage and self-confidence. What seems to stand out for many nurses is the sense of camaraderie and teamwork experienced between the nurses and the doctors while overseas.

The United States continues to be involved in conflicts, and nurses continue to serve this great country and care for soldiers as the need arises throughout the world.

◎ Try This

If you know someone who is serving or has served in the Afghanistan or Iraq war, ask him or her about his/her feelings about nurses serving in the military.

NURSE LEADERS IN U.S. GOVERNMENT

Several women currently serve in U.S. Congress, and others have recently held senior management positions in diverse public entities. As nurses have transformed from "doers" to "thinkers" over the last few decades, their emergence in policy development is logical and beneficial to the advancing of the health of the nation.

Their strategic positions can be a conduit for nurses to communicate their views regarding various issues that impact health care.

AMERICAN NURSES ASSOCIATION MOVEMENT TOWARD TWO LEVELS OF NURSING

In 1965, the American Nurses Association (ANA) presented a position paper outlining how to solve the issues of the different levels of the nursing profession. They recommended that all RNs graduate from a 4-year collegiate program and all LPNs graduate from a 2-year technical program. Many hospital-based RN programs closed during that time. In the 1980s, a resurgence of the ANA 1965 movement toward establishing two levels of nursing temporarily gained momentum. This original movement was reinterpreted by many stakeholders, resulting in a surge of 2-year Associate Degree in Nursing (RN) programs. However, some states did work towards adopting the ANA recommendations. Because a serious nursing shortage developed in the late 1980s, the ANA movement stalled in most states.

AMERICAN MEDICAL ASSOCIATION MOVES TO EASE NURSING SHORTAGE

With the goal of easing the nursing shortage, in 1989, the American Medical Association (AMA) proposed a new health care worker: the registered care technologist (RCT). The RCT was to be trained in 1- and 2-year programs. Because this new level of health care worker correlated with existing personnel, the practical nurse, and the associate degree nurse, the RCT proposal was not successful. This event is a gentle reminder for practical/vocational nurses to be strong, organized, and vigilant as a group. Changes in the health care system are occurring daily, as are opportunities for LPNs/LVNs. See Chapter 18 for a discussion regarding workforce trends.

UNLICENSED ASSISTIVE PERSONNEL

During the 1990s, unlicensed assistive personnel (UAP) were hired to give patient care. A major concern for LPNs/LVNs and RNs was their legal responsibility for the care given by the unlicensed caregivers. Meanwhile, primary employment for nurses, especially for the LPNs/LVNs, moved out of hospitals and into the community.

FIRST COMPUTERIZED TESTING: NCLEX-PN®

In 1994, the first computerized adaptive testing (NCLEX-PN® examination) became available for the practical/vocational nursing graduate. The computer format provided an individualized test for each graduate, based on the answer to the previous question. It also excluded questions that were not within the nurse's role, according to their state's Nurse Practice Act.

LONG-TERM CARE CERTIFICATION

In 1996, long-term care certification became available to LPNs/LVNs in some states. Since that time, other certifications have become available for LPNs/LVNs in some states (see Chapter 19).

TWENTY-FIRST CENTURY

Nursing organizations continue to define the responsibilities of the different levels of nursing. More remains to be resolved. Nursing shortages have created changes in nursing programs. Approximately 50 years ago, Associate Degree (AD) nursing programs were set up in technical schools, and they have flourished. Today, approximately 38% of the current RN workforce hold an Associate's degree as their highest nursing degree earned (HRSA, 2013). The goals of AD programs were to move nursing education out of hospital-based programs and to help ease the shortage by shortening the amount of time required to become an RN. However, the AD graduate, diploma graduate, and baccalaureate graduate all take the same licensing examination to become an RN. It was and continues to be confusing for those doing the hiring at a facility, because all RNs, regardless of their education, can legally assume the same responsibilities. Finances are always a major concern for health facilities. Years ago, when LPNs/LVNs earned much less than RNs, more LPNs/LVNs were hired. When salaries were narrowed and the difference in salary was considerably less, more RNs were hired.

Nursing organizations continue to work on resolving the issue of nursing levels and present new recommendations and position papers. Nursing shortages continue periodically. Changes in how health facilities are reimbursed for patient care have had major impacts on patient acuity, staffing ratios, overtime, patient care loads, and patient safety. The average age of the nurse workforce continues to increase.

In the last five years, fueled by the Institute of Medicine (2010) Report, *Future of Nursing: Leading Change, Advancing Health*, many stakeholders are again discussing the levels of the nursing profession, an age old debate that began in the 1960s. Given historical implications, such as the increase of Associate Degree in Nursing programs, the new discussion focuses on the need for Baccalaureate preparation as an entry point for RNs and a need for an increase in doctorally prepared nurses. In response, several states have introduced legislation to achieve these goals. However, the educational level of practical nurses has not been a focal point of the debate.

In 2014, the NLN released a Vision Statement titled, *Recognizing the Role of the Licensed Practical/Vocational Nurses in Advancing the Nation's Health*, supporting the critical role of LPNs/LVNs in providing quality patient-centered, evidenced-based care to vulnerable groups across the health care continuum. In addition, the NLN also developed a guiding curriculum framework for practical/vocational nursing programs aligned with LPN/LVN workforce trends. This support is timely as health care reform has created changing job roles for health care providers.

YOU HAVE COME A LONG WAY!

As a final note, it may be interesting to compare present practical/vocational nursing tasks with those that you would have been expected to perform in 1887. Practical/vocational nursing has indeed come a long way. The job description in Box 4-2 was given to floor nurses by a hospital in 1887 (author unknown).

Box 4-2 Hospital Nursing 1887

In addition to caring for your 50 patients, each nurse will follow these regulations:

- Daily, sweep and mop the floors of your ward, dust the patient's furniture and window sills. Maintain an even temperature in your ward by bringing in a scuttle of coal for the day's business.
- Light is important to observe the patient's condition. Therefore each day fill kerosene lamps, clean chimneys, and trim wicks. Wash the lamp windows once a week.
- The nurse's notes are important in aiding the physician's work. Make your pens carefully; you may whittle nibs to your individual taste.
- Each nurse on day duty will report every day at 7 AM and leave at 8 PM, except on the Sabbath, on which day you will be off from noon to 2 PM.
- Graduate nurses in good standing with the director of nurses will be given an evening off each week for courting purposes or two evenings a week if you go regularly to church.
- Each nurse should lay aside from each payday a goodly sum of her earnings for her benefits during her declining years so that she will not become a burden. For example, if you earn $30 a month, you should set aside $15.
- Any nurse who smokes, uses liquor in any form, gets her hair done at a beauty shop, or frequents dance halls will give the director of nurses good reason to suspect her worth, intentions, and integrity.
- The nurse who performs her labors and serves her patients and doctors without fault for 5 years will be given an increase of 5 cents a day, providing there are no hospital debts outstanding.

Get Ready for the NCLEX-PN® Examination

Key Points

- The nursing profession, including practical nursing, has experienced a history of transformation, emerging as a highly respected profession. Duties have changed according to the needs present at various times in history.
- Currently, practical/vocational nurses are taught both technical skills and critical thinking skills. This includes a focus on evidence-based (i.e., data-driven) decision-making, often described as critical thinking during their educational program.
- According to some states' Nurse Practice Act, LPNs/LVNs are allowed to perform more complex skills. LPNs/LVNs work under the supervision and collaboratively with the RN, physician, and physician extenders (i.e., Nurse Practitioner).
- Historical figures in nursing include Florence Nightingale, founder of modern nursing; Clara Barton, founder of the American Red Cross; Lillian Wald, founder of public health nursing; and Dorothea Lynde Dix, advocate for the mentally ill.
- Nurses have played a significant role in all wars, contributing positively to the development of the nursing profession.

Additional Learning Resources

evolve Go to your Evolve website (http://evolve.elsevier.com/Knecht/success) for the following FREE learning resources:
- Answers to Critical Thinking Scenarios
- Additional learning activities
- Additional Review Questions for the NCLEX-PN® exam
- Helpful phrases for communicating in Spanish and more!

Review Questions for the NCLEX-PN® Examination

1. Which statement relates to Florence Nightingale's contribution to nursing?
   a. She established the first visiting nurse service for the poor in the Lower East Side slum section of New York.
   b. She wrote the Nightingale Pledge in 1893 to set guidelines and inspire her nurses on graduation.
   c. She discovered antibiotic use during the Crimean War.
   d. She stressed environment, the need for careful observation, care of the whole person, and critical thinking.

2. Periodically, various organizations have suggested eliminating practical/vocational programs. Which statement objectively provides a reason for continuing the LPN/LVN programs?
   a. LPNs/LVNs possess the same level of skill in patient care as do registered nurses.
   b. RN education is more focused on nursing theory, relying on LPNs to perform all tasks.
   c. LPNs/LVNs are well prepared to provide evidenced-based care to vulnerable groups across the health continuum, collaborating with the RN as needed.
   d. Physicians prefer to work with LPNs/LVNs because they follow orders without question.

Alternate Format Item

1. Identify possible reasons why a nurse involved in care of soldiers in the war zone may develop PTSD. (Select all that apply.)
   a. Told to do tasks that are out of their scope of practice
   b. Long hours with limited sleep
   c. Faced with caring for patients with gruesome injuries
   d. Lack of essential items required to give safe care
   e. Adequate nutrition

2. Florence Nightingale's beliefs formed the basis of medical asepsis, which continues to be a critical concept in health care delivery today. The following were included in these beliefs: (Select all that apply.)
   a. brightly painted walls
   b. clean environment
   c. handwashing
   d. clean linens
   e. shades on windows

Critical Thinking: A Lifelong Journey

Objectives

On completing this chapter, you will be able to do the following:

1. Discuss the difference between nonfocused and directed thinking
2. Identify where to find evidence necessary for effective practical/vocational nursing decision making.
2. Discuss how to use evidence to assist in decision making.
3. Explain why critical thinking is essential to decision making as a practical/vocational nurse
4. Differentiate among the terms *knowledge, comprehension (understanding), application,* and *analysis.*

5. Evaluate your personal need for help in comprehending information.
6. Identify two new suggestions for increasing reading effectiveness that you will begin to apply immediately.
7. Develop a plan using critical thinking to increase your ability to think critically.

Key Terms

analysis (ă-NĂL-1-sĭs)
application (ĂP-lĭ-KĂ-shŭn)
attitude (ĂT-ĭ-ood)
capability (KĂ-pă-ĬL-ĭ-tē)
cognitive levels (KŎG-nĭ-tĭv)
comprehension (KŎM-prē-HĔN-shŭn)

critical thinking (KRĬT-ĭ-căl)
directed (or focused) thinking (dĭ-RĔCT-ĕd)
knowledge (NŎL-ĕj)
problem-oriented thinking (prŏ-blĕm ŎR-ē-ĕn-tĕd)
reflective thinking (rē-FLĔK-tĭv)

Keep in Mind

Become an active learner and critical thinker, and be successful in the practical/vocational nursing program, on the National Council Licensure Examination for Licensed Practical Nurses (NCLEX-PN®) and as a candidate for a job you will love as a Licensed Practical Nurse/Licensed Vocational Nurse (LPN/LVN).

As Kamy and Hilary are waiting for class to begin, you overhear them discussing the evolving role of the LPN/LVN from "doer" to "thinker." Kamy states, "Wow, it seems like the LPN/LVN has a much more challenging job today than they did 20 years ago. At first I thought, well I am a "doer;" that is why I chose this career. But now I realize how important it is to be a "doer" and a "thinker." Anyone can do but not everyone can use several pieces of evidence to think in a critical manner and arrive at the best decision for the patient's plan of care. This is exciting. I feel like we really are a critical member of the health care team. This role seems very different than my role as a pharmacy technician." Hilary agrees and states, "I was thinking the same thing. My role as a nursing assistant is heavily focused on "doing." Although a very important role, this "critical thinking" really changes our job as an LPN/LVN. I am excited to learn about simulation and all the other ways to begin to think in a critical manner. Class is about to begin. Talk to you tomorrow." You reflect on this conversation as class begins.

OVERVIEW OF CRITICAL THINKING

The following are the *Top 10 Reasons to Improve Thinking*, adapted for practical/vocational nurses:*

10. Things are not what they used to be, or what they will be, in this changing health care system.
9. Licensed practical nurses/licensed vocational nurses (LPNs/LVNs) frequently care for patients, as a member of the health care team, who are not yet stabilized and have multiple problems.
8. More patients and their families are involved in health care decisions.
7. LPNs/LVNs must be able to move from one health care setting to another.
6. Rapid change and information explosion requires LPNs/LVNs to develop new learning and workplace skills.

---

*Adapted with permission from Alfaro-Lefevre R. (2009). *Critical thinking and clinical judgement: a practical approach* (ed 4). Philadelphia:WB Saunders.

5. Patients, families, and insurance companies demand to see evidence of benefits, efficiency, and results of care given.

4. Today's progress often creates new problems that cannot be solved by old ways of thinking (e.g., ethical and legal issues involved in end-of-life decisions, questions regarding stem cell research, determining who is entitled to receive expensive medical care).

3. Redesigning care delivery and education programs is useless if students and nurses do not have the thinking skills required to deal with today's world.

2. Learning how to improve your thinking skills does not have to be difficult.

1. Your ability to focus your thinking on how to get the results you need can make the difference between whether you succeed or fail in the fast-paced health care system.

Years ago, nurses saw themselves as doers, not thinkers. Nurses were primarily told what to do, and they carried out the orders. Certainly there were exceptions, such as Florence Nightingale, a historical pioneer in nursing. By 1996, the National Council of State Boards of Nursing (NCSBN) included four phases of the nursing process in the NCLEX-PN® examination. Questions were at the cognitive level of knowledge, comprehension, and application (NCSBN, 1995). In 1999, the four phases were integrated throughout the test plan (NCSBN, 1998). By 2002, the NCSBN integrated all phases of the nursing process, as well as critical thinking, into the NCLEX-PN® examination. As a result, the cognitive level of analysis was added to NCLEX-PN® examination questions (NCSBN, 2001). Analysis is an essential component of critical thinking; likewise, critical thinking is an integral part of the nursing process. As a nurse, you have to think critically. It is part of the process of nursing. The 2014 NCLEX-PN Test Plan (NCSBN, 2014) indicates that critical thinking is essential to use evidence-based practice to provide nursing care. Evidence-based care is essential to everyday nursing practice. Thus, the ability to critically think is an essential job role as an LPN/LVN.

Professional Pointer

Critical thinking is a lifelong process (Alfaro-Lefevre, 2013).

WAYS OF THINKING

DEFINITION OF APPLIED CRITICAL THINKING

What exactly is *critical thinking*, and how does it relate to the nursing decisions you will make at school and during your career? Alfaro-Lefevre (2013) provides a definition of critical thinking and clinical judgment in nursing. **Critical thinking** in nursing, adapted

for practical/vocational nursing, is defined as the following:*

- Entails purposeful, informed, outcome-focused (results-oriented) thinking that requires careful identification of the problems, issues, and risks involved (e.g., deciding whether a patient needs one or more staff to move him from bed to chair in a manner that is safe for both patient and staff).
- Is driven by patient, family, and community needs. The licensed practical/licensed vocational nurse must be able to use knowledge to tailor approaches based on circumstances.
- Is based on the principles of the nursing process and on scientific methods; for example, making judgments based on evidence (facts) rather than guesswork. This is a major difference between LPNs/LVNs and unlicensed assistive personnel (UAPs).
- Uses both logic and intuition, based on knowledge, skills, and experience of the LPN/LVN.
- Is guided by professional standards, such as those developed for the LPN/LVN by the National Association for Practical Nurse Education and Service (NAPNES) (www.napnes.org), the National Federation of Licensed Practical Nurses (NFLPN), (www.nflpn.org), and the practical/vocational nursing code of ethics.
- Calls for strategies that make the most of human potential (e.g., using individual strengths) and compensates for problems created by human nature (e.g., overcoming the powerful influence of personal beliefs, values, and prejudices).
- Is constantly reevaluating, self-correcting, and striving to improve (e.g., practicing skills, learning new skills, and attending classes and workshops).

Thinking is divided into nonfocused thinking and **directed thinking**. At one time or another, most of us have used the following examples of thinking:

- **Nonfocused thinking:** You engaged your brain out of habit without much conscious thought.
- **Habitual thinking:** We get up to go to the bathroom, shower, dress, and so on. This type of thinking involves any routine we do that is important but does not require us to think hard about how to do it (automatic pilot).
- **Random thoughts:** Multiple short scenes and thoughts come and go through the mind and have no particular purpose or goal (mental channel surfing).
- **Ruminative thinking:** The same situation or scene is replayed in the mind over and over, without reaching an outcome (instant replay).
- **All-or-none thinking:** The mind is made up, and no additional facts will be considered (black-and-white thinking with no grays in between).
- **Negative thinking:** The mind is stuck on negative thoughts and blocks worthwhile thinking (emotional sabotage).

---

*Adapted for practical/vocational nurses with permission from Alfaro-Lefevre R. (2006). *Evidence-based critical thinking indicators*, www.alfaroteachsmart.com/.

- **Directed (or focused) thinking:** Purposeful and outcome-oriented.
- **Problem-oriented thinking:** Focus on a particular problem to find a solution (e.g., planning your school, work, and home schedule). This could involve collecting information on school and work schedules and schedules of family members who rely on you. It might include delegating tasks, requesting help, making your goals known, and listening for input from those involved in the immediate situation. Once the schedule is developed, no further attention is given to the situation until another problem emerges (problem solving).
- **Critical thinking:** Critical thinking is an advanced way of thinking, a problem-solving method, and more. It is used to resolve problems and to find ways to improve a situation even when no problem exists. Critical thinking involves collecting and analyzing data to make a decision. It answers questions such as: "How can we do this better?" and "How can we assist the patient in achieving the highest quality outcome; what resources are essential; and which can be eliminated to save costs?"

◎ Try This

Survey of your Current Level of Critical Thinking

Based on a scale of 0 to 10, with 0 as the lowest and 10 as the highest, rate each statement about thinking as it applies to you. Then list the items you rated starting with the lowest rated first.

___ I identify the purpose of my thinking.
___ My thinking is goal (or outcome) directed.
___ I have an organized method of thinking.
___ I question what I do not understand.
___ I continually question: What does this mean? Is this useful? Is it fact?
___ I question the reliability of sources and information available.
___ I keep an open mind.
___ My judgments are based on fact (evidence).

? Critical Thinking

Make a Personal Plan

1. Prioritize the critical-thinking items you need to work on from the previous learning exercise. Choose the items you think are most important to work on first.
2. Make a schedule and estimate the amount of time it will take to see progress. (We all need to work on critical thinking throughout our lives.)
3. Identify how you will determine what progress is being made.

CRITICAL THINKING AND LICENSED PRACTICAL/ LICENSED VOCATIONAL NURSING

Critical thinking involves questioning with meaning. This type of thinking involves examining personal thinking and the thinking of others. Judgments are made on facts (evidence), not assumptions. The critical thinker avoids criticizing just for the sake of having his or her own way. Decisions are based on the right thing to do rather than emotions or a need to save face. New ideas and alternatives are offered in a constructive way. The thinker is willing to consider other ideas and recognizes that there may be more than one right way to do something. The thinker realizes that a perfect solution may not be possible. The thinker realizes that collaboration is a key to effective critical thinking and decision making.

Critical thinking is at its best when you have your brain purposefully engaged; for example, while you listen to a minilecture, view a video, listen to a podcast, participate in a discussion or study group, or are being tutored. A critical thinker is paying attention to what the speaker is saying.

- Do I understand it?
- What does it all mean?
- Where does it all fit in?

You are examining your thinking and the thinking of others. Critical thinking is based on science and scientific principles. The principles include the following:

- Collecting data in an organized way
- Verifying the data in an organized way
- Arranging the data in an organized way; this is often referred to as trending data
- Looking for gaps in information
- Analyzing the data
- Testing it out (Is the data purposeful and outcome/ goal-oriented?)

These scientific principles align with the nursing process, as you will learn in Chapter 12. A major difference for the scientist is that a problem is identified and then data are collected. The nurse, using the nursing process, collects data first and then determines the nature of the problem (Ignatavicius and Workman, 2010). The critical thinker should routinely ask the following questions about the subject of the thinking task at hand (adapted from Alfaro-Lefevre, 2013):

1. What major outcomes (observable beneficial results) do you expect to achieve (e.g., when collaborating with the RN to develop a care plan for a newly admitted patient)?
2. What problems, issues, or risks must be addressed to achieve the major outcome (e.g., the hospital unit you are working on is short staffed)?
3. What is the circumstance or context (e.g., the LPN/ LVN is working in the patient's home and assesses the environment to determine if equipment will need to be improvised)?
4. What knowledge is required (e.g., clinical areas where you had limited clinical experience, such as mental health)?
5. How much room is there for error (e.g., the patient is positioned on his back as directed after surgery and begs to be on his side)?
6. How much time do we have (e.g., the patient who was just admitted is bleeding profusely)?

7. What human and professional resources can help me/us (e.g., the patient is acutely ill and refuses care because of lack of insurance or adequate personal funds)?

8. What perspectives must be considered (e.g., the patient has refused to be examined because of religious beliefs)?

9. What is influencing my thinking (e.g., you are against abortion and do not want to take care of a patient hospitalized because of self-induced abortion)?

10. What must we do to prevent, manage, or eliminate the problems, issues, and risks identified with question 2?

For each element, the thinker (in this case the LPN/LVN) must be able to reflect on the 10 key critical-thinking questions that shed light on the effectiveness of his or her thinking. In other words, is the thinking solving the problem or finding the answer you are looking for? Critical thinking is an essential part of nursing. The overall purpose of nursing is to assist people to stay well or regain their maximum state of health as quickly as possible. Both purposes are to be achieved in a cost-effective manner and in a manner that fits within their culture and their belief system. Nurses make decisions that affect both purposes. Nursing decisions must be accurate and based on evidence. As a nurse, your critical-thinking skill will vary according to your education and clinical experience. Box 5-1 lists suggestions to increase your critical thinking.

| Box 5-1 | Ways to Challenge Yourself to Think Critically |

- Anticipate questions that the patient or instructor might ask
- Ask for clarification of what you do not understand
- Ask yourself if there is more that you can do to improve the patient's outcomes
- Reword in your own words what you have read or been told (e.g., stating a nursing diagnosis as a nursing problem)
- Make comparisons with something similar to help you understand
- Organize information in more than one way to see if you have missed anything important; this is to avoid being impressed when the "facts" fall into place but you have missed the obvious
- Ask your instructor to check out your conclusions
- Strive for objectivity. Keep an open mind and avoid drawing conclusions in advance
- Review all your data again, especially after a period of time; trend the data as appropriate (e.g., how have the patient's vital signs and symptoms changed over time) because they may look different, and you may reach a different conclusion
- Get used to saying, "I don't know, but I will find out"
- Learn from your mistakes, fix them if you can, do not hide an error; someone's life may be at stake, and others can learn from your error
- Think about what you are reading about while you are reading it; ask your instructor or peer to challenge you to think critically while you are on the clinical area

---

WHAT YOU NEED TO THINK CRITICALLY

For the LPN/LVN to think critically, it will be necessary to do the following:

1. Access information.
2. Comprehend (understand) information.
3. Store comprehended information in long-term memory. This includes having strategies to move information to long-term memory.
4. Determine what you know and what you do not know.
5. Recall the comprehended information when needed. (You will need to have the most important information in your head for patient care on clinical.)
6. Know what to do when information is not in long-term memory. Where can you find the information needed?

As an LPN/LVN student, you will be exposed to a great deal of new knowledge during the year in the LPN/LVN program. You will gain knowledge, as stated in the course objectives. Your real test as an LPN/LVN will be your ability to access information, understand that information, recall it, and use it as the basis for critical thinking in the clinical area. Evidence needed to think critically is available in various sources, including the scientific literature and policy and procedure of the institution. Other members of the health care team can be a valuable source to assist in obtaining evidence for decision making.

FACTORS THAT INFLUENCE CRITICAL THINKING

Your current critical-thinking status is influenced by the following personal and situational factors:

- **Upbringing and culture.** Having family and teacher support and opportunities to learn to read well and understand the meaning of what you read; beginning to make simple, limited choices at an early age, which become more complex with consequences as you grow.
- **Motivation.** Whether you learned early to rely on others for motivation or decided you would learn in spite of the lack of external motivators, motivation determines in part the progress you have made in problem solving and critical thinking. You have the ability to think critically if you choose to do so. It is a preference on your part. Remember that the brain is like a muscle: The more you exercise it, the better it works.
- **Attitude influences thinking.** Critical thinkers are humble and recognize that they do not have all the answers and may be influenced by their beliefs and values. While in the process of patient care, it makes a critical difference whether a problem is recognized, missed, or ignored. Take time to collect some data on your **attitude** by completing the learning exercise in the Try This: Attitude Evaluation: My Attitude box.

Try This

Attitude Evaluation: My Attitude

Directions: On a scale of 0 to 10 (with 0 as the worst and 10 as the best), rate your attitude.

7 I am aware of the limitations of my knowledge.

10 I am aware that my dislikes, biases, and prejudices may influence my decisions.

10 I try to be fair-minded.

10 I am interested in understanding other people's thoughts and feelings.

10 I check to find out if my statements are clear.

7 I can be influenced by another person's conclusions, if based on fact.

5 I question other people's sources of information.

7 I acknowledge that what I have been thinking can be incorrect.

1 I question the availability of additional alternatives.

8 I listen to my intuition and compare it with my reasoning.

10 I am aware that perfect solutions are not always available.

10 I am willing to work as a team member.

5 I try to anticipate problems before they occur.

6 I am continually looking for ways to improve my thinking.

These items describe your strong attitudes for the development of critical thinking. The items are attitudes you need to improve to increase critical thinking.

? **Critical Thinking**

Attitudes to Work On

Prioritize the attitudes you choose to work on first to help increase your critical thinking. How will you recognize improvement in each item you listed?

 Try This

Bias

Personal bias can influence your critical thinking. In today's world, much of our bias occurs at the unconscious level but can influence our critical thinking. Psychologists at Harvard developed "Project Implicit" to measure unconscious bias. Go to https://implicit.harvard.edu/implicit/ to determine your unconscious bias. Categories include but are not limited to race, age, gender, and mental health.

ADDITIONAL FACTORS THAT INFLUENCE CRITICAL THINKING

Alfaro-Lefevre (2013) discusses the following personal factors that also influence critical thinking. These are summarized with some additional thoughts for LPNs/LVNs

1. Effective reading
   a. Effective reading, as you have learned, is more than reading with speed.
   b. It means that you are able to identify the significance and potential application of what you are reading.
   c. An effective learning skill means that you are able to organize the data you have so you can access them efficiently.
   d. Chapter 2 provides suggestions to make studying and comprehending information work for you. Remember that employers need more than someone with random-access memory.

2. Maturity
   a. Maturity most often comes with age; however, age does not determine maturity.
   b. Maturity provides past opportunities to have worked through problems. It becomes easier to see problems through someone else's eyes.
   c. Do you work to understand others before expecting them to understand you?

3. Problem solving and the nursing process
   a. Knowledge of problem solving and of the nursing process is based on many of the same principles as critical thinking.
   b. Do you use the problem-solving steps to work out problems now? Understanding and applying the problem-solving steps gives you a head start in thinking critically.

4. Communication skills
   a. Communicating effectively means being aware of the message you are sending verbally, in writing, and through body language. Are you willing to listen and consider ideas and views that are different from your own? Do you express yourself well in writing?

5. Self-confidence
   a. Self-confidence is often the personal characteristic that is the least available to a student.
   b. Without self-confidence, the student is wasting a lot of energy worrying that he or she will not "get it."
   c. It may help to remember that no one can give you self-confidence. You develop self-confidence as you succeed in your endeavors. This is where the saying "Self-confidence is earned, not learned" comes from.
   d. Overconfidence can make people assume they are correct even before data are available to back up what they believe to be correct. Do you acknowledge the limits of your knowledge and skills?

6. Moral development
   a. Moral development creates fair-mindedness, a strong sense of what is right and wrong and just. Have you examined your values, and can you separate them from the values held by others?

7. Capability in nursing
   a. **Capability** in nursing is essential. You must have nursing knowledge and skills to do the work of nursing and know how to access the resources.
   b. Nursing instructors have an enormous amount of factual information that they expect to

introduce to their nursing students. The amount is often overwhelming to both the instructor and the student.

c. Distinguishing what is absolutely necessary to know from what is nice to know is no easy task. The tendency is to hang onto what is fun to know and old information, just in case someone asks or it is in a test somewhere.

d. With the knowledge explosion, instructors are no longer able to infuse their students with all they need to know.

e. Have the tools for locating information and comprehending information, storing information in long-term memory, and recalling the comprehended information when needed. It is essential to evaluate whether or not a source of data (evidence) is reliable.

8. Collaboration

a. A collaborative effort has been shown to promote critical-thinking skills. Interprofessional education occurs in many schools and clinical sites promoting this type of learning. Students can also facilitate this type of learning by presenting the instructor with a well thought out collaborative plan (including observable, project outcomes/goals).

b. Occasionally, students become frustrated when he or she comes to class and discovers that lecturing is not the primary way of teaching. Remember that working in teams can be very beneficial to student learning. Challenging each other's ideas is a core component of critical thinking.

9. Anxiety

a. When anxiety overwhelms, it effectively stops critical thinking.

b. The same is true regarding a high level of fatigue. Adequate rest is essential to critical thinking.

10. Mentors and experience in nursing

a. Work experience and the guidance of nursing mentors, starting with your instructor, will assist you in learning to identify priorities in nursing care.

b. Depending on the work area, patients may be there to seek help for only a few hours or days (emergency or treatment) or for the rest of their life (nursing home).

CRITICAL THINKING AND THE NCLEX-PN®

The NCLEX-PN®, the national licensing examination for LPNs/LVNs, includes items that require various levels of thinking to answer a test item. These various levels are called **cognitive levels**. The cognitive levels used on the NCLEX-PN® examination, based on Bloom's taxonomy, are knowledge, comprehension, application, and analysis. The following definitions will help you understand the meaning of the words *knowledge* (knowing), *comprehension* (understanding), *application*, and *analysis*.

1. **Knowledge** refers to the ability to recall and repeat information you have memorized. *Memorizing is not the same as understanding a concept.* Knowledge is the lowest level of learning. Defining a concept as stated in a dictionary is an example of knowledge level. Knowing a normal lab value is another example.

2. **Comprehension** refers to the ability to basically understand information, recall it, and identify examples of that information. To comprehend is to *grasp the meaning* of the material. Comprehension is the lowest level of understanding. An example of the comprehension level is the ability to repeat information in your own words. This indicates that you understand the information.

3. **Application** means being able to *use learned material in new situations*. For example, you apply what is learned in class to your clinical work. Application involves being able to prioritize or determine what is most important, what comes first. Application is a higher level of understanding. *You must be able to use knowledge to tailor approaches depending on circumstances.* Clinical simulation is used extensively today in nursing education, allowing students to apply theory information in a "safe" setting. Clinical simulation can also involve a higher level of cognition, called analysis. At this level, the student or group of students are challenged to collect data, analyze data, and make collaborative patient care decisions based on evidence.

4. **Analysis** means to be able to *break down complex information into its basic parts* and relate those parts to the whole picture. An example of analysis is the ability to *organize and prioritize* (what is most important, most urgent) two or more pieces of information in a patient situation to *process a safe response*. Analysis is a higher level of application. Being able to identify the most important symptoms that a patient with a specific problem presents, including the initial nursing response, is an example of analysis.

Comprehension, application, and analysis are what employers expect of an LPN/LVN on the job. Your instructors will also expect this level of competence in the clinical area and in clinical simulation as you continue to develop your critical-thinking skills. Some previous students with college degrees have stated that the consistent requirement to apply and analyze both prior and newly learned information is the major point about LP/LV nursing that differs most from their college experience and creates a challenging educational environment.

The review questions for each chapter in this text will include items in multiple choice format, the same as in the NCLEX-PN® examination. These multiple choice items will test you at the knowledge, comprehension, application, and analysis levels. They will help you understand the four cognitive levels and help you prepare for testing. Most important, they will keep your focus on understanding information to be able to continue the development of your critical-thinking skills.

In April 2005, the National Council revised new format items on NCLEX-PN® examinations (first introduced in 2003). Called *alternate format items*, these items may include multiple response, fill-in-the-blank (e.g., calculation, ordered response), and hotspot (e.g., the place on a diagram that answers the question). All format items may have charts, tables, or graphic images. Alternate format items are included at the end of the chapter with review questions. Currently, test items are written at the application level and higher (2014 NCLEX-PN® test plan). You have access to more NCLEX-PN®–type questions in Evolve. Your school may also utilize an NCLEX success product throughout the program. It is essential that you complete all assignments as directed. This enhances your critical thinking and ability to succeed on NCLEX style questions.

Storing information in long-term memory and being able to recall the comprehended information when needed is discussed in Chapter 2. Your effort in this area will make a difference in all of your studies and in being prepared for the NCLEX-PN® examination.

MAKING IT WORK FOR YOU

This is a good time for you to be reminded that we all have special, although different, abilities in the area of thinking. The trick is to discover what those abilities are, embrace them, and make them work for you. You can choose whether or not to make the most of your abilities. However, not deciding is also a decision. There is also the tendency to be impressed by those who begin to speak immediately on an issue as though they have all the facts, when in truth their style of processing is outside of themselves. Perhaps your way is to process internally and not speak out until you have all the words in place. The one who processes externally may ask the questions you wish you had asked. This difference is related to their personality. Their verbalization sounds impressive and tends to frighten the person who processes internally before speaking. Both types can be equally effective in their ability to think critically. Each way is different; a difference in personality is all it has to be unless you allow yourself to begin thinking negatively about your abilities.

WHERE TO GO FROM HERE

This chapter is written as a critical-thinking primer, and it is limited to need-to-know information. The questions and suggestions offered are those that are within the scope of the LPN/LVN and the nursing program. **Reflective (critical) thinking** will assist you in determining if you need outside assistance from your school's study skills center or the instructor in setting up realistic observable goals/outcomes. You may even decide that the awareness of personal and situational characteristics is enough to get you started on your own. The critical-thinking exercises provide you with a practical framework for increasing your critical-thinking ability.

Get Ready for the NCLEX-PN® Examination

Key Points

- Thinking is divided into nonfocused thinking and directed thinking.
- Critical thinking answers the question "How can we do this better?"
- To think critically, it is necessary to access information, comprehend (understand) information, store comprehended information in long-term memory, and recall the comprehended information when needed.
- Comprehension, application, and analysis are what employers will expect from LPNs/LVNs on the job.
- The cognitive levels used in the NCLEX-PN® examination are knowledge, comprehension, application, and analysis. Most questions are written at the application or higher level of cognitive thinking.
- The ability to read with understanding is the cornerstone of critical thinking.
- Both personal and situational factors influence critical thinking.
- The decision is yours whether to use the abilities you already possess to enhance your critical-thinking ability.

Additional Learning Resources

evolve Go to your Evolve website (http://evolve.elsevier.com/Knecht/success) for the following FREE learning resources:
- Answers to Critical Thinking Scenarios
- Additional learning activities
- Additional Review Questions for the NCLEX-PN® exam
- Helpful phrases for communicating in Spanish and more!

Review Questions for the NCLEX-PN® Examination

1. Why did critical thinking become a necessary component of nursing education?
   a. To ensure that all health care team members could speak the same language
   b. To address the new acute disease processes that were emerging in the twenty-first century
   c. To assist the nurse in integrating knowledge (evidence) and skills and technology; resulting in data driven decision making
   d. To align the nurse with other professionals and elevate the nursing profession

2. Which of the following statements is most accurate?
   a. Knowledge is the ability to understand and apply information to a situation.
   b. Knowledge is the ability to explain information in your own words.
   c. Application is the ability to break down information into its component parts.
   d. Application is the ability to apply learned information in a new situation.

3. Which pattern shows the use of critical thinking?
   a. During report, you learned that the new patient is short-tempered. You decide you will humor her, do what is necessary, and give her plenty of space the rest of the time.
   b. Mr. Fodor has to have six small feedings each day, and although he can feed himself, you have decided to increase the intake by sitting on the bed and feeding him.
   c. Mrs. Still is crying when you arrive to give her a bath. She tells you her baby died after birth. You state "Oh, Mrs. Still that was forty years ago. You have 15 healthy grandchildren now."
   d. Charlie was admitted as an emergency admission. You are asked to hold him in position for a spinal tap. You hold him firmly in position and speak softly and reassuringly.

4. A friend of yours is attending an RN program. They state, "Only RNs use critical thinking to assist with decision making." You best response is . . .
   a. The RN is not the only member of the health care team.
   b. The LPN also learns to think in a critical manner, working collaboratively with the RN. A collaborative effort has been shown to promote critical-thinking skills.
   c. Critical thinking is really only done by the physicians.
   d. All members of the health care team, licensed and nonlicensed, are expected to engage in critical thinking as a key aspect of their job description.

Alternate Format Item

1. Which of the following statements support reasons for why the nurse must think in a critical manner? *(Select all that apply.)*
   a. The patient often has multiple diagnoses requiring complex treatment modalities.
   b. The way nursing has always been done is the best it can be for nurses and patients.
   c. Rapid change and information explosion create a need for new learning and skills.
   d. The interdisciplinary team collaborates to develop the best plan of care for the patient.
   e. Evidence is available from multiple sources.

2. If you are going to assist someone in learning to think critically, which statements most describe your planning process? *(Select all that apply.)*
   a. When you feel strongly about a situation, you are usually correct.
   b. Remind yourself that you are not always correct in your analysis.

c. Listen to another opinion even if it contradicts what you believe.
d. Remember that a patient can provide you with subjective information.
e. Collaborate with other health care team members to discuss complex patient diagnoses.

Critical Thinking Scenarios

Scenario 1

Carol, a vocational nursing student, is assigned to Veronica, a patient with the diagnosis of possible depression. The police brought Veronica to the hospital when a neighbor became alarmed by her attempt to cut her wrist. During the past 2 days since Veronica was hospitalized, the staff have seen no behaviors that alarm them. Veronica has showered every morning, fixed her hair, put on makeup, and wears nice clothes brought in by her family. Whenever the staff check on her at night, she appears to be sleeping. She eats modest portions of food at mealtimes and says she wants to keep her weight where it is. She greets staff with a smile and inquires what she can do to be of help.

Today, Veronica will go to court (which is held in the hospital) to determine if she will be committed for care. Carol will accompany her. What is troubling Carol is that Veronica swore her to secrecy and then told her she was using all effort to "hold it together" so she will be discharged after court. Once she gets home, she will kill herself, and this time she has a plan that is "foolproof." Carol feels torn between her promise of secrecy and her concern that Veronica will follow through with her plan for suicide.

As Carol sits in court and listens to Veronica tell her story, what critical-thinking steps will help her reach a decision of what to do?

1. Analyze the situation. Provide a rationale for what she is thinking.
2. Identify all possible alternatives. What is the rationale for each of the alternatives?
3. Choose the best alternative and provide the rationale.

Scenario 2

The correctional institution in your community has just begun hiring LPNs. You interviewed and were offered the job. As a new LPN, you are excited about this opportunity; however, you became concerned when you found out that you are the only nurse in the prison on night shift.

1. Identify what data you will collect to assist you in determining your best next steps.
2. Analyze the situation.
3. Discuss your options with a peer.
4. How would you proceed?

Ethics Applied to Nursing: Personal Versus Professional Ethics

Objectives

On completing this chapter, you will be able to do the following:

1. List four current ethical issues of concern in twenty-first century health care.
2. Explain the differences among ethics, morals, and values.
3. Differentiate between personal and professional ethics.
4. Identify ethical elements in your state's Nurse Practice Act.
5. Describe how the role of nursing has changed since the introduction of the nursing process and critical thinking into nursing curricula.
6. Discuss how nonmaleficence is more complex than the definition of "do no harm."
7. Differentiate between beneficence and paternal beneficence.
8. Explain the steps for an autonomous decision.
9. Describe how fidelity affects nursing care.
10. Discuss how a nurse applies the principle of justice to nursing.
11. Differentiate between ethical and legal responsibilities in nursing.

Key Terms

autonomy (Ăw-TŎN-ŏ-mē)
beneficence (bĕ-NĔF-ĭ-sĕns)
beneficent paternalism (bĕ-NĔF-ĭ-sĕnt-pă-TŬR-nă-lĭz-ŭm)
ethics (ĕ-THIKS)
fidelity (fĭ-DĔL-ĭ-t ē)
justice (JŬS-tĭs)

morals (MŎR-ăls)
nonmaleficence (nŏn-mă-LĔF-ĭ-sĕns)
nursing ethics (NŬR-sĭng ĕ-THIKS)
personal ethics (PĔR-sŭn-ăl ĕ-THIKS)
privacy (PRĪ-vă-sē)
values (VĂL-ū)

Keep in Mind

Nurses are challenged daily to make decisions in situations that are complex; ethical dilemmas complicate many scenarios.

Ed and Susan share with their clinical instructor a concern regarding a conversation they overheard while caring for their patient at the nursing home earlier in the week. Their patient's son, accompanied by his friend, had arrived to visit. The son was trying to convince their patient to sign a new will. The patient was asking questions, and her son stated, "Just sign right on the line, Mom, everything will be okay. Trust me." The students stated that the patient seemed very uncomfortable but did sign the will. They had not said anything to the staff, as they thought they were respecting the patient's autonomy. Thus they did not think it was their concern. However, after completing their reading for their ethics class today, they believe they may have made a mistake and should have reported this event. Their instructor indicates that this is an important issue, and she will notify the nursing home. She thanks the students for reporting their concern and directs them to report any ethical issues immediately in the future.

As you read this chapter, think about all of the ethical issues that can face a nurse on a daily basis.

The twenty-first century presents numerous ethical issues in health care, as reflected in agency policies and medical procedures that create life, prolong life, cure chronic diseases, ensure a peaceful death, and end life. Additional ethical issues will arise as scientific research continues to explore possibilities, the procedures are discussed, and, if procedures are legalized, people press for their right to make autonomous decisions. Students in practical/vocational nursing classes identified the following current ethical issues in health care: in vitro fertilization, artificial insemination, surrogate motherhood, cloning, organ donation (including cadaver donations), child organ donors, procedures that use fetal tissues (stem cells) or organs from aborted fetuses, conceiving a child to produce tissue for a sibling, abortion, experiments that destroy a human embryo, euthanasia, assisted suicide, advance directives (including living wills and durable power of attorney), and insertion and/or withdrawal of feeding tubes.

A clinical example of an ethical issue follows: A patient has verbalized to the physician the wish to avoid further heroic means to stay alive. Two adult children have arrived and insist that all means be used to maintain life, but the three children already at the bedside do not agree. The patient lacks a living will and durable power of attorney and is unconscious at this point.

You will encounter similar scenarios as a student participating in a clinical assignment. These learning experiences are instrumental to provide time for self-discovery, self-reflection, and self-analysis. Understanding your own ethics is a first step in providing unbiased ethical care to your patients.

> **? Critical Thinking**
>
> Where do nurses get their ethics and morals in terms of self-analysis?

DESCRIPTION AND SCOPE OF ETHICS

Ethics is a system of standards or moral principles that direct actions as being right or wrong. Ethics is concerned with the meaning of words such as *right, wrong, good, bad, ought,* and *duty.* Ethics is concerned with the ways people, either individually or as a group, decide the following:

- What actions are right or wrong
- If one *ought* to do something
- If one has the *right* to do something
- If one has the *duty* to do something

This basic definition is somewhat of an oversimplification. Ethics sounds like the words *morals* and *values,* but there are differences among them.

> **? Critical Thinking**
>
> How does the nurse avoid imposing his or her morals and ethics in a working situation?

MORALS AND VALUES

Morals are concerned with dealing with right or wrong behavior (conduct) and character. The terms *ethics* and *morals* are difficult to define separately. *Morals* comes from a Latin root, and *ethics* comes from a Greek root. Both words mean "customs" or "habits" and refer to the general area of rights and wrongs. The words are often substituted for each other. *Ethics* and *morals* are used in the same way in this chapter.

Values involve the *worth* you assign to an idea or an action. Values are freely chosen and are affected by age, experience, and maturity. A child usually embraces family values during childhood. The teen years are a time of trying out family values and either incorporating them or rejecting and replacing them with new values. Values continue to be modified throughout your lifetime as you acquire new knowledge and experience. Based on changes in values, one's code of ethics/morals can shift (e.g., organ transplants after you have learned about or cared for a patient who receives a transplant).

Law is thought of as a minimum ethic that is written and enforced. As a licensed practical nurse/licensed vocational nurse (LPN/LVN), the Nurse Practice Act in your state is your final authority on what you are legally obligated to do as a nurse regardless of where you are employed (see Chapter 7 for more about nursing and the law). It is essential to have a thorough knowledge of the Nurse Practice Act in the state in which you are employed.

COMPARISON OF LEGAL ASPECTS OF NURSING AND ETHICS

Nursing ethics are similar to, but also different from, the legal aspects that regulate your nursing practice. Table 6-1 presents a comparison of legal aspects and nursing ethics.

NURSING ETHICS

According to the *Miller-Keane Encyclopedia & Dictionary of Medicine, Nursing & Allied Health,* nursing ethics is described as "the values and ethical principles governing nursing practice, conduct, and relationships." Nursing ethics deals with the relationship of a nurse to the

Table 6-1	Comparison of Legal Aspects and Nursing Ethics	
	LEGAL ASPECTS	**NURSING ETHICS**
Definition	The state statutes that apply to licensed persons and the situations in patient care that could result in legal action	Set of rules of conduct (moral and practical) that guide decision making
Focus	Rules and regulations Obligations under the law Safe care	Ideal behavior of a group of licensed people Morality Higher standards
Applies to	Member of a professional/career group	Member of a nursing group
Participation	Mandatory	Voluntary but expected
Source	Your state's Nurse Practice Act	NFLPN and NAPNES codes, Florence Nightingale Pledge, PN Pledge

NAPNES, National Association for Practical Nurse Education and Service; *NFLPN,* National Federation of Licensed Practical Nurses; *PN,* practical nurse.

patient, the patient's family, associates and fellow nurses, and society at large. Nursing ethics attempts to look for underlying patterns or order in a large number of ethical decisions and practices of nurses, individually or as a group. Codes provide a guideline for what the LPN/LVN ought to do. However, codes do not carry the weight of law. It is interesting to note how many ethical items are actually found in the law, such as your Nurse Practice Act. When ethical items are included in a legal document, it places emphasis on the importance of these items. It also gives the LPN/LVN a source to fall back on to defend the choices in behavior they make in regard to patients and families; it is then a matter of law. Mosby Medical Dictionary (2012) describes ethics as "the science or study of moral values or principles, including the ideals of autonomy, beneficence, and justice." A discussion of all of these terms follows.

ETHICAL CODES OF THE NATIONAL ASSOCIATION FOR PRACTICAL NURSE EDUCATION AND SERVICE AND NATIONAL FEDERATION OF LICENSED PRACTICAL NURSES

Ethics that are adopted by nursing groups are in their codes of behavior. Both the National Association for Practical Nurse Education and Service (NAPNES) and the National Federation of Licensed Practical Nurses (NFLPN) have ethical codes for LPN/LVNs.

Try This

Ethical Issues and Your Nurse Practice Act

Discover how your state includes ethical issues (what you ought to do as an LPN/LVN) in the law, which is your Nurse Practice Act (what you must do as a licensed person).

- Read the ethical codes of the NAPNES (www.napnes.org) and NFLPN (www.nflpn.org).
- Use the NFLPN code as an example.
- Search for the elements of this ethical code in your Nurse Practice Act. Fill out the following worksheet.
- Summarize the ethical elements found in the Nurse Practice Act.

Ethical Area	Is this Ethical Area Addressed in your State's Nurse Practice Act?	If "Yes," Cite Section
1. Know and understand the scope of maximum utilization of the LPN/LVN, as specified by the Nurse Practice Act, and function within this scope.		
2. Safeguard the confidential information acquired from any source about the patient.		

Ethical Area	Is this Ethical Area Addressed in your State's Nurse Practice Act?	If "Yes," Cite Section
3. Provide health care to all patients, regardless of race, creed, cultural background, disease, or lifestyle (e.g., single parent, sexual orientation).		
4. Refuse to give endorsement to the sale or promotion of commercial products or services.		
5. Uphold the highest standards in personal appearance, language, dress, and demeanor.		
6. Adhere to a community standard of justice, honesty, and good morals.		
7. Stay informed about issues affecting the practice of nursing and the delivery of health care, and, where appropriate, participate in government and policy decisions.		
8. Accept the responsibility for safe nursing practice by keeping mentally and physically fit and educationally prepared to practice.		
9. Strive to deliver the highest quality of care keeping current with best practices and the use of information technology.		
10. Accept the responsibility for membership in NFLPN or the LPN/LVN organization of your choice, and participate in its efforts to maintain the established standards of nursing practice and employment policies that lead to quality patient care.		

YOUR PERSONAL CODE OF ETHICS

Practical/vocational nursing students and LPNs/LVNs also have **personal ethics** that provide personal guidelines for living. You ultimately chose what your personal code of ethics includes. Your personal code of ethics will influence your nursing ethics. Sometimes personal ethics conflict with the law (state's Nurse Practice Act). When this occurs, you have an obligation to follow the law. If you object to a medical procedure on religious or moral grounds, discuss this concern during the interview process. This objection may be incompatible with the job description and the mission and beliefs of the institution. In this case, you are not the right "fit" for the job. However, if an institution initiates a new procedure/service during your employment period that challenges your religious or moral beliefs, discuss and submit in writing your objections. Present the statement to your employer, including a possible solution to the issue. For example, you may be ethically opposed to abortion. Abortion in the United States is permitted under certain circumstances. You may ethically wish to refuse to assist with the abortion procedure. Proactively creating a plan may prevent an ethical dilemma for you. However, you cannot refuse to give nursing care if needed. Abandonment is a legal matter, and maintaining your license may be at risk. The best strategy is to seek employment in a health agency that does not participate in procedures or nursing care of which you do not ethically approve.

Some nurses have tried to opt out of caring for patients who have an illness that may be related to a lifestyle of which they do not approve. A nurse needs to separate personal ethics from nursing ethics. You are legally expected to care for a patient regardless of his or her lifestyle. For example, when caring for a patient with acquired immune deficiency syndrome (AIDS), use proper technique during care as you would with any patient with an infectious disease. You may not refuse to care for this patient. Ethically and legally this patient must receive the same level of care, with dignity and respect that other patients do. *Nursing is not about giving care selectively to those patients you approve of and refusing care to others you see as less deserving.*

[?] Critical Thinking

Personal Values

Write down your personal value system regarding health and illness. To get started, think about your family's value system. Be concerned with content, not form. What you write will be an ethical code in progress. You may want to add or subtract statements after you have completed this chapter. It will also be a code you can modify as your experience with patients increases.

ROOTS OF NURSING ETHICS

Years ago, nurses saw themselves as doers, not thinkers. Nurses worked only to serve the physicians' wishes. Before the nursing process and critical thinking were added to nursing curricula, those in the nursing profession did not see themselves as having something separate to contribute to patient care (in addition to the nurses' dependent role to physicians). Nursing ethics was primarily a modification of medical ethics and ethics of other professions at that time.

WHAT CHANGED?

Nursing education was initially disease oriented. Nursing textbooks focused on the disease process, including cause, signs, symptoms, treatment, prognosis, and nursing care related to the treatment. Physicians did the medical assessment and wrote orders for the nurse to carry out. The nurse reported on patient progress, based on physicians' orders. Nursing assessments did not exist. Additional concerns the patient might have had (e.g., spiritual, cultural, emotional, sexual) were not routinely assessed and addressed. Patients were expected to follow physicians' orders without question. The nurse's job was to see that the orders were carried out. The early nursing role was limited to the dependent relationship with the physician.

As nursing theories emerged, so did the nursing process and critical thinking, and nursing textbooks began to include these topics. Nurses discovered that in addition to their dependent role to physicians, they had something special to contribute to the patient. Finally, it was understood that the patient was a person, not just a disease. With the help of the nursing process, nurses had a way to identify additional needs that could be responded to through nursing care. Rather than expecting patients to blindly follow orders because "we know what is wrong with you and we can fix it" (benevolent paternalism), patients were encouraged to be an active part in planning and implementing their own nursing care plan (support of patient **autonomy**). Today, the availability of evidence based resources on the Internet has contributed to patient autonomy.

Despite what we observe today, changes in nursing did not happen easily. Many nurses were entrenched in their dependent role to physicians, and they believed that nursing was being ruined by the changes that were taking place. Nursing textbooks and curricula, however, both had to change to reflect the nursing process, critical thinking, and a focus on the total patient (not just the physically diseased or injured portion of the patient). Adding the nursing process and critical thinking changed the nursing role and changed nursing philosophy. Nurses, both LPNs/LVNs and registered nurses (RNs), are not just "doers" but also "thinkers." The nursing process and critical thinking empowered nurses. This in turn influenced a change in nursing ethics.

Ethical principles in this chapter are about application of nursing ethics to nursing decisions and action. You are encouraged to look at both sides of an ethical principle. Recognize that no principle applies in the same way to all patients and their unique situation. No principle is absolute.

Critical thinking (see Chapter 5) plays a major role in sorting out ethical choices and legal responsibilities in regard to the patient. The patient's knowledge of choices regarding care also affects ethical decision making.

ETHICAL DECISIONS IN HEALTH CARE

ETHICS COMMITTEES

Health agencies such as hospitals, hospice units, and long-term care settings have an ethics committee. This multidisciplinary team (e.g., nurses, physicians, clergy, social worker, and other allied health members) assists with difficult ethical decisions. Usually the discussions relate to new or unusual ethical questions. The recommendations of the ethics committee are expected to be given serious consideration by all stakeholders. In a faith-based organization, the principles of the faith can be anticipated to impact the decision making of this committee. However, if you think the ethics committee makes all the medical ethical decisions, you are only partially right. Patients arrive with their culture-based and/or religion-based ethics, which were often established long before they were born. What the person can and cannot do in regard to health care has already been established by the culture of which they are a part. See Chapters 10 and 11 for a discussion of cultural and spiritual needs, spiritual caring, and religious differences.

WESTERN SECULAR BELIEF SYSTEM

In the Western secular belief system, the emphasis is shifted from duties to the rights of the individual. This system has the following characteristics:
1. *Individual autonomy* means "self-rule." Individuals have the capacity to think and, based on these thoughts, to make the decision freely whether or not to seek health care (the freedom to choose).
2. *Individual rights* mean the ability to assert one's rights. The extent to which a patient can exert his or her rights is restricted (i.e., their rights cannot restrict the rights of others). For example, the patient's right to refuse treatment can be at odds with the health professional's perceived duty to always act in a way that will benefit the patient (do good and prevent harm). The individual's right has become a central theme of health care:
   a. Right to consent to care
   b. Right to choose between alternative treatments
   c. Right to consent or refuse treatment
   d. Women's rights over their own bodies
Numerous bills of rights have been written, and fierce debates have taken place at both state and national levels. The question of individual autonomy and individual rights is far from being settled. At the time of this writing, some laws based on individual autonomy and rights have been passed (e.g., Health Care Reform; Oregon, Washington, and Montana assisted suicide laws). However, attempts to rescind laws that have been passed continue. The question is, to what extent do one's individual moral decisions (rights) get in the way of another's moral autonomy?

Personal Beliefs That May Affect Medical Decisions

What cultural or religious values do you hold that may affect personal health care decisions?

Discuss with your significant other, family, coworkers, and peers your response. Reflect on how your discussion varied. Next, project to the future: Given the diverse patient populations you will encounter as a student and as an LPN/LVN, how often will you encounter personal beliefs that differ from your own? Think about how you will respect the patient's autonomy in these situations.

ETHICAL RESPONSIBILITIES OF NURSES

As the nurse's role has evolved from being simply a "doer" to being also a "thinker," it is logical that the number of ethical issues has also increased. Adding the nursing process and critical thinking to nursing curricula changed the nursing focus to the whole patient. Although the interdependent role to the health care team remains, responsibilities that are unique to nursing were added. The following responsibilities, both ethical and legal, emerged:
1. *Patient advocacy:* Patient advocacy is a key role of all nurses. Patients are often in a vulnerable state when they are in need of nursing care; vulnerable because of the symptoms of the illness and vulnerable because of the complexity of health care delivery. As a result, their need for advocacy often increases. Knowledge is power. Thus informing the patient of the plan of care is essential. This needs to be done at least every shift and more often if indicated by the patient's condition. Information, as simple as explaining the steps of a procedure, will empower patients. You also need to include a brief overview of the role of all the members of the health care team in the plan of care. At times, you may need to advocate ensuring the plan of care is not altered inappropriately because of an error or misjudgment. Advocacy is usually done in collaboration with the RN. Fully understand your advocacy role. In most states, the LPN/LVN's role is to support teaching done by the RN, physician, or other members of the health care team. If the patient has questions, and you are unsure about whether you should provide an answer, discuss with the RN your next steps. When the patient does make a decision, be supportive even though you might not agree with the decision. It is your job to ensure that the patient has enough knowledge and resources (evidence) to make an informed decision. If not, seek out the resources needed and provide them to the patient.
2. *Accountability:* The word *accountability* means that you are answerable to yourself, to your assigned patient and their family, to your supervisor, the health care team, and to your instructor who evaluates your work. As an LPN/LVN, accountability to

the instructor is replaced by accountability to the employing agency. You are held accountable for all the nursing actions that you perform or are assigned to perform. The measures of accountability are the nursing standards of practice; that is, what a nurse with your education and experience would do in a similar situation.

3. *Colleague reporting:* Report peers, supervisors, or any team members for behaviors that are potentially harmful to patients (e.g., impaired at work because of alcohol and/or other drug use, stealing patient's medication, substituting water or normal saline for injectable narcotics, leaving unstable patients unattended in the shower, sleeping while on duty, and verbal or physical abuse).

4. *System based issues:* Identifying system based issues is essential to providing safe high quality care (e.g., if new procedures are implemented without appropriate education and training on all shifts, you need to notify administration and suggest a plan to ensure safe practice).

PRINCIPLES OF ETHICS

As a nurse of the twenty-first century, you recognize there is something unique that a nurse has to offer patients beyond the dependent role to physicians. This realization places greater responsibility on student practical nurses/student vocational nurses (SPNs/SVNs) to learn all they can during the nursing program of study. For example, now you can add knowledge of basic ethics to critical thinking as you assist the RN with the nursing process. The data you collect will have an added dimension of ethics. It will make a difference in developing a quality care plan that considers the patient as a whole person and not just the part of his or her body that is sick.

At this level, you incorporate a basic understanding of how SPNs/SVNs and LPNs/LVNs practice nursing according to nursing codes. Learning about ethics is more than being able to recite the definition to pass a test; it means being able to help make ethical decisions when ethical dilemmas arise.

The following ethical principles are discussed in this chapter:

1. Nonmaleficence (do no harm)
2. Beneficence (do good)
3. Autonomy (free to choose)
4. Fidelity (be true)
5. Justice (fair to all)

NONMALEFICENCE (DO NO HARM)

In her book *Leadership and Management According to Florence Nightingale*, Nightingale said the following:

> *"It may seem a strange principle to enunciate as the very first requirement in a hospital that it should do the sick no harm. It is quite necessary nevertheless to lay down such a principle."*

Nightingale is referring to the ethical principle **nonmaleficence**, which comes from the Latin *primum non nocere*, meaning "first do no harm." Nonmaleficence is the basis of many of the "rules" promoted by your instructors, such as the following:

- Six rights for giving medications
- Use of SBAR (Situation Background Assessment Recommendation) in collaboration with the RN for interdisciplinary communication
- Checking the temperature of bath or shower water
- Checking the temperature of formula before feeding the patient
- Returning the bed to its lowest position after completing a treatment or preparing to leave the room
- Raising side rails after nursing care if it is in the plan of care
- Providing care for your patients when their ethical principles conflict with yours
- Performing only necessary procedures on patients, instead of unnecessary procedures just to gain additional experience
- Protecting those who cannot protect themselves; for example, mentally challenged, unconscious, weak, or debilitated patients

If the principle of nonmaleficence is taken to the extreme, however, SPNs/SVNs and LPNs/LVNs would not be able to perform many nursing duties. Few beneficial treatments are entirely without harm, including the following:

- Anytime you puncture the patient's skin with a needle, there is some tissue damage, a risk of infection, and the possibility of an untoward reaction to a solution if administered.
- All drugs have side effects: rare, serious, and not so serious.
- Anytime you put a tube into a bodily opening (e.g., catheterization, irrigating a colostomy), there is some trauma to surrounding tissue. There is the possibility of introducing infection and penetrating the tissue wall.
- Many procedures hurt physically in the process of performing them (e.g., positioning a patient properly after surgery, cleansing the mouth of an elderly patient who has not had proper mouth care for a period, irrigating a pressure ulcer, moving a patient with osteoporosis from bed to chair to toilet and back).
- Giving a vaccination carries the risk of the patient experiencing a side effect, but the overall effect for most people is the prevention of serious diseases.
- When you monitor an intravenous (IV) line, one thing to check is that the solution and additive, if any, are infusing, as compared with what the physician ordered. A common additive is KCl (potassium chloride). KCl within a narrow blood level range is necessary for proper heart functioning. If too little or too much is administered, it can result in heart dysfunction, sometimes resulting in death. (Jack Kevorkian, a physician who participated in several

assisted suicides, used KCl.) KCl can save lives, but it can also kill.

- Performing range of motion after a stroke can elicit some discomfort because of stiff and slightly contracted muscles.

Each of the preceding procedures has the potential for doing good and doing harm. The question always is how to do the least amount of harm when doing something that is expected to result in good. The obvious answer is to never knowingly participate in any action that will deliberately harm the patient. The patient must also have agreed to the procedure verbally or in writing, depending on the procedure (autonomy). This is a reason for practicing procedures in the nursing lab; preparing for nursing care; reviewing your nursing care plan with the instructor; and reviewing action, side effects, and dosage with the instructor before giving a medication.

The following are negative examples of nursing actions that were meant to do no harm but resulted in injury:

- Putting down a patient's side rail without first checking that the patient's arm is not hanging between the rail and the bed. The patient who immediately comes to mind is a woman in her eighties whose arm was fractured and who received several skin tears and bruises. The staff person who put the rail down was irritated because of "a bad night shift" and was hurrying to get off duty.
- Rapidly feeding large spoonfuls of food to a patient who has a dry mouth as a side effect of medication. Because of the lack of liquid before beginning to eat, large spoonfuls of food, lack of adequate time to chew, and lack of additional liquid before the next bite, the patient aspirated some of the food that accumulated in his mouth. The patient survived but refused future attempts to eat when he saw the same nurse come in with his food tray.
- Applying an external (Texas) catheter (condom like catheter applied to male's penis) incorrectly causing constriction of circulation resulting in gangrene of the penis. The patient's penis required amputation.

▣ Try This

Procedures and Their Effects

Think about procedures with which you are familiar. Review the procedure. List two procedures that "do good" but also have the potential to do harm. State both the good and potential harmful effects of each procedure.

BENEFICENCE (DO GOOD)

Beneficence means to "do good" with your nursing actions and is the basis of trust in nursing. It also involves preventing harm and removing harm. You have read how nonmaleficence and beneficence are often difficult to separate and may go hand in hand.

The following major nursing duties to the patient are associated with beneficence:

1. Put the patient's interests first; for example:
   - You do not go off duty until you hand over the care of the patient to equally skilled nursing staff to continue the nursing care. You are obligated to report to the nurse taking over the next shift what has transpired during the time you have been responsible for nursing care. This includes a situation such as: You receive an emergency phone call regarding a sick child and leave abruptly. This would be viewed as patient abandonment. You must always ensure that the patient receives adequate nursing care in your absence. Reporting off to a colleague who is capable/competent of receiving the assignment is essential.
   - If you give the wrong medication, report it as soon as you recognize the error. Your ethical concern is to "do good" and "prevent harm." Beneficence is a greater good than concern for self in regard to the error. In addition, your individual error may be related to a system error. Prompt reporting and investigation can minimize a similar event from occurring in the future.
   - You go to work even though you are tempted to call in sick because you want to go out of town for the weekend.

2. *Place the good of patients before your needs.* This is where interpretation of duty gets more complex. Does this mean that duty to the patient means utmost sacrifice? No, it does not, but it does mean that you sacrifice something. Here are some examples:
   - Patient needs are above organizational needs. You may have administrative responsibility (perhaps as a charge nurse) that must be completed by the end of the day or meetings you are expected to attend that day. If a patient needs your skill and expertise, as in an emergency situation, your first duty is to the patient.
   - Placing the good of patients before your needs does *not* mean that you behave as though no one in the world can assume the nursing care you give to a patient. Do not stay past your scheduled hours when there is someone ready to assume responsibility for nursing care. This also means that you do not call the patient from home, accept calls in your home from the patient, or visit the patient after hours. If you are doing any of this, you have just entered an unhealthy codependent relationship with the patient. These behaviors are usually prohibited by your employer.

❓ Critical Thinking

Ethical Obligations

When a patient is demanding, angry, or uncooperative and threatens to become violent, is the nurse obligated to put herself or himself in danger of serious harm? Are nurses ethically obligated to perform heroic acts of self-sacrifice?

Volunteer (pro bono) work is a professional obligation of beneficence for nurses. For example, a nurse may decide to volunteer some hours a week at a free clinic or children's center.

AUTONOMY (FREE TO CHOOSE)

Potter, Perry, and Stockert (2015) describe autonomy as respecting a patient's independence and right to determine a course of action. However, autonomy does not mean that patients can do whatever they want. Autonomy means the following:
- *Thinking* through all the facts
- *Deciding* on the basis of an independent thinking process
- *Acting* based on a personal decision
- *Undertaking a decision voluntarily* without pressure, direct or subtle, from anyone else

Rumbold (2002) states the following:

> *"Autonomy does not mean freedom to do as one wants or to act in accordance with one's desires. Autonomous action is based on rational thought or reason. It embodies the notion of freedom and liberty, but only within the constraints of reason."*

We expect people to respect our rights, and we respect their rights as long as their rights do not interfere with someone else's rights.

For patients to make an autonomous decision, they must have all the facts without leaving out information to influence the decision in a particular way. For example, the nurse may unintentionally (sometimes intentionally) influence the patient's decision by repeating what the physician has suggested is best for the patient ("The doctor would not have suggested the treatment if he/she did not think it best for you").

There is also a fine line between autonomy and abandonment. Excessive control means interfering too much in a patient's life. Not interfering enough results in neglect of the patient. Here are some examples:
- The right of the elderly to make decisions about their treatment
- A patient's right to be left alone or not treated

More information is needed in both situations to determine if more or less interference is recommended.

Role of Privacy in Autonomy

Privacy is both an ethical and a legal issue. Autonomy includes a patient's right to privacy. This is the reason your instructor asks a patient directly for permission to allow SPNs/SVNs to observe a particular treatment or to do a procedure. Similarly, the instructor checks with the patient before assigning a student to give nursing care. The patient has the right to refuse care from a student nurse. Privacy includes the right to choose care based on personal beliefs, feelings, or attitudes. It includes the patient's right to decide what is done to their body (accepting or rejecting treatment or exposure of the body). As an SPN/SVN, you respect the patient's

decision. When giving care, avoid exposing the patient needlessly in the course of care. *This is an invasion of privacy.*

Role of Culture, Religion, and Personal Values in Autonomy

Culture or a religion-based belief system may be contrary to the accepted medical ethics. Examples of decisions based on religion and culture include the following:
- The patient, a Jehovah's Witness, could benefit from a blood transfusion for severe blood loss. The adult patient has refused because a blood transfusion is forbidden by his religion (religion based).
- The patient, an underage child, parents forbade the blood transfusion on religious grounds. The physician might decide to go to court to ask the court to overrule the parents' decision. The physician can do this because parents cannot give *informed consent* for the treatment of underage children. An underage child is too young to understand all the facts to make a decision required for informed consent. Parents can *authorize treatment* for what is appropriate for their children up to a certain age. In this case the physician has decided that the value of beneficence is greater than the value of respect for the parents' autonomy. The court is the greater authority and will decide if the physician can transfuse the child.
- The patient, a young woman, is diagnosed with breast cancer. Her husband has received a complete explanation from the physician about her illness, alternatives for each treatment, anticipated effects, possible side effects, and prognosis with each treatment. Her husband will not permit any treatment to take place (culture based).

The patient's personal values may also be opposed to accepted medical ethics. The following is an example of a personal value-based decision:
- A man in his late sixties is diagnosed with advanced cancer of the colon. He has refused to have treatment, even though he understands that although not curative, the surgery could result in less discomfort for a period and more time to live (personal value based).

FIDELITY (BE TRUE)

Fidelity challenges each practical/vocational nurse to be faithful to the charge of acting in the patient's best interest when the capacity to make free choice is no longer available to the patient. This does not include rescuing behaviors and becoming paternalistic in making decisions for vulnerable patients (legal competency will be described in Chapter 7). As a nurse, you must *differentiate* between your feelings and choices regarding an issue and the feelings and wishes of the patient. These points are foremost in making a decision. Charting the patient's feelings and wishes as expressed, without your personal interpretation, provides information for the physician when important decisions need to be considered. Examples of breaching fidelity include the following:

- Discussing a patient in a public area such as the cafeteria, an elevator, at home, or when you are out with friends. Never mention a patient by name. In doing so, fidelity and confidentiality (a legal term) would both be compromised, as would the patient's dignity. The action says the patient has limited worth in the eyes of the nurse and chips away at the patient's dignity.
- You overhear LPNs/LVNs speaking disrespectfully about an obese patient and complaining about how difficult it is to move her. What will you do in response to this discussion? Explain why you will take the action you have chosen. Is it an ethical response?
- A student practical nurse shared a personal experience that sharpened her awareness of the meaning of fidelity. During her first day of the mental health rotation, she saw her neighbor, now a patient, in the day room. The SPN's husband worked with the patient. One day the patient did not come to work. The boss offered no information about what happened. Being a close-knit neighborhood, the SPN's husband, other workers, and neighbors speculated with great concern about the missing worker. Seeing him on the psychiatric unit was a shock, and the SPN did not know how to approach him. The SPN asked her instructor for assistance. The instructor suggested that the SPN approach the patient and let him know that she recognized him but reassure him that she would not tell anyone he was hospitalized. The SPN was also to tell the patient that not telling anyone outside of the hospital was part of her nursing education and duty. She must abide by the Health Insurance Portability and Accountability Act (HIPAA) guidelines. That took care of the discomfort for both the SPN and the patient regarding his hospitalization. The class after the clinical day was about fidelity and confidentiality (a legal concern). The SPN was sure she would never breach her promise not to talk about patients, except to the health care team and her instructor. That evening at dinner with her husband, she decided he should know because of his concern for his coworker. The SPN made her husband promise not to tell anyone about the patient, and the husband agreed. Later that evening, while they were grocery shopping, the SPN was in another aisle, and she heard her husband say to someone, "My wife ran into Joe at the psych hospital this morning. He's a patient, but don't tell anyone." The SPN breached confidentiality, an ethical and legal matter. She also started a chain reaction of "I'll tell you, but you can't tell anyone." This constituted both an ethical and legal breach of confidentiality. The patient's best interest (fidelity) was not served. You alone make the decisions regarding what you do when you are away from the clinical area and the

immediate support and supervision of the instructor. In a sense, fidelity sits on your shoulder, to ignore or to embrace. To ignore creates an ethical dilemma and a potential legal consequence. Dismissal from school or termination from a job can be the end result.

JUSTICE (FAIR TO ALL)

Justice means that SPNs/SVNs and LPNs/LVNs must deliver fair and equal treatment to all patients, recognizing and avoiding personal bias. For example, each patient with the same diagnosis should receive the same level of care. Being fair does not mean giving every patient the same things. It means treating them all the same (i.e., with dignity and respect). As a nurse, you make daily decisions to provide the highest quality of care possible. Personal bias can cloud our vision as nurses. Identifying hidden bias can assist the LPN/LVN in providing justice to all patients. For example, say the patients on your floor in the hospital represent different levels of wealth, social status, culture, religion, and moral and value systems, but all of them are acutely ill. The newest patient has Kaposi sarcoma, a defining component of AIDS. Do you classify AIDS as a life-threatening illness or as a retribution for behaviors you consider immoral? If your personal ethics interfere with the care you give, you may find yourself giving this patient more time than needed and doing less than needed for other acutely ill patients or providing minimal care for the patient and lavishing attention on those who "deserve the care."

Consider a young, single mother who has five children and just found out she is pregnant. How you proceed can be impacted by a personal bias, assuming that she should have prevented this pregnancy. All patients must be treated equally. This is your ethical duty.

It is within your power to make decisions about daily issues related to justice. Be careful to hear hidden bias within yourself: "He's so young; so much living left to do"; "She's had a full life already"; "She's an alcoholic; never took care of her kids;" and so on. Identifying a bias will assist you in providing "just" care. Visit the following web site to identify your hidden biases: https://implicit.harvard.edu/implicit/

[?] Critical Thinking

At the end of your next clinical day, take time to reflect on your reaction to patients and how it affected your patient care. Did the word *deserve* enter into your thoughts, or did you provide justice for all? Listen to the health care team. Did you hear any comments that would make you question if the quality of justice was met? If so, what did you do?

As an SPN/SVN, you report patients' comments regarding ethical matters to the RN. Final ethical decisions are not within the LPN/LVN scope of nursing practice. Recall also that ethics is what you *ought* to do; law is what you *have* to do.

ROLE OF BENEFICENT PATERNALISM

We are including beneficent paternalism because it continues to be confused with the ethic of beneficence (do no harm). **Beneficent paternalism** is a disrespectful *attitude* toward the patient and what the patient has to contribute to personal care and recovery. It is an "I know what's best for you" attitude that discounts the patient's knowledge of self. The following are examples of beneficent paternalism:

- When assisting to collect data, really *hear* what the patient is trying to tell you. If you have determined in advance that this patient fits into a "specific category," you will discount what the patient wants you to know. Many medication errors could have been avoided if the nurse listened to the patient when they stated, "That pill looks different to me." The error may occur in part because of beneficent paternalism.
- Assisting with developing the care plan without patient input will reflect the nurse's needs, not the patient's. Later on, you will complain that the patient is noncompliant and will not cooperate with the plan of care. Ask yourself: "Did the patient know what the alternatives were for treatment?" and "Did the patient have the opportunity to offer input into the plan and agree to what the care plan would be?" It is difficult for patients to cooperate when they are not empowered.
- If the patient has agreed to the patient care plan, then encouraging the patient to do what has been agreed upon is beneficence. However, if you are influencing the patient into choosing one alternative treatment over another, it is paternalistic beneficence. If you find yourself saying, "I overheard the doctor saying he thinks you should choose this treatment" or "My husband chose the treatment and he is doing great," you are actively influencing the patient's decision (paternalism).
- Perhaps the patient asks your opinion for the choice, and you respond with your choice ("Well, if I were you, I would . . .") instead of saying, "The doctor explained the alternatives for treatment and the possible side effects of each, and it is for you to decide what is best for you."

Beneficent paternalism is justified only in extreme circumstances and is most often a medical decision (e.g., a physician approaching the court to be allowed to do a potentially lifesaving procedure when parents have refused to sign an authorized treatment form for the child).

To avoid paternalism with new mothers, a lactation counselor at a public health nursing, seminar, knowing the evidence (i.e., Baby-friendly Hospital Initiative), presented the following method: "I wish all women would breastfeed their babies. The value to both mother and child is a scientific fact. I present the facts and respond to their questions, but the final decision belongs to the mother. I respectfully support their decision." As an LPN/LVN, evidence should always guide your decision-making and education strategies with patients and the community, while respecting individual autonomy and avoiding paternalism.

PATERNALISM AND WOMEN'S HEALTH

The issue of paternalism toward women in medical research and receiving health care is slowly changing through the efforts of women themselves and the advocacy of nurses. The term *paternalism* is derived from a Latin word that means "father" (i.e., father knows best). In the health care system, it is interpreted, as "doctors know best because of their superior knowledge." Because the word is derived from the Latin word *pater*, they believe that men know better than women. Physicians define what is considered ill health for women. Anything that is normally different from men is considered an illness and requires the physician's intervention. Because women are different from men biologically, medicine has defined what is normal for women as being abnormal. For example, menstruation, pregnancy, and menopause have been defined as ill health instead of normal, healthy processes. Many of these same attitudes toward women continue in the health care system.

Although this trend still can exist, great strides have been made in women's health care. Many factors have contributed, including the increase in female physicians and empowerment of nurses and females in general in the United States. Accomplishments have been realized; however, clear signs remain as women continue to average 82% of the total income of their male counterparts for similar jobs (BLS, 2014). Advocacy for women remains an important responsibility. As a nurse, speak up when you see decisions being made based on incomplete information (e.g., the physician or other health care worker not really listening to a female patient). Review Chapter 9 regarding assertiveness and your responsibility. It reminds you that an aggressive, rude approach does not gain you anything except a bad reputation among your peers and patients. Practice assertiveness, and remember that change will occur slowly. Many female patients are already experiencing a change and assertively stating their needs. Nurses who advocate for their female patients assist in this process of reducing a paternalistic attitude toward women, one patient at a time, as the need arises.

? Critical Thinking

Do I Respond Differently to Male and Female Patients?

Keep track of the differences in your responses to male and female patients for 2 or 3 days. Record your response to the male or female patient and what the patient said.

When you think you have enough examples, review the data you have collected. Use critical thinking to determine what differences you noted in your response to male and female patients. Because this is for your eyes only, be candid. Are there any changes that you recommend for yourself? If so, write them down.

Get Ready for the NCLEX-PN® Examination

Key Points

- Ethics is concerned with the meaning of words such as *right, wrong, good, bad, ought,* and *duty*.
- Nursing ethics provide guidelines for making ethical decisions in nursing.
- LPNs/LVNs need to be aware of the contents of their state's Nurse Practice Act regarding ethical issues.
- Ethics is something an SPN/SVN *should/ought* to do. However, ethics themselves do not carry the weight of law.
- Content of the law (state's Nurse Practice Act) is something the SPN/SVN must do.
- Both NAPNES and NFLPN provide an ethical code for SPN/SVNs and LPN/LVNs.
- SPNs/SVNs and LPNs/LVNs must know the nursing code of ethics and not confuse it with their personal code of ethics.
- The nursing role includes a dependent role to physicians but is now viewed as a collaborative role, providing nursing care to the whole patient and being a patient advocate.
- Encounters with ethical dilemmas have increased as the LPN transitions from a "doer" to a "thinker."
- Cultural and religious backgrounds and personal values may influence ethical decisions of patients seeking health care.
- Nonmaleficence means "do no harm." Few treatments are entirely without harm.
- Beneficence means to "do good" with your nursing actions and is the basis of trust in nursing.
- Autonomy means respect for a patient's right to choose, as long as the patient's rights do not interfere with the rights of others.
- Fidelity means to be true. It challenges SPNs/SVNs and LPNs/LVNs to be faithful to the charge of acting in the patient's best interests, even when the capacity of free choice is not available to the patient because of his or her condition.
- Justice means that the SPN/SVN and the LPN/LVN must give the same level of care to all patients, with dignity and respect.
- The LPN/LVN has an ethical objection to carefully evaluate a job role before employment and avoid employment where ethical issues will routinely occur. (e.g., working at Planned Parenthood although having a pro-life personal belief system).
- Beneficent paternalism is justified only in extreme circumstances and is most often a medical decision.
- Paternalism in women's health care is decreasing. Nurses' advocacy for women helps promote this change, one patient at a time.

Additional Learning Resources

evolve Go to your Evolve website (http://evolve.elsevier.com/Knecht/success) for the following FREE learning resources:
- Answers to Critical Thinking Scenarios
- Additional learning activities
- Additional Review Questions for the NCLEX-PN® exam
- Helpful phrases for communicating in Spanish and more!

Review Questions for the NCLEX-PN® Examination

1. Which of the following best defines your ethical responsibility as a nurse?
   a. An understanding of each person's legal right to access care.
   b. The worth assigned to an idea or an action, freely chosen, affected by maturity.
   c. Understanding the meanings of words such as *right, wrong, good, bad, ought*, and *duty* and their impact on clinical decision making.
   d. Customs, habits, and behaviors in a society that are approved by that society.

2. Select the statement that **best** describes how the nursing profession has evolved:
   a. Nursing discovered its unique role in providing care to the whole patient, not just the diseased part, using evidence to make decisions.
   b. Nurses now view themselves as independent practitioners, able to meet all of their patients' needs.
   c. Because of the implementation of the nursing process and critical thinking in nursing schools, nurses now need to think independently to develop the best patient plan of care.
   d. Nurses discovered that curricula and textbooks changed but not the work on patient care units.

3. How will you respond to the mother who has refused a blood transfusion for her 2-year-old son, but the doctor has asked the court to overrule her refusal?
   a. "In your son's case, beneficent paternalism (explain term) overrules respect for your autonomy."
   b. "In this hospital, the doctor knows best because of his/her superior knowledge."
   c. "We have saved many children by ignoring parents' religious beliefs and doing what is best."
   d. "He is too young to understand and make his own choice in something this serious."

4. After seemingly successful treatment for depression and a serious suicide attempt, a patient will be in court this morning to find out if she will be released. The patient tells the SPN/SVN, "As soon as I get out, I am going to kill myself. Promise me you won't tell anyone." What course of ethical action should the SPN/SVN take?

   a. The SPN/SVN promises not to tell anyone. His/her personal ethic is to never break a promise when one is made.

   b. Despite respect for the patient's autonomy, ensuring a safe environment is essential. The SPN/SVN reports the patient's comment to their supervisor.

   c. The SPN/SVN believes in waiting to see what will happen. He/she plans to do the same during the court hearing.

   d. The SPN/SVN keeps the promise made to the patient but checks on the patient very frequently.

Alternate Format Item

1. Which statements **best** describe steps in making an autonomous decision? *(Select all that apply.)*
   a. Voluntary without pressure
   b. Fair to all parties involved
   c. Doctor suggests his personal solution
   d. Nurse provides evidence to assist the patient in decision making
   e. Personal gain is achieved

2. Which statements best describe the difference between personal and professional ethics? *(Select all that apply.)*
   a. Personal ethics means the same as beneficent paternalism.
   b. Professional ethics sometimes conflict with the law.
   c. Personal ethics provide guidelines for one's life.
   d. Professional ethics means you cannot abandon the patient.
   e. Personal ethics can conflict with professional ethics.

Critical Thinking Scenarios

Scenario 1

You are currently at the Good Haven Nursing Home 3 days a week on a geriatric nursing clinical rotation. The instructor has talked to the class about being aware of sounds when walking in the halls. You see Mrs. Garnet being pushed to the shower room in a wheelchair by one of the nursing aides. On the way back down the hall, you hear a sound from the shower room and decide to open the door to the shower room. Much to your surprise, you see the aide putting a washcloth into the resident's mouth. The muffled sound from Mrs. Garnet is barely audible. The nursing assistant states, "She was screaming and disturbing Mr. Jones (in the room next door) who has pneumonia and is trying to rest. I am just doing this for a few minutes. She hates this part of the bath." What will you do?

Scenario 2

The instructor asked Shawn, a staff LVN, and the patient for permission to have Kathy, an SVN, observe Shawn insert a urinary catheter. Permission was granted (Kathy had already watched a catheter insertion and given a successful return demonstration in class).

Kathy watched Shawn open the "catheterization tray" and noted a couple of breaks in technique. Shawn contaminated her gloves when cleansing the patient's perineal area. Shawn then began to reach for the sterile catheter. What should Kathy do?

Nursing and the Law: What Are the Rules?

Objectives

On completing this chapter, you will be able to do the following:

1. Discuss the content of your state's Nurse Practice Act (NPA).
2. Describe the responsibilities of your state's board of nursing (or nursing regulatory board), including their number one mandate.
3. Explain the limits, including prohibited acts, of a Licensed Practical Nurse/Licensed Vocational Nurse (LPN/LVN) license within your state.
4. Compare and contrast the state regulations governing Registered Nurse (RN) practice versus LPN/LVN practice.
5. Discuss the impact of the Institute of Medicine (2010) *Future of Nursing Report: Leading Change, Advancing Health*'s recommendation for nurses to practice to the full extent of their education and training.
6. Discuss the use of evidence-based resources such as The Joint Commission's (2015) *National Patient Safety Goals* to assist LPNs/LVNs in delivering safe care and avoiding a potential lawsuit.
7. Define the nursing standard of care.
8. Differentiate between common law and statutory law.
9. Explain the difference between criminal and civil action.
10. Discuss the difference between intentional and unintentional torts.
11. List the four elements needed to prove negligence.
12. Discuss the typical steps in a lawsuit.
13. Differentiate between student practical nurses/student vocational nurses (SPNs/SVNs) and instructor liability in preventing a lawsuit.
14. Discuss the need for personal malpractice insurance even if provided by your employer.
15. Explain the nurse's role in disclosure (i.e., child abuse, elder abuse).
16. Describe the major focus of the Health Insurance Portability and Accountability Act (HIPAA).
17. Discuss the differences among general consent, informed consent, and authorized consent.
18. Differentiate between the living will and durable power of attorney.
19. Explain the difference between physician-assisted suicide and euthanasia.
20. Explain the key components of the Nurse Licensure Compact.
21. Explain how you would legally deal with two difficult situations that might occur in a clinical setting.

Key Terms

accountability (ă-kŏwn-tă-BIL-ĭ-tē)

advance directives (ăd-VĂNS dĭ-RĔCT-ĭvs)

assault (ă-SŎLT)

authorized consent (ĂW-thŏr-izd kŏn-SĔNT)

basic patient situation (PĀ-shĕnt sĭt-u-Ā-shŭn)

battery (BĂT-ĕr-ē)

breach of duty (brĕch)

civil action (sĭ-vŭl ĂK-shŭn)

common law (KŎM-mŏn)

complex nursing situation (KŎM-plĕks NŬR-sēng sĭt-u-Ā-shŭn)

confidentiality (kŏn-fĭ-dĕn-chē-ĂL-ĭ-tē)

criminal action (KRIM-ĭn-ăl ĂK-shŭn)

damages (DĂM-ăj-ĕs)

defamation (dĕf-ă-MĀ-shŭn)

delegated medical act (dĕl-ĕ-GĀ-tĕd)

depositions (dĕp-ō-ZISH-ŏn)

direct supervision (dĭ-RĔCT soo-pŭr-VI-shŭn)

do not resuscitate (DNR) (rĭ-SŬS-ĭ-tāt)

durable medical power of attorney

duty (DOO-tē)

end-of-life principles (EOL)

euthanasia (ū-thă-NĀ-zhē-ă)

felony (FĔL-ō-nē)

general (implied) consent (JĔN-ĕr-ăl kŏn-SĔNT)

general supervision (JĔN-ĕr-ăl soo-pŭr-VI-shŭn)

Good Samaritan Act

Health Insurance Portability and Accountability Act (HIPAA)

informed consent (ĭn-FŎRMD kŏn-SĔNT)

institutional liability (ĭn-stĭ-TOO-shŭn-ăl lī-ă-BIL-ĭ-tē)

intentional tort (ĭn-TĔN-shŭn-ăl tŏrts)

interstate endorsement (ĭn-tĕr-STĀT ĭn-DŎRS-mĕnt)

law

liability (lī-ă-BIL-ĭ-tē)

libel (LĪ-bĕl)

living will (lĭ-VING wĭl)

malpractice (professional negligence) (măl-PRĂK-tĭs)

misdemeanor (mĭs-dĭ-MĒ-nŏr)

multistate licensure (Nurse Licensure Compact) (LĪ-sĕn-shŭr)

negligence (NĔG-lĭ-jĕns)

Nurse Practice Act (NPA) (nŭrs PRĂK-tĭs ăkt)
nursing standard of care (NURS-ĭng STĂN-dĕrd)
Oregon Death with Dignity Act
patient competency (PĂ-shĕnt KŎM-pĕ-tĕn-sē)
Patient Self-Determination Act (PSDA)
personal liability (PĔR-sŭn-ăl lī-ă-BIL-ĭ-tē)
physician-assisted suicide (PAS) (fĭ-ZI-shŭn ă-SIS-tĕd SOO-ĭ-sīd)

preponderance (prĭ-PŎN-dĕr-ănts)
proximate cause (PRŎKS-ĭ-mĕt căws)
slander (SLĂN-dĕr)
statutory law (STĂ-chū-TŏR-ē)
unintentional tort (ŭn-ĭn-TĔN-shŭn-ăl tŏrts p.)
vicarious liability (vĭ-KĂR-ē-ŭs)

Keep in Mind

Ethics, workforce trends/demands, and law drive the practice of nursing. When there is a dispute, the law (the Nurse Practice Act [NPA] in your state) is the final authority. No one has the authority to expand your scope of practice, not even your employer.

Mary and David work as nursing assistants on the weekend at Stellaris Nursing Home. This past weekend they observed a Licensed Practical Nurse (LPN), Bryan, who struggled with a clinical decision. Bryan was working on a team with a Registered Nurse (RN), LPN, and two nursing assistants. The RN, Kelly, became acutely ill during her work shift. As a result, she left her shift early to go home. The evening shift RN was to arrive before Kelly left; however, he was stuck in traffic and did not arrive as anticipated. Kelly did leave and stated to the LPN, "Just keep things quiet until the RN arrives." Minutes after Kelly left, Bryan realized that Kelly had neglected to initiate an intravenous (IV) infusion on a patient who had been septic. Bryan had practiced in another state where IV therapy was within the Nurse Practice Act. Although Bryan realized that IV therapy was prohibited in this state, he thought this was an extenuating circumstance and, because he knew what to do, he would proceed and initiate the IV.

As you read this chapter, think about how Bryan's actions violated the Nurse Practice Act. What could be the result of these actions? Would you have proceeded differently?

As we just reviewed in Chapter 6, ethics in nursing deals with rules of conduct, what is right and what you should do in a particular situation. Ethical values, in turn, are the *basis* of nursing law. **Law** has to do with regulations that control the practice of nursing. Your state's NPA, discussed below, is your *legal* guideline in nursing. The state is the final authority.

Knowledge of your state's NPA is critical to making safe nursing decisions. This knowledge will protect you against acts and decisions that could involve you in lawsuits and criminal prosecution. Lawsuits are commonplace in health care today. Your goal is to implement all strategies to minimize malpractice claims (lawsuits) and decrease your personal chance of being involved in a lawsuit. An in-depth knowledge and understanding of your state's NPA coupled with your continued competency as a Licensed Practical Nurse/Licensed Vocational

Nurse (LPN/LVN) will provide a solid foundation to reach this goal.

NURSE PRACTICE ACT

The state **NPA** defines nursing practice and establishes standards for nurses in your state. Ignorance of your state's NPA is never a valid defense against any legal proceeding regarding your license.

BASIC TERMINOLOGY

Similarities in basic terminology in an NPA exist in many states. As you study the scope of practice for licensed (or trained) practical/vocational nurses (LPNs/LVNs) in your state, an understanding of the following terms is necessary:

- **Activities of Daily Living (ADL).** Basic self-care tasks that an individual performs on a daily basis. These include but are not limited to basic hygiene (body and mouth), grooming, dressing, eating, exercising, and toileting. The nursing staff assists patients and their families in meeting these needs.
- **Basic nursing care.** Nursing care that can be performed safely by the LPN/LVN, based on knowledge and skills gained during the educational program. Includes ADL activities and skilled nursing procedures. Modifications of care are unnecessary, and patient response is predictable.
- **Basic patient situation.** The patient's clinical condition is predictable. Medical and nursing orders are not changing continuously. These orders do not contain complex modifications. The patient's clinical condition requires only basic nursing care. The professional nurse assesses whether the situation is a **basic patient situation.** A basic patient situation can include a chronic stable patient with the need for skilled nursing procedures. However, the patient's condition is stable (e.g., a patient with chronic obstructive disease [COPD] who has a tracheostomy but whose disease process is currently stable. As a result, the physician orders do not contain complex interventions).
- **Complex nursing situation.** The patient's clinical condition is not predictable. Medical orders or nursing interventions are likely to involve continuous changes or complex modifications. Nursing care expectations

are beyond those learned by the LPN/LVN during the educational program. The professional nurse assesses whether the situation is a **complex nursing situation.**

- **Delegated medical act.** During a **delegated medical act**, a physician's order is given to a registered nurse (RN), an LPN, or an LVN by a physician, dentist, or podiatrist.
- **Delegation (nursing).** The nurse directs another person to perform nursing tasks and activities while the licensed person retains accountability and responsibility for the service provided. Consideration of the right person, right task, right education, and right experience should be reviewed before delegation (American Nurses Association [ANA] & National Council of State Boards of Nursing [NCSBN], 2005).
- **Direct supervision.** With **direct supervision**, the supervisor is continuously present to coordinate, direct, or inspect nursing care. The supervisor is in the building.
- **General supervision.** Under **general supervision**, a supervisor regularly coordinates, directs, or inspects nursing care and is within reach either in the building or by telephone.
- **Professional nurse.** In many states, the professional nurse is defined as the RN.

CONTENT OF NURSE PRACTICE ACTS

The NPA (rules and regulations) of each state commonly includes the following content:

- General provisions
  - Functions of the state's board of nursing
  - General procedures (e.g., fees)
  - Licensure process
  - Elements of unprofessional conduct
    - Information related to reasons for a suspended or revoked license
    - Impaired Professional Program
- Responsibilities
  - General functions of the licensed nurse (e.g., LPN/LVN, RN)
  - Definition of nursing (specific definitions for practical nursing [LPN/LVN] and professional nursing [RN])
  - Standards of nursing conduct
- Organization, approval, and administration of nursing programs
- Continuing education

◉ Try This

Get Familiar with Your Scope of Practice in Your State's Nurse Practice Act (NPA)

Find your state's NPA (or occupational title act) online (visit www.ncsbn.org for a list of links to NPAs). As you read it, note the major categories listed above.

What does it state about the following topics?
1. Definition of licensed practical/vocational nursing and professional nursing (RN) in your state
   a. Compare and contrast the definition of practical nursing (LPN/LVN) versus professional nursing (RN).
   b. What differences are important?
   c. How do these differences impact respective scope of practices? Seek assistance from your instructor to fully understand the differences, if needed.
2. Use of the titles *licensed practical nurse* and *licensed vocational nurse*
3. Specific functions of the LPN/LVN
4. Prohibited functions of the LPN/LVN
5. Elements of unprofessional conduct

STATE BOARD OF NURSING

All states and provinces have examining councils that provide nursing examinations for licensure and review complaints that can lead to revocation of a license.

FUNCTIONS OF THE BOARD

State boards of nursing (sometimes called nurse regulatory boards) can have a single NPA or two distinct NPAs that address both the LPN/LVN and RN scope of practice. The boards have committees or councils that decide whether specific activities are within the scope of LPN/LVN practice in their state. An activity that is legal in one state may not be legal in another state. See Box 7-1 for common board of nursing functions.

State nursing boards offer a variety of services that can be accessed/completed online through their websites (e.g., license renewal, application for licensure by examination, verification of licensure status of a state nurse, change of address/phone number/email address, downloadable forms, links to continuing education courses, the state's NPA). As a practical/vocational nurse, understand that you must limit your work to the area of nursing defined in the state's NPA.

Box **7-1** Common Board of Nursing Functions

- Licensing and certifying (specialty certifications may be from related associations, e.g., NFLPN, NAPNES) nurses
- Setting fees
- Establishing standards for educational programs
- Approving schools of nursing
- Determining duration and renewal of licenses (some boards require continuing education credits for renewal of license)
- Maintaining inactive status lists
- Carrying out disciplinary action for violators
- Developing programs for impaired nurses
- Suspending and revoking licenses and dealing with the appeal process

In 2014, the National League for Nursing released a vision statement, *A Vision for Recognition of the Role of the Licensed Practical/Licensed Vocational Nurses in Advancing the Nation's Health*. In addition, the National Association for Practical Nurse Education and Service Inc. (NAPNES) (2003) issued a professional guideline for LPNs/LVNs titled, *The LPN/LVN Fulfills the Professional Responsibilities of the Practical/Vocational Nurse*. These are examples of statements from national nursing organizations, but they do not carry the weight of law. These statements are useful as *guides* for behavior and recommendations regarding workforce trends and LPN/LVN job roles and may be used in a court of law as a point of reference. *The NPA in your state is always your final authority*.

DISCIPLINARY RESPONSIBILITY OF THE BOARD

Each state's NPA lists specific reasons for which they seek to discipline a nurse. Eight general categories of disciplinary actions can be taken against nurses. Brent (2001) lists them as "fraud and deceit; criminal activity; negligence; risk to patients because of physical or mental incapacity; violation of the NPA or rules; disciplinary action by another board; incompetence; unethical conduct; and drug and/or alcohol use." See Box 7-2 for the eight categories of disciplinary action.

DISCIPLINARY PROCESS AND ACTION

The disciplinary process is based on law and follows the rules of law. See Box 7-3 for the steps of a disciplinary process.

NURSING LICENSURE

It is nursing licensure that defines and protects the title of LPN or LVN. Some states (e.g., Minnesota) have amended their NPA to include the provision that only licensed practical or registered nurses may use the professional title "nurse." This prevents an unlicensed person in a health care setting from misrepresenting themselves and stating "Hi, I am your nurse Mary today." This is illegal in states where the title of nurse is protected. It is definitely also unethical.

On completion of a state-approved practical/vocational nursing education program, a graduate is eligible to apply for the National Council Licensure Examination for Licensed Practical Nurses (NCLEX-PN® examination). In some states, immediately upon completion of their practical nursing program, the graduate may apply for a temporary permit to practice nursing as a Graduate Practical Nurse/Graduate Vocational Nurse (GPN/GVN). Today, this is a less common

---

Box 7-2 **Eight Categories of Disciplinary Actions Taken Against Nurses**

1. **Fraud and deceit:** Most often, fraud and deceit involve a person using fake means to get a nursing license (e.g., forging documents).
2. **Criminal activity:** This includes conviction of a felony, such as murder; or conviction for gross immorality, such as theft, fraud, personal misrepresentation, or embezzlement.
3. **Negligence:** The nurse does not do what a reasonable, prudent nurse would do in a similar situation. Negligence includes serious risk to the health, safety, or physical or mental health of a patient. (This may include patient injury. Injury can be physical, emotional, or spiritual.)
4. **Violation of the NPA:** Some states' NPAs list specific violations (e.g., unprofessional conduct, such as becoming personally involved with a patient).
5. **Discipline by another jurisdiction:** In the past, it was difficult to find out if a nurse had been disciplined in another state. Now there are two national data banks that make it easier to track disciplinary action of LPNs/LVNs in other states. However, it is not mandatory for the disciplining authority to notify a data bank. The data banks are as follows:
   a. *National Practitioner Data Bank* (NPDB). The Medicare and Medicaid Patient and Program Protection Act of 1978 led to the establishment of the NPDB, creating a data management system to track unfit health care practitioners and restrict the ability of incompetent professionals to move from state to state without disclosure of previous incompetence. Another entity, Healthcare Integrity and Protection Data Bank (HIPDB),

was established in response to the Health Insurance Portability and Accountability Act of 1996. In 2013, authorized by the Affordable Care Act, the two data banks merged, resulting in one entity, the NPDB. All state board of nursing entities are mandated to report disciplinary actions including probation, suspension, and revocation of a nursing license to NPBD. The NPDB primarily contains disciplinary actions taken against health care practitioners, including nurses, and serves as a repository, providing access for various stakeholders.

6. **Incompetence:** Examples include failure to meet generally accepted standards of nursing practice; negligence; and a nurse's mental disability that would interfere with patient safety.
7. **Unethical conduct:** Examples include a breach of nurse-patient confidentiality; refusal to provide nursing care for someone because of race, creed, color, national origin, disease, or sexual orientation; violation of the ethical code for LPNs/LVNs; and failure to maintain nursing competence.
8. **Alcohol and/or other drug abuse:** Alcohol and other drug abuse by a nurse (e.g., diversion of drugs, such as controlled substances, for personal use) is a threat to patient safety. Some nurses steal and sell diverted substances and equipment such as syringes and IV tubing, falsify patient records, and deprive patients of their medication. The number of nurses disciplined for alcohol and/or other drug abuse is increasing. Various programs exist to assist professionals, such as the Impaired Professionals Program.

Box **7-3**	Disciplinary Steps

FILING A COMPLAINT (LICENSED NURSE OR LICENSURE APPLICANT)
- Evaluate the following:
  - Is the nurse's behavior unsafe, incompetent, or unethical?
  - Is alcohol, drugs, or other chemicals affecting the nurse's physical or mental condition?
  - Is there a violation of the NPA or other related law?

REVIEW OF COMPLAINT
- Verify if and in which state the nurse is licensed.
- Verify whether the act is regulated by the NPA (i.e., practice-related, drug-related, boundary violations, sexual misconduct, or abuse and fraud).
- Verify if there is a positive criminal background check.

INVESTIGATION
- Interviews
- Evidence

BOARD PROCEEDINGS (OPPORTUNITY FOR THE NURSE TO RESPOND TO ALLEGATIONS)
- Informal proceedings
- Formal administrative hearing
- Alternative to discipline programs (i.e., substance abuse monitoring programs)

BOARD ACTION
- Emergency action (i.e., immediate suspension to protect the public pending a complete investigation)
- Disciplinary action (i.e., fine or civil penalty, public reprimand with no license restriction, limitation of practice, suspension, revocation, provisions for remediation, education, or monitoring)
- Remediation

REPORTING AND ENFORCEMENT
- NURSYS (National database for verifying license and discipline actions for nurses)

Data from National Council of State Boards of Nursing. (2015). *Discipline.* www.ncsbn.org/discipline.htm.

practice as technology has improved the speed of scheduling and confirming successful completion on the NCLEX-PN®. Thus the temporary permit has become less necessary for most graduates because the graduate receives prompt notification of successful completion of the examination and a nursing license is issued promptly. If the graduate nurse fails the NCLEX-PN® examination, the temporary permit is revoked. The graduate is responsible for reporting their unsuccessful exam immediately to their employer. Until successful completion of the NCLEX-PN® examination, the temporary permit remains revoked and the graduate cannot work as a GPN/GVN. The graduate has an opportunity to retest at a later date for an additional fee. The number of allowable retests and length of time between each exam is dictated by each state's NPA and varies across the United States.

Issuance of an LPN/LVN license can also be impacted by a previous criminal or child abuse history. In many states, each individual situation is reviewed on a case by case basis and recommendations to issue a license are made by the state board of nursing legal counsel. This also remains true throughout a nurses' career as their license is renewed. Drug and alcohol violations, fraud, theft, and other infractions can result in license suspension or revocation or denial of renewal. Your license is essential to your profession. Be sure to protect it accordingly.

WORKING IN OTHER STATES

States have arrangements for **interstate endorsements** for nurses who choose to work in other states. This means that it is possible to work in another state without repeating the NCLEX-PN® examination, after you meet that state's criteria for licensure by endorsement. Thus, you can breathe a sigh of relief that once you pass the NCLEX PN exam you will not need to retake the exam if moving to another state.

Some states are involved in **multistate licensure**: a mutual recognition model for nursing regulation. The Nurse Licensure Compact allows LPN/LVNs and RNs to have one multistate license. The National Council of State Boards of Nursing (NCSBN) adopted the Nurse Multistate Licensure Mutual Recognition Model in 1997. Utah was the first state to adopt the NCSBN Nurse Licensure Compact language that took effect in 2000. The Nurse Licensure Compact allows a nurse to have one license in his or her state of residency and practice in other states, depending on each state's NPA and legislation (www.ncsbn.org). To become law, each state must pass the law as part of their state NPA. As of 2015, 25 states are members of the Nurse Licensure Compact. Eligible nurses must legally reside in a Nurse Licensure Compact state to participate. You cannot experience the benefits (Box 7-4) of the Nurse Licensure Compact unless you declare a Nurse Licensure Compact state as your primary residence. Check the NPA of the state in which you will be working to find out if it is a compact state or if any other special considerations with border states exist.

Try This

Compact States and the Nurse Practice Act

Obtain and read the NPA of a compact state online. If approved to work in a compact state, the LPN/LVN must know the contents of the NPA of the compact state. Confirm the residency requirements to participate in the Nurse Licensure Compact.

Keep in Mind

If you do not have legal residence in a Nurse Licensure Compact state you cannot experience the benefits of the Nurse Licensure Compact. Thus you can apply for licensure in a Nurse Licensure Compact state; however, you will receive a single state license for that state, not a multistate license.

Box 7-4   Benefits of the Nurse Licensure Compact

- Ease of LPN/LVN or RN work mobility: Ability to practice across state lines.
- Increased cooperation and collaboration between states Boards of Nursing.
- Public receives safe nursing care protected by licensure laws across state boundaries.

Modified from National Council of State Boards of Nursing. (2015). *Nurse licensure compact.* www.ncsbn.org/nurse-licensure-compact.htm.

VERIFICATION OF LICENSURE

Most boards of nursing have instituted online verification of nursing licensure. The board provides public information about nurses who have current licensure. The verification system enables potential employers to use an online database confirming a nurse's license number, registration expiration date, and whether any board action (disciplinary) has taken place. The service is available 24 hours a day, 7 days a week. Check your state's board of nursing site to find out if this service is available.

Employers are able to use this option to comply with requirements for written verification of a nurse's registration by The Joint Commission (TJC) and other accreditation agencies.

UNLICENSED ASSISTIVE PERSONNEL

The use of unlicensed assistive personnel (UAP) to provide patient care has grown dramatically in recent years. It is expected that the trend will continue. These unlicensed persons are trained to perform a variety of nursing tasks. Licensed nurses need to be aware of specific training that UAPs have had and facility job descriptions so they can safely make assignments. Supervision of UAPs by the RN and the LPN/LVN charge nurse in long-term care to ensure safety of patient care is a major concern. There is apprehension that because of the lack of licensed nurses in an agency, duties might be delegated and/or assigned inappropriately to UAPs. It is the RNs and LPNs/LVNs who stand to lose their jobs and licenses if the care provided by UAPs does not meet the standards of safety and effectiveness. The training program for UAPs does not provide the same in-depth education and experience that programs for student nurses provide. Licensed nurses are accountable to both their employers and their state nursing boards (see Chapter 17). Providing safe, high quality care is always the focus. Working conditions that prohibit safe care need to be reported to employers, state boards of nursing, and accreditation agencies.

NURSING STANDARD OF CARE

The **nursing standard of care** is your guideline for good nursing care. The phrase "you are held to the nursing standard of care" has important legal implications. The

Box 7-5   Resources for the Nursing Standard of Care

- **NPA:** Identifies the minimum level of competency necessary for a person to function as an LPN or LVN or RN in a particular state.
- **Nursing licensure examination** (NCLEX-PN® examination): Tests for minimum competence.
- **Practical/vocational nursing programs:** Based on guidelines provided by the board of nursing, these programs guarantee a minimum knowledge base and the clinical practice necessary to provide safe nursing care. Curricula, textbooks, and instructors are resources for information about the standard of care.
- **Written policies and procedures:** The agency that employs the individual provides a standard of nursing care that must be followed. Read the policies of the agency to find out whether or not verbal directions are supported by written policies. If a question about care ever comes up in court, a lawyer will use the agency's policy and procedure manual as one guide to expected behavior. Remember that policies and procedures do not overrule the state's NPA and educational preparation. However, institutional policies may be stricter than state law.
- **Custom:** An unwritten, usually acceptable way of giving nursing care. Expert witnesses, not coworkers, would be called to testify to "the acceptable way."
- **Law (precedent):** Decisions that have been arrived at in similar cases brought up before a court (judge-made law).
- Statements from the NAPNES and NFLPN.
- Nursing texts and journals.
- Administrative rules of the board of nursing.

standard is based on what an ordinary, prudent nurse with similar education and nursing experience would do in similar circumstances. Resources for the nursing standard of care are found in Box 7-5. Note that health care institution routine ("I know you studied how to do this in nursing school, but this is how we do it here") is not on the list. All clinical decisions made must be based on evidence.

Keep in Mind

Accurate documentation is an important part of nursing care. In the eyes of the law, if it was not documented, it was not done.

HOW THE LAW AFFECTS LICENSED PRACTICAL NURSES AND LICENSED VOCATIONAL NURSES

COMMON LAW VERSUS STATUTORY LAW

The legal system in both the United States and Canada originates from English common law. **Common law** is called *judge-made law* because it originates in the courts. Common law is one way of establishing standards of legal conduct and is useful in settling disputes. Once the judge has made a decision, this decision *sets the* *precedent* for a ruling on a case with similar facts in the future. Thus, common law can change over time, based on precedent. **Informed consent** and a patient's right to refuse treatment are examples of common law.

Statutory law is law developed by the legislative branch of the state and the U.S. Congress of the federal government. The NPA, which governs the practice of nursing, is an example of a statutory law. State boards of nursing can make nursing laws as long as the items in their laws do not conflict with any federal statutes. Because the NPA is statutory law, governed by states, differences exist across the United States.

CRIMINAL VERSUS CIVIL ACTION

The two classifications of legal action are criminal action and civil action. A **criminal action** involves people and society as a whole. It involves relationships between individuals and the government. It is unlikely for nurses to be involved in criminal action. A criminal action is classified as follows:

- **Misdemeanor:** A **misdemeanor** is the least serious charge and can result in a fine or prison sentence of generally no more than 1 year. This criminal act might include taking a narcotic intended for the patient's pain relief and giving the patient another substance in its place.
- **Felony:** A **felony** is a serious offense with a penalty that usually ranges from more than 1 year in prison to death; for example, when the nurse injects a patient with a lethal drug to hasten death or removes life support before the patient has been pronounced dead by the physician.

Guilt on the part of the nurse needs to be established by producing proof *beyond a reasonable doubt*. Regardless of the outcome of the criminal case, when a criminal case is completed, it is also possible to be sued in a civil court.

A **civil action** protects individual rights and *results in payment of money* to the injured person (e.g., a back injury was sustained during a fall because spilled urine was not wiped up. This injury caused the patient additional treatment time, including physical therapy, pain, suffering, and loss of time from work). A civil action involves a relationship between individuals and the violation of those rights. A *tort* is a civil wrong. The two kinds of torts are intentional and unintentional, which are described as follows:

- **Intentional:** An **intentional tort** is intended to cause harm to the patient (e.g., threat or actual physical harm).
- **Unintentional:** An **unintentional tort** did not mean to harm the patient. "I did not mean to hurt the patient" is no defense if you did not use the "Six Rights" and gave the patient an incorrect medication, which caused injury.

Guilt on the part of the nurse can be established by a **preponderance** (majority) of the evidence. Table 7-1 provides a comparison of criminal and civil law.

INTENTIONAL TORTS

Tort law is based on the premise that in the course of relationships with one another there is a general **duty** to avoid injuring one another. A tort is a wrong or injury done to someone that violates his or her rights.

Intentional torts require a specific state of mind; that is, that the nurse intended to do the wrongful act.

Table 7-1	Comparison of Two Basic Classifications of Law	
	CIVIL LAW	**CRIMINAL LAW**
Who the law generally applies to	Relationships between private individuals and infringements on individual rights	Relationships between individuals and the government (state)
Who is affected?	Individuals	Society as a whole
Sources of law	U.S. Constitution, state and federal legislatures	U.S. Constitution, state and federal legislatures
Punishment for breaking the law	Generally payment of a monetary compensation. Other settlements could include a public apology or implementation of new safety standards	Death, imprisonment, fines, restrictions
How guilt is established	Proof by a preponderance of the evidence	Proof beyond a reasonable doubt
Examples of nursing liability	Contract Tort Unintentional Intontional Negligence	Murder, rape, larceny, homicide, manslaughter, assault and battery, embezzlement
Criminal infraction	None	Felony/misdemeanor/summary

Common law is judge-made law. A trial judge's ruling lays down a legal principle and sets a precedent. These principles are used to decide future cases. This type of law is continually adapted and expanded.
Statutory law is formal legislative enactment. Law passed by Congress or enacted by state government. May be amended, repealed, or expanded by the legislature. The NPA is an example of statutory law.

Assault and battery, false imprisonment and use of restraints, **defamation** that includes both libel and slander (discussed later), and physical and emotional abuse are examples of intentional torts. Not all insurance companies cover intentional torts in their malpractice insurance policies, so you should check your policy.

Assault and Battery

Assault is an unjustified attempt or threat to touch someone. **Battery** means to cause physical harm to someone. (Students often confuse these two terms. To avoid this, remember that assault and attempt both begin with the letter "A"). When a patient refuses a treatment or medication, forcing the patient to take medication could result in an assault and battery charge against you. The patient gives *implied consent* (permission) for certain routine treatments when entering the institution. Patients retain the right to refuse any treatment verbally and may leave the institution when they choose, unless they are there for court-ordered treatment. Nurses can also protect themselves from assault by a patient but can use only as much force as is considered reasonable for self-protection.

Treating a patient without consent is battery even if the treatment is medically beneficial. A physician might go to the court to attempt to get a court order to allow a blood transfusion for someone who opposes it on religious grounds. If the patient is fully competent, is not pregnant, and has no children, the court is likely to rule for the patient even if a blood transfusion would save his or her life. When faced with a similar situation, the practical/vocational nurse respects the patient's belief system and notifies the RN and/or supervisor for further advice or interpretation.

False Imprisonment and Use of Restraints

False imprisonment is keeping someone detained against his or her will. It can include the use of restraints or seclusion in a room without cause and without a physician's order. Restraint by verbal threats or physical harm is also included in this category. Chemical restraint (with medication) is defined as administering a PRN (from Latin, pro re nata meaning "as needed") medication with a sedating side effect every 4 hours to keep the patient tired and in his or her room. In this situation, the intent is to keep the patient quiet and out of the way. The intended use of the medication has been circumvented to meet the nurse's need.

Defamation

Defamation means damage to someone's reputation through false communication or communication without their permission. Libel and slander are included in this category and are described as follows:

- **Libel** is defamation through *written* communication or pictures.
- **Slander** is defamation by *verbalizing* untrue or private information (gossip) to a third party.

The patient has the right to expect you to speak the truth. Additional unnecessary conversation with coworkers and those outside the agency can result in a charge of defamation. The same is true for taking unwanted photographs or showing a patient's injury, cancerous growth, or gunshot wound to others, students included, without the patient's permission. Social media has escalated issues related to defamation. Posting any patient information or "patient story" on any type of social media site is prohibited unless written permission is obtained from the patient and approved by your employer. Posting your clinical day experience, even without using patient names or specific information is prohibited. Review the pamphlet created by NCSBN, *A Nurse's Guide to the Use of Social Media* (https://www.ncsbn.org/NCSBN_SocialMedia.pdf).

Consider also that you often are privy to information about the personal lives of other nurses, physicians, and other coworkers; and they are privy to information about you. Although the desire to repeat the information you hear may be tempting, it is best left unsaid. Later in the chapter, you will learn about HIPAA and how that law defines privacy.

Physical and Emotional Abuse

Physical abuse is generally easier to identify, although the victim may find creative ways to hide the injuries for a period of time. Emotional abuse is more difficult to identify. The person doing the abusing may be very personable and attentive to the victim when out in public. A former student described how everyone thought her husband loved her and how fortunate she was. When they were alone, he would tell her she was ugly, worthless, and no one else would ever want her or love her. When she became pregnant, he would always take her to her doctor appointment. He would answer the doctor's and nurse's questions for her, and when she tried to speak, he would take over in gentle terms, doing the explaining. At no time was she alone with a doctor or nurse.

In the course of your career in practical/vocational nursing, you will probably suspect or actually see the results of some types of abuse. As a practical/vocational nurse, you have a legal responsibility to report your suspicions or observations of abuse by following your facility's abuse policy. Note that a "suspicion" is a nagging doubt. Be empathetic (as opposed to sympathetic) so that your observations or report will be as objective as possible. Becoming a part of the patient's emotions may lead you to jump to conclusions or accept a particularly convincing but untrue explanation. Whether the patient is a child, woman, man, or elder, reputations are at stake. Once an accusation has been made, it is difficult to be truly free from it, even when it is proved groundless.

Refer to your state's abuse laws for specific rules that govern your responsibility for reporting abuse. Remember that you are a mandated reporter. You must report any suspected or observed physical or emotional abuse. Some state's laws may include a mandate that the individual who is suspicious of abuse contact the government authority directly, or at a minimum, ensure the supervisor reported the event and follow up has occurred. It is not sufficient to report to your supervisor and then move on, unsure if any investigation occurred. In addition, child abuse training or like training may be mandated for licensure and licensure renewal in your state. Follow your facility's policy for reporting abuse. The social services department can help you report abuse. Offer concrete, specific observations. Quote the statements made, and avoid offering a personal interpretation. Let the facts speak for themselves.

UNINTENTIONAL TORTS

An unintentional tort holds that the nurse did not intend to injure the patient. However, the nurse did not maintain the nursing standard of care and did not do what a prudent nurse with comparable education and skills would do in a similar situation. Negligence and malpractice (professional negligence) are examples of unintentional torts.

NEGLIGENCE

Brent (2001) defines **negligence** as "conduct that falls below the standards established by the law for the protection of others against the unreasonable risk of harm." A common type of negligence is personal injury. For example, say your town has a law stating that sidewalks must be shoveled within 24 hours after a snowstorm. Your sidewalk has not been shoveled within the 24 hours, and your neighbor falls in front of your house and breaks her arm. The neighbor sues you for negligence. Remember that in negligence the property owner did not intend to cause the injury to the neighbor, but knowing the risks and the law, he or she should have guarded against the injury. Good intentions do not enter in. It is your conduct, not your intent that is the issue.

MALPRACTICE (PROFESSIONAL NEGLIGENCE)

Malpractice, the legal name for professional negligence, means negligence by a professional; in this case a LPN/LVN. The most common type of negligence in practical/vocational nursing relates to action or lack of action, not what you intended to do. These are often referred to as Acts of Commission or Acts of Omission. For example, you can give the wrong medication (commission) or forget to give a medication (omission). Box 7-6 lists the most common sources of malpractice, according to Watson

---

Box **7-6**   **Some Common Sources of Malpractice**
• Medication errors • Working while impaired • Failure to follow standards of care • Lack of observation and timely reporting about the patient • Failure to use a medical device accurately • Failure to communicate • Failure to properly supervise a patient • Negligent delegation and supervision • Failure to act as a patient advocate • Failure to get informed consent

Modified from Watson, E. Nursing malpractice: Costs, trends, and issues, *Journal of Legal Nurse Consulting*, 25(1), 26-31, 2014.

(2014). The top three closed claim sites per practice setting for the LPN/LVN are Hospital-Inpatient Surgical Service, Patient's Home, and Hospital-Inpatient Medical Service (Watson, 2014). In addition, the LPN/LVN had an average paid indemnity of $83,213 (Watson, 2014). The charges of professional negligence (malpractice) listed could be avoided by good nursing practice (i.e., what a reasonable, prudent nurse would do in a similar situation). This includes knowing strategies to minimize errors required by entities such as The Joint Commission (e.g., creating an institutional list of drugs based on TJC's published list of commonly confused look-alike, sound-alike drug names). The student practical/vocational nurse is held to the level of a licensed practical/vocational nurse's performance. Know your state's NPA and know essential standards of care.

There are occasions when the evidence is overwhelming and indicates the accused nurse is responsible for the patient injury. Such an occasion is called *res ipsa loquitur*, meaning "the evidence speaks for itself." For example, a patient develops a drop in blood pressure immediately after the nurse administered an injection improperly.

MALPRACTICE INSURANCE FOR NURSES

More nurses are being named in lawsuits. Nurses assume **liability** for their own acts. Although the employing agency may assume responsibility for the nurse during a lawsuit, the agency can then turn around and sue the nurse. You can also be held responsible for the "neighborhood advice" you give; for example, telling a neighbor how to care for her sick child or emergency aid you provide in the community.

Each nurse must carefully consider whether or not it is necessary to purchase a malpractice insurance policy. Incidents of suing for malpractice continue, although your chances of being sued as an LPN/LVN compared with other health care providers, is minimal. Given the inexpensive cost of malpractice insurance (approximately $100.00 per year for a recommended policy) for

Box 7-7	Reasons for Your Own Malpractice Insurance

- The jury's award could exceed the limits of your agency's coverage.
- Your *employing agency* could pay out an award to a plaintiff and then countersue you.
- You acted outside the scope of employment, and the agency argues it is not liable.
- Your employer's policy covers you only on the job.
- An agency might carry a policy that covers you only while you are employed by that institution. A suit may come up years after you have stopped working for the employer. It is suggested that nurses purchase occurrence coverage if malpractice coverage is desired and not claims coverage. Occurrence coverage protects the nurse for each incident regardless of the present employer.
- The agency may decide to settle out of court. The plaintiff could then pursue a case against the nurse.
- Employer lapses in payment or renewal of policy.
- After a settlement, *insurers* could turn around and sue the nurse.
- If you have your own coverage, you will have your own lawyers, not the lawyers who are also defending the agency.

Box 7-8	Four Elements Needed to Prove Negligence

1. Duty refers to the nurse's responsibility to provide care in an acceptable way. The nurse has a duty based on education, as well as the policies and standards of the place of employment.
2. Breach of duty means that the nurse did not adhere to the nursing standard of care. What was expected of the nurse was not done (omission) or was not done correctly (commission). An expert nurse witness establishes the standard of care.
3. Damages mean that the patient must be able to show that the nurse's negligent act injured him or her in some way. The patient must prove actual damage.
4. Proximate cause means that a reasonable cause-and-effect relationship can be shown between the omission or commission of the nursing act and the harm to the patient. Did the nurse's negligent act cause the injury in question? For example, a member of unlicensed assistive personnel bumps the patient's toe in the shower. The patient has a history of diabetes mellitus. Despite prompt reporting, observation, and care of the toe, the toe becomes gangrenous and the foot requires amputation. The cause of the amputation was from the original "bump" of the toe.

LPNs/LVNs, it is an important consideration. Malpractice insurance is provided for you as a student nurse, generally included in your total costs of attendance. Consider purchasing your malpractice insurance immediately upon graduation. Some reasons for having your own malpractice insurance are found in Box 7-7.

Try This

Malpractice Coverage

If you are currently assigned to a clinical area, find out what the agency policy is on malpractice coverage for practical/vocational nurses. If not required by the employer, consider reasons why an LPN/LVN working there should purchase malpractice insurance.

FOUR ELEMENTS NEEDED TO PROVE NEGLIGENCE

Duty, **breach of duty, damages,** and **proximate cause** are the four elements that must be present to cause an action for negligence against a nurse. Each of the four elements must be proved by the patient to receive compensation. Box 7-8 explains the four elements needed to prove negligence.

Critical Thinking

Develop a scenario of an LPN/LVN who is being sued. Use the four elements needed to prove negligence as the basis for the suit.

STEPS FOR BRINGING LEGAL ACTION

Legal actions follow an orderly process. Remember that the nurse also has rights and is not considered guilty simply because someone filed a complaint. Steps for bringing a legal action by a patient are found in Box 7-9.

DEPOSITIONS

Depositions are used to gather information under oath (fact finding). Once the deposition is scheduled, provide information on where and how you can be reached. The deposition usually takes place in an attorney's office. You may be able to request that it be in your attorney's office. (It will be helpful to have an attorney who understands nursing and is familiar with legal action against a nurse.) Opponents' attorneys may also be present. However, only one of the opponent's attorneys should be permitted to ask questions so as not to "tag team" (multiple attorneys firing questions at the nurse). A court reporter or stenographer will record your testimony.

Dress professionally, as you would for a job interview. Do your utmost to be calm and polite no matter how rude others, including the opposing attorney, seem to you.

ATTORNEY PROCEDURES

In preparation for a deposition, your attorney will do the following:
- Provide a checklist of basic instructions for the deposition.
- Practice likely questions that may be asked and critique your responses.

| Box **7-9** | **Steps for Bringing a Legal Action by a Patient** |

- The patient believes that the nurse has violated his or her legal rights.
- The patient seeks the advice of an attorney.
- The attorney has a nurse expert review the patient's chart to see whether the nurse has violated the nursing standard of care. If it is determined that a standard of care has been violated, a lawsuit is filed.
- The patient (the plaintiff) files a complaint that documents the grievance (violation of rules). This is served to the defendant (the nurse).
- The defendant responds in writing.
- The discovery period (pretrial activity) begins. Statements are taken from the defendant nurse, witnesses, nurse expert, patient (plaintiff), and other caregivers. Policies and procedures of the health care facilities are reviewed.
- During the trial, important information is presented to the judge or jury. A verdict (decision) is reached. The plaintiff (the patient) has the burden of proof (evidence of wrongdoing) during the trial. The award in a malpractice case is to make the aggrieved person whole. There is generally a monetary settlement. In addition, an apology or a safety initiative could be mandated by the court.
- An appeal (request for another trial) can be made if either the plaintiff or the defendant does not consider the verdict acceptable.

- Prepare you for types of questions that may slant your testimony.
- Suggest appropriate ways to respond, but not tell you what to answer.
- Use a practice deposition video (usually, not always).
- Meet with you in advance on the day of the deposition to answer any last-minute questions.

GIVING TESTIMONY

Here are some basics to keep in mind during a deposition:

- It is important to tell the truth, *always*. Avoid trying to be clever.
- A court reporter or stenographer can only record words, so questions must be answered verbally.
- Listen carefully to the question. If you do not understand the question, ask that the question be repeated or rephrased.
- Before answering, pause. This will give you an opportunity to consider the question. Think about what is being asked and how you will answer.
- Be specific in answering a question: If it is a "yes" or "no" question, then answer it that way. *Resist the urge to say more.* If you do not know the answer to a question, say so, and do not speculate. If you do not remember, say, "I do not remember."
- If your attorney instructs you to not answer a question, do not answer. Instruction to not answer a question is permitted under certain circumstances.

- Be careful not to reveal the content of any conversation with your attorney.
- Ask for a break, especially if you are tired or not thinking clearly. If there is a question pending, you will be expected to answer it before taking a break.
- You will not be permitted to take any notes during the deposition.
- A few weeks after the deposition, you and your attorney may be able to review the testimony and make corrections. You may be asked about the corrections during the trial.

LIABILITY

KINDS OF LIABILITY

Personal liability holds us responsible for our own behavior, including negligent behavior. This rule makes it impossible to completely shift responsibility onto someone else. **Vicarious liability** means responsibility for actions of another because of a special relationship with the other. The term *respondeat superior*, Latin for "let the master speak," is based on vicarious liability. It is applied in the following two ways:

1. *Borrowed servant doctrine* (e.g., the master/servant relationship between an employer [hospital] and an employee [nurse]). The employer (master) is assumed to be better able to pay for the injuries than the employee (servant). The employer may also be held responsible in a suit for the negligent acts of the employee performed during the time of employment. This provides incentive for health care agencies to hire carefully, as well as orient and supervise the work of the employee.
2. *Captain of the ship doctrine* (e.g., in an operating room). A nurse becomes the temporary employee of the physician doing the surgery. This doctrine assumes that in this situation the surgeon exerts control of the nurse in relation to specific conduct that caused patient injury in the operating room.

Institutional liability is vicarious liability. It assumes that the health facility provides certain safeguards to keep the patient from harm. This includes a safe facility to prevent physical harm (e.g., adequate supervision of staff, adequate staffing, and safe equipment).

COMMON CAUSES OF NURSING LIABILITY

Many of the errors leading to common nursing liabilities can be avoided by following the guidelines you learned in nursing school. The major areas of liability (responsibility/accountability) can be categorized as lack of safety, knowledge, skill, observation and reporting, documentation, and acceptance of responsibility for nursing actions, all of which are part of the usual clinical evaluation. The most common errors are drug errors, most of which can be avoided if you follow the guidelines you learn in basic nursing and practice in the clinical areas. One of the best defenses for prevention of legal liability is development of rapport with the patient. If you treat patients with courtesy and respect, they are less likely to sue (unless you provide care below the nursing standard of care). Be honest, be nice, and be thorough. The very best defense is not to make a mistake in the first place. If you do err, the second best defense is to immediately admit that you made an error and communicate freely all steps taken to prevent or minimize harm. Transparency is a must!

Professional Pointer

Ignorance of nursing law is no excuse.

RESPONSIBILITY AND ACCOUNTABILITY IN NURSING

Nursing demands that you be responsible. This means being reliable and trustworthy. At no time can you expect a peer, supervisor, or patient to say to you "it's okay that you didn't come to work today because your car wouldn't start;" or "it's okay if we talk about just your problems today instead of the patients;" or "it's okay that you didn't do the work you were assigned because you're having a bad day." Nursing says, "I'm sorry that you have personal problems that are distracting you, but you have to deal with them because your priority in this profession is the patient."

The word *accountability* means that you are answerable. As a nursing student, you are answerable to yourself, to your assigned patient, to the team leader, to the preceptor, to the physician, and to your instructor who constantly evaluates your work. As an LPN/LVN, accountability to the instructor is replaced by accountability to the employing agency. You are held accountable for all the nursing actions that you perform or are assigned to perform. The measures of accountability are the following nursing standards of practice:

- NPA of the state
- NAPNES Standards and Educational Competencies of Graduates of Practical/Vocational Nursing Programs (see www.napnes.org)
- NFLPN Nursing Practice Standards for the Licensed Practical/Vocational Nurse (see www.nflpn.org)

They recommend minimal acceptable standards of nursing behavior for the SPN/SVN and the LPN/LVN.

LIABILITY OF STUDENT NURSES AND INSTRUCTORS

Student nurses are held accountable for the nursing care they give. They are held to the standards of a licensed practical/vocational nurse. This emphasizes *the necessity to prepare for providing care for assigned patients in the clinical area.* The instructor has the responsibility to make patient assignments based on the

---

Box 7-10 SPN/SVN Responsibilities for Patient Care

- Prepare by reading the assigned patient's chart, patient profile, and established plan of care, and develop your own plan of care for the patient to whom you are assigned.
- Look up action, safety of ordered dose, side effects, and nursing considerations for the assigned patient's routine, PRN medications, and IV additives.
- Review how to perform ordered treatments.
- Compose a time sequence for care during your time with the patient.
- When you arrive on the clinical unit, review your plan of care with the instructor before you begin your nursing care.
- Identify a need for and request additional help or supervision.
- Comply with agency and school of nursing policies.
- Document appropriately.
- Maintain patient confidentiality.

---

student's knowledge base and ability to give safe nursing care. The instructor is also expected to provide reasonable supervision for the care given by a student. A list of your responsibilities is found in Box 7-10.

FUNCTIONING BEYOND THE SCOPE OF PRACTICE AND EXPERIENCE

As an LPN/LVN, you might be asked by an RN or physician to perform nursing duties that are beyond your scope of practice or experience. It is up to you to speak up. Box 7-11 contains examples of responses

Box 7-11 Possible Responses When Asked to Perform a Nursing Task Unfamiliar to You or Beyond Your Scope of Practice

- "I am not legally able to do something beyond the LPN/LVN NPA."
- "I need to have an RN immediately available for collaboration as the patient's condition is unstable and changing."
- "I have never done this before. I will be glad to learn if you teach me, watch me demonstrate in return, and write a memo for my file that you have taught me to do this and watched a satisfactory return demonstration."
- "I was taught to do this while in school but did not have a chance to catheterize a real person. I observed the educational skills demonstration video on the Internet. Please observe me perform a catheterization, and intervene if necessary."
- "My orientation here did not include how to make daily assignments according to the skill level of staff. I need to be shown. Will you show me how to make assignments? I learn quickly, so it will be time well spent."
- "You have provided a detailed orientation, but I do not feel ready (or qualified) to assume a charge nurse position. I think I need more experience as a staff nurse so I can function effectively and within my NPA."

when asked to perform beyond your scope of practice. When seeking employment, check out the philosophy, mission statement, and policies of your potential place of employment. Ask what is included in your job, the period of orientation you will receive, what the orientation will cover, and who will do the orientation. If you discover during your inquiry that your work will cover more than you have learned or tasks that are beyond your scope of practice, say so. Listen also to your affective response: What is your intuition saying? Getting a job just to get a job may result in your being fired or losing your license. You may end up losing your job for something that was not your fault. The ideal is that everyone around you shares your ethics and demonstrates fairness, but the reality of ethics is sometimes quite different. Institutional policy and procedure is a critical resource for safe practice. Your employer can limit your scope of practice based on policy and procedure, but may not expand it. For example, if you are employed in a state where LPN/LVNs are not permitted to administer intravenous medications via a central access device, then despite in-depth education and approval by your supervisor and institution, you may not perform that procedure.

SPECIFIC PATIENT SITUATIONS

A professional relationship between the nurse and the patient is essential for the provision of nursing care. Legal precedent has established that the health care agency also has a responsibility to the patient. Patients have become increasingly concerned and vocal about the quality of care they expect to receive. Many of the issues are directly related to privacy, confidentiality, and safety. These are also concerns of health agencies and health care workers, including nurses.

PRIVACY AND CONFIDENTIALITY

Privacy in health care means the right to be left alone and free from intrusion, including the right to choose care based on personal beliefs, feelings, or attitudes; the right to govern bodily integrity (accepting or rejecting treatment or exposure of the body); and the right to control when and how sensitive information is shared. **Confidentiality** in health care refers to the nondisclosure of information regarding patients.

INFORMATION THAT MUST BE REVEALED

Some laws require that certain patient information must be reported without the patient's consent. The purpose is to protect the public. Examples of patient information that must be revealed are listed in Box 7-12.

PATIENTS' RIGHTS

Patients' rights in all types of institutions are mandated by the U.S. Constitution and by state and federal laws.

Box 7-12 Patient Information That Must Be Revealed

In all situations the supervisor (RN), director of nursing, and policy set by the facility are resources.

- **Communicable disease:** To the local health department or the Centers for Disease Control and Prevention. This includes AIDS, but the nature of the disclosure varies according to state law.
- **Vaccine-related adverse reactions:** To the Department of Health and Human Services. (Reporting of some reactions is mandatory; for others it is voluntary. Call (800) 822-7967 for the U.S. Food and Drug Administration's reportable events table.)
- **Criminal acts:** All states mandate reporting of rape cases. Some mandate reporting of injuries by gunshot or sharp instruments. Some states require reporting of blood alcohol levels (BAL) beyond the legal limit. Clarify your state's specific mandates. The local police department is a good place to clarify what is reportable *before* an incident occurs.
- **Equipment-related injuries:** When use of a medical device results in injury or death, it is reported immediately to your supervisor and physician. If emergency first aid is called for, follow the procedure you have been taught.
- **When there is a clear and present danger:** HIPAA laws, for instance, mandate reporting of patient mistreatment or professional misconduct. Report immediately to your supervisor or follow the policy manual for an emergency course of action.
- **Abuse and neglect of a patient (child or elderly):** Report the incident immediately to your supervisor or director of nursing. He or she will usually follow up by reporting to police and/or social services. It is your responsibility in many states to ensure a report has been made. Thus be sure that the required reporting has occurred.
- **Incompetence (including alcohol or drug impairment) or unprofessional acts:** As defined by state law. Facilities have policies for how to report and to whom. Report immediately to your supervisor, your director of nursing, or as directed in the facility's policy manual. Violation of nursing law will be reported to the state board of nursing.

Legal rights vary depending on the health care agency and the patient's competency. The American Hospital Association (AHA) developed *The Patient's Bill of Rights* in 1972. It was revised in 2003 and renamed *The Patient Care Partnership: Understanding Expectations, Rights, and Responsibilities*. This is an ethical, rather than legal, document for hospitals recommending ways to guarantee patient rights. It is intended as a model for states to develop rights statements. Some state legislatures have adopted patient rights statements. Additional bills of rights have been developed for pregnant patients, nursing home residents, and mental health patients. The document is reviewed and revised yearly as needed. Box 7-13 provides *The Patient Care Partnership* recommendations.

Box 7-13 *The Patient Care Partnership* Recommendations: What to Expect During a Hospital Stay

- High quality hospital care
- A clean and safe environment
- Involvement in your own care
  a. Discussing your medical condition and information about medically appropriate treatment choices
  b. Discussing your treatment plan
  c. Getting information from you
  d. Understanding your health care goals and values
  e. Understanding who should make decisions when you cannot
- Protection of your privacy
- Help when leaving the hospital
- Help with your billing claims

From American Hospital Association (2003). *The patient care partnership.* www.aha.org/advocacy-issues/communicatingpts/pt-care-partnership.shtml.

◎ Try This

Patients' Rights

Obtain a copy of your state's or health facility's patient rights statement. Briefly explain what is meant by each of the main topics. Identify the topics that are a part of what you have already learned in nursing.

HEALTH INSURANCE PORTABILITY AND ACCOUNTABILITY ACT

The U.S. **Health Insurance Portability and Accountability Act (HIPAA)** rules took effect on April 14, 2003, for health insurance companies, hospitals, clinics, doctors, pharmacies, and other health groups throughout the United States. The original intent of HIPAA was portability of insurance for employees from one job to the next. Portability is addressed in the law, but the main focus of the law is privacy. Changes to modify HIPAA privacy, security, and enforcement of rules are updated as technological advances dictate. The law gives patients rights over their health information. Basic HIPAA terminology is provided in Box 7-14.

Basics of the Health Insurance Portability and Accountability Act

The following are the three basic parts of HIPAA:

1. **Protection of privacy.** HIPAA provides a guide for health-related facilities and individuals to establish privacy standards based on the HIPAA model. This is intended as a national privacy standard throughout the United States. When discussing privacy, HIPAA uses the term *protected health information* (PHI) when referring to patient information that should not be revealed. Proposed are rules to increase efficiency of the health care system by creating standards for use and dissemination of health care information.

Box 7-14 Basic Health Insurance Portability and Accountability Act Terminology

- **HIPAA:** Passed in 1996. Enforcement began April 14, 2003.
- **Portability:** Original intent of HIPAA was portability of health insurance for employees from one job to the next.
- **Protection of patient privacy:** Main focus of HIPAA is protection of patient health information.
- **Covered entity:** Health facilities that provide, bill, or receive payment for health care as a normal part of business.
- **Health care:** Any care, services, or supplies related to the care of a patient.
- **Privacy officer:** HIPAA requirement that all covered entities designate a privacy officer.
- **Notice of privacy practices:** Each covered entity must develop a document, written in plain language that explains the facility's privacy practices. It is distributed to all patients. The notice must also be posted in a prominent place to be read by all interested parties.
- **Department of Health and Human Services (DHHS):** The federal agency that oversees HIPAA.
- **Mandatory law:** Law that must be followed or penalties will be involved.

---

2. **Administrative simplification.** The overall goal of administrative simplification is to reduce paperwork related to health care reimbursement (e.g., a goal is to develop a universal insurance claim form).
3. **Security standards.** The overall goal is to establish security standards for the protection of electronic (computer and fax) transmission of PHI (e.g., encrypted password protection when using a computer is a HIPAA requirement). Confidentiality and complete security requirements have increased since February 2010, including having a small health plan use a single national provider identifier.

The Department of Health and Human Services is the federal agency that oversees HIPAA. It has emphasized reasonableness as a guide to applying HIPAA regulations. Depending on the facility with which you are involved, interpretation of HIPAA ranges from reasonable to very strict. HIPAA rules and regulations have been reviewed and updated yearly since 2003.

? Critical Thinking

Patient Privacy

List some examples of patient information that could compromise patient privacy if revealed.

The Notice of Privacy Practices

The main focus of HIPAA is protection of privacy. Each covered entity (health facility) must develop a written

"Notice of Privacy Practices." The notice is made available to all patients, employees, and health-related companies with whom the facility does business (e.g., health insurance companies, medical equipment companies). The patient receives a personal copy to read and sign. Signing the copy denotes understanding of, and agreement with, the use and disclosure of PHI for treatment, payment, and facility operation. This is not the same as consent for treatment. If the patient is incompetent, state laws are followed. This usually means that the patient's health proxy is treated as though he or she is the patient.

What the Notice of Privacy Practices Addresses

The Notice of Privacy Practices must address the following in plain language:

1. **Access to medical records.** Patients have a right to a copy of their medical records and to review the records upon request. The facility determines under what conditions the records can be reviewed. Generally, this means reviewing the records with an RN or a physician present to translate medical terminology and answer questions. At no time does an SPN/SVN or LPN/LVN provide the records, or any part of them, to the patient. The request must follow the protocol set up by the facility. The Notice of Privacy Practices must clearly state how to access the records. HIPAA provides up to 30 days for a facility to provide medical records for a patient. A patient may be charged for being provided PHI as hard copies or on electronic media; for example, the cost of a CD or flash drive.

2. **Amendments to medical records.** According to HIPAA, patients have the right to request changes in their medical records. All covered entities must appoint privacy officers. It is the job of the privacy officer to process a request for change in a patient's medical records. The facility is obligated to consider the request and then notify the patient of the final decision.

3. **Restrictions on the use of protected health information.** Patients can restrict use of their PHI as long as the requested information does not interfere with activities related to treatment, payment, or facility operation. The privacy officer usually makes the final decision. Rules include prohibition of the sale of PHI (without authorization) for use in marketing and fund raising.

4. **Access to an accounting.** Patients can request a list of the people, companies, or agencies that have received their PHI. The Notice of Privacy Practices lists steps for requesting an accounting on written request from a patient. Rules exist restricting certain types of information to health plans.

5. **Confidential communications.** Patients may request that PHI be delivered in such a way that the sender cannot be identified. For example, the patient may request that blood test results be mailed in a plain envelope without the agency's return address.

6. **Complaints about violations of privacy.** Patients can file a complaint if they think their privacy has been violated. The Notice of Privacy Practices tells them how to contact the privacy officer, as well as how to file the complaint. The Notice also provides information on how to contact the Department of Health and Human Services (DHHS), the federal oversight agency for HIPAA. If a patient is not satisfied with the outcome of filing a complaint with the facility's privacy officer, he or she may choose to contact DHHS. If DHHS determines there is reason to investigate, it will do so and impose a fine on the covered entity if it has violated HIPAA law.

7. **Minimum necessary rule.** This rule assists you in making an on-the-spot decision about how much patient PHI you need to divulge. For example, if you are ordering a special bed for a patient, you will need to include the patient's height and weight. You will usually have no reason to include diagnosis, among other information.

8. **Telephone requests for PHI.** Nurses are often faced with telephone inquiries about a patient. It is difficult to identify who is really making the inquiry and for what purpose. Ecker (2003) states the following:

   "HIPAA suggests that whenever a caller asks for a patient, the provider can verify whether that person is in the hospital, but only if the caller asks for the patient by name. If the caller asks for specific information about the patient, the new guidelines recommend that only minimal information about general status be communicated. The caller should be directed to speak to the patient or family for further details.

   Exceptions to this rule include clergy who ask for all people of a certain faith or a patient who requests anonymity on admission. A parent, for example, may request anonymity regarding his or her child's hospitalization when there is concern of the child being abducted by the other parent."

9. **Email and faxes.** To reduce the possibility of error during electronic transfer of information, the "minimum necessary" rule applies. Perhaps you have experienced sending an email or fax to the wrong person. Think about the possible consequences of this happening with PHI. One safety feature is a disclaimer on an email or fax that identifies the mail as confidential and explains how to notify the sender in case of error.

? **Critical Thinking**

Medical Records

Think of one or more reasons why if a patient removes or changes information in a medical record, it can affect a pending legal case.

Box 7-15   **Additional Concerns Not Addressed by HIPAA***

- PHI not meant for the chart includes daily patient assignments, nurse's personal notes about the patient (used as the basis for charting), and anything else that could identify the patient that is crumpled up and thrown in the wastebasket at the end of the shift. Many facilities have dealt with this by identifying a specific disposal area where the notes ultimately get shredded.
- Hallway conversation remains a problem. For example, a conversation about a patient might not be overheard by the patient involved but is often overheard by other patients or visitors. The same is true with conversation in lunchrooms, nursing desk areas, waiting rooms, and elevators.

Concerns That the Health Insurance Portability and Accountability Act Does Not Address

Additional concerns that the HIPAA does not address include discarding PHI that is not meant for the patient's chart and hallway conversations (Box 7-15).

◎ Try This

Maintain Patient Confidentiality

Keep confidential the conversations you overhear in the clinical area that include personal information about a patient and those that include more than the "minimum necessary" about a patient. List one time that you were trapped into providing confidential information to an unauthorized person about a patient.

Expect to find differences in interpretation of the HIPAA law. Find a copy of the facility privacy policy during each clinical rotation, and do the same with each job you have after graduation. Note the differences and adjust to them. Question your employer if you do not understand why the differences exist. Seek to understand how the differences still meet HIPAA requirements.

PATIENT COMPETENCY

You can expect to hear increased use of the term *competency* in both a legal and a clinical sense. The following details provide a brief framework to help you use this term correctly.

Patient competency has both a legal meaning and a clinical meaning. Some patients' rights issues are based on proof of competence or incompetence within the court system. *Legal* competency refers to a patient who is:

- Eighteen years old or older.
- A pregnant or married woman.
- A self-supporting minor (referred to as a legally emancipated minor).
- Competent in the eyes of the law (incompetence is determined by the court).

Clinical competency refers to a patient who is able to do the following:

- Identify the problem for which he or she is seeing the physician.
- Understand the options for care and the possible consequences.
- Make a decision.
- Provide sound reasons for the option he or she chooses.

PATIENT'S RIGHT TO CONSENT

The patient's right to consent to or refuse treatment is a significant example of patient autonomy (right to choose). It is advisable for a patient to be accompanied by someone he or she trusts whenever he or she goes to a health agency for care. Patients are often stressed to the point that they do not "hear" what is being said to them. Words such as "cancer" and "heart attack" can cause sheer terror. Furthermore, some patients still are afraid to question the physician and therefore agree to procedures that they do not understand: "whatever you think is best" is a frequent response.

General (Implied) Consent

General (implied) consent for treatment is obtained on admission. It may be obtained by the LPN/LVN or by an admission clerk during a routine admission. The fact that a person has voluntarily sought admission to a health care agency and willingly signs a general admission form is an example of general consent. A patient may revoke this permission verbally or in writing (e.g., you walk into a patient's room with a syringe and explain that the doctor has ordered Demerol for pain relief; the patient might say, "I don't want a shot; I'm going home"). Institutional policy and procedure will confirm if the LPN/LVN can obtain general consent.

? Critical Thinking

Resolve Consent Issues

What steps will you take in the case of a patient refusing to be turned every two hours?

Informed Consent

Informed consent must be obtained for invasive procedures ordered for therapeutic or diagnostic purposes (e.g., surgery). Informed consent means that the patient is told the following in nonmedical language:

1. Diagnosis or suspected diagnosis
2. Purpose and description of treatment (some surgeons send the patient home with a video or provide instructions to access a web site that shows the surgery being performed before asking them to sign a consent form)
3. Expected outcome, expected benefits, and possible side effects or complications

4. Explanation of alternative treatments and their benefits, possible side effects, or complications
5. Names and qualifications of the people who will perform the procedure (treatment)
6. Prognosis if treatment is not done (when known)
7. Answers to questions patient wants clarified
8. Explanation that the patient has the right to revoke written permission at any time

The patient must indicate comprehension (understanding) of the information. This means considerably more than just nodding the head. For example, have the patient explain in his or her own words what he or she thinks is going to happen and the benefits and risks involved. Document the patient's understanding of the information.

Informed consent is the responsibility of the physician because he or she must explain the implications and complications of the procedure to the patient before written permission is obtained. *It is never the responsibility of the LPN/LVN.* If you are in the room when the physician is obtaining informed consent, you might be asked to witness the signing. Sullivan (1998) explains:

> "Being asked to witness a patient's signature on a consent form is no small responsibility. Your signature attests to three things: that the patient gave his consent voluntarily, that his signature is authentic, and that he appears to be competent to give consent."

If the LPN/LVN is present when the treatment is being explained and the informed consent signed, in most states the LPN/LVN may support the teaching that has taken place by the physician. Be sure to check your state's NPA and employer's policy.

Authorized Consent

Parents cannot give informed consent for the treatment of their children, but they can authorize treatment for their children up to a certain age; this is called **authorized consent**. Courts of law recognize that parents generally authorize what is appropriate for their children. In most states, "minor" is defined as younger than age 18. Some states allow minors to give their own consent for treatment of substance abuse, mental health problems, and sexually transmitted diseases (STDs). Emancipated minors (legal mechanism) are defined as those living on their own and managing their own finances or who are married and have children. They are competent to give their consent.

END-OF-LIFE ISSUES

PATIENT SELF-DETERMINATION ACT

The **Patient Self-Determination Act (PSDA)** (ACS, 2015) is an amendment to the Omnibus Budget Reconciliation Act (a federal law). The PSDA requires many Medicare and Medicaid providers (e.g., hospitals, nursing homes, hospice programs, home health agencies, and health maintenance organizations [HMOs]) to give adult individuals, at the time of inpatient admission, certain information about their rights under state laws governing **advance directives**, including the following:

- The right to participate in and direct their own health care decisions
- The right to accept or refuse medical or surgical treatment
- The right to prepare an advance directive
- Information on the provider's policies that govern the utilization of these rights.

ADVANCE DIRECTIVES

Two types of written advance directives are available to patients giving direction to health care providers about treatment choices in certain circumstances. The two types of advance directives are a living will and a durable power of attorney for health care. A good advance directive describes the kind of treatment that is desired by the person depending on how sick he or she is. Usually the advance directive indicates what type of treatment is not desired. However, it can indicate that the person wants all possible measures used to prolong life. Information on advance directives can be found at MedlinePlus at www.nlm.nih.gov/medlineplus/advancedirectives.html.

Living Will

A **living will** is a legal document that describes the kind of medical treatments or life-sustaining treatments the person would want if seriously or terminally ill. There are many issues that can be addressed, including the following:

- Transfusion of blood or blood products
- Cardiopulmonary resuscitation (CPR)
- Diagnostic tests
- Administration of drugs
- Tissue or organ donations
- Dialysis
- Use of respirator
- Tube feeding
- Surgery
- Hydration, pain medication, food, and other comfort measures.

A living will does not let the person select someone to make decisions for them. An attorney is not required to draft a living will. The living will is filled out by the individual and witnessed by a person who will not benefit by the death of that individual.

Living wills are recognized as legal documents in most states in the United States, the District of Columbia, and Guam. A few states do not recognize a living will as binding. The individual generally is advised to give a witnessed copy to the health care provider and a trusted friend or relation and to keep one copy in a location that is easily accessible. If a person is moving to or spending time in another state, he or she is advised to determine whether or not the living will is considered legal in that state. Otherwise, the person may discover too late that the written directive may not be honored. Blank forms are available from hospitals, other health care agencies, age-related organizations such as the American Association of Retired Persons (AARP), and attorneys' offices. Living wills can be revoked in writing or orally.

Durable Medical Power of Attorney (Advanced Health Care Directive)

A **durable medical power of attorney** (DPOA) is a legal document that is valid in all 50 states. It names a health care proxy (anyone at least 18 years old) to make medical decisions if that person is no longer able to speak for himself or herself. The DPOA is generally more useful than a living will. It becomes active anytime the person is unconscious or unable to make a medical decision. The DPOA may not be a good choice if the person has no one he or she trusts to make these decisions. There are some differences in various states; for example, the title of the document (AARP, 2015).

⊚ Try This

Legal Directives

Discuss the difference between a durable medical power of attorney and a living will.

DO-NOT-RESUSCITATE ORDER

A **do-not-resuscitate (DNR)** order is an advance directive based on the Patient Self-Determination Act that gives a physician legal permission to write such an order. The physician may also write a DNR order for a patient who no longer has decision-making ability but does not have personal advance directives written and signed. Commonly called a "no-code" order, it is a legal order to not resuscitate a patient. The DNR order does not have to be updated unless the patient changes her or his mind. If a written DNR order does not exist and the nurse does not try to resuscitate the patient, the nurse is in effect making a medical decision. The nurse is essentially practicing medicine without a license and may be subject to a lawsuit. In addition, occasionally you may hear terms used such as "partial" or "slow" code. Generally, these terms may not be legal and are viewed as unethical. All caregivers must know when a written DNR order exists. Check your state and agency policies regarding DNR orders because they vary considerably among states.

Sometimes providers ignore patient advance directives. The patient's instructions may be too vague, or the physician might assume that the patient did not know about an available treatment, or simply defers to the wishes of family members. Sometimes patients have not discussed advance directives with their physician, or a facility has a policy that a written physician's order of DNR must be in the chart to comply with the patient's wish. A survey by the California Health Care Foundation (2012) showed that only 7% of the respondents had spoken to their provider regarding end of life wishes, despite the fact that 80% wanted to have a conversation. In the same survey, only 23% had put their end of life wishes in writing. Thus end of life dilemmas will occur in your practice. For your legal protection, find out about your state's and facility's policies and if the patient has a written advance directive of which the physician is aware. Do-not-hospitalize (DNH) orders may be more effective than DNR orders in limiting treatment and preventing unnecessary or unwanted patient transfer *from* long term care *to* an acute treatment facility. Most important for you, as an LPN/LVN, is to know your agency's policy. The Conversation Project provides a wealth of resources to assist people in having end of life conversations. More information can be found at http://theconversationproject.org

REMOVAL OF LIFE SUPPORT SYSTEMS

The physician must pronounce the patient dead and document this status before the nurse turns off a ventilator. In many states the RN can also pronounce the patient dead; however, this is beyond the scope of practice for the LPN/LVN. If the nurse removes a life support system before the physician pronounces the patient dead, it can be considered an act of murder.

PHYSICIAN-ASSISTED SUICIDE AND EUTHANASIA

Physician-assisted suicide (PAS) and **euthanasia** are not the same. "Physician-assisted suicide refers to a physician providing the means for death, most often with a prescription. The patient, not the physician, will ultimately administer the lethal medication. Euthanasia generally means that the physician would act directly (for instance, by giving a lethal injection) to end a patient's life" (Starks, Dudzinski & White, 2013).

Both are different from the DNR order that a physician writes based on an agreement the physician makes with the patient or the patient's family. A DNR order is a passive action, with the goal of avoiding prolonging life unnecessarily, not actively ending it. Table 7-2 provides a comparison of active and passive euthanasia.

The following practices are also different from PAS:
- Terminal sedation that refers to sedating terminally ill persons to the point of unconsciousness and allowing them to die. If the person has made the decision to refuse further treatment, the law and medical profession respect this.
- The practice of administering pain medication that may hasten death and relieve suffering for a

Table 7-2	Active and Passive Euthanasia
ACTIVE (actions that speed the process of dying)	**PASSIVE** (do nothing to preserve life)
Actively end a person's life	Avoid prolonging a person's life
Initiate the dying process	Allow to continue a process that causes death
Morally wrong	Morally permissible
Legally not allowed	Legally allowed
Forbidden by professional organizations	Approved by professional organizations

Try This

Terminally Ill Patients

Divide into three groups. Choose a viewpoint about the terminally ill from the following descriptions. Be prepared to present reasons for the viewpoint. Choose a spokesperson to summarize the group's views.

- Group 1: Terminally ill patients have the right to choose death by physician-assisted suicide.
- Group 2: Terminally ill patients must wait to die of natural causes.
- Group 3: The nurse's personal ethics conflict with the decision of groups 1 and 2. Discuss the nurse's rights, roles, and responsibilities to the patient.

Refer to the critical thinking steps in Chapter 5 to assist you in making your decision.

terminally ill person has been held justifiable by courts (as long as the intent is to relieve suffering).

- The ANA (2013) position statement, *Euthanasia, Assisted Suicide, and Aid in Dying* states, "The ANA recognizes that assisted suicide and euthanasia continue to be debated. Despite philosophical and legal arguments in favor of assisted suicide it is the position of the ANA as specified in the Code that nurses' participation in assisted suicide and euthanasia is strictly prohibited."

There is continual draft legislation regarding these controversial topics. Be sure to keep abreast of the changes in your state. This information is often posted on your state board of nursing website.

Oregon Death with Dignity Act

The **Oregon Death with Dignity Act** allows terminally ill Oregonians to end their lives through the voluntary self-administration of lethal medications that are expressly prescribed by a physician for that purpose. Death with Dignity Act information is available at http://public.health.oregon.gov/ProviderPartner Resources/EvaluationResearch/DeathwithDignity Act/Pages/index.aspx. The Death with Dignity Act legalizes physician-assisted suicide but specifically prohibits euthanasia; see www.deathwithdignity.org. Only six places in the world openly and legally authorize active assistance in dying patients:

- Oregon (since 1997, physician-assisted suicide only)
- Washington State (since 2009)
- Vermont (2013)
- Montana (not illegal because of Supreme Court ruling)
- Switzerland (1941, physician-assisted and non-physician-assisted suicide only)
- Belgium (2002, permits "euthanasia" but does not define the method)
- Netherlands (voluntary euthanasia and physician-assisted suicide since April 2002, but permitted by the courts since 1984)

ORGAN DONATION

Organ donations are voluntary. At this time organs cannot be bought or sold. Although many patients and families give permission for organ donation after death, the demand for organs far exceeds the supply. You may have been asked to agree to personal organ donation when you received/renewed your driver's license. Many states participate in this effort. To increase the number of donors, it has been suggested that money be allocated to cover the donor's funeral expenses.

Body tissues that can be donated include skin, corneas, bone, heart valves, and blood. One example of a successful body tissue transplant was the transplantation of umbilical cord blood for a rare genetic bone disease at the University of Minnesota in Duluth in 1995. Approximately one cup of blood, taken from a newborn's discarded umbilical cord and placenta, was donated. Donated body organs include the heart, liver, kidneys, lungs, and pancreas. Organ donation has raised both ethical and legal questions in some instances; for example, having a baby so that select organs or body tissues can be used to save a sibling.

END-OF-LIFE CARE

Many organizations and projects are devoted to establishing **end-of-life (EOL) principles**. Numerous organizations, including the American Medical Association, TJC, National Hospice and Palliative Care Organization (NHPCO), and the National Association for Home Care and Hospice (NAHC) have adopted or support core principles for end-of-life care. The NHCPO describes hospice as focusing on caring, not curing when patients face a life limiting illness (see http://www.nhpco.org/about/hospice-care for more details). The Center to Advance Palliative Care defines palliative care as "specialized care for people with serious illness" (see https://www.nahc.org/assets/1/7/NAHCPCWhitePaper.pdf for details). Palliative care can be provided aside curative procedures. Palliative care and hospice care are common care modalities today. LPNs/LVNs are employed in home care and hospice units where this care is provided.

The National Association for Home Care and Hospice provide related resources at their website www.nahc.org/haa/consumer-information.

GOOD SAMARITAN ACT

The **Good Samaritan Act** stipulates that a person who renders emergency care in good faith at the scene of an accident is immune from civil liability for his or her action while providing the care. Details of each state's Good Samaritan laws vary. The state statutes are of particular interest to nurses and physicians who provide emergency care when they are not in their employment setting. Check with your state's board of nursing or agency risk manager for information about your state's Good Samaritan laws. For example, in some states a nurse has a choice of whether or not to give aid to someone during an emergency outside of a health care setting. A few states obligate health care professionals to assist at a scene of an accident requiring medical help. If, for instance, you provide pressure to stop severe bleeding and the patient develops complications, you will not be held responsible as long as you acted without gross negligence. The law also permits the nurse to give aid to a minor at a sports event or accident scene before getting authorized consent from the parents. The LPN/LVN must have permission to treat the person, and verbal permission must be obtained from the victim. The person has the right to refuse. Once first aid is initiated, the nurse is obligated to continue until the victim can be turned over to someone with comparable or better training (Christensen and Kockrow, 2011).

◎ Try This

Good Samaritan Act

Explain the protection that your state's Good Samaritan Act provides for the LPN/LVN.

Get Ready for the NCLEX-PN® Examination

Key Points

- The state's NPA is the most definitive legal statute or legislative act regulating nursing practice. It governs what you can and cannot do as a nurse.
- Student nurses are held to the standard of an LPN/LVN, working under the supervision of the clinical instructor.
- Basic terminology in the NPA is standard in many states; however, scope of practice differs.
- Eight general categories of disciplinary action by the board of nursing include fraud and deceit, criminal activity, negligence, incompetence, violation of the NPA or rules, disciplinary action by another board, unethical conduct, and alcohol and/or other drug use.
- Disciplinary action is based on rules of law. If guilty, the board may issue a public or private reprimand, such as probation, nonrenewal of license, suspension of license, revocation of license, or instruction to enter into a voluntary diversion rehabilitation program if the issue is alcohol and/or other drugs.
- After successful completion of the NCLEX-PN® examination, the LPN/LVN may practice in the state of licensure. Some other states accept licensure through interstate endorsement or the Nurse Licensure Compact.
- The nursing standard of care is what an ordinary, prudent nurse with similar education and experience would do in a similar situation.
- Ethics deals with rules of conduct; law provides regulations that control the practice of nursing.
- Common law is judge-made law that is useful in settling disputes such as tort law.
- The legislative branch of the state and federal government develops statutory law: The NPA is a statutory law.

- Civil action is related to individual rights; criminal action involves persons and society as a whole.
- Tort law has to do with a wrong or injury to someone that violates his or her rights.
- Intentional torts involve intended harm by the nurse, such as assault and battery; false imprisonment and use of restraints; defamation; and physical and emotional abuse.
- Unintentional torts mean no harm was intended by the nurse (e.g., professional negligence [malpractice]).
- Elements necessary for negligence are duty, breach of duty, damages, and proximate cause.
- Personal liability holds us responsible for our behavior, including negligent behavior.
- Depositions are used to gather information under oath.
- When giving testimony, take your time; say "yes" or "no" when possible, *without adding details*; stick to the facts; and correct mistakes and misconceptions.
- Documentation is a legal expectation in nursing regardless of the method used. If it was not charted, it was not done or it did not happen.
- Medication errors are among the most common errors related to nursing liability.
- Patient competency has both a legal and a clinical definition.
- A patient's right to consent is general, informed, or authorized, depending on the situation.
- Patient rights include *The Patient Care Partnership: Understanding Expectations, Rights, and Responsibilities;* the HIPAA Privacy Rule; and the Patient Self-Determination Act.
- The Patient Self-Determination Act includes advance directives (living will and durable power of medical

attorney), written and signed by a patient to state his or her wishes for end-of-life care.

- DNR orders written by a physician are legal orders to not resuscitate a patient and are made possible because of the Patient Self-Determination Act.
- Nurses may not remove a life support system until a patient is declared dead by the physician, or RN where allowed.
- Physician-assisted suicide involves a patient voluntarily ending his or her life by self-administering lethal medication prescribed by a physician, especially for that purpose. In the United States this is legal in Oregon, Washington State, and Vermont.
- Active euthanasia entails physicians directly administering a lethal medication to end a patient's life. This is not legal in the United States or Canada.
- The ANA and AMA oppose nurse or physician participation in assisted suicide.
- Organ donation has cultural, religious, legal, and ethical constraints. In the United States, you can note on your driver's license if you wish to donate your organs.
- Good Samaritan Acts hold that a person who gives emergency care in good faith at the scene of an accident is immune from being successfully sued. Some states have laws that make it mandatory to assist at the scene of an accident. A victim has the right to refuse aid.
- Incident reports should be legible, factual, specific, objective, and not worded to place blame.

Additional Learning Resources

evolve Go to your Evolve website (http://evolve.elsevier.com/Knecht/success) for the following FREE learning resources:

- Answers to Critical Thinking Scenarios
- Additional learning activities
- Additional Review Questions for the NCLEX-PN® exam
- Helpful phrases for communicating in Spanish and more!

Review Questions for the NCLEX-PN® Examination

1. Which of the following is your legal guideline for all you can do as an LPN/LVN?
   a. Institutional policy and procedure
   b. State NPA
   c. Employee handbook
   d. School of nursing
2. Which situation most clearly illustrates negligence?
   a. The nurse became angry when the patient would not stop screaming and slapped the patient's face.
   b. The nurse inserted the urinary catheter, despite the patient's refusal, because their bladder was visibly distended.
   c. The nurse decided to restrain an elderly female patient to prevent her from falling out of bed.
   d. The nurse forgot to lower the patient's bed after completing colostomy care, and the patient fell when he tried to get out of bed.

3. A student nurse is assigned to a drug and alcohol rehabilitation unit. The preceptor recommends that the two students review several charts to compare various treatment strategies. While reviewing, the student nurse realizes that one of the charts is her ex-husband's chart. She did not know he was admitted to this institution. However, he is the father of her children and they are on friendly terms. She decides to go visit him before she leaves for the day. This action is:
   a. Permissible as long as you do not look at his confidential records.
   b. A violation of the Affordable Care Act.
   c. A violation of HIPAA.
   d. Unacceptable because he is father of your children.
4. How should you answer the lawyer's questions when asked to give testimony during a legal action?
   a. Offer to tell what you believe really happened when the wrong medication was given.
   b. Avoid referring to any documents to show how well you recall the incident.
   c. Fill in silences with information about the physician who ordered the medication.
   d. Be specific, answering "yes" or "no" whenever possible, without adding details.

Alternate Format Item

1. Which of the following are legal patients' rights? (Select all that apply.)
   a. The right to revoke a signed informed consent verbally on the way to surgery.
   b. The right to take their medical records with them when they leave the hospital.
   c. The right to designate who will make decisions for them should they become incapable.
   d. The right to ask their physician to inject them with lethal drugs that will end life.
   e. The right to file a suit for injury that they see as being the result of negligence.
2. Which of the following are needed to prove negligence? (Select all that apply.)
   a. Deposition
   b. NPA
   c. Duty
   d. Proximate cause
   e. Damages

Critical Thinking Scenarios

Scenario 1

You walk in the day room on a psychiatric unit and there is a patient on the floor, profusely bleeding from the facial area. A nursing assistant indicates that another patient hit the injured patient. Two other patients contradict this statement and state, "the nursing assistant pushed the patient when she would not start walking back to her room and the patient fell."

You are the LPN in the scenario described. Explain all actions you will immediately implement and all related follow up. Explain your actions/provide rationales.

Scenario 2

Julia, an RN, works nights on the neurology unit in a small private hospital. During the night, George, a patient who had cranial surgery, began to have a great deal of pain. Julia called George's physician and gave her a brief review about George, his surgery, and his recent medications. Julia asked the physician if she could come to the unit to evaluate George's condition. The physician told Julia to give George morphine sulphate. The dose was large, and Julia repeated the order and asked if she really meant the amount she stated. The physician became angry, insisted that Julia immediately give George the dosage instructed and to repeat the dose in an hour, and threatened to lodge a complaint against Julia if she did not follow instructions. Julia gave George the morphine as directed, and George died. Julia was charged with negligence, and at the trial, the physician testified that Julia had never called. What could Julia have done to protect both George and herself?

Effective Communication: Health Care Team, Patients, Faculty and Peers

Objectives

On completing this chapter, you will be able to do the following:

1. Explain how communication strategies affect your everyday practice of nursing.
2. Describe essential characteristics of effective communication.
3. Discuss the difference between one way and two-way communication.
4. Self-evaluate your usual communication style, identifying areas for growth.
5. Discuss various modes of communication, including social media.
6. Discuss potential barriers to therapeutic communication.
7. Discuss how nonverbal and affective communication can support, or cancel the meaning of, verbal communication.
8. List two common differences in male/female communication, supported by evidence.
9. Give an example of a cultural communication difference in the area in which you live.
10. List two common factors related to role change for a hospitalized patient that can create distress, impacting communication.
11. Identify a communication difference for patients in two separate age groups.
12. Compare and contrast ways to resolve conflict depending on the participants and setting.
13. Identify the four steps of situation, background, assessment, and recommendation (SBAR) and give an example of how it can be used for health care team communication.

Key Terms

active listening (ĂK-tĭv)
affective communication (ă-FĔK-tĭv)
belittling (bĕ-LĬT-lĭng)
closed-ended questions (KLOZD-ĔN-dĕd)
commitment (kŏ-MĬT-mĕnt)
communication blocks (kŏm-U-nĭ-kā-shŭn blŏks)
empathy (ĔM-pă-thē)
false reassurance (RĒ-ă-shŭr-ĕns)
feedback (FĒD-băk)
focused questions (FO-kŭsd)
giving advice (GĬV-ĭng ăd-VĪS)
honesty (ŎN-ĭs-tē)
humor (HU-mŏr)
judging
knowledge (NŎL-ĕj)
message (MĔS-ĕj)
nonverbal communication (nŏn-VĔR-băl)

one-way communication (wŏn-wăy)
open-ended questions (O-pĕn ĕn-dĕd)
simple answers
patience (PĀ-shĕnts)
probing (PRO-bĭng)
purpose (PĔR-pŭs)
receiver (rĕ-SĒ-vĕr)
respect (rē-SPĔKT)
self-esteem (SĔLF-ă-STĒM)
sender (SĔN-dĕr)
sensitivity (SĔN-sĭ-TĬV-ĭ-tē)
situation, background, assessment, and recommendation (SBAR)
therapeutic communication (THĔR-ă-pū-tĭk)
trust (trŭst)
two-way communication (TOO-wăy)
verbal communication (VĔR-băl)

Purposeful communication is an integral part of your personal and professional world. Take time to learn, and know that language is powerful, resulting in a positive or negative outcome. This includes verbal and written language. Social media presents new challenges to communication.

Kamy and Hilary are frustrated with their clinical instructor. Kamy states, "She is never consistent. Her communication is confusing. We are never sure what is really expected until we are reprimanded for not meeting the clinical objectives. I wish she could be more like Professor Shelly." Hilary agrees, stating, "Professor Shelly is tough and has high expectations; however, her communication is clear. Anytime I have been confused, she paraphrases and then asks a focus question. This helps me clarify my thinking. She then listens to my plan of care, summarizing as needed, to be sure that I know the plan of care before entering the room. This really decreases my anxiety and improves my learning. I think Professor Shelly should teach the entire faculty how to communicate. Our lives would be much easier!" As you read this chapter think about why Professor Shelly's communication was so effective. How can you implement similar strategies in your professional and personal life to improve your communication?

COMMUNICATION PROCESS

Sara walked into a patient's room without knocking on the door. "I'm going to measure your blood pressure. Give me your arm," she said. The patient gave her a quizzical look, but he put out his arm. This was Sara's first contact with the patient. When she finally got the cuff on, her face was flushed, and her own heart was beating so hard that she could not hear the patient's heartbeat.

◎ **Try This**

Communicating with Your Patient

1. What kind of communication did Sara engage in with the patient?
2. Who was Sara's focus?
3. What steps did Sara skip that resulted in showing disrespect for the patient?

Sara engaged in **one-way communication**, in which the **sender** (Sara) controlled the situation by telling the **receiver** (patient) what she was going to do (the **message**). Sara offered no opportunity for **feedback** (response) from the patient. Feedback would have provided the patient an opportunity to question, agree, or refuse the procedure. Sara was so focused on herself that she omitted common courtesies: a knock on the door, addressing the patient by name, and introducing herself, her position, and reason for being there. Best practice requires using two patient identifiers to ensure safe practice. Sara created an unsafe environment by not using two patient identifiers when engaging in the interaction. The patient's unspoken response may have increased Sara's discomfort.

ONE-WAY VERSUS TWO-WAY COMMUNICATION

One-way communication is used to give a command, as in military service, or information with no expectation of feedback. There are rare occasions when one-way communication is acceptable. An imminent or real disaster could be an example. Even during an urgent patient situation, two-way communication generally creates a safer environment. A doctor's oral order is repeated by the nurse, thus verified for accuracy. **Two-way communication** is the usual form of conversation. Each person contributes equally, and feedback is both expected and respected.

ESSENTIAL COMPONENTS OF THE COMMUNICATION PROCESS

There are five essential components to effective communication (Cherry and Jacob, 2014):

1. Source/sender
2. Message
3. Method of transmission
4. Receiver
5. Feedback.

All five components are required for effective communication. In Figure 8-1 you can see that communication is a circular process. Feedback is received by the sender, which often triggers the sender to send another message, prompting the receiver to give additional

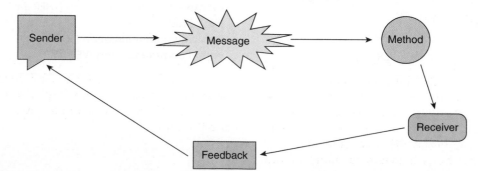

FIGURE 8-1 Communication. (From Cherry, B., & Jacob, S. [2014]. *Contemporary nursing: Issues, trends, and management* [ed 6]. St. Louis: Mosby.)

feedback. The circle of communication continues. There are multiple factors that can affect communication at any point in the process. A discussion of those factors follows.

FACTORS THAT AFFECT COMMUNICATION

Some common factors that can influence communication include the following:

1. Personal characteristics of both the sender and receiver
2. Cultural characteristics
3. Situational influences
4. Context in which the message is sent and received.

Personal characteristics can include such things as age, gender, income, and marital status. Life experiences, attitude, personal opinions and bias are other personal characteristics. *Cultural characteristics* can involve personal space and distance, language and dialect, use and meaning of touch, values, meaning of gestures, and time of day. *Situational influences,* sometimes referred to as *noise,* can include the physical and emotional state of the patient and nurse, the room temperature, interruptions, background noises, odors, and environmental distractions. *Context* can include the appropriateness or inappropriateness of the communication. "What can I do to make you more comfortable?" is an appropriate question directed to a dying patient. Discussion by the family about who gets what after the patient dies, within earshot of the patient, is inappropriate communication. As a student it is easy to forget context as you are focused on your own learning. Be sure to stop and think before you speak.

TYPES OF COMMUNICATION

The three types of communication are **verbal** (spoken or written word), **nonverbal** (body language), and **affective** (feeling tone). They may or may not all occur at the same time. When they do occur together, all three must mirror one another (be congruent) for the communication to be honest. This is the ideal but often does not occur. We frequently send mixed messages. For example, your patient has diarrhea and is incontinent for the third time that evening. They apologize to you. You state, "No problem," however the patient notes a sense of frustration in your voice. As a result, they feel more embarrassed and depressed.

VERBAL COMMUNICATION

The spoken word is powerful. A patient may accept what you say as an absolute fact, clear evidence. Know in advance what you can or cannot discuss with a patient and when you should refer to an established fact (evidence). Sometimes your response will be: "I do not know, but I will find someone who does." Evidence provides answers to many of our patient's questions. Be sure to use a valid source when answering patient's questions. Collaborate

with the Registered Nurse (RN) to ensure communication is accurate and appropriate.

Speak as clearly as possible, using proper grammar. Slang is usually not appropriate and may have a different meaning to different people. Depending on age and culture, the patient may not understand slang. Using out-of-date slang also can make you come across as unprofessional or silly, or worse yet, the slang word may be considered no longer culturally acceptable.

Medical jargon is rarely helpful. If you truly understand the medical terms, you can translate the words into everyday language. The use of colloquial (common) expressions will be appropriate with some patients. For example, the word "urinate" may be understood by some as pass water, tinkle, or pee-pee. Use the word that the patient understands. Remember that the patient needs a professional he or she can look up to and one who will respect his or her individual differences; the patient does not need the nurse to be a buddy.

Maintain professional boundaries. A patient will respect you and is more likely to follow the directions you are giving than if you are trying to be "familiar" with him or her. Be careful about your conversation with colleagues when caring for your patient. The focus is on the patient not your child's crisis at school or an argument with your classmate.

Some illnesses also affect a patient's interpretation of verbalization. Patients with neurological disorders can experience diverse communication issues. Both expressive and receptive aphasia can occur. Expressive aphasia will contribute to the patient's difficulty finding and saying the right word, phrase, or sentence. They will have great difficulty sending a message. Receptive aphasia can prohibit the patient from understanding the spoken word. Thus their ability to receive a message is adversely impacted. They may be completely unable to understand the message sent. Patients with Alzheimer disease also experience communication issues caused by memory impairment. Patients diagnosed with schizophrenia interpret words concretely (literally). They experience difficulty with abstract (inferred) meanings. For example, after using a stationary bicycle, a patient was asked by the nurse, "How do you feel now?" He grabbed his buttocks and responded, "My butt is numb; that's how." The nurse had been trying to determine change in his stress level. Instead, his response was based on literal interpretation of the question.

As you can see, communication will be a challenge in many patient care settings. Well-developed communication strategies and the ability to try multiple approaches will enhance communication with the patient and their family.

NONVERBAL COMMUNICATION

Commonly known as body language, nonverbal communication either supports or cancels out verbal communication. Expressions, posture, movements, and gestures, whether they are your own or the patient's, give important clues to the truth of the verbalization. Careful observation of body language may clue you in to patient discomfort, even though pain has been denied verbally. Gathering additional data will help clarify the real issue creating the discomfort. Use of Telehealth and social media communication modalities, can further limit nonverbal communication, eliminating this potential piece of data. Be sure to implement all strategies to ensure a minimal impact to nonverbal behavior.

Verbal communication works both ways. Patients tend to observe you closely as well; looking for clues regarding the seriousness of their illness. For example, a patient carefully watching you review results of his diagnostic tests may conclude erroneously that he is acutely ill, because of a distressed look on your face. How is he to know that you just received a text from your child's school informing you of a verbal altercation involving your son?

Physical appearance is a part of nonverbal communication. The patient's appearance on admission provides signs of personal care plus important clues about the illness. Patients also quickly evaluate you and, based on what you project and even before you speak, will draw conclusions about your competence as a nurse. Arnold and Boggs (2003) explain, "Clothing communicates a nonverbal message about competence and professionalism to a patient, which can influence the nurse-patient relationship." This is a major reason why most nursing schools continue to have a dress code. It is also the reason why your instructors model appropriate dress and behavior for their students.

◉ Try This

Appropriate Dress Code and Behavior

Observe a patient's response to different members of the health care team, based on their dress and behavior. What do you observe?

AFFECTIVE COMMUNICATION

"Affect" refers to mood or emotion. The feeling tone that you pick up on as you approach a person or step into a room is real. For every thought you have, there is a physiologic response in your body. The same is true for the patient and others you encounter. We are made up of energy, so we emit energy. The tendency may be to ignore this level of communication because we cannot see, hear, or read it. Affective communication is as significant as verbal and nonverbal communication. Truly honest communication integrates verbal, nonverbal, and affective communications so they all express the same message.

❓ Critical Thinking

Affective Communication

1. Give an example of a time that you stepped into a room or approached a person and, before anyone spoke a word, experienced a feeling of excitement, happiness, sadness, anger, tension, or some other emotion. What was the outcome?
2. Think of a time when you were angry and tried to hide the feeling. Did anyone pick up on your feeling tone and ask you if you were angry? How did you deal with the question?
3. Give examples of how you try to be congruent (together) verbally, nonverbally, and affectively in your communication. What do you need to improve to achieve more congruency?

COMMUNICATION STRATEGIES

There are many strategies suggested to improve communication skills. Research agrees on some key strategies, such as active listening (Cherry and Jacob, 2014). Effective communication cannot exist without active listening. How do we become and strive to be a great active listener?

ACTIVE LISTENING

Active listening is probably the most important part of communication, particularly **therapeutic** (health-related) **communication**. Key factors in active listening include purpose, disciplined attention, and focus. **Purpose** refers to the health-related reason for gathering data or giving information. *Disciplined attention* means that you do not assume accuracy of information without checking it out. Clarify what you think you understand the patient is saying and ask further questions as needed. This applies both to gathering data and giving health-related information. *Focus* means that all your senses are alert to clues that the patient may be communicating. A common mistake in listening is to listen to the words but not really hear the words (i.e., comprehend [understand] the meaning).

ACTIVE LISTENING BEHAVIORS

The most commonly used active listening behaviors include restating, clarifying, reflecting, paraphrasing, minimal encouraging, remaining silent, summarizing, and validating.

- **Restating** refers to repeating in a slightly different way what the patient has said as in the following example:
  Patient: "My chest hurts. I can't sleep at night."
  Nurse: "You've been unable to sleep at night because of chest pain."
- **Clarifying** is asking a closed-ended question in response to a patient's statement to be sure you understand such as in this example:
  Patient: "My chest hurts."
  Nurse: "Exactly where does your chest hurt?"

- **Reflecting** is putting into words the information you are receiving from the patient at an effective communication level. Here is an example:

  Patient: "I'm sick of seeing doctors and not getting answers."

  Nurse: "You are upset with the lack of answers to your health problems."

- **Paraphrasing** refers to expressing in your own words what you think the patient means; for example:

  Patient: "I don't think I'm being told the truth about my condition."

  Nurse: "You believe you have not received all the important information about your health condition."

- **Minimal encouraging** involves using sounds, words, or short phrases to encourage the patient to continue as in this example:

  Patient: "It just happened so fast . . . "

  Nurse: "Yes . . . go on . . . and then what . . . hmmm . . . uh huh . . . "

- **Remaining silent** involves using pauses effectively. The normal tendency is to fill silence with chatter or your speculation. This may cause the patient to "turn off" or change the story. Maintaining disciplined attention and focus during silence lets patients tell the story in their own way. Avoid making interruptions and doing busywork while the patient is speaking. Even five seconds of silence can seem like forever. Practice using silence as a communication strategy.

- **Summarizing** means briefly stating the main data you have gathered such as:

  Nurse: "This is what I heard you say. Is that correct?"

- **Validating** provides the patient with an opportunity to correct information, if necessary, at the time of summary shown in the following example:

  Patient: "That is correct" or *"No, you got this part wrong . . . "* (This allows the patient to correct the information.)

TYPES OF QUESTIONS

The three types of questions that are commonly used in therapeutic communication are open-ended, closed-ended, and focused questions. **Open-ended questions** permit the patient to respond in a way that is most meaningful to him or her. The questions often begin with what, where, when, how, or why. For example, the nurse might ask, "What happened to your leg?" **Closed-ended questions** require a specific answer. For example, the nurse might ask, "When did you first notice the pain?" **Focused questions** provide even more definitive information. For example, the nurse might ask, "On a scale of 1 to 10, with 10 as the worst possible pain, how do you rate your pain right now?"

NURSE-PATIENT COMMUNICATION EVALUATION

Communication is far more complex than just talking. Some of the many contributing characteristics are listed in this section, with a brief description in the following learning exercise. Evaluate the characteristics of your communication that are working for you and those you need to work on.

◎ Try This
Self-Evaluation of Personal Characteristics

CHARACTERISTIC	DESIRABLE	SELF-EVALUATION
Eye contact	Usually 3-5 seconds. Cultural variations exist.	_____
Respect for personal space	Approximately 1.5 feet, except for personal care. Cultural variations exist.	_____
Appropriate touch	Gentle, but firm. Cultural variations exist.	_____
Attitude	Nonjudgmental. Practices unconditional love.	_____
Voice/tone	Moderate or according to growth and development needs. For example, newborns.	_____
Rate	Paced according to patient's ability to comprehend.	_____
Appearance	Models positive nursing image. Looks healthy and ready to deliver high quality care.	_____
Posture	Open, without folded arms or hands on hips. Stands or sits upright to increase confidence.	_____
Gestures	Moderate to enhance conversation. Consistent with conversation.	_____
Language	Speaks effectively and at patient's level of understanding. Correct grammar.	_____
Expression	Congruent with topic. Nonjudgmental.	_____

? Critical Thinking

A Plan for Change

List the personal characteristics that are impacting your communication. Develop a plan for change and measuring improvement, using the phases of the nursing process.

BLOCKS TO COMMUNICATION

Communication blocks occur daily. Often we are not even aware of the impact. Perhaps the patient's visual image, voice, or behaviors trigger a sad thought or biased experience. Workload, stress, and exhaustion can create blocks to effective communication. Imagine it is a snowy night, three people call off and you are literally trying to survive, performing priority tasks only. A patient is silently sobbing and starts talking to you as you are administering medications and you are already beyond the state-allowed time period for safe practice. In addition, the patient reminds you of your whiney mother-in-law. As you can see, multiple blocks are present. It is unlikely, despite the issue, that real communication will occur. As a nurse you want to continue to give every patient the best care possible, regardless of your personal response and the given circumstance. You are not a Magician, however careful planning can minimize communication blocks even in difficult situations. Common **communication blocks** involve false reassuring, probing, judging, belittling, giving advice, providing simple answers, and acting disinterested.

AVOIDING BLOCKS

- "Why" questions can put the patient on the defensive.
- **False reassurance** involves making statements to the patient such as "Everything will be okay," or "You'll be just fine," or "Don't worry about anything," or "We'll make sure you get well," or "This experience will make you stronger," or "You'll see the good in this someday." There is no way you can guarantee what you have just told the patient.
- **Probing** means pushing for information beyond what is medically necessary to know. Curiosity takes over, and the patient's privacy is no longer respected. Ask yourself about the value of the information and how you will use the information once you have it. Think twice before continuing with statements such as "Let's get to the bottom of this once and for all."
- **Judging** patient behavior, such as smoking, is of limited value to the patient with severe emphysema or lung cancer (or perhaps the patient never smoked). Your information is hardly an "alert." You can be sure that she or he has heard the message over and over. Without supporting the behavior, you can continue to be therapeutic to the patient.
- **Belittling** involves mimicking or making fun of the patient in some way. It may include downplaying the importance of the symptoms; for example, "You could be having heart surgery! This is just wart removal." As a physician pointed out, "If you have a tonsillectomy, it's minor surgery; if I have a tonsillectomy, it's major surgery." It is all a matter of perspective.
- **Giving advice** when you know what someone else should do is very tempting. Unsolicited advice is rarely beneficial and closes the door to having the patient solve the problem himself/herself. A more beneficial response, even when the patient asks what you would (or he or she should) do, is "What ideas do *you* have? I'm sure you've thought of ways you might solve this problem." This also gives you an opportunity to review any evidence to assist them with decision making. Listen carefully, summarize what the patient has said, and then support the patient in identifying next steps, suggesting available resources as needed. Since the initiation of the Affordable Care Act in 2010, transitions in care are a critical communication issue. Following the steps outlined above will assist in maintaining the patient's autonomy and providing seamless quality care.
- **Simple answers** such as "Everyone feels this way" come so easily, but they make patients feel dismissed and misunderstood. Patients do not really care if everyone else feels this way. As far as they are concerned, these feelings are theirs, they are different from everybody else's, and they need a comforting touch or reassuring words. If you can, offer something you know you can deliver, such as "I'll be with you the entire time you are having your bone marrow drawn" or "I'll be in the room when you return."
- Acting disinterested with comments such as, "I have several other patients who are very sick tonight, what do you need?" can negatively impact communication, even if it is true. The patient needs to know that their issues are important.

MALE/FEMALE DIFFERENCES

Being equal does not mean being the same. Men and women communicate differently for biological reasons. Although there are examples of similarities between the sexes, most males and females follow certain patterns. According to Sieh and Brentin (1997), four areas that relate to nursing communication are conversation patterns, head movements, smiling, and posture.

CONVERSATION

Men tend to approach a conversation with an eye to maintaining status and independence, to report or to get information, and to provide a solution. They use few words, share less feelings and are analytical in their approach. In contrast, women use conversation to work through a problem. They are sensitive to everyone's feelings and build consensus while working towards a solution. Thus, male opinions are sometimes valued more highly without validation. Women seek to establish intimacy and develop rapport, share feelings, and establish relationships. Men ask fewer questions, but they may readily interrupt during conversations without apology. Women often use questions to encourage conversation. They wait for a pause to seek clarification and apologize for the interruption. Men apologize for a wrong, whereas women say "I'm sorry" to indicate regret, sympathy, or concern. Men rarely say, "I don't know;" women often phrase ideas as questions, such as "Have you thought of . . . ?" Men make demands more often, whereas women express preferences with reasons. Men's sentences are shorter and fewer; women create longer, more complex sentences, linking more ideas together. Men make declarations; whereas women often end a statement with a question, such as "Don't you think so?" (Tannen, 1990; Gray, 1992).

OTHER DIFFERENCES

A rounded posture with the chest in and chin down gives an appearance of being threatened. Standing tall, with shoulders back and head held high, speaks of confidence and control. Confidence is important in therapeutic communication. The patient is in a vulnerable state and needs a confident nurse. Communication can be influenced by confidence. Research has demonstrated a relationship between positive thinking, posture, and confidence (Cuddy, 2012). How the patient perceives your level of confidence could impact communication.

Looking at differences in the way men and women communicate has important implications in working with patients, staff, and instructors. Smiling and nodding by a woman does not have to mean she understands the instructions. A lack of questions from a male patient may not mean he knows what the surgery entails. Gather all three types of communication data. Ask the patient to tell you what he or she understands, then summarize and validate. *Use the skills you are learning* to communicate effectively.

◎ Try This

Power Pose

According to Cuddy (2012) a power pose can boost self-confidence. Visit https://www.ted.com/talks/amy_cuddy_your_body_language_shapes_who_you_are and discover how to improve your confidence resulting in more effective communication.

CULTURAL DIFFERENCES

Members of diverse cultures within our dominant culture embrace and value their beliefs and practices. You need to be respectful of these beliefs and practices and respond therapeutically. Know about cultural differences in communication. Individual patient differences need to be identified. Be sure to read Chapter 10 for a more complete understanding of cultural diversity. Mark the chapter and use it as a reference for the Learning Exercise.

◎ Try This

Cultural Differences

List and discuss two cultural differences of someone in the area in which you live that could impact communication.

1. _____
2. _____

Communication patterns change with time, vary with the situation, and differ in public or private settings. Learn as much as possible about the cultures frequently served where you work. Be mindful also that families may have been in this country for generations, and differences may be nonexistent regardless of ethnic background.

ROLE CHANGES FOR THE PATIENT

What happens to patients who find themselves in a dependent position after having always been in charge of their lives? The concerns they have go beyond the physical realities into areas we consider in the next section.

❓ Critical Thinking

Immediate Concerns upon Hospitalization

Imagine yourself being hospitalized. List four immediate concerns you would probably have. Discuss how these concerns relate to your various roles in life.

1. _____
2. _____
3. _____
4. _____

🖐 Professional Pointer

Best practice requires using two patient identifiers (e.g., name and birth date) to ensure safe practice. After the patient states their name, ask the patient what they prefer to be called and address the patient consistently thereafter, as desired. However, always be sure to verify their formal name and utilize two patient identifiers when required.

IT BEGINS WITH "HELLO, MY NAME IS . . . "

Whatever you communicate verbally, nonverbally, and affectively sets the tone for rapport with the patient. You have some preliminary information (a name) even when the patient is just being admitted. Knock on the door; pause briefly to collect data *before* walking in. You begin to pick up nonverbal and affective communication clues. Address the patient as Mr., Mrs., Miss, or Ms., or by a professional title if it applies. Extend your hand (unless culturally improper). Give your name; identify yourself as a student practical nurse/student vocational nurse (SPN/SVN), the name of your school, and your purpose for being in the room.

It may sound something like this "Mrs. Hill, my name is Mr. Fry. I am a student practical nurse from the Middle American Technical College. I am here to measure your blood pressure, pulse, and respiration. It is a part of the admission procedure. Would you please confirm your name and date of birth?" Two patient identifiers are minimum safe practice standards for all patient interactions. The patient may request that you address him or her by his or her first name, but do not assume this without permission. Your hospital or other health agencies may have a policy regarding how employees introduce themselves. This will dictate your actions.

NURSING JARGON

Remember how time consuming it was to learn all those medical terms? Using the terms may sound impressive to you now and involve a feeling of having arrived, but using unfamiliar terminology can increase patient fears and cause misunderstandings, "What does it mean that I will have an IV started, have a WBC stat, and you'll be doing vitals q2h for now?" When you really know something, you can explain words and symbols in terms the average layperson can understand. Now *that's* impressive!

FEAR OF THE UNKNOWN

Patients often have numerous unspoken fears about tests, procedures, and possible outcomes. These include, but are not limited to, pain, sleep, needle sticks, thirst, hunger, and being treated respectfully. A **simple answer** of "Everything will be fine" displays a lack of understanding of the depth of patient fears. Patients may not ask questions because they think it might sound silly or that they are bothering the staff. An open-ended question from you, such as "What questions do you have? If I don't know the answer, I'll try to find out for you," can open the way for expression of fears.

PERSONAL FACTORS

A patient's illness rarely affects the patient alone. Thoughts and concerns may extend to family, work, finances, and so on. For example, the mother of a newly hospitalized child was irritable and inattentive when the nurse was explaining the unit rules. Finally, the nurse stopped midsentence and said to the mother, "Tell me what is troubling you." The mother looked at her and then blurted out that she had another sick child

at home, her husband worked nights and slept days, and she had been up most of the last three nights. "Where should I be? Both kids need me, and my neighbor can only come in for two hours a day. I'm at my wits' end!" The mother could not begin to focus on the unit rules until there were solutions to the problems at home. You may not have a solution, but you can be a catalyst to make needs known to the instructor or assigned nurse. They are aware of additional resources.

ENVIRONMENTAL FACTORS

Health care settings (whether clinics, hospitals, rehabilitation centers, or nursing homes) are very different from home. There is no true opportunity for privacy. A variety of staff show up at different times throughout a 24-hour period; lights are on day and night; the staff make more noise than they realize; machinery is humming, buzzing, or beeping; staff check out different parts of your body, picking and poking; you get the picture. The patient may have put the light on because of a need to go to the bathroom *now*. By the time someone arrives, it may be too late, much to the patient's embarrassment.

Advance communication and planning does not take as long as it sounds. Make sure the patient knows their plan of care and who are their caregivers, including their title and explanation of their role in the patient's care. You may find out that the patient always has a snack of toast and tea at 9 PM, always gets up to go to the bathroom at 11 PM, always has bran cereal and a banana at 6 AM. Notes of this nature in the patient's care plan can assist in the continuity of communication and care.

COMMUNICATING WITH INSTRUCTORS AND STAFF

Good communication involves respect, trust, honesty, empathy, **sensitivity**, humor, knowledge, **patience**, commitment, and self-esteem. These characteristics are equally important in communicating with patients, instructors, and staff.

RESPECT

Respect involves both self-respect and respect for others. You communicate self-respect by doing your best each day. When you treat yourself with self-respect, it becomes easy to extend respect to your instructors, staff, and patients. Patients quickly pick up on whether or not they are being respected during conversation and physical care (e.g., verbal and nonverbal communication, such as eye signals between staff). In-depth personal conversation with peers while delivering care is a sign of disrespect to the patient.

TRUST

Trust begins with confidence in your ability to make decisions. You communicate this to instructors and staff by consistently doing the required preliminary preparation for assignments. This preparation and knowledge, along with the willingness to seek out information when needed, contributes to creating a trusting relationship with the patient.

HONESTY

Honesty implies that you will not deliberately deceive to present yourself in a more favorable light. Arranging a time with the instructor for you to repeat a procedure for more practice is an example of this characteristic in communication.

EMPATHY

Empathy is the ability to understand and appreciate what someone else is feeling without experiencing the emotion itself. When you are sympathetic, as you would be with a family member or dear friend, you actually experience the emotion. Being empathetic permits you to understand how someone is feeling and why he or she feels that way, to maintain control of your emotions, and to think clearly. For example, you might offer to help a staff member who is having a bad day do patient care (a practical intervention), instead of getting pulled into an "Isn't it awful?" conversation.

SENSITIVITY

Tuning in on nonverbal and affective communication helps you to verify verbalization or a lack thereof. Picking up at nonverbal and affective levels permits you to check them out with the staff or instructor: "Is there something else I need to know?"

HUMOR

Healthy **humor** at the patient's level of appreciation can help "lighten up" a situation. Offensive humor and poking fun at the patient or at other cultures or races is unacceptable. The staff sometimes privately gets involved in "gallows humor," which is laughing at something very serious or medically gross. Look for examples in movies and television programs with medical themes or examples observed while at your clinical rotation. Reflect on how these behaviors impact patient care and job satisfaction.

KNOWLEDGE

The cornerstone of gathering data and other health-related communication is **knowledge**. Instructors and staff quickly determine your level of knowledge. Instructors communicate the significance of this characteristic by making assignments early enough for you to research the information. You communicate back to the instructor (and staff) by preparing for patient care.

PATIENCE

In this modern world we are often accustomed to instant results and gratification. It is sometimes difficult to provide the time needed to learn, receive explanations from instructors, or follow staff orders. This extends to our work with patients, in whom illness and growth and development levels dictate the need to slow down or repeat directions. The patient (or you) may be tempted to say "I know" when such is not the case. The characteristic of patience takes time to perfect. You may initially feel like you are moving backward in your communication attempts with patients.

COMMITMENT

Commitment means incorporating all the previous characteristics into your nursing communication practices. Decide that you are in nursing because you really want to be here. Then do the work that needs to be done. It shows, and it pays off. Take time to appreciate the uniqueness of each patient (see Chapter 10).

SELF-ESTEEM, THOUGHTS, AND STRAIGHTFORWARD COMMUNICATION

Self-esteem is earned, not learned. No one can give it to you or take it away! It is that special sense that it is okay to receive credit for something you did well. Self-esteem also gives you permission to recognize that you have something very special to offer in nursing communication; such as being able to communicate effectively with patients and the health care team.

What kinds of thoughts do you have?

- Are they positive or negative when you think about yourself?
- The two basic types of thought are random and active. Random thoughts just show up, but you initiate active thoughts. Random thoughts usually pass through, unless you pick a thought and change it into an active thought.
- What do your active thoughts say about you and the person you are? Do they support your sense of self, or do the thoughts tear you down?
- If your thoughts are not serving you, change them. If you have made a mistake, learn from it and let it go. Do not continue to punish yourself.
- Every day, look for what you have done well and give yourself a cheer for a job well done!
- Compliment your peers for a job well done! It can be contagious.
- Thoughts also set the feeling tone for how you communicate with patients and other staff. How you feel about something creates actions that bring about results.
- Remember as Socrates stated, "The unexamined life is not worth living".

Practice makes your conversation meaningful. Make peace with silence. If you find yourself talking just to fill in the silence, *stop!* Learn to say what you mean. Be direct in your conversation, remembering that language is never innocent. Listen, before you speak. When you give patients information or directions, avoid medical jargon. Being long-winded just means that you do not know how to express yourself clearly. Ask the patient what they think you said as a way to avoid misunderstanding. If you are on the receiving end of a lengthy conversation, remember that you can take control. Check out what it is the person really wants you to know and set a time limit if needed: "I have to go in __ minutes."

"I" MESSAGES

Remember to use "I" messages whenever possible. Self-confidence will assist you in using "I" messages effectively. "I" messages are effective in communication as they allow the receiver time to respond without becoming defensive. Messages that begin with "you" often cause the receiver to become immediately defensive.

◎ Try This

"I" Messages

Discuss how your immediate feelings differ if you received each of the following messages:

"You make me want to scream when you do not answer the patients' call lights immediately."

"I am trying to understand why the call lights are not answered in a timely manner. Can you help me understand what the issue is?"

SITUATION, BACKGROUND, ASSESSMENT, RECOMMENDATION

Nurses are taught to be objective and detailed when providing information. Physicians generally are brief and to the point: They are more interested in the "bottom line." The situation, background, assessment, and recommendation (**SBAR**), was first developed in the military and has been adopted by many health care institutions to facilitate clear communication. For example, if you are calling a physician because of concern about a patient, SBAR can be useful following these guidelines:

- **S.** Situation (about 10 seconds). Identify the following about the situation:
  1. Who you are
  2. Your unit
  3. Patient name and room number
  4. What the problem is (briefly), when it started, and how severe it is.
- **B.** Background
  1. Patient's admitting diagnosis
  2. Date of admission
  3. Information related to current status, such as:
     a. Recent mental status
     b. Vital signs
     c. Oximetry
     d. Oxygen device and flow rate
     e. Current medication
     f. Allergies
     g. Intravenous (IV) fluids, lab results
     h. Code status.

- **A.** Assessment includes the following (collaborate with the RN as needed):
  1. What you think is going on based on the evidence
  2. If appropriate, based on the signs and symptoms, if you believe the problem is life threatening.
- **R.** Recommendation involves what you need from the physician. Terms like "could be" and "might be" are usually effective; for example:
  1. Do you want the physician to come and see the patient?
  2. Do you want the physician to give an order for a medication?
  3. Do you want to transfer the patient to a higher level of care?
  4. Do you need a patient consult with another member of the health care team?

SBAR FOR THE SHIFT REPORT

SBAR is also a useful tool for the shift report, reporting off when you leave the clinical unit, or transferring a patient to another unit. The process will have some differences, such as the following:

Situation: Include the admission date, chief complaint, and diagnosis.

Background:
1. Patient's medical and social history
2. Allergy status
3. Code status
4. If patient is in isolation
5. Pain management strategies and response to interventions
6. Imaging studies
7. Lab results
8. Location of peripheral or central venous line access devices.

Assessment: Provide relevant information in a systematic manner using a systems approach (collaboration with RN as needed).
1. Vital signs and range of vital signs since admission
2. Pain assessment and patient's pain goal
3. If patient has diabetes, how frequently monitored and readings since admission
4. Diagnostic studies and results
5. If patient needs turning or other therapeutic/preventative measures, how often and whether patient can turn self
6. Fall risk if it applies and any other precautions specific to this patient.
7. Medications prescribed and patient response

Recommendations:
1. The patient's goals of care
2. What needs to be done on the next shift
3. Any procedures that must be done
4. Patient's education and discharge needs.

Both the Joint Commission and the Institute for Healthcare Improvement support the use of SBAR in health care facilities.

Using the SBAR Method

Write an example of how you will use the SBAR method with a patient you are assigned to when you are on clinical rotation. Identify differences compared with the way you made reports in the past.

Go to the National Council of State Boards of Nursing website (www.ncsbn.org) and access the Transition to Practice (TTP) Toolkit and the Communication and Teamwork Module (TEAMSTEPPS). Review the I PASS the BATON strategy to improve team communication. Think of a recent clinical scenario when this strategy would have assisted in making your communication complete, brief, clear and timely; ultimately improving patient safety.

LIFE SPAN COMMUNICATION

Growth and development levels, male/female differences, and medical conditions all affect communication with patients. Each age group (whether infant, preschool, school age, teenage, adult, or elderly) has somewhat different communication needs.

INFANTS

Infants' communication includes crying, cooing, and body language. They act out their feelings with total body language. As their recognition of words grows, certain words act to soothe or trigger a reaction. Up to that time, infants are most influenced by the sound of voices. As one father pointed out, "I used to put my baby to sleep each night by rocking her and reading *USA Today* aloud in a soothing voice." Newborns respond favorably to a high-pitched voice, but this changes by the end of the first month; after that, calm, low tones are more soothing.

Parents (caretakers) are the best source for learning the meaning of different cries. They learn quickly to differentiate among wet, hungry, and uncomfortable. Rely on them for specific information on communication style.

PRESCHOOLERS

We are including toddlers in this category as early preschoolers. They are usually known for magnificent tantrums, and it is no wonder: they have learned some words, but when frustrated, they may not be able to put them together effectively. Thus the body acts out what the words cannot tell. Laughing at or trying to reason with the preschooler is counterproductive.

When a child has a tantrum, he or she should be removed from the immediate situation and audience. Once preschoolers are more composed, they can communicate by pointing or by showing on their bodies or in a picture what they are upset about. During procedures, explain briefly and simply what is going to happen. Tell them what they can do to help. For example, preschoolers will often assist and cooperate with receiving injections if they are patiently coached on exactly what to do (e.g., position, what to do with their feet and hands, how long they need to stay still, and what to expect during the injection).

SCHOOL-AGE CHILDREN

The vocabulary of school-age children has increased considerably. They are ready to be a part of most (but not all) discussions with their parents. Drawings or pictures can be used to explain an illness or procedure. Ask for feedback to avoid misconceptions: "Tell me in your own words what . . . ." The child may not be privy to all information. In that case, go with the parent to a separate area so the child will not overhear the conversation or parts of it. Whispering and misinterpretation can evoke new problems.

TEENAGERS

Teenagers can be either the easiest or the most difficult to communicate with, depending on your perspective. When ill, they need to believe that someone knows more than they do, and that someone is in charge. Deal with them with the same courtesy that you extend to adults. Have similar expectations of them. Encourage expression of feelings, fears, and concerns. Their sense that nothing will happen to them has been shaken. Answer questions within your role. Seek out answers as appropriate. Avoid hiding behind nursing jargon. Using teen slang generally does not work out. Without real knowledge of the meaning, you may end up looking foolish instead of "cool."

ADULTS

Many of the issues discussed in this chapter apply to adult communication. Collecting data at all three levels of communication is essential. Remember to limit your questions to areas that are medically or safety (e.g., abuse) related. Pushing and probing based on curiosity may open a Pandora's box (i.e., painful issues that have been suppressed). It does not work to probe and then leave the patient to pick up the pieces of what he or she revealed to you under pressure. If you are concerned about conversation shared by a patient, collaborate with the RN or physician to obtain an appropriate consult.

Patients with diminishing memory seem to have a relatively preserved reading ability. Visual information seems to be more permanent. The health care worker or family member can try writing the information in a size that is easy for the patient to read. Written information seems to be more neutral and does not evoke the emotional reaction that words can have.

GENERATIONAL DIFFERENCES

Be careful to note generational differences that may occur among adult patients. Most importantly, note what mode of communication they use. For example, it is unlikely that Millennials (see Chapter 1) will return phone calls or possibly even e-mails. Their preferred mode of communication is texting. Thus, if a nurse is attempting to contact a Millennial, a phone message may be ineffective. Conversely, a Baby Boomer would probably return a voice mail message and appreciate the phone call.

ELDERS

How do you picture elderly people in your mind? Unresolved parental issues, for example, can get in the way of quality care. If you can see aging as just another part of the life cycle, you will be able to work effectively with elderly patients. Assume that elderly patients can hear and communicate effectively. If your assessment produces different results, then accommodate as needed. As the elderly can tire towards the evening, plan detailed conversations to occur earlier in the day if possible.

Hearing can be impacted as we age. When hearing begins to diminish, it is easier for both men and women to hear lower-frequency sounds. Be sure to assess if hearing loss is present, and as importantly, if it occurs only in one ear, then plan your interactions accordingly.

Communication is essential to ensure a smooth transition in care for the elderly. Preparing for discharge begins on admission. The nurse takes advantage of teachable moments to interject information, demonstrate techniques, and have the patient repeat the demonstrations. Be sure to respect the elderly person's autonomy while carefully evaluating who can assist them in understanding important directions regarding their health care. Always speak directly to the patient, unless the patient requests otherwise. Listen carefully when the patient describes their home environment and available resources. Will adaptive equipment be necessary? Will other health providers have to be involved in making the transition between this facility and home? As a student, be sure to collaborate with your instructor and staff nurses to meet your patient's needs effectively. See the National League for Nursing (NLN) Advancing Care Excellence for Seniors (ACES) information for more information regarding care of the elderly (www.nln.org).

CONFLICT RESOLUTION

In the health setting, conflict can be related to diversity; English as a second language, differences in gender or generation, and personality. Doctors and nurses often provide information in different formats. According to Paolini (2009), "nurses are trained to communicate in narrative form, providing all details about a patient. Physicians are trained to communicate in bullet points, providing key information." Differences can be magnified in high-stress situations. Problems can translate into medication errors, patient safety, and even patient

mortality. Individual or team communication issues can be a sign of a system based issue. Many health facilities and educational institutions have developed educational programs to improve interdisciplinary communication and collaboration. Keep the following basic steps in mind, and try to focus on a mutually beneficial solution based on shared interests.

1. Accept conflict as a natural part of life. Different points of view, needs, and beliefs are often involved.
2. Temper your own attitude and behaviors. Be aware of your initial reaction, and take a deep breath. (Your automatic defense system wants to dig right in and fight.)
3. Take time to think critically before reacting. For example, did you think through beforehand what you were going to report, or did you come off as rambling?
4. Treat conflict as an opportunity to voice your own opinion and listen to the other side of the story. Know that you may have to take the initiative to approach the health care team member regarding what you are seeing as a conflict. They may not be aware of how you are being affected, and ultimately feelings may escalate, job satisfaction will be negatively impacted, and patient care will suffer.
5. Choose your approach. A win-lose approach will only escalate the intensity of the feelings involved. The best choice for a solution depends on the situation. There is no "blanket" correct way. A win-win approach often involves active listening, creative thinking, and compromise.
6. Listen and learn. Conflicts are often based on assumptions and a lack of information. If you did happen to be entirely wrong, apologize, and find out how to correct your mistake in future incidences. Do not dwell on the mistake, move on.
7. Discover what is important; that is, the core issue. It can range from hurt feelings to unmet needs. Getting to the root of the problem assists in resolving the conflict.
8. Respect one another. Conflict can be very emotional. Show respect despite the anger and hurt feelings. Stay away from name calling and blaming. Using "I" statements (for example, "I don't understand what you mean") lets you own your own statements.
9. Find common ground to create the highest common denominator. In this case, it is generally for the patient's highest good (see Chapter 17).

◎ Try This

Resolving Conflicts

Think of a time recently when you experienced a conflict with someone. What was the outcome? Are you still upset with the other person, or was the issue resolved in a mutually beneficial way? What part of your behavior are you especially pleased with? What, if anything, would you do differently the next time?

ELECTRONIC COMMUNICATION

Electronic documentation, including e-mail and texting are valuable modern methods of communication when used effectively and appropriately. Electronic documentation (Electronic Health Record [EHR]) ideally provides a location where all agency professionals involved in patient care enter the most recent information. Electronic documentation will be part of your basic education for learning to document medications and treatments and obtaining patient information. Each facility may have slightly different protocols; however, the underlying concepts are similar. E-mail is a popular way of communicating with administration, within departments, and with other departments. Before getting involved in sending e-mail, review the basics of e-mail etiquette. Some people e-mail things they would never write in a memo or say directly to someone. Box 8-1 lists some e-mail essentials suggested by Lauchman (1999) and Pagana (2008). Lastly, be sure to adhere to the electronic communication policies of your employer. These policies will outline steps to enhance secure communication, thus protecting the patient's and employee's private communication and private information.

CELL PHONES AND TEXT MESSAGING

You are sitting in class or watching a clinical demonstration, when someone's cell phone rings. It certainly disturbs the chain of thought for both the students and the instructor. Although the phone can be set to vibrate, the shuffle to see who called is annoying. Who knows; you may have missed something essential for the care of a future patient.

Text messaging has been integrated into student life with astonishing momentum. Some students continue to text during class, providing a distraction to their peers. An additional concern is that some students are using it as a way to cheat on exams.

Box 8-1	E-mail Etiquette

- Determine whether or not e-mail is the best way to send your message.
- Consider the content of the e-mail message and to whom you are sending it.
- Be sure to use the subject line. People read this first to decide whether the message is worth opening.
- Use effects, such as boldface and underlining to emphasize points.
- Keep your sentences and paragraphs short.
- Skip a line to separate topics.
- Send your message to the right person. Determine if you wish to respond to all or just the sender.
- Be specific. Avoid useless information.
- Avoid using inappropriate language.
- Be cautious with humor. The person sees only the written word.
- Check your spelling and punctuation. Proofread all messages before sending them.
- Avoid typing an entire e-mail in uppercase or "red;" both "scream" at the recipient.
- Use capitalization. Lowercase letters make you look sloppy and lazy.
- Avoid sending confidential information unless the e-mail system is encrypted. Verify policy and procedure.

Many programs have adopted a rule of shutting off cell phones during class and clinical. As a matter of etiquette, it is considered disrespectful to your classmates and instructor to text during class. Cell phone access is restricted during any testing situation.

Be careful if using your personal cell phone to send or retrieve confidential information related to clinical or employment in the future. Your cell phone may be an unsecure network and patient or employee personal information may be at risk. It is generally prohibited to use a personal cell phone at a clinical site or for any related activity.

Get Ready for the NCLEX-PN® Examination

Key Points

- The communication process has five essential components: sender, message, method of transmission, receiver, and feedback.
- Communication involves verbal, nonverbal, and affective communication.
- The most important part of therapeutic communication is active listening. It involves purpose, focus, and disciplined attention.
- Common active listening behaviors involve restating, clarifying, reflecting, paraphrasing, minimal encouraging, remaining silent, summarizing, and validating.
- Common blocks to communication involve false reassuring, probing, judging, belittling, giving advice, providing simple answers, and acting disinterested.

- Male/female differences do exist. Some differences are believed to be "hardwired" biologically. Characteristics can be modified, if desired.
- Cultural differences in communication exist, especially with individuals who are new to the country and/or maintain their strong cultural beliefs and customs.
- Role changes for the patient during an illness experience can be distressing. Staff attitude, nursing jargon, fear of the unknown, and personal and environmental factors are all involved.
- Communicating with the instructor and staff involves the same characteristics as communicating with a patient. They include trust, honesty, empathy, respect, sensitivity, humor, knowledge, patience, and commitment. Self-worth is earned as your knowledge and skill in application grow.

- SBAR is a way to give precise information when communicating to other members of the health care team or providing shift report.
- Life span communication differences are related to developmental and other issues, male/female differences, and medical problems.
- Be alert to what your thoughts are saying, and if they help you or hinder you.
- Take your conversation seriously: Practice saying what you mean, and know that your thinking affects your feelings and the way you communicate with patients and staff.
- Successful conflict management is based on a mutually beneficial solution through direct interaction among both parties.
- E-mail etiquette is essential for effective and efficient electronic communication.
- Many programs have adopted a no private cell phone or text messaging policy during class or clinical.

Additional Learning Resources

evolve Go to your Evolve website (http://evolve.elsevier.com/Knecht/success) for the following FREE learning resources:

- Answers to Critical Thinking Scenarios
- Additional learning activities
- Additional Review Questions for the NCLEX-PN® exam
- Helpful phrases for communicating in Spanish and more!

Review Questions for the NCLEX-PN® Examination

1. What is the primary reason for basic male/female differences in communication?
   a. Socialization
   b. Environment
   c. Acculturation
   d. Biology
2. The communication process is circular to ensure . . .
   a. the patient receives feedback on a daily basis
   b. verbal, nonverbal, and affective communication is used.
   c. that feedback is received from the receiver, potentially prompting the sender to send a new message
   d. that all team members are aware of the patient's needs.
3. Which is an appropriate response to the patient when you pick up affectively and nonverbally on the patient's anger?
   a. Leave the room and report your observations to the team leader immediately.
   b. Lighten up the situation by sharing some funny e-mail jokes with the patient.
   c. Provide observations of nonverbal behavior and encourage the patient to talk about their feelings.
   d. Continue what you came in to do silently and leave as soon as you are through.

4. Which statement most accurately reflects a nursing communication difference that is age related?
   a. Speaking in a loud, high voice makes it easier for an elderly patient to hear you.
   b. Discussing with school-age patients their illness in age appropriate terms.
   c. Giving a toddler having a tantrum a special treat.
   d. Using medical jargon and current slang to help a teenager to see you as human.

Alternate Format Item

1. Marty has arrived for her first clinical experience in the nursing home. She wants to do everything right and feels she is ready because she has an elderly grandmother. What tips will you give her for getting acquainted with the residents? *(Select all that apply.)*
   a. Walk in with great enthusiasm and say, "Hi, Grandma, how are you doing?"
   b. Talk loudly in the resident's left ear to be sure the resident can hear her.
   c. Say, "Good morning. My name is Latoya. I am a student nurse from the college. Can you confirm your name and birth date?"
   d. Knock on the door before entering. Take time before moving into the patient's personal space.
   e. Quietly enter the room and touch the person's shoulder while saying "hello".
2. A physician has reprimanded you at the patient's bedside. You feel an instant flash of anger, but you say nothing. When the physician leaves the room, you follow quickly to catch up before he moves on to another room. What might you say? *(Select all that apply.)*
   a. "Dr. Jones, I wish to speak with you privately."
   b. "How dare you shame me in front of a patient?"
   c. "Please explain what you wanted me to know."
   d. "In the future, talk to me privately, not at the bedside."
   e. "I am going to report you to my nursing supervisor."

Critical Thinking Scenarios

Scenario 1

The instructor has discussed using SBAR when reporting off clinical. You have had a chance to practice this in class using a case study provided by the instructor. The case study indicates that Mrs. Dithers is 78 years old and has a diagnosis of exacerbation of congestive heart failure. She is short of breath when speaking. Her husband died four weeks ago. She is crying as you enter the room. Discuss your approach to Mrs. Dithers.

Scenario 2

Mrs. Rotherham is used to having things her own way and is critical of everything the staff are doing to deal with her illness. Neil, a student nurse, has been assigned to give her medication this morning. When Neil enters the room, Mrs. Rotherham demands to know what he is doing there. What might Neil say?

Assertiveness: Your Responsibility

Objectives

On completing this chapter, you will be able to do the following:

1. Explain why assertiveness is a nursing responsibility.
2. Differentiate among assertive, aggressive, and nonassertive (passive) behaviors.
3. Maintain a daily journal that reflects your personal interactions and responses.
4. Self-reflect on daily interactions and create a personal plan to improve your assertiveness.
5. Discuss positive manipulation as a cultural choice.
6. Discuss how codependency can be an attempt to find relief from unresolved feelings.
7. Differentiate between lateral violence, bullying, and vertical violence in nursing.
8. Discuss dealing with sexual harassment in nursing.
9. Explain why insidious aggression is difficult to deal with.
10. List two to three behavioral changes in an individual that may be a sign of potential employee violence.
11. Identify steps you can personally implement to improve your job satisfaction, while creating a safer work environment.

Key Terms

aggressive (ă-GRĔSĭv)
assault (ă-SÖLT)
assertiveness (ă-SŬR-tĭv-nĕs)
automatic responses (ĂW-tŏ-MĂTĭk)
bullying
choice (chŏys)
compensation (KŎM-pĕn-SĂ-shŭn)
denial (dē-NĪ-ăl)
insidious aggression (ĭn-SĬD-ē-ŭs ă-GRĔ-shŭn)

lateral violence
manipulation (mă-NĬP-ū-LĀ-shŭn)
nonassertive (passive) (nŏn-ă-SŬR-tĭv)
problem solving (prŏ-blem sol-ving)
projection (prŏ-JĔK-shŭn)
rationalization (RĂSH-ăn-ă-lĭ-ZĀ-shŭn)
sexual harassment (HĂR-ăs-mĕnt)
vertical violence (horizontal hostility)

💡 Keep in Mind

Assertiveness is an expectation in nursing, a responsibility for you as a patient advocate.

❓ Critical Thinking

Personal Expectations

Imagine for the next few minutes that the nurse-patient roles are reversed and that you are the patient. What are your expectations of the nurse assigned to you? List the rationale for each expectation you identify.

Expectations	Rationale
_____	_____
_____	_____
_____	_____

The exercise in the Critical Thinking: Personal Expectations box should give you some insights into why a nurse must be assertive. At the end of this chapter you are encouraged to do this exercise again. Evaluate any changes in your expectations.

Verbal, nonverbal, and affective communication translates into three major behavior patterns. You will *hear, see,* and *feel* the message acted out. The most effective communication style is open and honest. It promotes positive relationships, a healthy sense of self, and establishes trust. Ineffective communication or behavior is hurtful. It blames, attacks, or denies and is harmful to the self as well.

The three major behavior styles are nonassertive (passive), aggressive, and assertive. An *assertive* style separates the person from the issue. Most importantly, you speak out of **choice**. An emotional hook catches you when you use either an *aggressive* or a *nonassertive* (passive) style of communication. Both types of responses are **automatic responses**.

121

NONASSERTIVE (PASSIVE) BEHAVIOR

Nonassertive (passive), fear-based behavior, is an emotionally dishonest, self-defeating type of behavior. Nonassertive nurses attempt to look the other way, avoid conflict, and take what seems to be the easiest way out; they are never full participants on the health care team. Nonassertive individuals do not express feelings, needs, and ideas when their rights are deliberately or accidentally infringed on. There may be a lack of eye contact, swaying and shifting from one foot to the other, and whining and hesitancy when speaking. The overall message is "I do not count. *You* count." This personal pattern of behavior is reflected in their nursing as well. Consequently, they are unable to recognize and meet patient needs. Here are some examples of nonassertive behavior, with the type of behavior in parentheses:

- Telling another nurse how "stupid" the doctor is for ordering a certain type of treatment (indirect, nonassertive behavior).
- Limiting contact with a patient he or she is uncomfortable with to required care only (indirect nonassertive behavior).
- Routinely telling patients who ask questions about their illness, test, medications, or treatment to "Ask the doctor" or "Ask the RN." Although this answer is advisable some of the time, it certainly can be a form of brush-off (taking the easy way out). Part of nursing responsibility is to seek answers for the patient.
- Experiencing an inability to continue with a necessary, uncomfortable treatment ordered for a patient (interpreting the patient's expression of discomfort personally: "The patient will not like me if I do this").
- Assuming, without checking, that the patient wants to skip daily personal care when a visitor drops in (avoiding conflict).
- Experiencing a feeling of being "devastated" when a patient, doctor, nurse, or other staff person criticizes his or her work (interpreting criticism of work as criticism of self).
- Responding to a patient's in-depth questions about own personal life and that of other staff (afraid of not being liked). The nurse is leaving the professional role and is assuming a social role instead.
- Patient asks the nurse to pick up some personal items on the way home. The nurse frowns but agrees to do so (communicating the real message nonverbally). This may be a violation of institutional policy.
- Becoming angry with the team leader and dropping hints to others about own feelings (communicating the real message indirectly).
- When asked by another nurse to assist with the care of assigned patients, responding by saying, "Well, uh, I guess I could," although already too busy (hesitating, repressing own wishes).

- Needing help with an assignment but saying nothing (refrains from expressing own needs).
- After making an error, overexplains and continually apologizes (is unaware of the right to make a mistake; should take responsibility for it, learn from the error, and go on). Points blame on staffing pattern, when an error is made.
- Following completion of an error, plans on finding a new job because of fear of the outcome and administrative response (avoiding conflict).
- Getting angry when "chewed out" by the doctor in front of a patient, but not saying anything (refraining from expressing own opinion, internalizing anger).

◎ Try This

Nonassertive Behavior

Identify nonassertive behaviors in which you have been involved. Describe how each behavior worked or did not work for you or the patient.

Observe the health care team during a clinical assignment. Determine assertive, nonassertive, and aggressive behavior in different members of the health care team. Do you notice any trends?

By not taking risks and not being honest, nonassertive nurses typically feel hurt, misunderstood, anxious, and disappointed, often feel angry and resentful later. Because they do not allow their needs to be known, they are the ones who lose out. Their patients can also be impacted adversely.

? Critical Thinking

Nonassertive Behavior

Develop a plan for change for each one of the nonassertive behaviors that you identified as having unsatisfactory outcomes.

AGGRESSIVE BEHAVIOR

Outspoken people are often automatically considered assertive, when in reality their lack of consideration for others may be a sign of **aggressive** behavior. Aggressive (anger-based) behavior violates the rights of others. It is an attack on the person rather than on the person's behavior. The purpose of aggressive behavior is to dominate or put the other person down. This behavior, although expressive, is self-defeating because it quickly distances the aggressor from other staff and patients. Examples of aggressive body language include leaning forward with glaring eyes; pointing a finger at a person to whom you are speaking; shouting; clenching fists; putting hands on hips; and shaking the head. The overall message is *"You do not count. I count."* The following examples show how aggressive behavior can be recognized. An explanation of the rationale is included in parentheses.

- You have asked to go to a workshop, and the supervisor says, "Why should you go? Everyone else has worked here longer than you have" (attempting to make you feel guilty for making a request).
- Another nurse points out your error in front of other staff and adds, "Where did you say you graduated from?" (attempting to humiliate as a way of controlling).
- A peer approaches you with a problem. You don't want to listen and say, "If it isn't one thing, it's another for you. Why don't you get your act together?" (disregarding others' feelings).
- A new rule is instituted without requesting input from or informing those it will involve. You protest but are told, "That's tough; this is the way it's going to be from now on" (disregarding others' feelings and rights).
- The patient has had his call light on frequently throughout the morning. You walk in and say, "I have had it. You have had your light on continuously for nothing all morning. Do not put your light on again unless you are dying, or I will take it away" (hostile overreaction out of proportion to the issue at hand/verbal abuse).
- You attempted to express your feelings to a peer about his or her behavior toward you. Today the peer greets you with an icy stare when you say hello (hostile overreaction).
- A patient tells you, "I thought this was a pretty good hospital, but none of you seem to know what you are doing" (sarcastic, hostile).
- You park in a handicapped parking spot because it is raining and you do not want to be wet all day (rudeness).
- You ask the nurse manager a question. Instead of answering, he just stares at you with lips curled slightly upward (attempting to make you uncomfortable, a put-down).

◎ Try This

Aggressive Behavior

Circle the aggressive behaviors in the previous example that are similar to behaviors you have experienced. How could you address these scenarios?

❓ Critical Thinking

Aggressive Behavior

Develop a plan for dealing with the aggressive behaviors you identified in the previous learning exercise.

Aggressive behavior certainly is a way of saying what you mean at the moment, and it does produce temporary relief from anxiety. The feeling, however, does not last. Very often the aggressive person is left with residual angry feelings that simmer until the next stressful situation or person comes along. It is interesting to note that sometimes an aggressive person was once passive and made a decision that "no one will ever step on me again." However, instead of practicing assertiveness, such a person practiced and became involved in another form of destructive, self-defeating behavior. Aggressive nurses, like nonaggressive nurses, are unable to function as true advocates for the patient because they are too busy taking care of what they perceive to be their personal needs.

ASSERTIVE BEHAVIOR

Assertiveness is another name for "honesty"; that is, it is a way to live the truth from your innermost being and to express this truth in thought, word, and deed. The concept seems simple enough, but it is another thing to be truthful all the time. According to *Webster's Dictionary*, *assertiveness* means "taking a positive stand, being confident in your statement, or being positive in a persistent way." You, the nurse, work in a setting that requires speaking frankly and openly to others in such a way that their rights are not violated. *Assertiveness is a tool, not a weapon.* As with any new behavior (or skill), becoming truly assertive will take practice and time. Avoid being harsh with yourself or giving up just because old behaviors emerge when you are under pressure. Resolve to try again until assertive behavior is integrated as a part of your being. Although it is not the nurse's right to hurt others deliberately, it is unrealistic to be inhibited to the point of never hurting anyone. Some people are hurt because they are unreasonably sensitive, and some people use their sensitivity to manipulate others. Assertiveness is not only what you say but how you say it. Examples of assertive body language include standing straight, steady, and directly facing the people to whom you are speaking while maintaining eye contact; speaking in a clear voice, loud enough so the people to whom you are speaking can hear you; and speaking fluently without hesitation and with assurance and confidence. Practicing your assertive response in the mirror can be very beneficial. Asking a colleague for feedback will also improve the effectiveness of your assertive approach.

Nurses have a right to express their own thoughts and feelings. To do otherwise would be insincere. It would also deny patients and other staff the opportunity to learn to deal with their feelings. Assertiveness, then, is a way of expressing oneself without insulting others. It communicates respect for the other person, although not necessarily for the other person's behavior. The overall message is *"I count, and you count too."* Being assertive does not guarantee that you will get your way. What it does guarantee is that you will experience a sense of being in control of your emotions and your responses. Win or lose, you gave it your best shot. The real bonus is freedom from residual feelings of fear and anger. Later in this chapter, we will deal with exceptions when you are faced with a potentially violent situation.

The following examples, with the rationale in parentheses, are expressions of assertive behavior. As an assertive nurse, you claim responsibility for your own feelings, thoughts, and actions. Using "I" in your statements shows acceptance of responsibility for your thinking, feeling, and doing.

- The doctor orders a medication or treatment that seems inappropriate. You request to talk to the doctor privately and ask about expected outcomes. You present evidence that may potentially affect the decision to continue with the order (direct statement of information).
- The patient has been giving you a difficult time. Pulling up a chair and sitting down, facing the client, you say, "Mr. Smith, I would be interested in knowing how you are feeling. I have noticed that whatever I do, you are critical of my work." Then you listen attentively and with understanding (comprehension) and respond nondefensively (direct statement of feelings; does not interpret patient's criticism as a personal attack).
- When the patient requests information you are unfamiliar with regarding the illness and treatment, you say, "I do not know, but I will find out for you." You follow through by checking with appropriate staff. You determine who is to inform the patient (respect for the patient's right to know).
- The doctor has ordered the patient to walk for 10 minutes out of each hour. The patient complains that it hurts and asks to not be required to walk. You respond by saying, "I know it is uncomfortable, but I will walk along beside you. We can stop briefly any time you like. I will also teach you how to do a brief relaxation technique that you can use while you are walking." If pain medication is available, you will also make sure that this is given before walking and in enough time for the medication to take effect (respects patient's feelings but supports the need to carry out doctor's orders).
- Unexpected visitors arrive when it is time for you to help the patient with personal care. You ask the patient directly if care should be done now or postponed briefly. You state the time that you will be available to assist with care (respects the patient's autonomy [right to choose] and does not compromise the care).
- You have just been criticized for your work. You respond by saying, "Please clarify. I want to be sure I understand." If the error is yours, ask for suggestions to correct it or offer alternatives of your own (separates criticism of performance from criticism of self).

- A patient asks for personal information about you (or another staff member). You respond by saying, "That information is personal, and I do not choose to discuss it" (stands up for rights without violating rights of others).
- A patient asks you to pick up some personal items from the store. This would mean doing it on your own time, which is already very full. You respond by saying, "I will not be able to do the errand for you" or "Our institution policy will not allow me to assist you in this manner. Can I call the case manager for you to see if she can assist?' (direct statement without excuses).
- The team leader has been "on your case" constantly and, you think, unfairly. You approach the team leader and say, "I would like to speak with you privately today before 3 PM. What time is convenient for you?" (direct statement of wishes).
- You are being pressed by other staff members to help with their assignments but you are also very busy. You say, "I am also busy today. Let's discuss all of the patient's priorities and come up with a plan to deliver the best possible care together to all of the patients" (compromise).
- Your day is overwhelming. You approach your team leader and say, "I know you would like all of this done today. There is no way I can get it all done. What are your priorities?" (direct statement of information and request for clarification).
- The doctor has criticized your work in front of a patient. You feel embarrassed and angry. You approach the doctor and ask to speak privately. Using "I-centered" statements, you begin by saying, "I feel both embarrassed and angry because you criticized me in front of a patient. Next time, please ask to talk to me privately." (stands up for your rights without violating the rights of others).
- You are ready to leave work, when a peer approaches you about a personal problem. You respond by saying, "I have to leave now, but I'll be glad to listen to you during our lunch break tomorrow" (compromise).
- Another staff person moves into the cafeteria line ahead of you with a nod and a smile. You are in a hurry, too, and feel this is an imposition. You say firmly, "I am not sure you realize that the line begins at the entrance to the coffee area" (stands up for your rights).

Now complete the exercise in the Try This: Identify Assertiveness box.

◎ Try This

Identify Assertiveness

List examples of assertiveness you can identify in your own behavior or in people around you. If the situation changes, do you see a change in behavior? Reflect why, and think of strategies to remain assertive.

The following three rules are helpful overall in being assertive:

1. Own your feelings. Do not blame others for the way you feel.
2. Make your feelings known by being direct. Begin your statements with "I."
3. Be sure that your nonverbal communication matches your verbal message.

NEGATIVE INTERACTIONS: USING COPING MECHANISMS

With so many types of preparation for a career in nursing and the lack of differentiation in roles based on preparation, nurses sometimes experience insecurity in their role and the worth of the role as they understand it. As a licensed practical nurse (LPN) you may experience role confusion between the LPN and registered nurse (RN) role, particularly in the community and long-term care setting. This may contribute to the LPN's sense of job worth/job satisfaction. In these types of ambivalent situations, humans often use coping mechanisms. A discussion follows regarding types of common coping mechanisms used by nurses.

Projection is a coping mechanism during which individuals attribute their own weaknesses to others. The interaction can be characterized as "My education is better than yours" or "I'm more competent than you are" or "You're only a practical nurse." Unfortunately, this negative, aggressive interaction wastes energy that could be used to provide patients with the care that is being alluded to. Nurses who are confident and assertive enhance one another's knowledge base and legal responsibility. The patient benefits from assertiveness.

Another negative interaction is based on a previous unresolved incident between the patient and the nurse. The nurse uses the coping or mental mechanism of **rationalization**, in which a logical but untrue reason is offered as an excuse for the behavior. The nurse quickly informs others that this patient is a "troublemaker" or a "manipulator" or "uncooperative." This is a nonassertive, indirect type of behavior on the part of the nurse. Obviously, if other nurses incorporate this information into their transactions with the patient, the patient will never be seen as his or her true self. Anything the patient does can be interpreted within the context of the label given by the nurses. A vicious circle can ensue. If the patient's needs are not met because of this labeling, this increases his or her frustration. This in turn is a threat to self, resulting in anxiety. Depending on the patient's personal strength at this time, the situation can lead to problem solving, the use of coping/mental mechanisms, or symptom formation.

An honest, assertive response on the part of the original nurse involved would consist of dealing with the patient directly in regard to the previous situation. It would not involve other nurses as allies in "getting this patient." An example of an extreme situation resulting from just such a seemingly innocent rationalization occurred at a nursing home.

A young man who was paralyzed from the waist down as a result of a car accident was being transferred from one nursing home to another. A transfer form arrived before he did. The information on the form created immediate anxiety for the nurses involved before they had even met the man. The form labeled the man as "manipulative." It stated, "He will be pleasant and polite at first, but watch out because it is a trick. When he has won you over, you will see his 'true colors.'" The nurses discussed the prospective admission. They expressed gratitude that their colleagues in the other nursing home had warned them. After all, that is what colleagues are for. They felt, "forewarned is forearmed." When the patient arrived and attempted to get acquainted, he was dealt with coldly and abruptly and made to wait. The nurses intended to show him that he could not manipulate them. As his frustration and discomfort increased, he began to demand that his treatments be done on time. He shouted angry comments at the nurses when they finally arrived to assume his care. The nurses called him "demanding" and "hostile." The original label of "manipulative" was supported when the patient asked his roommate to put on the call light to get help to take him to the bathroom. Each day seemed worse than the day before.

The showdown finally came when a longtime nurse employee left, saying that she would not come back until the patient was transferred to another facility. She would even volunteer to do the transfer note. Other nursing staff threatened to follow suit. Finally, the administrator gave in. The patient was transferred, and the nurses congratulated one another for having worked together! Complete the exercise in the Critical Thinking: Negative Interactions box.

? **Critical Thinking**

Negative Interactions

1. What factors contributed to the patient's behavior?
2. What factors contributed to the nurses' response to the patient?
3. How could this situation have been handled differently?
4. Was the behavior of the nurses passive, aggressive, or assertive? Explain your answer.
5. Is it ethical or a legal risk to "label" patients?

Another negative transaction involves the patient's right to know (for example, a patient being transferred from a skilled nursing home facility to an intermediate nursing home facility). This transaction can be known by many titles, depending on the issue. It can be called "I've got a secret" or "It is not my responsibility" or "She will be upset" or "She is too weak to figure out what is going on." The responsibility of informing the patient about his or her condition or transfer plans is not carried out just so the present staff does not have to deal with the full impact of the patient's reaction to the information. The coping or mental mechanism used is **denial**. The nurse refuses to recognize the existence and significance of the patient's personal concerns. The nurse also uses denial as a way of excusing personal responsibility: "The doctor should tell him" or "It's the team leader's responsibility." Although the decision may not be entirely yours, it is clearly your responsibility to check out what portion of the information is yours to give. You also have the responsibility to check out who is going to present the information and when. Complete the exercise in the Try This: Identify If Behavior Is Passive, Aggressive, or Assertive box.

⊚ Try This

Identify If Behavior Is Passive, Aggressive, or Assertive

Is the nurse's refusal to take responsibility to seek out the information the patient needs to know a passive, aggressive, or assertive transaction? Explain your answer.

GOSSIP HURTS

Although it has many possible negative interactions, certainly the passive or aggressive game of gossip; for example, "Did I tell you?" or "I just found out," is a destructive interaction that has the potential to ruin the reputations of both patients and personnel. The coping or mental mechanism is **compensation**. The nurse is covering for real or imagined inadequacies in his or her work by developing what he or she considers desirable traits of observation, listening, and reporting. The energy is misguided because reputations are at stake, and time spent socializing while at work is time away from providing quality patient care. A listener can squelch this game by saying assertively, "I will work on a good relationship between you and me, but I would prefer you do not talk to me about others." Instead, if the listener, while calling the other nurse a gossip, listens with interest, continuation of this behavior is supported. Today, gossip can also be accomplished through social media. Complete the exercise in the Critical Thinking: More Damaging Interactions box.

❓ Critical Thinking

More Damaging Interactions

1. What other damaging interactions among staff or between patients and staff do you know about?
2. Provide examples of how continuation of this type of interaction is supported by others.
3. What can you do or say to avoid being drawn into these interactions?
4. Think about a recent scenario in your class when a peer tried to engage you in gossip. Self-reflect how you responded to the situation. How should you change your behavior to avoid nonassertive behavior in the future?
5. How does social media contribute to gossip? Remember that all patient information is confidential!

GUIDELINES FOR MOVING TOWARD ASSERTIVENESS

Read the poem *"Myself"* in Box 9-1. It captures the reason for working toward assertiveness and being able to feel good about yourself as you continue to grow as a person. Changing behavior is difficult. After all, the behaviors have been practiced and perfected for years. It is so much easier to tell others what *they* should do to change. The decision to change must come from inside you so it becomes yours alone.

THE PROBLEM-SOLVING PROCESS

The **problem-solving** process is a series of steps used to solve problems long before the nursing process was developed. You will note similarities between problem-solving and nursing processes. The nursing process is a more focused method of using the problem-solving steps. We reintroduce you to problem solving in this chapter because of its continued usefulness in dealing with self.

It is easier to begin the problem-solving process before feelings and behaviors about a troublesome problem become deeply rooted. A common response to unresolved problems is the cycle of worry → fear → anger → rage. This cycle can be interrupted and resolved at any stage, but it requires different levels of nursing skill. When dealing with the underlying problem, ask the person, "What do you want?" Putting the problem-solving steps into action is work! Without resolution, the cycle continues and intensifies with time. This behavior, for example, can be seen in the nursing home patient who strikes out, seems calm for a period, gets irritable, and eventually strikes out again. If the underlying problem is not resolved, the cycle continues. The person gets labeled as one who strikes out without warning, so "Watch out." Ask a more skilled staff member to do the behavioral intervention if you are uncomfortable. You must not contribute to an unsafe environment and possible harm to you or the patient.

Box 9-1   Myself

I have to live with myself and so,
I want to be fit for myself to know.
I don't want to stand with the setting sun
And hate myself for the things I've done.
I want to go out with head erect.
I want to deserve all men's respect.
But here in this struggle for fame and self,
I want to be able to like myself.
I don't want to look at myself and know
That I'm bluster and bluff and empty show.
I never can fool myself, and so
Whatever happens, I want to grow
More able to be more proud of me,
Self-respecting and conscience free.

Edgar Albert Guest

The self tries to find relief of unresolved feelings through behavior such as codependency, self-medicating with alcohol and/or other drugs (or food), and projecting the anger toward patients and others (burnout). Prolonged, unresolved negative emotions such as worry, fear, and anger create changes in the body at a cellular level and can result in physical illness. We first get clues in our thoughts of how we will become ill. Listen to your self-talk: "I'm sick of this!" or "I feel like I have the weight of the world on my shoulders" or "He's a pain in the neck" or "Oh, my aching back!" or "I'm so upset I can't speak" or "I can't take this much longer" and so on. If your self-talk is negative, pay attention. These statements give clues to potential areas of physical involvement. We also read or hear news almost daily of mild mannered, nice people who suddenly acted out because of rage. No one wants to get there. Rage can be turned against others (including homicide), or it can be turned against oneself. Active rage against self includes the extreme act of suicide. In extreme situations, such as suicide, undiagnosed or improperly treated mental health issues existed before the actual event. Passive means of rage turned against oneself include adopting personal habits that are damaging to one's health. The risk of suicide for nurses is real.

? Critical Thinking

Plan for Living

Begin a plan for living in a personal, confidential journal. Include specific examples of positive health habits that you currently practice and how you can improve these resources. See Chapter 3 for potential community resources.

The problem-solving process is a conscious growth-producing method of dealing with challenges in your life. Note that problem solving is an active process and is more than simply developing an intellectual awareness of the challenge at hand.

PROBLEM-SOLVING STEPS

Step One: Define the Problem

Sometimes what is perceived as the problem is not really the problem. For example, you may have been blaming another individual for talking you into behaviors of which you do not approve. Before making a commitment to change, look objectively at the gains and losses associated with the present behavior. For example, blaming someone else for your behavior may get you sympathy and concern from your friends. However, you lose by not taking responsibility for your own behavior and dealing with it in a growth-producing way. Your present way of responding to others developed as a response to anxiety-producing situations in life. The behavior usually has its roots in childhood. Complete the exercise about

gains and losses in the Critical Thinking: Gains and Losses box.

? Critical Thinking

Gains and Losses

Answer the following questions in your confidential journal: What are you gaining from maintaining your nonassertive/aggressive behavior? What are you losing from maintaining your nonassertive/aggressive behavior?

Another consideration is that when you change the way you act toward others, you change the way they act toward you. What has been a predictable reaction will no longer be predictable. Initially the "others" will test you. They will increase their old way of behaving as a way of getting you to give up the new behavior. If you persist with your new way of dealing with and responding to situations, their behavior toward you will gradually change. *This is the only way to influence change in anyone's behavior.* No amount of "telling" or "scolding" makes a difference as long as others can count on you to continue behaving in the old, predictable way.

Defining the problem depends on collecting data for two or three days and writing your problem statement based on this information. Collecting data needs to be done in an objective manner, as though you were observing someone else. Asking colleagues or family to assist you in identifying behaviors can be very helpful. However, you need to be ready to listen with an open mind.

◎ Try This

Keep a Daily Journal

Maintain a daily confidential journal to help pinpoint specific situations that create worry, fear, anger, and rage in you. Track the following:
1. What happened.
2. When it happened.
3. How you felt physically.
4. How you felt emotionally.
5. What you would have liked to have done instead.
6. What kept you from doing it.

Step Two: Decide on a Goal

Review the problem statement and write it out, applying the nursing process. Ask yourself what you want to do differently. This can be stated as a single goal. Often it is more useful to break the goal down into a long-term goal (what change or outcome you want) and several short-term goals (steps needed to attain the desired long-term goal). All goals must be realistic (attainable), measurable (how you will know the goal has been attained), and time-referenced (an educated guess on when you will see results). Before you read further, complete the exercise in the Critical Thinking: Deciding on a Goal box.

? Critical Thinking

Defining the Problem

Review the data you have collected for two or three days in your daily journal. It will give you an insight into the pros and cons of your current behavior. Develop a problem statement that is personal and specific for you. Before writing the problem statement, read the following:

SAMPLE

I am afraid to say what I mean for fear that others will get angry with me.

This behavior is demonstrated in the following situations:

- Saying "yes" to requests to babysit or go out with friends when I need the time for homework.
- Not asking for help with household chores, even though I am a full-time student plus a homemaker.
- Saying "yes" to added requests not related to responsibilities for school that I must complete on my own time.
- Feeling tired and resentful much of the time and eventually blowing up over something insignificant.

? Critical Thinking

Deciding on a Goal

Write a goal about assertiveness for yourself. Before you write the goal, read the sample that follows.

SAMPLE

Long-Term Goal	Short-Term Goal
Within six months I will say what I mean without fear that others will be angry with me (give an actual date—this is your best "guesstimate").	Within two weeks I will say "no" to babysitting requests or going to a family event when I need the time to do homework (give actual date—this is your best "guesstimate").

As you read each of the goals you have written, ask yourself whether they are realistic. Are they reasonable to attain? Next, review each goal and ask whether or not it is measurable. Are they so specific that you can use the senses to detect the change? Note that each goal begins with the phrase "I will." This phrase signals a personal commitment to work on the goal. Note that the goals are to be attained within a designated period; that is, they are time-referenced. This is also the only way to give yourself a push to get started.

All the changes are not going to occur exactly by the projected date. You will have to revise the goal dates from time to time. Most importantly, they provide target dates to strive for. As you accomplish each short-term goal, cross it out, and then go on to the next one. Do not be alarmed if you find yourself working on more than one goal at a time. This is possible and even desirable when the opportunity presents itself. Continue recording your progress in the confidential journal that you began initially to obtain data. Its value now lies in keeping a record of the process you are going through and seeing the changes taking place. Unless you do this, you may not fully appreciate your work and its progress. Many changes will be subtle and will not be accompanied by bells and claps of thunder.

Step Three: Choose Alternatives

Alternatives are the approaches that you will be using to attain each of the established goals. When you make a list of alternatives in your journal, let your imagination run wild. Consider all the possible solutions, from serious to humorous. This may even provide some comic relief from the serious challenge with which you are dealing. Remember to include "do nothing" in the list of alternatives. Doing nothing is a *choice* and therefore an alternative. Look at each of the goals and think of specific things you can do or say to help support the goal. Complete the exercise in the Critical Thinking: Personal Alternatives box.

? Critical Thinking

Personal Alternatives

Write alternatives to support the short-term goal(s) you chose in the Deciding on a Goal exercise. Before you write in your journal, read the sample that follows.

SAMPLE

Approach: Practice in front of a mirror. In an even tone of voice, say, "No, I will not be able to babysit tonight, but try again another time." If the person persists, say, "No, I do not have the time tonight." Repeat as needed until heard. Compliment yourself for not giving in.

How does the approach (alternative) correspond specifically to the short-term goal from the assertiveness exercise?

Step Four: Try Out the Alternatives

The initial plan has been made. It is now time to put the plan into action. For many of you, the paperwork is far easier than taking the first step to make the "paper trip" a reality. You may also have discovered that it is far easier to offer ideas to peers than to take the first step into action with your own plan.

It is a good idea to build in an incentive to continue using the new assertive approaches. Promise yourself something that is worthy of you (a worthy goal). As you go along, you will sometimes slip back into old familiar ways of behaving. Do not be dismayed. This is normal. Simply reinstitute the newly planned approaches immediately and continue. The more you practice the new approaches, the more they will become part of you. Ultimately, new assertive behaviors will replace old nonassertive or aggressive behaviors. Identifying a mentor or peer, who can provide feedback and assist you in debriefing situations, can assist you in this goal.

◎ Try This

Celebrate Attaining Your Goals

Identify a worthy incentive to celebrate attaining your goal. To make it work, the goal must be within your budget and not create a new problem for you to solve!

Step Five: Evaluate the Effectiveness of Your Approach

The evaluation mechanism is built into the overall plan for change by making the goals time-limited. This tells you that each goal, along with the alternatives you have chosen, will be evaluated at the time indicated. Do not change a goal or approach it too quickly. Give it at least two to three weeks. You need to do this for two reasons: the negative behaviors of other individuals toward you will increase initially as they attempt to resist the change created by the change in you, and it takes a minimum of three weeks for the new behavior to catch on. (It takes approximately a year for a new behavior to become part of you.)

◎ Try This

Review Your Journal

As a part of the evaluation process, review your entire confidential journal. This is an excellent source of information for what happened, how you dealt with it, and whether the present course was, and continues to be, effective.

Step Six: Repeat the Process if the Solution is not Effective

Step five gave you information about whether or not to pursue the established course of action. If changes are needed, go back to step three, identify additional alternatives, or perhaps choose alternatives that you originally identified but did not use. Then go through the rest of the steps as before.

As you pursue an assertive way of behaving, monitor your nonverbal messages. The nonverbal communication you provide is even more powerful than your words. It is possible to have the words just right but to sabotage the words by hesitation, a sarcastic tone of voice, or emphasis on certain words. Practice in front of a mirror. If you feel like you don't have time, practice while taking your shower, waiting to pick up your child, or waiting on a bus. Listen to the way you sound. You can also ask a friend to videotape you or record on your phone and then review and critique the tape. Try changing the tone and monitoring the level of your voice. Be sure that the last word of a sentence is no higher than the one before it. Listen for this in others. It can make a statement sound like a question.

Posture plays an important role: sit up straight; walk with the shoulders back and a confident stride. Make eye contact when speaking. If this is new and difficult for you, look at the area between the eyes of the person you are addressing. This provides an illusion of eye contact. Periodically look away so that it does not look as though you are staring. Avoid annoying habits such as staring, nail biting, finger or foot tapping or jiggling, playing with your hair, chewing on a pencil or glasses, nervous laughter, putting hands in and out of pockets, and so on. Sometimes it can help to determine a certain spot on your body to keep your hands (e.g., folded on your lap, or lightly sitting on your hip). Amy Cuddy in a 2012 TED talk emphasizes how "power posing" can impact your confidence. Visit the website and view the talk. It only takes two minutes to benefit from the "power pose." (www.ted.com/talks/amy_cuddy_your_body_language_shapes_who_you_are?language=en).

When someone asks you what you think of an issue or what you would like to do, answer the person. Instead of saying, "I really do not know" or "Whatever you like" or "It does not matter," take the risk and express your opinion. Life is an adventure. Your ideas count, and the more you express your opinion, the easier it becomes.

Lack of autonomy has been reported by some LPNs working in long-term care (Knecht, 2014). They report feeling unvalued and often not requested to participate at patient care meetings, despite their in-depth knowledge of the patients. Be assertive and request to attend related meetings. Include the value you will bring as part of your request.

NEGATIVE MANIPULATIVE INTERACTIONS

Manipulation is considered maladaptive if the feelings and needs of others are disregarded or other people are treated as objects to fulfill the needs of the manipulator. The following examples of negative manipulative interactions show a lack of consideration for others' feelings and needs:

- The *seducer* initiates a relationship with someone (e.g., a nurse with a supervisor). They share what seem to be common goals and insights. Ultimately, the seducer asks for special favors or privileges. If denied, the seducer pushes the guilt button, saying, "I thought you liked me" or "I thought we understood each other." The other person is left feeling guilty, angry, or both.
- The *passive-aggressive* manipulator focuses on the other person's weaknesses. He or she uses this knowledge to exploit or create anxiety for the victim. For example, a physician might point out a nurse's errors or personal or professional problems in front of a patient or other staff. The nurse is left feeling guilty, angry, embarrassed, or all of these emotions.
- The *divide-and-conquer* manipulator "confides" half-truths, rumors, gossip, and innuendo. A skilled manipulator can sever work relationships by sowing seeds of distrust. As the staff squabbles, there is less energy to unite and focus on common patient issues.

For example, a divide-and-conquer manipulator who is an established member of the community might "confide" to another department head that a newer employee cannot be trusted. By the time this information proves to be untrue, valuable time has been lost in patient planning and care. Meanwhile, the divide-and-conquer manipulator has continued to tell the same story to other listeners. Because the feelings and needs of others are not considered, they are left with anger and seeds of distrust.

Dealing with a negative manipulator is difficult. An assertive approach is the best recourse. This will, however, be met with resistance and resentment. You may end up backing off if the problem cannot be worked out. Set limits on any inappropriate manipulative behavior toward you. Refuse to play the game anymore.

As a nurse, you must learn to take care of yourself. In turn, you will be more effective in meeting patients' nursing needs. In taking care of yourself assertively, you serve as a positive role model for your coworkers, those you lead and manage, and your patients. How you view and deal with an event determines the outcome for you.

AGGRESSIVENESS AND WORK-RELATED ISSUES

ASSAULT

Workplace violence has always existed in nursing facilities. It is the increase in violence, however, that is making nurses take notice. Nurses are frequently targets of violence, hostility, sexual harassment, and discrimination. In a recent study of acute care nurses, Speroni et al. (2014) found that 54.2% of nurse participants experienced verbal abuse by patients whereas 29.9% experienced physical abuse by patients. A nurse's response to a patient can decrease the potential for violence. Being assertive but not aggressive can deescalate a patient or peer.

According to the Bureau of Labor Statistics (BLS), 27 out of the 100 fatalities in health care and social service settings occurring in 2013 were because of assaults and violent acts. According to the Occupational Safety and Health Administration (OSHA, 2015) **assaults** comprise 10% to 11% of workplace injuries involving days away from work for health care workers. This is more than triple the amount of injuries of all private sector employees. Inpatient and acute psychiatric settings, emergency room, geriatric long-term care, and residential and day social service settings are at high risk for assault (OSHA, 2015). In March 1996, OSHA released its first *Act of Violence Prevention Guidelines* (1996) geared toward protecting health care and social service workers on the job. Unfortunately, incidences of work related assaults continue to exceed the overall industry norm. As a result, in 2015, OSHA published *Guidelines for Preventing Workforce Violence for Health Care and Social Service Workers* to improve the safety of the workplace (Box 9-2).

Box 9-2 Occupational Safety and Health Administration Guidelines for Preventing Workforce Violence for Health Care and Social Service Workers

VIOLENCE PREVENTION PROGRAMS:
- Management commitment and worker participation
- Worksite analysis and hazard identification
  - Record analysis and tracking (identify patterns of assaults or near misses and how controls can decrease)
  - Job hazard analysis
  - Employee surveys*
  - Client patient surveys*

*Help identify new or previously unnoticed risk factors and deficiencies or failures in work practices
- Hazard prevention and control
  - Substitution (substitute hazard with a safer work practice)
  - Engineering controls and workplace adaptations to minimize risk (e.g., physical barriers, door locks, panic buttons, metal detectors, better/additional lighting, more accessible exits)
  - Postincident procedures and services (identify "root cause")
  - Investigation of Incidents
- Safety and health training
  - Understand the concept of "universal precautions for violence"
  - Training topics
  - Training for supervisors and managers
  - Training for security personnel
  - Evaluation of training
- Recordkeeping and program evaluation

Source: OSHA (2015). Occupational Safety and Health Administration Guidelines for Preventing Workforce Violence for Health Care and Social Service Workers. Retrieved from https://www.osha.gov/Publications/osha3148.pdf

Not all agencies have complied with the OSHA guidelines, but some State Nurses' Associations are working toward increased penalties against those guilty of assaulting a health care worker or to establish task forces to study workplace violence. A recent New York Senate bill made an assault against an RN or LPN on duty a class C or class D felony. Although this law applies to physical abuse and does not include verbal abuse, it is a step in the right direction in protecting nurses.

⊚ Try This

The American Nurses Association Bill of Rights

The American Nurses Association (ANA) *Bill of Rights for Registered Nurses* states, "Nurses have the right to a work environment that is safe for themselves and their patients." Research what your State Nurses Association is doing to minimize risks of violence in the workplace.

CONTRIBUTING FACTORS

Many of the findings regarding factors contributing to violence apply to all of nursing.

Personal Factors

Personal factors include verbal, nonverbal, and affective communication, including nurses' attitudes and behaviors. Attitude and body language are considered more significant than the sex and age of the nurse. The manner of approaching a patient, such as with respect and confidence, emerged as important.

Workplace Practices

Workplace practices aimed at improving safety for health care workers are critical. The quality, performance, and availability of security personnel is a key strategy. Officers convey authority in uniform more so than when they wear a customer-friendly jacket and tie, a nonverbal form of communication. Incidents are also more common when nurses and security personnel lack aggression management skills. Finally, not all administrators back nurses on reporting incidents of physical and verbal abuse, including those involving supervisors and physicians. Nurses should document the key objective information immediately following an incident. This information may be needed if the perpetrator denies the abuse. Nurses may also be able to elicit the support of their union representative to enhance the safety of the workplace and address any current issues.

Environmental Factors

The type of patient seen and the location of the care facility (for example, high-crime risk area) determine the type of patient admitted to a hospital. An important risk factor at hospitals and psychiatric facilities is the carrying of guns by patients, family, or friends of the patient. Other issues include early release of acute or chronic mentally ill, the right to refuse psychotropic medication, the inability to voluntarily hospitalize mentally ill persons unless of immediate danger to self or others, and the use of hospitals for criminals instead of incarceration. In 2013, according to the BLS, psychiatric aides reported the highest rate of violent injuries that resulted in days away from work.

Risk Diagnosis

The majority of all assaults are perpetrated by a minority of persons. A history of previous violence is a strong indicator, but sometimes this information is not available to the staff. Although patients suffering from dementia and mental crisis commit some of the assaults, a 2014 survey indicated that almost 50% is accounted for by patients and family members affected by alcohol or drugs. In addition, some people simply report being frustrated when they assault a nurse (Jacobson, 2014). Patients are placed in a vulnerable position by virtue of entering the health care system. This may elicit unwarranted behaviors that the patient normally is able to control through coping mechanisms.

Nurses need to learn how to read cues for potential risk of violence in the patients (and others) with whom they are dealing. Some diagnoses that can cue you to possible risk include affective disorders, paranoid delusions, chemical abuse/dependency, dementia, impulse control disorders and personality disorders, and patients/family undergoing extreme stress.

If you find yourself in potential danger, take the following immediate steps:

- Have an escape route in mind.
- Stand at the side of the door; do not block a door. Always keep your back to a door.
- Maintain an open position: hands out of pockets, uncrossed arms and legs, hands visible.
- Call the person by name.
- If the person's voice is raised, speak softly and maintain a quiet, controlled voice.
- Remain calm; sit or stand still; do not fidget.
- Keep five to seven feet of distance between you and the person.
- Do not touch, point, order, challenge, argue, plead, belittle, threaten, or intimidate the person.
- Never turn your back on the person.
- Match eye contact.
- If overtly threatening, some people will respond to being told firmly, "You may not harm me" or "You do not want to harm me" or "It's against the rules."
- Enroll in a workshop aimed at teaching staff how to deescalate a patient and/or includes instructions on using self-defense techniques in a health care setting.

Many other practical suggestions are available from experienced nurses like your instructor and are based on tools such as those developed by osha.gov. These tools and resources can be found at https://www.osha.gov/dsg/hospitals/workplace_violence.html. This is a time to keep a cool, calculating head (function now, shake later). Complete the exercise in the Try This: Evaluate Protection Against Potential Dangers box.

◎ Try This

Evaluate Protection Against Potential Dangers

Do the health care agencies where you receive your clinical experience educate their employees in management of assault behavior and/or gentle self-defense? Are assaults at this facility reported to the police? Under what circumstances are charges pressed against the perpetrator?

Investigate where in your nursing program you learn about identifying signs of possible danger to you and techniques of gentle self-defense to protect yourself.

? Critical Thinking

Preventing Possible Assault

Depending on what you discovered in the previous learning exercise, make a plan for learning what you need to know to better protect yourself from possible assault.

◄ Professional Pointer

If you feel unsafe, follow your intuition and remove yourself from the situation. Immediately notify your supervisor and provide for the patient's safety.

EMPLOYEE VIOLENCE

Workplace violence is defined by four categories (Romano et al. 2011):

1. Label 1: Criminal (perpetrator has no relationship to the workplace)
2. Label 2: Client-customer (involves abuse by a patient, family member, or visitor)
3. Label 3: Coworker (current or former employee)
4. Label 4: Domestic violence

The most common category is Label 2: client-customer. Most abuse reported by nurses has involved a patient, family member, or visitor (Romano et al. 2011).

Signs of Workplace Violence

Be alert to signs of violence in your patients, family members, visitors, and coworkers. Early signs of workplace violence might include the following:

- Unusual behavioral change
- Lack of cooperation with nurses, other patients, or family members
- Cursing and other hostile forms of communication
- Short fuse and frequent arguments
- Spreading gossip or rumors to harm others deliberately
- Uninvited sexual remarks
- Hostile responses to other nurses, patients, or family members
- Sleep disturbances mentioned at work
- Increased irritability and anxiety

The next stage of violence might include the following signs:

- Conversation focused on "poor me, the victim"
- Notes with threats, violent, or sexual content
- Verbalization that includes plans or a desire to harm someone
- Stealing workplace property
- Less interest in work and workplace assignments
- Increased arguments
- Increased physical accidents or injuries

As the anger intensifies, and if conflicts remain unresolved, the result can be violence against oneself or others:

- Behaviors directed toward oneself might include depression or suicidal threats
- Behaviors directed toward others might include physical fighting, property destruction, or use of a weapon to harm others

Prevention of Workplace Violence

Prevention entails management commitment and employee involvement. Prevention begins when each nurse:

- Makes a personal commitment to follow prevention guidelines
- Participates in the training and refresher courses offered by the health care agency
- Takes advantage of programs offered by the police department or other agencies
- Remembers that his or her focus is on *gentle self-defense*, not offense
- Is prepared before workplace violence becomes an issue
- Is familiar with his or her workplace policies that cover forms of violence, as well as harassment
- Is alert to warning signs and has thought through what he or she can do to prevent an escalation
- **Takes all threats seriously,** reports them to management, and encourages others to do the same
- Advocates assertively for implementing prevention guidelines in the facility (Box 9-3)

Box 9-3   Some General Safeguards for Preventing Workplace Violence

- Do your part to promote a supportive, congenial, yet professional work environment.
- Whenever possible, resolve conflicts as they arise. Know that there are times when you have to back off. However, most of the time people want to have their point of view heard. A technique called *creative communication* encourages you to do the following:
  - Listen carefully to the other person's point of view.
  - Ask questions to clarify what you do not understand. (Remember that this step is not a sneaky way to argue or interject your own opinion!)
- Tell the person what you think he or she said and what you think he or she is feeling. If your version is inaccurate, have the person repeat the explanation. When you can repeat back accurately what the person thinks and feels, then it is your turn to present your view.
- Use these steps as well when you present your point of view.
- Deal directly with unwanted or unwelcome behavior, including uninvited sexual advances.

- Review your own behavior to determine whether:
  - A clarification of the person's signals is in order.
  - Limits must be stated clearly and firmly on what you consider unacceptable behavior.
  - Supervisor or management intervention may be needed.
  - Get to know your fellow workers, and look out for one another.
- Promote workplace integrity. Treat one another, your patients, and their families with respect, courtesy, and professionalism. Negative comments by patients and relatives usually are a response to their fear of the unknown. Rarely are the comments meant to be personal. Check out the fear. What are the questions? What can you do to help find answers?
- Be alert to changes in behavior that may signal violence.
- Avoid putting yourself in obvious danger. Make use of security guards for escorts to parking lots and out-of-the-way areas. Listen to your intuition. This is making conscious use of affective communication.

? Critical Thinking

Personal Violence Prevention Plan

What additional ideas do you have to put into action to defuse or prevent violence of any kind in the workplace? Create an assertive approach.

SEXUAL HARASSMENT

Sexual harassment is about abuse of power. It is not about sex or passion. Out of the four world regions (Anglo, Asia, Europe, and Middle East), Spector et al. (2014) found that the rate of sexual harassment was highest in nurses who work in the Anglo region, with a report rate of 38.7% versus Europe (16.2%). Most nurses do not report the incidents, mostly from fear of losing their job, embarrassment, or fear that he or she will not be believed. According to the Equal Employment Opportunity Commission (EEOC), sexual harassment includes unwanted sexual advances or other verbal or physical conduct of a sexual nature, such as a condition of employment or advancement, or a hostile environment where the advances intimidate, offend, or interfere with the nurses' ability to do their work. The keyword is "unwanted." A distinct difference is made between consent and unwanted.

If you are the target, confront the person who is harassing you. Your assertive response is to tell the person clearly what he or she is doing, that this behavior is offensive to you and is unwanted. Be sure that your response is firmly assertive. Your message must be congruent so that the verbalization, body language (nonverbal), and affective communication all say the same thing. Mere words do not justify a physical response on your part. Document for yourself what happened, as well as what you said and did. Employers have the responsibility to correct unwanted (unwelcome) behavior that they know about or should know about in the workplace. If the unwanted behavior does not cease, report it to your supervisor, union representative, or department head, as needed, until you are heard. Take along your documentation. If the employer is convinced that someone is harassing you, they can reprimand, require counseling, demote, transfer, deny a promotion or raise, or dismiss the harasser. The seriousness of sexual harassment can no longer be ignored. The nurse's work is usually affected, and some will even leave their jobs to get away from it. For others, their emotional and/or physical health is affected, sometimes with long-term consequences. Complete the exercises in the Try This: Sexual Harassment Policy, and Critical Thinking: Personal Plans for Safety boxes.

◎ Try This

Sexual Harassment Policy

Locate your school policy regarding sexual harassment. Discuss with a peer common types of sexual harassment in a workplace setting.

? Critical Thinking

Personal Plans for Safety

Make a plan for yourself on how you will deal with any harassment attempts during future employment.

COUNSELING AND FILING CHARGES

Levine et al. (1998) concluded that assault-related injuries are preventable. Often only physical injuries are treated; all employees who have been verbally or physically assaulted should be referred for postincident debriefing. Hospital managers should implement violence prevention programs as recommended by OSHA (2015). If you are harmed or threatened by a patient or a patient's family member, you have the option to file charges. Some agencies will do this for you after a review board hearing, or they will support you if you file charges yourself.

LATERAL VIOLENCE

Some of the worst attacks on nurses are from within their own medical community. The attacks range from nasty words and vicious threats to physical assaults. Many nurses accept the violence as the norm and do not report an attack to their supervisor.

Lateral violence occurs between nursing colleagues. It includes both overt and covert physical, verbal, and emotional abuse by one nurse against another. These are the most common forms of lateral violence:

- Nonverbal innuendo such as eye rolling or eyebrow raising intended to belittle another nurse
- Verbal affronts
- Undermining activities
- Withholding information
- Sabotage
- Infighting
- Scapegoating
- Backstabbing
- Failure to respect privacy
- Broken confidences (Jahner, 2011).

Bullying is described as acts perpetrated by one in a higher level of authority. It includes behaviors such as the following:

- Intimidation, malice, or insults
- Abuse of power by an individual or group against others.

The behaviors are humiliating and threatening, and they can undermine self-confidence. Visit http://stop-bullyingtoolkit.org for resources to implement strategies aimed at decreasing bullying in your institution.

Vertical violence (horizontal hostility) occurs between persons of unequal power. For example, it might occur between a staff nurse and a student; a nurse manager and a student; an instructor and a student; or a new nurse and a seasoned staff nurse. The behavior humiliates and undermines confidence. The person who is bullied ends up feeling fearful and unsafe. Incivility is a common terminology used to describe hostility among nurses. Cindy Clark writes extensively on civility in nursing. Visit her blog at http://musingofthegreat blue.blogspot.com for details.

INSIDIOUS AGGRESSION

Insidious aggression, which is aggressive behavior in the workplace, is more harmful than sexual harassment. A study presented at the 2008 International Conference on Work Stress and Health (Health Day, 2008) reviewed 110 case studies over 21 years. According to the study:

- Agencies are more aware of sexual harassment, and it is lessening.
- Measures are being taken to recognize and prevent sexual harassment.
- Victims of sexual harassment find it easier to report incidences.
- Help is available to victims of sexual harassment.
- Insidious aggression is not against the law.

Issues of insidious aggression involve incivility, interpersonal issues, and hostile acts that are not obvious to others. For example, nurses do not generally report that they are being ignored by several staff members or that a staff member is not speaking to them. This can result in more job stress, less job satisfaction, less job commitment, less satisfying relationships, higher levels of anger and anxiety, and lower levels of overall well-being. Individuals who are subjected to insidious aggression are more likely to quit their job.

A lack of action on the part of the nurse gives approval and permission for the perpetrator to continue the behavior. As a nurse, you have the responsibility to act assertively, with the cooperation of other nurses, to advocate for a safe workplace.

? Critical Thinking

Think of a time that you might have experienced insidious aggression. What were your feelings during that time? Did your quality of work suffer? Did the experience affect your health? How did you ultimately resolve the situation?

Get Ready for the NCLEX-PN® Examination

Key Points

- Communication translates into behavior.
- Assertiveness is honest and open behavior. It considers others' feelings and needs. It is based on choice.
- Nonassertive (passive) and aggressive behaviors are based on emotional hooks. These styles are ultimately damaging to both parties involved. Be alert to unresolved feelings leading to a cycle of worry → fear → anger → rage.
- Using the steps of the problem-solving process can change undesirable behaviors and interactions. Verbal, nonverbal, and affective interactions must be dealt with during this change.
- Violence in the workplace has always been present. Health care institutions are not an exception.
- OSHA (2015) has established national guidelines to deter violence toward health care workers.
- Violent incidents are more common when nurses and security lack assertive management skills.
- Some patient diagnoses provide clues to potential violence.
- Legal redress is available to nurses who are injured during physical violence on the job.
- Both female and male nurses report sexual harassment as a condition for employment or advancement.
- Insidious aggression on the job includes incivility, interpersonal conflict, and bullying.
- Focusing on learning to be assertive in nursing benefits both you and the patient.

Additional Learning Resources

evolve Go to your Evolve website (http://evolve.elsevier.com/Knecht/success) for the following FREE learning resources:

- Answers to Critical Thinking Scenarios
- Additional learning activities
- Additional Review Questions for the NCLEX-PN® exam
- Helpful phrases for communicating in Spanish and more!

Review Questions for the NCLEX-PN® Examination

1. What is assertiveness?
   a. A level of communication that few nurses attain
   b. Outspoken, anger-based, honest communication
   c. An indirect method of getting others to do what you wish
   d. Taking a positive stand without violating others' rights

2. Which of the following best describes sexual harassment?
   a. A coworker and you have been sharing sexual jokes since you started working.
   b. The immediate supervisor has asked you (alone) to meet for dinner at his house.
   c. A patient asks you if you are willing to go out on a date after he is discharged.
   d. Your coworker is upset as a peer has refused to meet him socially for a drink.

3. What is an assertive response to a boss who is beginning to talk to you about problems with another nurse on the unit?

a. I am honored that you trust me to try to resolve this issue with you.

b. Maybe you and I can meet over coffee after the shift so it will be more private.

c. I am happy to assist in problem solving the broad issue, but I am uncomfortable discussing my peer's behavior with you, without them present.

d. If you don't tell anyone of our conversation, I'll tell you what I know.

4. Which of the following recommendations will you offer the unit's safety committee to promote a safe workplace?

a. We need to examine how staff attitude, body language, and the environment can impact unit/institution safety.

b. Safety is an issue that must be placed solely in the hands of nonuniformed, outside security staff.

c. It is necessary to go back to the strict visiting rules and limit hours and visitors to family.

d. Violence is a part of our current culture, and there is very little you can do to effect change.

Alternate Format Item

1. Which of the following is an example of an "I"-centered statement? *(Select all that apply.)*

a. I feel you are not quite working up to your potential.

b. I think that you could improve the accuracy of your work.

c. I feel that you are concerned for your safety.

d. I will watch you demonstrate inserting a catheter today.

e. I hope that you will be able to work tomorrow.

2. Which of the following are likely examples of insidious on-the-job aggression? *(Select all that apply.)*

a. Another nurse interrupted me to tell the physician about my patient.

b. I am routinely assigned the heaviest patient on the unit for morning care.

c. One group of nurses is bullying the new nurses on the unit.

d. When I am asked to go to lunch with someone, I explain that I must study for my classes.

e. A nurse is busy providing care to her patients and cannot assist another nurse when requested.

Critical Thinking Scenarios

Scenario 1

Pat is an associate's degree (AD) RN who had recently been appointed as unit manager in the Susan B. Nursing Home. The staff thought they had a winner: he is smart and outwardly charming to visitors and physicians. One day, Sara, an LPN, opened a door to a resident's room and heard Pat telling Mrs. B. in a sharp voice, "You are so stupid, and either you do as you're told or I will see to it that you are put out of the home." Neither Mrs. B. nor Pat heard her open the door, so Sara backed out quietly, unsure of what she should do. What are Sarah's options and the rationale for each option?

Scenario 2

Caroline is a newly licensed LPN. She is eager to do well in her new job at Dr. Smith's Medical Clinic. She is also trying hard to fit in with the rest of the staff (an advanced practice registered nurse [APRN] and a medical technologist). Caroline is responsible for greeting the patients, getting a brief statement of why they came in, measuring vitals and weight, and remembering to place the chart in the slot outside the door. What suggestions do you have as a former office nurse to help Caroline get started?

10

Cultural Uniqueness, Sensitivity, and Competence

Objectives

On completing this chapter, you will be able to do the following:

1. Define in your own words the following terms: culture; cultural competence; cultural diversity; cultural uniqueness; ethnocentrism; cultural bias; cultural sensitivity; stereotype.
2. Explain in your own words nine basic daily needs of all persons.
3. Describe your culture in the areas of: family; religion; communication; educational background; economic level; wellness, illness, birth, and death beliefs and practices.
4. Identify how all persons are unique and similar using Giger and Davidhizar's Transcultural Model (2008).

5. Explain in your own words the philosophy of individual worth as it applies to health care.
6. Describe general differences and stereotypes among cultural groups frequently served in your geographic area that may have importance in patient care situations.
7. Explain the importance of awareness, knowledge, information, and collaboration in developing an ability to provide culturally competent care.

Key Terms

assimilation (ă-SĬM-ă-LĀ-shŭn)
biomedicine (BĪ-ō-MĔD-ĭ-sĭn)
complementary and alternative medicine (CAM)
(KŎM-plĕ-MĔN-tĕ-rē, ăl-TŬR-nă-tĭv)
cultural bias (BĪ-ăs)
cultural competence (KŎM-pĭ-tĕns)
cultural diversity (dĭ-VŬR-sĭ-tē)
cultural sensitivity (SĔN-sĭ-TĬV-ĭ-tē)
culture
customs
discrimination (dĭ-SKRĬM-ĭ-NĀ-shŭn)
enculturation (ĕn-KŬL-chŭr-Ā-shŭn)

ethnic groups (ĔTH-nĭk)
ethnocentrism (ĔTH-nō-SĔN-TRĬZ-ĕm)
melting pot
naturalistic system (NĂCH-ŭr-ăl-LĬS-tĭk)
nonjudgmental (NŎN-jŭj-MĔN-tăl)
personalistic system (PŬR-sŏ-năl-LĬS-tĭk)
prejudice (PRĔJ-ŭ-dĭs)
repatterning
stereotype (STĔR-ē-ō-TĪP)
wellness and illness
worldview

💡 Keep in Mind

With knowledge comes responsibility. With knowledge of cultures, that responsibility entails a respect for differences.

You have chosen a career that will give you an opportunity to meet people who are different from you.
- Some of these people will be your patients.
- Some will be your peers at school.
- Some will be your coworkers.
- Some will be a different age than you.
- Some will belong to a different social class.
- Some will have disabilities.
- Some will have different health care beliefs about what causes them to get sick.
- Some will have different values.
- Because of ethnic group status, some of your patients and coworkers will have different cultural backgrounds.

- Regardless of cultural background, some differences will be the result of a growing diversity in individual and family lifestyles.

You will discover that people think, feel, believe, act, and see the world differently from you and your family and friends. Log on to www.minoritynurse.com/about/index.html to check out featured articles about issues facing nurses and to sign up for the free quarterly e-mail newsletter.

Review the standards of the National Association for Practical Nurse Education and Service, Inc. (NAPNES) at www.napnes.org, and the National Federation of Licensed Practical Nurses (NFLPN) at www.nflpn.org. You will note that both organizations have embraced statements that describe the need of the licensed practical nurse/licensed vocational nurse (LPN/LVN) to provide health care to all patients regardless of race, creed, cultural background, disease, or lifestyle. This is an ethical expectation. Review your state's Nurse Practice Act (NPA). You will find that failing or refusing to render nursing services to a patient because of the patient's race, color, sex, age, beliefs, national origin, or handicap is listed as unprofessional conduct. The ethical expectation now becomes a legal mandate. Nurses could risk legal suits because of their ignorance of the **culture** of the patient and resulting poor nursing judgment.

Not only do LPNs/LVNs need to provide care for all persons, but they also need to provide culturally competent care. **Cultural competence** is the *continuous* attempt of LPNs/LVNs to gain the knowledge and skills that will allow them to effectively provide care for patients of different cultures. Cultural competence is not gained by reading a chapter in a textbook or by looking up a culture in a reference book. It is developing an awareness of different cultures (**cultural sensitivity**) and continually learning about people who are different from you. Giger (2013) describes cultural competence as "a dynamic, fluid, continuous process whereby an individual, system, or health care agency finds meaning and useful care delivery strategies based on knowledge of the cultural heritage, beliefs, attitudes, and behaviors of those to whom they render care (p. 6)."

When differences are identified in a health care situation, the LPN/LVN needs to suggest adaptations to the plan of care so the plan recognizes these differences. In doing so, the patient will be encouraged to follow suggestions, avoid treatment failures, and return to health as quickly as possible. Practical/vocational nurses will then be able to say that they have truly met the patient's needs.

DEFINITION OF CULTURE

Culture is a way of life. It is the total of the *ever-changing* knowledge, ideas, thoughts, beliefs, values, communication, actions, attitudes, traditions, customs, and objects that a group of people possess and the ways they have of doing things. Culture also includes standards of behavior and sets of rules to live by. **Customs** are the generally accepted ways of doing things that are common to people who share the same culture.

CHARACTERISTICS OF CULTURE

An important point about culture is that it is *learned behavior*. The culture of a group is passed on from generation to generation. From the moment you were born, you began to learn about the culture of the group into which you were born. The process of learning your culture (the way your group does things) is called **enculturation**. A result of enculturation is a **worldview** that is generally shared by persons with the same cultural background. The worldview, or similar ways

of seeing and understanding the world, becomes the reality of the group. This reality fills every aspect of life. It is a **cultural bias** (a mental leaning) that is never proved or questioned by the individual. The worth of everything, either within or outside the group, depends on whether or not it fits the worldview of the cultural group. One's worldview can lead to ethnocentrism, prejudice, and discrimination, unless modified by knowledge and experience.

Socialization is the process by which a person of one culture learns how to function in a larger culture. Right now you are being socialized into the career of practical/vocational nursing. You are learning how to think and act like an LPN/LVN.

DANGER: ETHNOCENTRISM, PREJUDICE, AND DISCRIMINATION

People who belong to the same cultural group may develop the attitude, through their worldview, that their way of doing things is superior, right, or better than that of groups with different cultures (**ethnocentrism**). The group uses its culture as the norm against which to measure and evaluate the customs and ways of others. The group is uncomfortable with people who display customs and behaviors that differ from their cultural group. Ethnocentrism is common to all cultural groups. When intolerance of another cultural group occurs, **prejudice** results. When rights and privileges are withheld from those of another cultural group, this is called **discrimination**.

AVOIDING FALSE ASSUMPTIONS

Nursing students sometimes think that somewhere there is a manual that will tell them how to care for people who are different from themselves. This type of approach can lead to false assumptions, which are called **stereotypes**. A stereotype is an assumption used to describe all members of a specific group without exception. It is an expectation that all individuals in a group will act exactly the same in a situation just because they are members of that group. Stereotypes ignore the individual differences that occur within every cultural group. Members of any culture may have modified the degree to which they observe the values and practices of the culture.

[?] Critical Thinking

Example of a False Assumption

While speaking about a particular function at a seminar on business practices, the presenter singled out an engineer in the group who was of Japanese descent. He used the engineer as an example of someone who thinks differently from "Americans" because he is Asian. The engineer was a third-generation American and had no clue what the presenter was talking about.

How did the presenter in this situation go wrong in his assumption?

THINK LIKE AN ANTHROPOLOGIST!

Anthropologists are scientists who study physical, social, and cultural characteristics of human groups. It is helpful to understand how these scientists conduct their studies:

- Anthropologists start the study of cultural groups by identifying common trends in a cultural group.
- These common trends found in the group are called "generalizations."
- Then anthropologists gather data to determine if the common trends (generalizations) apply to all individuals within that cultural group.

Automatically generalizing cultural information about a group's health practices to one person in that group might be drawing a wrong conclusion. Does the individual follow the traditional practice of the group? Has the individual rejected the practice? Does the individual use the practice only in certain situations? If so, what situations? Is the person an immigrant? How recently? When people immigrate to a new country, culturally different groups do adopt some of the culture of the new country. The process of giving up parts of their own culture and adopting parts of the culture of the dominant group is called assimilation. Complete assimilation, however, rarely occurs. Members of the generations that follow the original immigrants may retain some elements of their original culture in addition to assimilating parts of the new culture. For these reasons, generalizations help explain observed behavior, but they do not *predict* behavior.

EACH CULTURE AND PERSON IS UNIQUE

Remember that each individual is unique and a product of their experiences, cultural norms, and beliefs (Giger, 2013). Giger and Davidhizar's Transcultural model (1991) provides a framework for caring for clients in a variety of settings focused on their unique personal identity. Giger and Davidhizar (1991, 2008) describe six cultural phenomena that are critical to the assessment of patients in providing data necessary for decision making in providing culturally competent care. See Figure 10-1 for details. These six phenomena include communication, space, social organization, time, environmental control, and biological variations. A brief discussion follows.

COMMUNICATION

Communication differences include language spoken, verbal behaviors (i.e., voice quality and pronunciation), nonverbal behaviors (e.g., direct eye contact, touching), and the use of silence. Communication is a cornerstone to effective patient care. Thus research supports the critical need for an interpreter, when a nurse and patient speak a different language. Communication and language assistance is listed as one of the National Standards for Culturally and Linguistically Appropriate Services in Health and Health Care (U.S. Department of Health and Human Services, 2013). The standards highlight the need to ensure the competence of an interpreter. Potential Health Insurance Portability and Accountability Act (HIPAA) violations should be

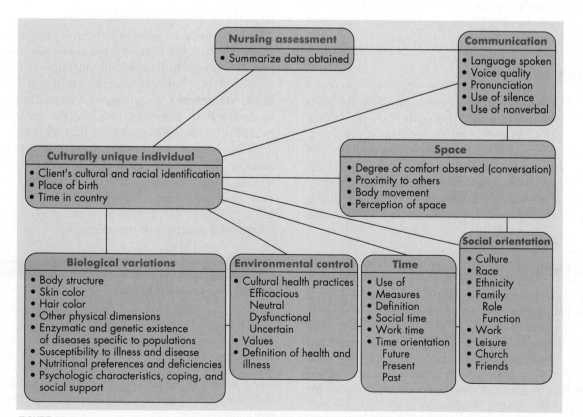

FIGURE 10-1 Schematic of Giger and Davidhizar's Transcultural Assessment Model. (From Giger J. [2013]. Transcultural nursing, assessment & intervention [ed 6]. St. Louis: Elsevier.)

considered if asking family to assist. In most cases, children should not be used as interpreters; women may also not be acceptable because of the cultural view of women in some cultures (Cherry & Jacob, 2014). Your local community may offer interpreter services. In addition, entities such as language line exist to meet this need (www.languageline.com). The LPN/VPN should review institutional policy and procedure for process and resources and implement accordingly.

SPACE

Space refers to the degree of comfort when speaking or interacting with people around us in a two person or a group setting. For example, Anglo Americans generally feel comfortable with a small space zone of 0 to 18 inches (Cherry & Jacob, 2014). This can vary significantly in other cultures. Some Asians would feel uncomfortable at this space range with strangers, such as an unfamiliar health care provider.

SOCIAL ORGANIZATION

Social organization refers to the family unit, the patient's affiliated religious or ethnic groups, and their political views. Family can be interpreted differently across cultures. For example, you may have heard an African American call someone their sister, even though they may not be related by blood but instead by friendship or experience.

TIME

Time orientation differs across cultures. People and cultures can be described as present, past, or future oriented. People who live in the present, live in the "moment." They move on to the next task when the time is right (Cherry & Jacob, 2014). This can contrast greatly with someone who lives in the past or future. People living in the past often look to their ancestors for wisdom and guidance and value previous experiences. Punctuality is often not a priority for those who have a past oriented time reference. Lastly, those who live in the future are generally punctual and strong planners. Long-term health care goals are important.

ENVIRONMENTAL CONTROLS

Environmental controls refer to whether the person has an internal (power is within them) or external locus of control (fate plays a large role in outcomes). The person's belief or lack of belief in supernatural forces can also vary across cultures.

BIOLOGICAL VARIATIONS

Biological variations across cultures can be visible or invisible. Genetic tendencies related to body build and body structure, hair type, eye shape, and skin characteristics can be easily visible. In contrast, nutritional variations and incidence of specific diseases can be invisible. For example, rates of cardiac disease can differ across cultures.

These six cultural phenomena should be an important component of a health care team's assessment of all patients, given our diverse society. Box 10-1 provides a detailed assessment model (Giger & Davidhizar, 1991) for the LPN/VPN to use. This will assist in providing data needed by the health care team to develop a culturally competent plan of care.

Box 10-1 Giger and Davidhizar's Transcultural Assessment Model

CULTURALLY UNIQUE INDIVIDUAL
1. Place of birth
2. Cultural definition
   What is . . .
3. Race
   What is . . .
4. Length of time in country (if appropriate)

COMMUNICATION
1. Voice quality
   A. Strong, resonant
   B. Soft
   C. Average
   D. Shrill
2. Pronunciation and enunciation
   A. Clear
   B. Slurred
   C. Dialect (geographical)
3. Use of silence
   A. Infrequent
   B. Often
   C. Length
      1) Brief
      2) Moderate
      3) Long
      4) Not observed

4. Use of nonverbal
   A. Hand movement
   B. Eye movement
   C. Entire body movement
   D. Kinesics (gestures, expressions, or stances)
5. Touch
   A. Startles or withdraws when touched
   B. Accepts touch without difficulty
   C. Touches others without difficulty
6. Ask these and similar questions:
   A. How do you get your point across to others?
   B. Do you like communicating with friends, family, and acquaintances?
   C. When asked a question, do you usually respond (in words or body movement, or both)?
   D. If you have something important to discuss with your family, how would you approach them?

SPACE
1. Degree of comfort
   A. Moves when personal space invaded
   B. Does not move when space invaded
2. Distance in conversations
   A. 0 to 18 inches
   B. 18 inches to 3 feet
   C. 3 feet or more

Continued

Box 10-1 **Giger and Davidhizar's Transcultural Assessment Model—cont'd**

3. Definition of space
   A. Describe degree of comfort with closeness when talking with or standing near others
   B. How do objects (e.g., furniture) in the environment affect your sense of space?
4. Ask these and similar questions:
   A. When you talk with family members, how close do you stand?
   B. When you communicate with coworkers and other acquaintances, how close do you stand?
   C. If a stranger touches you, how do you react or feel?
   D. If a loved one touches you, how do you react or feel?
   E. Are you comfortable with the distance between us now?

SOCIAL ORGANIZATION
1. Normal state of health
   A. Poor
   B. Fair
   C. Good
   D. Excellent
2. Marital status
3. Number of children
4. Parents living or deceased?
5. Ask these and similar questions:
   A. How do you define social activities?
   B. What are some activities that you enjoy?
   C. What are your hobbies, or what do you do when you have free time?
   D. Do you believe in a Supreme Being?
   E. How do you worship that Supreme Being?
   F. What is your function (what do you do) in your family unit/system?
   G. What is your role in your family unit/system (father, mother, child, advisor)?
   H. When you were a child, what or who influenced you most?
   I. What is/was your relationship with your siblings and parents?
   J. What does work mean to you?
   K. Describe your past, present, and future jobs.
   L. What are your political views?
   M. How have your political views influenced your attitude toward health and illness?

TIME
1. Orientation to time
   A. Past-oriented
   B. Present-oriented
   C. Future-oriented
2. View of time
   A. Social time
   B. Clock-oriented
3. Physiochemical reaction to time
   A. Sleeps at least 8 hours a night
   B. Goes to sleep and wakes on a consistent schedule
   C. Understands the importance of taking medication and other treatments on schedule
4. Ask these and similar questions:
   A. What kind of timepiece do your wear daily?
   B. If you have an appointment at 2 PM, what time is acceptable to arrive?

C. If a nurse tells you that you will receive a medication in "about a half hour," realistically, how much time will you allow before calling the nurses' station?

ENVIRONMENTAL CONTROL
1. Locus-of-control
   A. Internal locus-of-control (believes that the power to effect change lies within)
   B. External locus-of-control (believes that fate, luck, and chance have a great deal to do with how things turn out)
2. Value orientation
   A. Believes in supernatural forces
   B. Relies on magic, witchcraft, and prayer to effect change
   C. Does not believe in supernatural forces
   D. Does not rely on magic, witchcraft, or prayer to effect change
3. Ask these and similar questions:
   A. How often do you have visitors at your home?
   B. Is it acceptable to you for visitors to drop in unexpectedly?
   C. Name some ways your parents or other persons treated your illnesses when you were a child.
   D. Have you or someone else in your immediate surroundings ever used a home remedy that made you feel sick?
   E. What home remedies have you used that worked? Will you use them in the future?
   F. What is your definition of "good health"?
   G. What is your definition of "poor health"?

BIOLOGICAL VARIATIONS
1. Conduct a complete physical assessment noting:
   A. Body structure (small, medium, or large frame)
   B. Skin color
   C. Unusual skin discolorations
   D. Hair color and distribution
   E. Other visible physical characteristics (e.g., keloids, chloasma)
   F. Weight
   G. Height
   H. Check lab work for variances in hemoglobin, hematocrit, and sickle cell phenomena if black or Mediterranean.
2. Ask these and similar questions:
   A. What diseases or illnesses are common in your family?
   B. Has anyone in your family been told that there is a possible genetic susceptibility for a particular disease?
   C. Describe your family's typical behavior when a family member is ill.
   D. How do you respond when you are angry?
   E. Who (or what) usually helps you to cope during a difficult time?
   F. What foods do you and your family like to eat?
   G. Have you ever had any unusual cravings for:
      1) White or red clay dirt?
      2) Laundry starch?
   H. When you were a child what types of foods did you eat?
      I. What foods are family favorites or are considered traditions?

Box 10-1   Giger and Davidhizar's Transcultural Assessment Model—cont'd

NURSING ASSESSMENT

1. Note whether the client has become culturally assimilated or observes own cultural practices.
2. Incorporate data into plan of nursing care:
   A. Encourage the client to discuss cultural differences: people from diverse cultures who hold different world views can enlighten nurses.
   B. Make efforts to accept and understand methods of communication.
   C. Respect the individual's personal need for space.
   D. Respect the rights of clients to honor and worship the Supreme Being of their choice.
   E. Identify a clerical or spiritual person to contact.
   F. Determine whether spiritual practices have implications for health, life, and well-being (e.g., Jehovah's Witnesses may refuse blood and blood derivatives; an Orthodox Jew may eat only kosher food high in sodium and may not drink milk when meat is served).

   G. Identify hobbies, especially when devising interventions for a short or extended convalescence or for rehabilitation.
   H. Honor time and value orientations and differences in these areas. Allay anxiety and apprehension if adherence to time is necessary.
   I. Provide privacy according to personal need and health status of the client (Note: the perception of and reaction to pain may be culturally related).
   J. Note cultural health practices:
      1) Identify and encourage efficacious practices.
      2) Identify and discourage dysfunctional practices.
      3) Identify and determine whether neutral practices will have a long-term ill effect.
   K. Note food preferences.
      1) Make as many adjustments in diet as health status and long-term benefits will allow and that the dietary department can provide.
      2) Note dietary practices that may have serious implications for the client.

From Giger J. (2013). Transcultural nursing, assessment & intervention (ed 6). St. Louis: Elsevier.

KNOWING YOURSELF

According to the Standards of Practice for Culturally Competent Nursing Care (Douglas et al., 2011), critical reflection is defined in the following way: "Nurses shall engage in critical reflection of their own values, beliefs, and cultural heritage to have an awareness of how these qualities and issues can affect culturally congruent nursing care" (p. 318). Thus knowing yourself is a critical step in providing culturally competent care.

WHAT MAKES YOU UNIQUE?

To become aware of different cultures, you need to be aware of yourself as a person. Several activities are included in this chapter to help you with cultural self-awareness. The exercises also help you develop an awareness of cultural differences with peers.

◎ Try This

What Makes You Unique?

Let your uniqueness show! Divide the class into small but equal-sized groups. Find one item that makes you unique from other members of the group using Giger and Davidhizar's Transcultural Model (2008) as a reference. Share with your class the item that makes you unique.

HOW MANY HATS DO YOU WEAR?

Most people have several roles in life. People speak of "wearing many hats" or "having a full plate." Some of these roles are played out individually, one at a time, and others are performed simultaneously. The exercise in the

Try This: Identifying the Roles You Play in Your Life box gives you the opportunity to identify your roles.

◎ Try This

Identifying the Roles You Play in Your Life

The following categories describe the roles you play in several areas in your everyday life.

CATEGORY 1: ECONOMIC STATUS ROLE

Although standards are available to assign persons to each of the following economic classes, people generally place themselves in one of the following categories by how they perceive their economic status.

Place a check mark next to the economic class that best describes you.

I am in the

_____ Lower economic class
_____ Middle economic class
_____ Upper economic class

CATEGORY 2: POLITICAL ROLE

Put a check mark next to the word(s) that best describe(s) the political role you play in society.

I am

_____ Republican
_____ Democrat
_____ Libertarian
_____ Independent
_____ Liberal
_____ Conservative
_____ Moderate
_____ Indifferent
_____ To the left of liberal
_____ To the right of conservative

Other _____

Continued

(◎) Try This

Identifying the Roles You Play in Your Life—cont'd

CATEGORY 3: RACIAL OR ETHNIC ROLE

Place a check mark beside the racial or ethnic terms that best describe you.

I am

Black or African American/ non-Hispanic	Hispanic
White/non-Hispanic	Asian
American Indian or Alaska Native	Native Hawaiian or Pacific Islander
Of multiple races	Other

CATEGORY 4: SOCIAL ROLE

Circle the social roles that describe you.

I am (a)

Female/Male	Stepsister/Stepbrother
Married/Single	Half-sister/Half-brother
Separated/Divorced	Godmother/Godfather
Blended family	Godchild
Wife/Husband	Grandmother/Grandfather
Significant other	Granddaughter/Grandson
Mother/Father	Aunt/Uncle
Daughter/Son	Niece/Nephew
Sister/Brother	Cousin
Stepmother/Stepfather	Other_____
Stepdaughter/ Stepson	

CATEGORY 5: WORK ROLE

Place a check mark beside each work role you play in your life.

I am (a)

Blue-collar worker	Student
Businessperson	Technician
Laborer	Unemployed
Professional	White-collar worker
Service provider	Other
Skilled worker	

Summarize the hats you wear by listing the items you have checked and circled in the five categories.

Category 1: Economic status role _____

Category 2: Political role _____

Category 3: Racial or ethnic role _____

Category 4: Social role _____

Category 5: Work role _____

(◎) Try This

Who Am I Based on My Roles?

Make up a sentence using all the words you listed in the five role categories. This sentence describes you by the roles you play in your life. Working in groups of four to six, have each student type their sentence on a word document. Next, project the sentences for each member of the group on the screen/whiteboard in the classroom. Have students in the class vote for which member of the group the information describes. Particularly if there are different responses, discuss why. Could stereotyping be occurring? (A student response system [clickers] can assist in this exercise.)

WHAT WE SHARE IN COMMON

Because of our genes, each of us is different from every other person in the world. (The only exception is identical twins.) Before you start to think about the differences among people, it is a good idea to think about what people have in common.

(◎) Try This

What We Have in Common

When you are among a group of your peers (e.g., eating lunch in the cafeteria or walking to the parking lot), take a few minutes to play the "What We Have in Common" culture game. Excluding sex, age, marital status, and culture group, try to find five items you share in common with each member of the group. This activity is especially helpful when the group includes classmates you perceive as "different" from you.

1. _____

2. _____

3. _____

4. _____

5. _____

- In a class situation, discuss the items you have in common. Did any items you share in common with other members of the group surprise you?
- Did you discover any stereotyping in *your* thinking regarding your peers?

KNOWING OTHERS: CULTURAL DIVERSITY

In the nineteenth century, waves of immigrants from all over the world came to the United States. The United States was eventually called a **melting pot**, meaning that these immigrants had given up their native cultures and adopted the culture of the American people.

The 2010 U.S. Census included the categories of Hispanic/Latino/Spanish origin (if so, indicate if Mexican, Mexican American, Chicano, Puerto Rican, Cuban, Argentinean, Colombian, Dominican, Nicaraguan, Salvadoran, Spaniard, and so on), white, black, African American or Negro, American Indian or Alaska Native, Asian Indian, Chinese, Filipino, Japanese, Korean, Vietnamese, other Asian (Hmong, Laotian, Thai, Pakistani, Cambodian, and so on), Native Hawaiian, Guamanian or Chamorro, Samoan, other Pacific Islander, or other race. If the current trends continue, the U.S. Census Bureau predicts that minorities will make up 55% of the U.S. population by 2025 (U.S. Department of Health and Human Services, 2010). Thus minorities will be the majority in the United States. This has impacted our society. Today, the melting pot is more like a "casserole," with each ingredient (i.e., different culture) adding to the quality of the whole. The concept of the melting pot has been replaced by the concept of **cultural diversity**, which refers to the many differences in the elements of culture in groups of people in American and Canadian society.

Cultural diversity goes beyond racial and **ethnic groups**. As an LPN/LVN, you need to define this concept more broadly so culturally diverse groups can also mean single parents, people who live in poverty, homosexuals, bisexuals, the wealthy, the poor, the homeless, the elderly, and people with disabilities.

The concept of race as a means of categorizing people by biologic traits has come under attack by social scientists. These scientists suggest using ethnicity as a more accurate means of capturing the great diversity found in over 7.1 billion people in the world (World Bank, 2015) Members of ethnic groups are a special type of cultural group, composed of people who are members of the same race, religion, or nation, or who speak the same language. They derive part of their identity through membership of the ethnic group. Examples of ethnic groups in the United States include Irish Americans, African Americans, American Indians, Asian Americans, German Americans, Mexican Americans, Jewish Americans, Arab Americans, Greek Americans, Finnish Americans, and many more.

IMPORTANCE OF CULTURAL DIVERSITY

Health care today and into the future needs to be able to accommodate patients of many different cultural backgrounds. Failure to develop sensitivity to and competence in handling this diversity could lead to misunderstandings between you and the patient, resulting in stress for both. The plan of treatment for the patient could fail. You could make false assumptions based on generalizations. You might label patients as difficult or uncooperative when their lack of cooperation with the plan of care could be related to a conflict with their personal health belief system. Patients may experience less-than-adequate care when cultural diversity and the differences it represents are overlooked or misinterpreted.

Philosophy of Individual Worth

The philosophy of individual worth is a belief shared by all members of the health care team. The philosophy includes the uniqueness and value of each human being who comes for care, regardless of differences that may be observed or perceived in that individual. LPNs/LVNs need to realize that each individual has the right to live according to their personal beliefs and values, *as long as they do not interfere with the rights of others.* Each individual deserves respect as a human being.

Professional Pointer

Respect cultural differences.

Many factors are responsible for differences in patients. They may think and behave differently because of social class, personal income, religion, ethnic background, or personal choice. Regardless of these differences, all patients have the right to receive high-quality nursing care. As an LPN/LVN you cannot decrease the quality of the care you give because of differences you observe or perceive.

LPNs/LVNs need to guard against making judgments about people who are culturally different. This does not mean you must adopt differences as part of your behavior. It means being open-minded and **nonjudgmental**. It means taking the difference at face value, accepting people as they are, and giving high-quality care. Be aware of your own attitudes, beliefs, and values and hidden biases as they affect your ability to give care. If you do identify biases, see them for what they are. Become sensitive to cultural differences, and acknowledge that they exist. Gather knowledge about them so you can work on trying to modify your biases and provide more culturally competent care. Visit https://implicit.harvard.edu/implicit/takeatest.html to take a test to uncover your hidden bias.

LEARNING ABOUT CULTURAL DIVERSITY

How to Begin

You have been given exercises that help you to discover your own uniqueness and that of others, as well as similarities. Unless you understand your own culture, it will be difficult to understand the culture of others. You need to look inside yourself to learn about your own cultural beliefs, values, and worldview and the influence they have on how you think and act. Some elements of your culture are obvious, such as your language, celebrated holidays, and how and what you eat. However, other aspects of your culture are hidden. Elements such as aspects of communication, beliefs, attitudes, values, sex roles, use of space, concept of time, structure of the family, and family dynamics may be more difficult to recognize and discuss. Some areas of cultural diversity may be taken for granted in patient situations. Examples include food preferences, religion, educational background, economic level, wellness and illness beliefs and practices, the birth experience, and terminal illness and death beliefs and practices.

The first step to developing knowledge about patient differences in these areas is to become aware of and explore *your* cultural patterns in these areas. Read the general information about each area below. Develop an awareness of your own cultural patterns in these areas by answering the group of statements or questions included with each area. Sharing this information with peers will highlight the cultural diversity that exists in your nursing class, regardless of cultural background. The questions also provide examples of areas to be discussed with patients when collecting data about their personal beliefs and health practices.

AREAS OF CULTURAL DIVERSITY

Family Structure

No matter what culture is being discussed, the family is the basic unit of society. The role of the family is to have children, if desired or as they come, and to raise them to be contributing members of the group. Actual child-rearing practices vary from culture to culture. Families generally socialize the young to the culture of the group. They meet the physical and psychological needs of the young in culturally specific ways. Some cultures expect only the nuclear family (mother, father, and children) to live in the same house. Others may expect the extended family (the nuclear family plus the grandparents and other relatives) to do so. Some Vietnamese families are examples of extended families, with three or more generations living in the same house. In many of these families, ties are strong. Behaviors that enhance the family name are encouraged, such as obedience to parents and those in authority.

The single-parent family continues to challenge the traditional nuclear family as the typical family structure. A parent may become a single parent on the death of a spouse, by electing not to marry at the time of pregnancy, or by divorce. The blended family and same sex parent families represent a growing trend in our society. Health care workers who have not been in the same situation may be unaware of, and insensitive to, the way of life of these various types of family.

⊚ Try This

Cultural Patterns: Family

Respond to the following statements. Your responses will help you discover your own cultural patterns in regard to the family.
1. Describe your family structure (nuclear, extended, or alternative lifestyle).
2. Describe the role of children, if any, in your family.
3. Discuss who gives permission for hospitalization in your family.
4. List factors that influence the decision of your family members to visit or not visit the hospital when a member is ill. If visiting is acceptable, how long does your family think it is appropriate to visit?
5. Describe the effect that your hospitalization today at 4 PM for emergency surgery would have on you and your family.

Food Preferences

All cultures use food to provide needed nutrients. However, what they eat, when they eat, and how they eat differ vastly by cultural group. Knowledge of nutrition as a science differs by culture. It is interesting that the soil of some cultures (e.g., Mexico) encouraged the growth of two complementary foods that together make up a complete protein source (corn and beans) and became a staple of that culture's diet. Specific foods in different cultures have different meanings. All cultures use food during celebrations. Through generations of experience, different cultures have learned to use different foods to promote health and cure disease.

⊚ Try This

Cultural Patterns: Food

To assist you in identifying your own cultural patterns with regard to food preferences, respond to the following statements or questions.
1. What is your favorite food?
2. Identify one special occasion in which your cultural group participates. What foods, if any, are part of this celebration?
3. Describe your favorite recipe or meal from your mother and from your grandmother. What special ingredients or techniques are used to make the recipe? Is there a written recipe?
4. Discuss with a classmate food preferences that are unknown to you in your culture. Learn from each other.

Religious Beliefs

Religious beliefs are personal to the individual. Religion is an important aspect of culture. Religion can have different meanings in people's lives. For some, religion is a brief, momentary, and sporadic part of daily life. For another person, it may influence every aspect of life and have a profound effect on personal outlook and on how one lives his or her life. For others, religion may not play a part in their lives at all. Chapter 11 deals with spirituality and religious differences. There is a close relationship between religious beliefs and the concept of wellness and illness in some groups. LPNs/LVNs need to be aware of their own religious beliefs, obligations, and attitudes. They need to know whether or not these beliefs and attitudes influence the care that is given to patients.

Concept of Time

Some people follow clock time. An hour has a beginning and an end (after 60 minutes). People who follow clock time eat, sleep, work, and engage in recreational activities at definite times each day. Other people live on linear time. For them, time is a straight line with no beginning and no end. People who follow linear time eat when they are hungry and sleep when they are tired.

⊚ Try This

Cultural Patterns: Time

The questions that follow give you an opportunity to discover your own cultural patterns in regard to time.
1. What determines when it is time for you to eat or sleep?
2. When you are not in the clinical area, do you keep track of time?
3. Are you on time for appointments?

Communication

Chapter 8 introduced you to the types of communication and potential barriers to the communication process. As mentioned earlier in this chapter, a major barrier to communication in health care is when the patient or nurse speaks a different language. A person's language gives a view of reality that may differ from yours. For example, in English, the clock "runs," but in Spanish, it "walks." This illustrates the different concept of time between the two cultures. For a person who speaks English as a first language, time could move quickly, and there may be a rush to get things done. For some who speak Spanish as a first language, time may move more slowly. The following is a list of areas of communication that may vary for people who are culturally different.

Forms of hellos and good-byes
- You may greet your patient and want to get right down to business.
- The patient might expect some light conversation before getting to the matter at hand.
- In some cultural groups, people take an hour to say good-bye, whereas people from other cultures may get up and leave without saying anything.

Appropriateness of the situation
- Some groups prefer people to sit, not stand, while they converse.
- In some groups the sharing of food is a good way to relate to others and get them to verbalize.

Confidentiality
- All information the patient gives the nurse is considered confidential.
- Some patients do not want their spouse questioned or informed about their problems of the reproductive organs. They fear the spouse may think they are less desirable sexually.

Emotions and feelings and their expression
- Emotions are universal, but the cues to those emotions vary considerably. A lack of awareness of this fact can cause unnecessary stress between the patient and the nurse.
- In some cultural groups, people cannot display affection in public, show disapproval or frustration, or vent anger.
- Some members of cultural groups cannot take criticism.
- You may show dissatisfaction with other members of the health care team by approaching them directly, whereas some team members may show dissatisfaction with you by being polite to your face but then complaining about you to the rest of the staff. The same applies to your peers.

Pain expression
- Pain has two parts: sensation and response. All individuals experience the same sensation of pain.
- One's culture influences the definition of pain and the response to the sensation.
- Pain is whatever the person says it is. It exists whenever the person says it does.
- One's culture provides guidelines for approved ways of expressing one's response to the pain sensation and ways to relieve the pain.

- Some cultures teach individuals that it is acceptable to cry, moan, and exhibit other behavior that calls attention to the pain. These behaviors may be considered a cure for pain in their culture.
- Other cultures encourage uncomplaining acceptance of pain and passive behavior when pain is experienced (stoic behavior).

Tempo of conversation
- You may tend to speak quickly and expect a quick response.
- The patient may be accustomed to pausing and reflecting before giving a response.

Meaning of silence
- Silence can mean anything from disapproval to warmth, but generally it does not indicate tension or lack of rapport.
- Silence can be difficult for some nurses to tolerate. Resist the temptation to jump in at a pause in the conversation by forcing yourself to concentrate on listening.

[?] Critical Thinking

Stoic Behavior in Patients

Discuss some nursing situations in which a stoic (seemingly unaffected by pain) reaction to pain could have negative consequences if an LPN/LVN lacked knowledge of cultural differences in pain expression (e.g., a woman in labor or a patient having a heart attack).

[◎] Try This

Cultural Patterns: Communication

Develop an awareness of your own cultural patterns in communication by answering the following questions:
1. What is your first (native) language?
2. Do you speak additional languages?
3. What facial or body habits are you aware of in yourself while you are talking?
4. How do you greet people, and how do you say good-bye?
5. How do you express the following emotions?
   a. Love
   b. Hate
   c. Fear
   d. Excitement
   e. Disappointment
   f. Dissatisfaction
   g. Humor
   h. Anger
   i. Sadness
   j. Happiness.
6. Do you make eye contact when talking to people?
7. Do you touch people while talking?
   a. If so, how do they react?
   b. How do you react when people touch you while they are talking to you?
8. How do you express pain? How do you react to pain?

Educational Background

The 2003 National Assessment of Adult Literacy assessed the English health literacy of adults in the United States and found that 14% do not have basic health literacy skills (able to understand a simple health pamphlet), whereas 22% have these skills (able to understand a more complex health pamphlet). Adults assessed got most of their information about health issues from radio and television (Kutner, 2006). Differences in educational background and literacy need to be taken into consideration when teaching patients. When in the clinical area, try to adapt your explanations to the patient's level of understanding.

◎ Try This

Cultural Patterns: Education

Your responses to the following statements will help you identify your own beliefs and practices in regard to education.

1. Calculate the number of years of education you have.
2. State your ultimate educational goal.
3. Discuss the role education plays in your life.
4. Describe your feelings toward a person who has less education than you.
5. Describe your feelings toward a person who has more education than you.
6. Describe your feelings if you were referred to your school's tutor/skills development center/remediation center.
7. Discuss the effect of your cultural background on your values and practices with regard to education.
8. Who in your family has graduated from high school, technical school, junior college, or a college or university?

Economic Level

Economic level is often related to educational background. Sociologists use these two factors to determine the social class of individuals. You will meet patients who are very wealthy and patients who are at or near the poverty level. Others have midlevel incomes. Patients' annual incomes determine the type of house they live in, the neighborhood where they live, the availability of food, and the ability to participate in certain types of preventive health care. LPNs/LVNs need to take economic level into consideration while reinforcing patient teaching and should adapt their approach accordingly when needed.

◎ Try This

Cultural Patterns: Economic Level

Identify your personal patterns in regard to economic level by responding to the following statements or questions.

1. Describe how your economic background affects your daily life in the following areas:
   a. Availability of food
   b. Availability of shelter
   c. Availability of clothing
   d. Amount and type of recreation.

2. Discuss your feelings toward a person who has less money than you.
3. Discuss your feelings toward a person who has more money than you.
4. Describe how these feelings fit with those of your cultural group.
5. Discuss your ability to afford to go to a physician when you get sick.
6. If you work, do you have health insurance benefits?
7. Discuss the implications as they relate to Maslow's hierarchy of needs theory.

Wellness and Illness Beliefs and Practices

Wellness and illness can have different meanings for persons who are culturally different. *Wellness* and *illness* are relative terms. What is good health to one person can be sickness to another. Wellness may not be a high-priority matter to some patients.

Preventing illness. Some patients believe that illness can be prevented; they practice elaborate rituals and engage special persons to carry out those rituals in an attempt to prevent disease. Other patients look at prevention as an attempt to control the future; they may consider this an impossible feat in the way they view their lives. They may wonder about the necessity of making a trip to a health care provider for preventive care, such as immunizations. Others may think prevention is tempting fate and following through with prevention is risky.

Curing illness. When disease does strike, some people blame pathogens (germs), some blame spirits, and others blame an imbalance in the body. Some cultural groups have folk medicine practices, such as rituals, special procedures (e.g., rubbing the skin with the edge of a coin to release the toxins causing illness), and special persons in the group to cure disease (e.g., physician, herbalist, shaman). Some groups believe that special foods or food combinations (e.g., "cold" foods for "hot" illness) and herbs (e.g., Echinacea and Feverfew) can prevent or cure illnesses. Others see no relationship between diet and health.

Complementary and alternative medicine. The dominant health system in the United States is biomedicine (Western medicine). Biomedicine focuses on symptoms, with the goal of finding the cause of a disease and then eliminating or relieving the problem. Over 50% of Americans seek methods that avoid side effects from medications and treatments and/or that focus on the whole body and not just symptoms when treating disease. They are spending billions of dollars a year, mostly out of pocket, on complementary (used in conjunction with biomedical treatments) and alternative (a substitute for conventional medicine) medicines. **Complementary and alternative medicine (CAM)** focuses on assisting the body's own healing powers and restoring body balance. The diversity of non-Western health care practices among the many cultural groups in the United States has helped increase the interest and use of CAM. The National Center for Complementary and Alternative Medicine (NCCAM) of the National Institutes of Health conducts research and evaluates the effectiveness and safety of CAM. NCCAM's website (http://www.nccam.nih.gov) provides information about CAM.

Modesty. Individuals in some cultures are embarrassed when they have to discuss bodily functions or allow certain body parts to be examined. Hygiene practices vary according to beliefs, living conditions, personal resources, and physical characteristics.

Mental illness. Some cultural groups attach a stigma to mental illness and psychiatrists but are accepting of impairments to physical health. Other groups believe that the mental symptoms manifested are a healthy reaction to an emotional crisis. Yet others believe that the mind and body are united and are not separate entities. These cultures may have traditional healers who are experts at healing both the mind and the body. Some people may seek out traditional healers to heal the mind, while at the same time consult Western medicine to heal the body.

◎ Try This
Cultural Patterns: Wellness Beliefs and Practices

To assist you in identifying your own cultural patterns in regard to wellness beliefs and practices, respond to the following statements and questions.
1. Describe what it means to you to be in good health.
2. What are some of your own practices or beliefs about staying well?
3. Describe what it means to you to be sick.
4. List some foods in your diet that you believe help prevent illness.
   a. How does eating these foods prevent illness?
   b. What are some foods you must avoid to prevent illness?
5. List some foods in your diet that help you recover when you are sick.
   a. What illnesses do they cure?
   b. How do they cure illness?
6. Discuss CAM used by your family.
7. If you use CAM and biomedicine, do you inform the physician of CAM use, including herbs, during a clinic visit?
8. Describe your attitude toward mental illness.
   a. Describe what you think causes mental illness.
   b. Who do you think should treat mental illness?
   c. How do you believe mental illness is best treated?

Pregnancy and Birth Beliefs and Practices
Different cultures welcome a new member into the world in different ways. The Try This: Cultural Patterns: Pregnancy and Birth Beliefs and Practices box helps you to identify your own beliefs about pregnancy and birth.

◎ Try This
Cultural Patterns: Pregnancy and Birth Beliefs and Practices

To assist you in identifying your own cultural patterns in regard to birth beliefs and practices, respond to the following statements and questions about your family's customs regarding pregnancy and birth.
1. Do the women in your family receive prenatal care?
2. How is "discomfort" expressed during labor?
3. Who attends the birth?
4. Where does birth take place?
5. Who delivers the baby?
6. Is bonding encouraged?
7. What special practices take place after birth and during the postpartum period?
8. Are there special practices regarding the placenta and umbilical cord?
9. Is breastfeeding encouraged?
10. Are there precautions regarding breastfeeding?
11. Is birth control encouraged? Is it permitted?

Terminal Illness and Death Beliefs and Practices
Generally, death and terminal illness bring out strong emotions in most people. Be aware that some cultures have special taboos and prohibitions when a death occurs. Roles that family and friends carry out at the time of death may vary. There are many differences in the way different cultures handle terminal illness for a member. When death does occur, the rituals practiced are numerous and varied.

◎ Try This
Cultural Patterns: Terminal Illness and Death Beliefs and Practices

To assist you in identifying your own cultural patterns in regard to terminal illness and death beliefs and practices, respond to the following statements and questions pertaining to a death in your family.
1. Is it acceptable to tell a terminally ill family member the diagnosis? If yes, who tells the family member?
2. Would your family engage in palliative or hospice care for themselves or their loved one?
3. Where does an anticipated death usually occur (at home, in a hospital)?
4. Who should be present when the death occurs?
5. Does your family require specific treatment of the body after death?
6. Does your family permit/encourage autopsy or organ donation?
7. Who makes the burial arrangements?
8. Describe what you believe happens to you after death.
9. Does your family permit cremation?
10. Does your family have a funeral or memorial service?
11. Do you have a get-together after the burial? If so, for whom? What occurs during the get-together?
12. How does your family remember the dead?

◎ Try This

Areas of Cultural Diversity

With your peers, discuss your answers to statements and questions about various areas of cultural diversity, especially wellness and illness, birth, and death practices.

Regardless of which cultural group you belong to, these exercises about cultural diversity have given you the opportunity to think about the many ways you and your peers differ. You will observe some of these differences in patients in the clinical area and learn from them. Along with that awareness of and sensitivity to differences, a tolerance may develop for ways of doing things that may be different from yours.

INCREASING YOUR KNOWLEDGE OF CULTURALLY DIVERSE GROUPS

No one can be an expert on every culture in the world. Even those who are experts on a particular culture do not like being labeled as such. These people are aware of the ever-changing nature of cultures and of the important individual variations that occur within any cultural group. Experts are always cautious about stereotyping persons in any particular cultural group.

CATEGORIES OF MAJOR HEALTH BELIEF SYSTEMS

Anthropologists have developed a helpful framework for generally discovering and understanding health belief systems of groups. They divide health beliefs into three major systems: biomedicine, personalistic, and naturalistic.

- **Biomedicine** is the primary belief system of the United States and is also called "Western medicine." There is an effort to transform nursing curriculums so they reflect multicultural concepts in nursing. However, it is possible that the curriculum of your school of practical/vocational nursing is set up to reflect biomedicine (Box 10-2).
- The **personalistic system** is found among groups native to the Americas, as well as those south of the Sahara (e.g., Chad and Niger) and among the tribal peoples of Asia (Jackson, 1993) (Box 10-3).
- The **naturalistic system** of beliefs developed from the traditional medical practices of the ancient civilizations of China, India, and Greece (Box 10-4).
- Rarely does a group ascribe to all the beliefs in one system. You might see elements of each of the three systems at work in one individual. For example, a Hispanic patient with a strep throat might take an antibiotic as prescribed by the medical doctor, drink herbal teas as suggested by the curandero, and say prayers as suggested by the religious authority.

Box 10-2   Biomedical Health Belief

CAUSE OF DISEASE
- Abnormalities in structure and function of body organs, bacteria, viruses, biochemical alterations, immune system disturbance, environmental factors

HOW DISEASE IS DIAGNOSED
- Physical exam, x-ray, CT scan, MRI, identification of pathogens by lab studies

HOW DISEASE IS TREATED
- Drugs, surgery, diet

WHO CURES THE DISEASE
- Physician

HOW DISEASE IS PREVENTED
- Hand washing, covering mouth when sneezing, lifestyle (diet, exercise, etc.), immunizations

Adapted with permission from Jackson L. Understanding, eliciting, and negotiating patients' multicultural health beliefs. *Nurse Practitioner* 18(4):30-32, 1993.

Box 10-3   Personalistic Health Belief

CAUSE OF DISEASE
- Punishment by a ghost, god, evil spirit, sorcerer, ancestor spirit, witch
- Breach of taboo, sin, evil eye, curse
- Above results in loss or theft of soul, possession of spirit, poisoning, curse

HOW DISEASE IS DIAGNOSED
- By a person with magic or supernatural powers

HOW DISEASE IS TREATED
- Counteract cause with herbs, prayer, rituals, laying on of hands

WHO CURES THE DISEASE
- Shaman, diviner, herbalist, magic/religious specialist

HOW DISEASE IS PREVENTED
- Faithful observance of rituals (e.g., honor ceremonies for ancestors), protective spells, wearing objects that have magic properties against evil eye or injury (amulets)

Adapted with permission from Jackson L: Understanding, eliciting, and negotiating patients' multicultural health beliefs. *Nurse Practitioner* 18(4):30-32, 1993.

DIVERSITY PROFILES OF PREDOMINANT CULTURAL GROUPS IN THE UNITED STATES

At the beginning of the twentieth century, the majority of immigrants to the United States were of European ancestry. According to preliminary reports of the 2010 Census, the total population of the United States can be broken down as white: 65%; Hispanic: 16%; Asian: 5%; African American: 12%; and American Indian/Alaskan Native: 1.4% (Yen, 2011). If current immigration and birth trends continue, it is projected that by the year 2050, non-Hispanic whites will become a minority (Yen, 2011). Box 10-5 provides profiles of these culturally diverse groups.

| Box **10-4** | Naturalistic Health Belief |

CAUSE OF DISEASE
- Imbalance of body elements
- Yin (cold)/yang (heat)
- Wet/dry
- Emotions
- Bad luck

HOW DISEASE IS DIAGNOSED
- Cause of excess heat or cold identified

HOW DISEASE IS TREATED
- Regain body balance, foods, acupuncture, coining, cupping

WHO CURES THE DISEASE
- Physician or herbalist; no supernatural or magical powers

HOW DISEASE IS PREVENTED
- Maintain balance of hot and cold in body, mind, spirit, and environment

Adapted with permission from Jackson L: Understanding, eliciting, and negotiating patients' multicultural health beliefs. *Nurse Practitioner* 18(4): 30-32, 1993.

DEVELOPING CULTURAL COMPETENCE IN HEALTH CARE SITUATIONS

You have started the long road to becoming an LPN/ LVN who gives culturally competent care. Up to this point, participating in this chapter has given you the opportunity to do the following:
- Identify your culture and its strengths and limitations.
- Recognize how your culture affects your thinking and behavior.
- Discover how persons are similar despite their cultural group.
- Discover how persons are unique despite their cultural group.
- Gain knowledge of the three major health belief systems to increase your awareness of different worldviews about the cause, treatment, and prevention of disease.
- Gain awareness of ethnocentrism that can help you respect the health beliefs and practices of others when they are different from your own.
- Learn to be flexible when your values and assumptions differ from those of your patients.

| Box **10-5** | Diversity Profiles of Predominant Cultural Groups in the United States |

These profiles are intended to be a general sketch of the culture of the group.

AFRICAN AMERICANS
- **Origin:** From Africa as slaves
- **Family structure:** Matriarchal, nuclear and extended family, fictive kin (not really relation; for example, "Aunt" Bessie)
- **Religion:** Protestant denominations, Catholicism, and Islam
- **Food preferences:** Chicken, fish, leafy greens, yams, grits, and cornbread
- **Illness beliefs:** Illness results from bad spirits, a hex, a spell, as punishment from God. May treat illnesses with home remedies, teas, herbs, compresses. May wait until illness becomes serious before seeking medical care. May visit a spiritualist or folk healer.

HMONG
- **Origin:** Vietnam, Laos, Thailand, Burma
- **Family structure:** Patriarchal. Nuclear family plus extended family (father, mother, brothers, sisters, uncles, aunts, nieces, and nephews) considered one family.
- **Religion:** Animism (worship of deceased ancestors). This may be replaced by or combined with Catholicism and Buddhism.
- **Food:** Rice the main food and served at each meal. Noodles, rarely eat fruit, adults rarely consume dairy products.
- **Illness beliefs:** Imbalance between spirit and the body. Natural and supernatural causes of illness. Natural plants, roots, and herbs used to cure a sick person. Shaman may be called to visit sick person in hospital. Healing rituals performed at home. May use cupping, coining, and pinching of skin as cure.

HISPANICS
- **Origin:** Mexico, Puerto Rico, Cuba, Spain, Central America (El Salvador, Guatemala, Honduras, Nicaragua, Panama, Costa Rica, Belize), South America (Colombia, Ecuador, Peru, Argentina, Venezuela, Chile, Bolivia, Uruguay, Paraguay).
The following information may vary by country.
- **Family structure:** Nuclear, extended, and patriarchal. Family not always defined by blood or marriage.
- **Religion:** Catholic but changing to various Protestant Evangelical religions, Pentecostal and other sects/groups, African spirit religion, voodoo, or a combination of these.
- **Food:** Rice, beans, spices; food choices vary because of socioeconomic status, country of origin, and location within country. Many have "hot" and "cold" foods. Some think American food is bland.
- **Illness beliefs:** A punishment from God for bad behavior or God's will, evil eye (*mal de ojo*), evil spells, fright (*susto*), magic, "hot" and "cold" imbalance, lack of cleanliness, humoral (body fluids) imbalance.

AMERICAN INDIANS/ALASKAN NATIVES
- **Origin:** North America. The U.S. Federal Government recognizes 550 tribes, bands, and nations, with an additional 200 tribes not federally recognized. This population is very diverse, and retention of traditional customs and the level of acculturation are vastly different. Tribes in different geographic areas differ, as do people in tribes (Lipson & Dibble, 2006).
- **Family structure:** Matriarchal, patriarchal, kinship roles extensive and fictive at times.
- **Religion:** Traditional beliefs, Christian, combine different religious practices.
- **Food:** Diet high in fat, salt, and sugar.
- **Illness beliefs:** Violation of taboos; body, mind, or spirit out of harmony with God or nature. May use native

Continued

Box 10-5   Diversity Profiles of Predominant Cultural Groups in the United States—cont'd

healers and ceremonies to restore harmony in conjunction with Western medicine. Sacred objects should not be touched or moved by staff.

ARAB AMERICANS
- **Origin:** The Arab world consists of 22 countries and territories, and as with other cultural groups, there is great variation based on country of origin, social class, education, urban or rural origin, and time in the United States. Most of the people in these countries are Muslim (Lipson & Dibble, 2005). Approximately 128 countries have people of the Muslim religion. Not all of these people are Arab, but the culture of the Islam religion links people from these various countries.

NOTES
Information about "yin" and "yang" can be accessed at www.taopage.org/yinyang.html.
Information about coin rubbing cupping can be accessed at www.dimensionsofculture.com/2010/10/traditional-asian-health-beliefs-healing-practices/.
Information about "evil eye" can be accessed at www.dimensionsofculture.com/2010/10/folk-illnesses-and-remedies-in-latino-communities/.
Information about curanderos can be accessed at http://www.ioufoundation.org/press/health-science/187-curanderismo-spirituality-and-healing-in-oaxaca-mexico.

Adapted from Reinhardt E: *Through the eyes of others—intercultural resource directory for health care professionals.* Minneapolis: University of Minnesota School of Public Health 1995:pp. 5-6, 8-14; Lipson J, Dibble S: *Culture and clinical care.* The Regents, University of California School of Nursing, 2006, UCSF Nursing Press.

Your next step to cultural competence is to develop a knowledge base for a few cultures that are different from yours.

IDENTIFY YOUR AGENCY'S CULTURAL GROUPS

Identify the cultural groups in your community that are served by local health care agencies. Use the following blank lines to list the groups. It is necessary to be knowledgeable about the cultural groups that you frequently come across in your community.

_____
_____
_____
_____

Try This

Your Area's Cultural Groups

1. A helpful learning activity is to hear reports from peers about various cultural groups.
2. Remember to think beyond the more traditional cultural groups, based on ethnicity. Include the disabled, elderly, single parents, alternative lifestyles, and so on.
3. Read about the different cultures that are served in your area. Use the References and Suggested Readings for this chapter, Internet sources in the text, and the resources of your learning resource center (LRC) as suggested in Chapter 2 to find texts and articles about specific cultural groups. Google a specific group to obtain information (www.google.com), and remember to verify your sources.
4. View documentaries on television or on the Internet about cultural groups.
5. Attend community events sponsored by cultural groups.
6. Attend graduations, weddings, birth celebrations, and funerals of different cultures when the opportunities present themselves.
7. Attend a religious service of a cultural group.
8. Read novels involving different cultures.
9. Attend seminars about cultural groups.

10. Invite a member of a cultural group to class to talk about the health/illness beliefs of the group of whom he or she is a member.
11. Participate in diversity training or an international type of club, if offered by your university or clinical affiliate.

MODIFY YOUR WORK SETTING

The health care environment can be made more "welcoming" to culturally diverse patients. Many of these changes require little cost or time to implement, but the results can promote better health and compliance among culturally diverse patients. Box 10-6

Box 10-6   Modifying the Environment to Accommodate Culturally Diverse Patients

- Identify the various cultural groups that use the health care facility.
- Post welcome signs in the languages of the groups you serve.
- Arrange for messages on answering machines to include the languages of the patients you serve. Place magazines in waiting rooms that reflect the diversity of the patients you serve.
- Include background music that reflects the diversity of the patients you serve.
- Provide handouts, appointment cards, and patient education materials in the languages of the patients you serve.
- Decorate the environment (pictures, posters, objects, etc.) to reflect the diversity of the patients you serve.
- Stock adhesive bandages that do not match any specific skin tone; for example, Walt Disney characters for children and fluorescent or varied colors for adults.
- In waiting areas, provide books, toys, and multicultural videos for children that promote acceptance of diversity. Sesame Street and SpongeBob SquarePants themes are especially effective and accepted.

Adapted from Reinhardt E: *Through the eyes of others—intercultural resource directory for health care professionals.* Minneapolis: University of Minnesota School of Public Health, 1995, pp. 19-20.

presents suggestions for modifying the workplace environment for the practical/vocational nurse working in health care agencies with culturally diverse patients.

CARE PLANNING FOR CULTURALLY DIVERSE PATIENTS IN YOUR SERVICE AREA

Imagine this scenario: A 60-year-old Hmong female requires an urgent surgical procedure. The physician is frustrated as the consent form still is not signed and surgery is imminent. This patient speaks limited English. You are struggling to determine why the consent is still not signed. Through research, using the Dimensions of Culture website (www.dimensionsofculture.com), you conclude that Hmong people often need extra time to sign consent forms, as discussion with Hmong elders and the family (clan) needs to occur. Given this information, you assist the patient in contacting their elders, the physician obtains consent, and surgery occurs as planned.

Each patient of a different culture needs to have data gathered regarding activities of daily living (ADLs) and personal health beliefs and practices. Develop a fact sheet for collecting data for each patient (Box 10-7). Use your culture resources and select topics and questions from the exercises found in this chapter. Clarify ADLs and health beliefs and practices for your patient.

Use web sites such as http://www.dimensionsofculture.com and www.thinkculturalhealth.hhs.gov/Content/clas.asp to access general information about caring for different cultural groups. This information is helpful when you are dealing with a patient from a culture with which you are not familiar because they offer general information about, for example, wellness and illness beliefs and practices, nutritional preferences, and communication issues. These quick sources of generalities of various cultural groups are a starting point for learning which topics to include when collecting data (assessing) that must be clarified and validated with the individual patient. Remember that general group behavior *sometimes explains* observed behavior but it is *not predictive* of individual behavior. For example, not all Native Americans will avoid eye contact. Assumptions based on generalizations should not be made. When using this information, avoid stereotyping your patient. Use Box 10-8 as a guide to help you avoid falling into the stereotype trap.

Suspect cultural differences when a patient is not following the plan of care, refuses treatment, is a "problem" patient, and so on. Question the patient about his or her ADLs and wellness and illness beliefs. When cultural differences are identified, follow Jackson's (1993) suggestions for negotiating patient care with culturally diverse patients. Doing so will result in fewer dissatisfied patients and more compliance with the plan of care.

Box 10-7 Sample Data-Gathering Sheet Using a Traditional Hmong Patient as an Example

The following are 12 assessment items for all patients. In parentheses are generalizations from the text about traditional Hmong culture that explain the data collected for this patient. The explanations are applicable to the culture of the traditional Hmong group only.

Patient: Culture: Traditional Hmong

1. What language do you use to speak/read? (The Hmong written language developed in the 1950s. Most elderly Hmongs are illiterate in their own language.)
2. Observe eye contact during questions. (Consider prolonged, direct eye contact rude.)
3. Observe the reaction to a handshake when introducing yourself. (Handshakes are appropriate.)
4. How long have you lived in the United States? (Assimilation may occur the longer a person is in the dominant culture.)
5. What is your religion? What is its importance in your daily life? (May have animistic beliefs in which spirits inhabit objects and natural settings. Worship ancestors with ceremonies so ancestors will bring good fortune and protect the family from harm. Buddhism.)
6. What caused your present illness? (Traditional causes of illness might be soul loss or illness caused by an ancestral spirit.)
7. How can your illness be best treated? (In traditional religious/spiritual beliefs, a shaman is necessary to communicate with the spirit world to learn why the person is ill and what sacrifice is required to make the person well.)
8. Do you use home remedies to cure illness? (Cupping, coining, and pinching are used to release evil spirits or illness-causing toxins from the body.)
9. What is your usual meal pattern at home? (Hmong usually eat two to three meals a day. If two meals are eaten, the first meal is usually eaten at 9 AM or 10 AM.)
10. What foods are in your usual diet? (Rice with small amounts of meat, fish, and green vegetables. Fruit is rarely eaten.)
11. Will you accept visitors while in the hospital? (Visitors are welcomed and helpful in recovery.)
12. Who in your family has decision-making authority? (Women are allowed opinions; father/husband makes final decisions.)

Topics and explanations for this data-gathering sheet were taken from Lipson and Dibble: *Culture and nursing care: a pocket guide.* San Francisco: UCSF Nursing Press, 2006, pp. 250-263.

Box 10-8   How to Avoid Stereotyping Culturally Diverse Patients

- Avoid automatically applying the information you gain to all individuals in a cultural group. Doing so is called the "cookbook method" of learning about different cultures.
- Applying information with the cookbook method makes you guilty of stereotyping individuals; that is, assuming that everyone in that cultural group is the same.
- You have learned that classifying people as being the same just because they share the same religion, lifestyle, or ethnic background is stereotyping.
- Expect personal variations in each cultural group about which you gather information.
- Behaviors found in articles, reference books, and on the Internet containing culture and nursing care for various cultural groups can be applied generally to cultural groups as a whole but cannot automatically be applied to every individual in that group.
- Variable, individual differences exist because of the changing nature of the culture, the patient's personal life experiences (including hospitalization), age, religion, and adaptation to a new culture.
- No individual is a stereotype of one's culture of origin. Individuals are a unique blend of the diversity found within each culture.
- Gather cultural data for each patient. Discover the behaviors in your culture guide that apply to your patient.
- Look at information about cultural groups as explaining behavior in patients, not predicting behavior.

Adapted from D'Avanzo and Geissler: *Pocket guide to cultural assessment.* St. Louis: Mosby, 2008.

ADAPTING PLANS OF CARE FOR CULTURALLY DIVERSE PATIENTS

Jackson (1993) offers suggestions for finding out about patients' health beliefs, along with guidelines for developing plans of care that incorporate those beliefs through a process of negotiation with the patient. Jackson points out that discovering specific health beliefs is easier if the nurse is familiar with a specific culture, but this is not absolutely necessary. Jackson suggests ways of negotiating a treatment plan with culturally diverse patients. The LPN/LVN can collaborate with the professional nurse to incorporate these beliefs into the patient's plan of care:

1. *Discover the health beliefs of the individual.* Be respectful and open minded when you question the patient about the cause of the health problem, when it started, its severity, its course, the problems it has caused in the patient's life, and the treatment the patient thinks will cure the disease. *Avoid assuming anything.* When you are unsure of anything, ask! In situations of cultural diversity, our patients are the teachers and we are the students.
2. *Co-create treatment plans with the patient.* Avoid trying to change patients' beliefs. Cultural health practices are deeply ingrained. Tradition means more than your word does, even though you are a representative of a health profession. Instead, involve the patient in making decisions about his or her own care. Do so in a way that does not threaten the patient's beliefs and practices or conflict with them. Explain from the biomedical point of view the cause of the disease, how the disease alters the body, the role of treatment, and the expected outcome. Then compare the patient's belief system with that of biomedicine. All patients need to have this information to help ensure their cooperation with the plan of care. See Box 10-9 for an example of negotiating treatment plans with the patient.
3. *Preserve the beliefs and practices that are helpful to the patient.* Starting in 1993, the Office of Alternative Medicine of the National Institutes of Health began to identify, study, and bring together the best healing practices of other cultures with those of Western medicine. In 1998, the National Center for Complimentary and Integrative Health was established to focus on determining the usefulness and

Box 10-9   Co-Creating Treatment Plans with the Patient

SITUATION
Nancy Thai, a Cambodian refugee, resides in Chicago with her husband and three children. She delivered an 8-pound boy early this morning at St. Mary's Hospital. The LPN/LVN who was assigned to Mrs. Thai on the day shift reported to the evening staff that the patient was "uncooperative." Specifically, Mrs. Thai refused to eat and take her pills. In frustration the nurse said, "I just don't know what to do with her."

CULTURAL HEALTH BELIEFS IN THIS SITUATION
Mrs. Thai's health beliefs include the belief that pregnancy and birth weaken the body. Also, blood loss during delivery is considered a yin (cold) condition. Mrs. Thai believes that for one month after delivery, a mother must have a yang (hot) diet to restore strength, keep the stomach warm, counteract heat loss, prevent incontinence, and prevent itching at the site of the episiotomy. "Cold" refers to foods that are cold in their physical form as well as considered cold in nature. "Cold" foods (e.g., salt, crab, salad, bananas, sour foods

[e.g., tomato, tangerine, plum, lemon, grape, vinegar, grapefruit, olives]), as well as cold water, are viewed as bad for the stomach and the teeth. "Warm" refers to foods that are warm in their physical form as well as considered warm in nature. Among preferred "warm" foods are rice, fish, and chicken.

CO-CREATING TREATMENT PLANS
The nurse assigned to Mrs. Thai on the evening shift informed her that the doctor had ordered pills to help prevent bleeding after delivery. After discussing this, Mrs. Thai agreed to take her pills with warm water. In a respectful manner, the evening nurse asked Mrs. Thai if she did not like the hospital food. Mrs. Thai smiled and explained her need for a yang diet. The evening nurse said that she could arrange to have the dietary department send rice, chicken, or any other food Mrs. Thai would find helpful after childbirth. Mrs. Thai said her husband would bring rice and chicken from home. The nurse canceled Mrs. Thai's food order but requested a pot of hot water, silverware, and napkins for her use.

safety of complementary and integrative health interventions and their roles in improving health and health care. Many of the beliefs and practices of non-Western systems of health beliefs have proved beneficial. Acupuncture and acupressure are now a common practice in the United States and many more alternative treatment modalities continue to emerge. Collaborate with your professional nurse about patients' practices that have not yet been researched or found effective. If the practices seem to help the patient and do no harm, include them in the plan of care, regardless of your ability to see the benefit of the practice. These practices have special significance and meaning to some individuals, despite the fact that you may be unable to see how or whether they help. Box 10-10 provides an example

of preserving the beliefs and practices that are helpful to the patient.

4. *Repattern harmful practices.* Harmful practices that are prevalent in Western society include smoking, diets high in fat, refined grains, and refined sugar, and lack of exercise. In Burma, when a woman is pregnant, extreme dietary restrictions are imposed. In Cambodia, mud is placed on the umbilicus of newborns. These practices are dangerous and if followed could lead to health problems and complications. Smoking, diets high in fat, refined grains, and refined sugar, and lack of exercise can cause high blood pressure and heart disease. Extreme dietary restrictions during pregnancy can lead to maternal toxemia and poor fetal development; and mud placed on the umbilicus can cause tetanus in the newborn. Explain your reasons for opposing a harmful practice, and offer alternatives. Box 10-11 provides an example of **repatterning** harmful practices.

When LPNs/LVNs demonstrate awareness of and respect for the many cultural groups in their service area, knowledge about these cultural groups, and skill in applying their knowledge in a caring manner, they are on the road to delivering culturally competent care.

Box 10-10 Preserving the Beliefs and Practices that are Helpful to the Patient

SITUATION

Ted Washington, a 72-year-old African American, lives in a rural area of South Carolina. He was admitted to Brent Hospital with pneumonia and advanced osteoarthritis. John, an LPN, is his nurse. John cannot understand how anyone can get to such a state of ill health without seeing a doctor. John is especially upset because Mr. Washington could have prevented much of his disability from arthritis if he had followed a preventive program when he first developed symptoms of this disease.

CULTURAL HEALTH BELIEFS IN THIS SITUATION

Mr. Washington has lived in poverty for his entire life. As with any person in this situation, his main concern in life has been the present and getting through his problems on a day-to-day basis. Mr. Washington's time orientation is the moment (present), not the future; therefore, preventive regimens have not been central to his way of thinking. Persons with similar backgrounds and situations delay care until the disease interferes with their ability to work or results in a disability.

It cannot be said that Mr. Washington ignored his condition. He participated in self-treatment by using cultural health practices in the form of topical application of oils and ointments to his aching joints. These self-treatments helped Mr. Washington deal physically and psychologically with his condition. Mr. Washington looks at his disability as a punishment from God, who let something get into his joints. His belief stems from the wellness and illness beliefs brought to this country from Africa. These beliefs center on wellness as a state experienced when one is in harmony with nature. Illness is experienced as a state of disharmony with nature.

PRESERVING THE BELIEFS AND PRACTICES THAT ARE HELPFUL TO THE PATIENT

John supported Mr. Washington's application of oils and ointments. He applied massage lotion to Mr. Washington's joints at bedtime. John arranged for Mr. Washington's friend to bring his ointment from home. After clarifying self-treatment with the patient, John realized that such applications could give psychological comfort to the patient, as well as relieve pain. In the future John will make it a point to ask all newly admitted patients about self-treatment for their diseases.

Box 10-11 Repatterning Harmful Practices

SITUATION

Over a 2-month period during the summer, a Chinese infant was seen in a New York clinic for diarrhea that did not respond to treatment. Stool cultures showed no unusual organisms. A change in formula did nothing to stop the diarrhea. During a home visit, the visiting nurse found a hot apartment with several bottles of home-prepared formula on the windowsill. Several other full bottles were in the refrigerator.

CULTURAL HEALTH BELIEFS IN THIS SITUATION

The child's mother explained that she had recently given birth. Because of this, she had to avoid cold. To avoid her exposure to the cold of the refrigerator, her husband would remove the bottles from the refrigerator that she needed during the day before he left for work and line them up on the windowsill.

REPATTERNING THE PATIENT'S HARMFUL PRACTICES

The visiting nurse explained that by being exposed to the heat of the day, the formula would grow germs that could cause diarrhea. She asked if there was a way that the bottles could be kept cold until needed. After some thought, the mother said she could put on a hat, coat, and gloves before removing the bottles from the refrigerator. The nurse agreed with this plan. The baby had no further episodes of diarrhea.

Reproduced with permission from Jackson L: Understanding, eliciting and negotiating patients' multicultural health beliefs. *Nurse Practitioner* 18(4):30-32, 37-38, 41-43, 1993.

Get Ready for the NCLEX-PN® Examination

Key Points

- A good place to start learning about how people are different is to remind yourself that all persons are unique but have similarities as well.
- Giger and Davidhizar (1991) describe six cultural phenomena: communication, space, social organization, time, environmental control, and biological variations that are critical to the assessment of patients and provision of culturally competent care.
- One guideline in health care is the philosophy of individual worth; that is, the confidence that all persons are unique and have value regardless of the way they view their world and that they deserve the best nursing care you can give.
- Awareness of cultural diversity is important for LPNs/LVNs so they can avoid false assumptions and misunderstandings about the patients in their care.
- The first step in understanding other people's culture is to understand your own culture. Be aware of your personal beliefs and practices in the areas of family, religion, communication, educational background, economic level, pregnancy, wellness and illness beliefs and practices, and death and dying.
- Some ways to learn about cultural diversity include reading about different cultures, especially those found in your geographic area, and actively listening to reports from your peers and patients who are culturally different.
- Cultural characteristics of groups are not predictive of behavior of individuals in a group. They are generalizations. *Always allow for individual variations within specific groups*.
- Understanding your own culture, attaining sensitivity to cultural diversity, gaining knowledge about other people's cultures, and adapting the plan of care to reflect the patient's health and illness beliefs put you well on the road to providing culturally competent nursing care.
- Visit The Joint Commission website to access accreditation requirements related to cultural competence and health equity. www.jointcommission.org/Advancing_Effective_Communication/.

Additional Learning Resources

evolve Go to your Evolve website (http://evolve.elsevier. com/Knecht/success) for the following FREE learning resources:

- Answers to Critical Thinking Scenarios
- Additional learning activities
- Additional Review Questions for the NCLEX-PN® exam
- Helpful phrases for communicating in Spanish and more!

Review Questions for the NCLEX-PN® Examination

1. Select the term LPNs/LVNs need to avoid when studying different cultures:
   a. Stereotyping
   b. Socialization
   c. Enculturation
   d. Assimilation

2. Select the statement that best illustrates the philosophy of individual worth:
   a. All individuals are unique and have value regardless of their differences in how they meet daily needs.
   b. People who belong to ethnic groups have different daily needs in most needs categories.
   c. People of different cultures need to be approached as if their culture is the best of all culture groups in the area.
   d. Empowerment is culturally dependent.

3. An Asian-American resident in a nursing home does not want to follow the nursing care plan regarding diet. The best course of action for the nursing staff would be to:
   a. Insist the resident accept the diet as ordered.
   b. Document the stubbornness of this resident.
   c. Avoid making an issue of his noncompliance.
   d. Consider the possibility of cultural differences.

4. Mr. Metoxen, a member of the Oneida Tribe of Indians, was admitted to the medical floor with a diagnosis of angina. He is to receive nitroglycerin PRN (as needed) for chest pain. Select the priority cultural concern of the LPN/LVN for administering pain medication to a patient whose culture values stoic behavior:
   a. That the drug be kept in a dark container to protect it from light
   b. That the drug is always kept with the patient when he is walking
   c. That nonverbal signs of pain should not be overlooked in this situation
   d. That the patient's pain level be assessed at the beginning of the shift

Alternate Format Item

1. LPNs/LVNs use culture and nursing care guides to gather information about different cultures. Which of the following suggestions apply to the use of culture reference guides and other electronic resources (Select all that apply.)
   a. Avoid applying information automatically to all members of a culture.
   b. Variation in any member of the same cultural group does not occur.
   c. Assume that all members of a cultural group are the same in all aspects.
   d. Information obtained explains behavior but does not predict behavior.
   e. Once you gather data for one patient, this information can be applied to others.

Critical Thinking Scenario

Hector Santiago, a legal Mexican immigrant, has been in the United States for only a short time. He was admitted to the hospital after experiencing 3 days of intermittent chest pain. He is not taking well to bed rest and has attempted to walk down the hall several times when he should stay in bed. Using gestures only, Mr. Santiago has been indicating that he is in pain, but he consistently refuses drugs. During visiting hours, Mr. Santiago's wife, children, sisters, brothers, and parents visit. Dr. Jones plans to order a diagnostic study to evaluate Mr. Santiago's coronary arteries. He asks Mr. Santiago's wife for permission, and she refuses. Mr. Santiago has a stroke, and after a few days, the doctor tells Mrs. Santiago that he must go to a nursing home. Mrs. Santiago is horrified to hear this news. Why did Mr. Santiago wait 3 days to get care? Why did he attempt to walk down the hall when he knew he was on bed rest? Why did he refuse drugs for pain? Why did he have so many visitors? Why did Mrs. Santiago refuse coronary artery studies for her husband? Why did she become upset when nursing home placement was suggested for her husband?

Spiritual Needs, Spiritual Caring, and Religious Differences

Objectives

On completing this chapter, you will be able to do the following:

1. Differentiate between spirituality and religion.
2. Identify the difference between the spiritual and emotional dimensions of individuals.
3. Discuss the role of the licensed practical nurse/licensed vocational nurse (LPN/LVN) in providing spiritual care to the patient and the family as a member of the health care team.
4. List members of the health care team who can help provide spiritual care for patients.
5. Discuss key nursing interventions to meet the spiritual needs of patients.
6. Discuss personal religious and/or spiritual beliefs, or the absence of them, and how these beliefs will influence nursing practice.
7. Discuss the general beliefs and practices that account for the differences among various Western, Middle Eastern, and Eastern religions, philosophies, and groups in the United States and Canada.
8. Describe nursing interventions/considerations of patients of various religions, philosophies, and groups.

Key Terms

agnostic (ăg-NŎS-tĭk)
Allah (ĂL-ă)
atheist (Ā-thē-ĭst)
Buddha (BŪ-dă)
emotional needs (ē-MO-shŭn-ăl nēds)
Jesus Christ (krīst)
parish nurse (PĂR-ĭsh)
pastoral care team (PĂS-tĕ-RĂL)
reincarnation (RĒ-ĭn-kăr-NĀ-shŭn)

religion (rē-LĬ-jŭn)
religious denomination (dĕ-NŎM-ĭ-NĀ-shŭn)
rituals (RĬ-choo-ăls)
spirit (SPĬ-rĭt)
spiritual caring (SPĬR-ĭ-chūăl CĀR-ĭng)
spiritual dimension (SPĬR-ĭ-chūăl dī-MĔN-shŭn)
spiritual distress (SPĬR-ĭ-chūăl dis-TRĔS)
spiritual needs (SPĬR-ĭ-chūăl nēds)
spirituality (SPĬR-ĭ-chū-ĂL-ĭ-tē)

💡 Keep in Mind

If you were hospitalized, is it important to you that the staff be informed of your spiritual practices?

Jan, the evening nurse, found Thomas Bernes, age 32, sitting up in bed, crying and moaning with what she interpreted as pain after a testicular biopsy that was positive for cancer. After assessment, she volunteered to get Thomas some pain medication, but he refused. Thomas shouts, "Why did I have to get cancer? Why me?" Then he says, "Oh, I'll be fine. Just leave me alone, and I will get rid of the pain myself." Jan quickly and quietly leaves the room so Thomas can be alone.

In its *Nursing Diagnoses: 2015–2017* edition, the North American Nursing Diagnosis Association (NANDA) includes a nursing diagnosis related to spirituality and a separate diagnosis related to religiosity. In the foregoing patient situation, Thomas was in spiritual distress. A minister or priest might have been able to address Thomas's problem, but Thomas needed immediate spiritual care. It would have been helpful to Thomas if his nurse had offered to spend time with him and encouraged him to talk about what he was thinking and feeling at that time. Nursing has always embraced a holistic approach to patient care: care of the body, mind, and spirit. Despite the NANDA-I diagnosis, some nurses are uncomfortable with matters of the spirit. Some have not had adequate education in how to deal with patients in this aspect of care.

SPIRITUALITY AND RELIGION

Spirituality is an essential part of being human. The word comes from the Latin word *spiritus*, which means "breath" or "air." The **spirit** is the very essence of a person, the innermost part of a person that provides animation. The spirit is a life force that penetrates a person's entire being. It includes the beliefs and value systems that give people strength and hope. The spirit gives meaning to life. It is hoped that the spiritual self grows and matures throughout one's life.

The terms *spirituality* and *religion* are related, but they have different meanings. **Religion** may be a spiritual experience that contains specific beliefs and rituals. It can include spirituality, but spirituality, one's life force, does not necessarily include religion. Participation in a religion may include spirituality, but spirituality does not necessarily include participation in a religion. According to LeGere (Carson, 1989), spirituality is not a religion. Spirituality is related to experience, but religion has to do with giving form to that experience. Spirituality focuses on what happens in the heart, and religion tries to make rules and capture that experience in a system.

SPIRITUAL VERSUS EMOTIONAL DIMENSION

Meeting the spiritual needs of patients through spiritual caring differs from providing emotional support. The **spiritual dimension** of a person gives insight into the meaning of life, suffering, and death. This dimension refers to the relationship of an individual to a higher power. **Emotional needs** include how people respond and deal with feelings of joy, anger, sorrow, guilt, remorse, and love. The spiritual dimension of a patient's life requires the same emphasis that other daily needs receive. When **spiritual needs** of patients exist and are met, licensed practical nurses/licensed vocational nurses (LPNs/LVNs) can say they have directed care to the total person.

IMPORTANCE OF SPIRITUAL CARE

Spiritual care involves helping patients to develop an awareness of and maintain the following:
- Inner strength
- Self-awareness
- Life's meaning and purpose
- Relationship to others
- Relationship to a higher power

Florence Nightingale encouraged nurses to be instruments of **spiritual caring** in all situations. Nurses should avoid waiting for crisis situations to occur before they become concerned about spiritual care. The Joint Commission (TJC) requires that spirituality is assessed for all patients; however, TJC does not define exactly what should be included. TJC suggests questions such as the following when accessing spirituality (2008): "Who provides you strength and hope?" "How do you express your spirituality?" "What are your spiritual goals?" "What does suffering mean to you?" Spiritual care is mandated by organizations worldwide. The International Council of Nurses (ICN) (2015) states, "We are determined that science and technology remain the servant of compassionate and ethical caring that includes meeting spiritual and emotional needs." As an LPN/LVN, you have the responsibility to provide spiritual care to patients and families.

WHO NEEDS SPIRITUAL CARE?

An individual's spiritual dimension is a very private and personal area. Although all people have a spiritual dimension, needs that arise in this area depend on a variety of situations and the individual's ability to cope with them. An example of nurses who routinely recognize spiritual needs are nurses who work with patients in various church settings in a health ministry. The goal of these **parish nurses** is to keep their groups happy and healthy by treating the whole person: body, mind, and spirit. Parish nurses recognize the relationship between spirituality and health and encourage spiritual growth in their patients.

Crisis situations occur in all health care situations, but they especially arise in acute health care. Patients' beliefs and values can profoundly affect their response to these crises, their attitude toward treatment, and their rate of recovery. Be alert for the following patient situations that may intensify the need for spiritual care for patients and families:
- Hospitalization
- Patients who are in pain
- Patients who have a chronic or incurable disease
- Patients who are dying
- Families who have experienced the death of a loved one
- Patients who are facing an undesirable outcome of illness, such as an amputation
- Patients who have emotionally lost control of themselves

According to Delgado (2013), nurses in the last decade felt ill prepared to discuss spirituality with their patients. Contrary to these previous studies, Delgado (2013) found that nurses felt confident to discuss spiritual aspects of care with their patients, particularly when they noted spiritual distress. However, the nurses reported favoring spiritual interventions that were less religious in nature. Knowing yourself is an important step in providing spiritual care to patients.

GATHERING DATA FOR SPIRITUAL ISSUES

The first step to providing spiritual care for patients is to strive to become comfortable dealing with spiritual matters. The second step is to become aware of your own spirituality and the spirit that is the essence of *you*. Gather data about your spiritual self. The exercise in the Try This: Your Personal Spirituality box can help you increase awareness of your personal spirituality.

◎ Try This

Your Personal Spirituality

1. How do you cope?
2. Who is your source of support?
3. Who are the significant people in your life?
4. With whom do you laugh?
5. Do you feel loved?
6. Do you have someone with whom to cry?
7. What gives your life meaning?
8. What brings joy to your life?
9. Do you believe in the power of prayer?
10. What are your beliefs about a higher power?
11. Do you have a relationship to a higher power?
12. Do you have a religious affiliation? If so, how do your religious beliefs affect your spirit?
13. What is your philosophy about life and death?

? Critical Thinking

My Spiritual Sensitivity

Have you ever said or heard others say, "My spirit is broken"? What does this remark mean to you? Talk to a peer and discuss similarities and dissimilarities.

MEETING THE SPIRITUAL NEEDS OF PATIENTS AND THEIR FAMILIES

Once you know your spiritual self, you will be better able to help others meet their spiritual needs. When you acknowledge that your beliefs are effective for you but not necessarily for others, you will be able to set your beliefs aside when helping patients and families meet their spiritual needs. The questions in the Your Personal Spirituality box can also be used to gather data for patients' spiritual condition. Respect for the belief system of patients and families can give strength, hope, and meaning to their lives. When working with patients and families, try to do the following:

- Ask questions to help patients and families verbalize beliefs, fears, and concerns, such as "What do you think is going to happen to you (your father/mother)?" and "Who is your source of support?"
- Show interest through supportive statements (see Chapter 8).
- Listen with an understanding attitude. Be sure your body language and affective response reflect what you are saying.
- Respond as naturally to spiritual concerns as you do to physical needs.
- Help patients face the reality of a terminal illness without abandoning hope.
- Encourage the patient's active involvement in self-care, which can help uphold hope.
- Allow families to participate in caregiving (e.g., offering fluids/ice chips, when allowed; wiping the patient's brow).
- Avoid false assurances such as "Everything will be okay."

- When a patient faces death, you can help to make the remaining days meaningful by attending to needs, respecting their beliefs and death practices, and approaching the patient in a supportive and empathetic manner. Feeling loved helps bring peace to the dying.

Box 11-1 lists spiritual care interventions that can be used by LP/LV nurses.

PASTORAL CARE TEAM

The **pastoral care team** is made up of ministers, priests, rabbis, consecrated religious women (i.e., nuns/sisters), representatives of other religious organizations, and laypersons. All are educated to meet spiritual needs, in addition to religious needs, in a health care setting. The members of this team are allies with nurses in providing spiritual care. You can notify this team if a patient requests a visit. When members of the pastoral care team come to the unit to fill the request, inform them of the patient's background and condition. Describe the interventions you have incorporated into the patient's care to provide spiritual care. Remember that the pastoral care team does not relieve you of your responsibility to provide spiritual care.

By visiting, talking, and listening, the pastoral care team explores the patients' fears, hopes, and sources of strength. Because of federal privacy standards (see the Health Insurance Portability and Accountability Act [HIPAA] in Chapter 7), the health care facility may not make a patient's name available to church representatives without the patient's permission. Before being hospitalized/admitted, patients can personally notify their clergy regarding a planned hospitalization and desire for a visit. If an admitted patient requests a visit

---
Box 11-1   Spiritual Care Interventions

- Ask open-ended questions.
- Actively listen to the patient. Sit beside the patient. Make eye contact.
- Expect to learn from patients.
- Be nonjudgmental of patients and their responses.
- Avoid giving advice or a lecture to the patient.
- Avoid being a proselytizer (i.e., a person who tries to convert another person to one's religion).
- Be aware of nonverbal messages from the patient.
- Understand the feelings of the patient, but avoid adopting those feelings for yourself. (See Chapter 8 for a discussion of sympathy versus empathy.) Stay with the patient after the person has received an unfavorable diagnosis.
- When patients request help with prayer, offer to pray with them.
- When a patient requests help with specific readings, offer to read to him or her.
- Help the patient to participate in desired religious/spiritual rituals.
- Protect the patient's religious/spiritual articles.

---

of personal clergy, follow the facility directive for arranging this request. Agency policies vary.

HOW PATIENTS MEET SPIRITUAL NEEDS

PATIENTS' SPIRITUAL PRACTICES

Regardless of religious beliefs, or lack of them, *all* patients have a spiritual self. They also have spiritual needs and personal spiritual practices to meet those needs. Spiritual practices help individuals to develop an awareness of self, an understanding of the meaning and purpose of life, and an appreciation of their relationship to a higher power. Examples of personal spiritual practices may include gardening, reading inspirational books, listening to music, meditating, watching select TV shows and movies, communing with nature, walking a labyrinth, practicing breathing techniques, enjoying art, enjoying fresh flowers, volunteering, expressing gratitude, counting blessings, walking, talking with friends and relatives, and participating in crafts and hobbies.

◎ Try This

My Spiritual Practices

Identify the spiritual practices that you use to meet your spiritual needs.

RELIGION AND THE PATIENT

The religious self refers to the specific beliefs an individual holds in regard to a higher power. Some patients help to meet their spiritual needs by belonging to a specific religious denomination. A **religious denomination** is an organized group of people who share a philosophy that supports their particular concept of God or a higher power, as well as worship experiences.

Agnostics hold the belief that the existence of God can be neither proved nor disproved. **Atheists** do not believe that the supernatural exists, so they do not believe in God. Christians may find comfort and solace in their refuge in God, including passing into another life after death. The atheist does not have this belief. It may be difficult for the nurse who believes in the supernatural to relate to a person with atheistic beliefs. The nurse may feel unsuccessful in meeting the total needs of the patient who is an atheist because atheists do not believe in the supernatural. The spiritual aspect, however, is present in all individuals. Spiritual assessment and interventions are appropriate for agnostic and atheist patients. Encourage these patients to express personal feelings about life, death, separation, and loss.

👆 Professional Pointer

Avoid imposing your personal beliefs and values on the patient. Reexamine your personal beliefs at least yearly. Knowing your own personal beliefs is critical to providing unbiased spiritual and religious focused care.

VALUE OF RITUALS AND PRACTICES

The different rituals and practices of a religion are stabilizing forces for the patient. **Rituals** are a series of actions that have religious meaning. They can bring the security of the past into a crisis situation. Concrete symbols such as pictures, icons, herb packets, rosaries, statues, jewelry, and other objects can affirm the patient's connection with a higher power.

The value of patients' rituals and religious practices is determined by their faith. Value is not determined by scientific proof of their benefit. However, studies have shown that negative outcomes following surgery are impacted positively when patients employ prayer (Ai et al., 2010). As an LPN/LVN, you need to develop an awareness of the general religious philosophy of the patient's belief system. If membership is claimed in a specific denomination, question the patient about the rituals and exercises that the patient believes in and practices. **Spiritual distress** can be observed in patients who are unable to practice their religious rituals. It also can be observed in patients who experience a conflict between their religious and spiritual beliefs and the prescribed health regimen (e.g., a Catholic patient who has been raped and is considering an abortion).

THE PATIENT AND PRAYER

Prayer is a spiritual practice of some individuals whether or not they are members of an organized religion. Prayer can put a patient in touch with a personal higher power. Sometimes prayer can decrease anxiety as effectively as medication. Prayer helps some patients cope with their illness or situation. Honor the request of the patient who wants to pray privately. If the patient requests prayer, the nurse needs to assist the patient or seek assistance in this matter. When patients express an interest in praying, ask what prayer they would like to say. Try to accommodate the request.

In her book *Spiritual Dimensions of Nursing Practice* (1989), Carson comments on conversational prayer, one of the many forms that prayer can take. In this type of prayer, the specific concerns and needs of the patient are included in the prayer. Carson provides the following interaction between a patient awaiting a cesarean section and a nurse who noticed the patient had been crying. It is an excellent example of the simplicity and effectiveness of conversational prayer.

Nurse: You have been crying. What's wrong?

Patient: I wanted to see my minister this morning, but he will not be able to get here before my surgery. I wanted him to pray for me and my baby.

Nurse: Well, I'd be happy to pray for you and the baby. Would that be okay?

Patient: Oh, yes, would you please? This surgery really scares me.

Nurse: Dear God, please comfort this mother as she enters surgery. Lift her fear, and in its place give her peace and strength. Let her know that you are with her and the baby.

Patient: Thanks so much. That really means a lot to me.

THE RELIGIOUS AMERICAN

Examples of the religious American include Hindu, Jew, Buddhist, Muslim, Lutheran (Evangelical Lutheran Church in America, Wisconsin Synod, Missouri Synod, and English Synod), Catholic (Roman Rite, Eastern Rite as Ukrainian Catholic, and Greek Catholic), Eastern Orthodox (Russian Orthodox and Greek Orthodox), Quaker, Presbyterian, Methodist, Church of Christ, Mennonite, Seventh-Day Adventist, Assembly of God, Mormon, Baptist (Independent and Southern Baptist Convention), Wiccan, Jehovah's Witness, Episcopalian, African Methodist Episcopalian, Christian Science, United Church of Christ, Moravian, Evangelical, Salvation Army, and nondenominational.

The First Amendment of the U.S. Constitution allows the free exercise of religious choice. Starting with the Pilgrims, America has a long history of religious freedom and tolerance. As the preceding list shows, the United States is religiously diverse.

RELIGION IN THE UNITED STATES

There are 215 distinct church traditions in the United States (Giger, 2013). Thus as an LPN/LVN it will be impossible to know the key beliefs of each of these entities. However, only Christianity (76.7%) and Judaism (1.2%) represent greater than 1% of the total population (Religious Identification Survey, 2009). Other large organized religions in the United States include: Islam (0.6%), Buddhism (0.5%), Hinduism (0.4%), Unitarian Universalist (0.3%), and Wiccan/Pagan/Druid (0.1%) (Religious Identification Survey, 2009). The Roman Catholic Church, a Christian faith, is the largest denomination, estimated to include 57,199,000 families in the United States, followed by Baptist at 36,148,000, and Methodist at 14,174,000 (Religious Identification Survey, 2009). According to Giger (2013), Islam is one of the fastest growing religions in the United States and is estimated at six to seven million and growing.

AVOIDING FALSE ASSUMPTIONS AND STEREOTYPES

The suggestions presented in Chapter 10 regarding the avoidance of false assumptions and stereotyping when caring for culturally diverse patients also apply when caring for patients of different religions. Some nursing students may think there is also a guidebook that supplies nursing interventions when caring for patients who belong to different religions. As with different cultures, this type of approach can lead to false assumptions and stereotyping. Not only is there diversity among religious groups, but there is also diversity among members of a specific religion or group. It is a false assumption to expect that all individuals of a specific religion or belief system will believe exactly the same just because they are members of that religion or belief system. Avoid assuming that all Protestants, Catholics, Jews, Muslims, Buddhists, and Hindus, for example, believe in and follow all the aspects of their formal religion/belief system. *Individual differences occur in every religious or belief systems group.* Members may have modified the degree to which they observe the practices of their religion or belief system based on age, experience, education, socioeconomic, and social group. Avoid judging patients if their religious beliefs do not conform to the traditional ones for that religion. Data must be gathered about each patient's specific beliefs and religious practices (Box 11-2).

The nursing interventions provided in Boxes 11-3 to 11-8 and Tables 11-1 and 11-2 will serve as a reference to be used in meeting the religious needs of specific patients during your time as a student practical nurse/student vocational nurse (SPN/SVN). This information can also be used in your nursing career after you graduate. Each religion has specific beliefs and practices. Sometimes an individual will adapt them to fit his or her own circumstances. Clarify with the patient the specific beliefs and practices that offer comfort to them and that they prefer. Develop an awareness of health issues and decisions that may involve religious or philosophical beliefs.

WESTERN AND MIDDLE EASTERN RELIGIONS IN THE UNITED STATES AND CANADA

Judaism, Christianity, and Islam are examples of monotheistic (belief in one Supreme Being) Western and Middle Eastern religions found in the United States.

JUDAISM

Judaism is the oldest of faiths that have a belief in one deity. There are approximately 2.7 million Jews living

---

Box 11-2 **Gathering Data for Religious Beliefs and Practices of Patients**

- Do you have a religious affiliation? If so, state it.
- What role does religion play in your life?
- Is prayer helpful to you?
- What is your source of strength and hope?
- What brings you comfort and joy?
- What religious rituals or practices are important to you?
- What symbols or religious books are helpful to you?
- What dietary inclusions or restrictions are a part of your religious beliefs?
- How does your religion view the source and meaning of pain and suffering?
- When ill, does your religion prohibit people of the opposite sex from giving care?
- Does your religion have special days when certain behaviors are mandatory or prohibited?
- If a death is imminent, does your family have any special practices at the time of death?

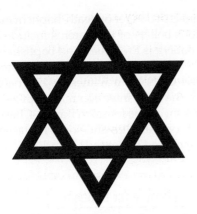

FIGURE 11-1 Star of David. This is a generally recognized symbol of Judaism.

in the United States (Religious Identification Survey, 2009). The prophet Abraham founded Judaism in approximately 2000 BC. The holy books of the Jews are the Torah and the Talmud. The Torah contains the written teachings, laws, and stories of Judaism. The Talmud contains the oral teachings and explanations. Followers of Judaism are called Jews, and Jewish clergy are called rabbis. Jews worship in buildings called temples or synagogues, and a common symbol of the Jewish faith is the Star of David (Figure 11-1). The following are the major divisions of Judaism:

- **Orthodox Judaism:** Orthodox Jews follow the traditional faith and strictly adhere to rituals, including a kosher diet (see Box 11-3) and keeping of the Sabbath. They consider the Torah and the Talmud as revealed by God and do not believe in completely integrating into modern society. Hasidism is an ultraorthodox form of Judaism.
- **Conservative Judaism:** Conservative Jews follow most traditional practices but adapt traditions to the modern world.
- **Reform Judaism:** Reform Jews stress the ethical and moral teachings of the prophets and autonomy of the individual. Rituals are performed that will promote a Jewish, God-filled life. Reformed Jews regard Judaism as evolving and subject to change. Reform Judaism does not accept the binding nature of Jewish law and believes that the Torah was written by human sources rather than by God. Traditionally, Jewish identity is considered to be passed on through the mother. Reform Jews accept Jewish identity passed on through the father. Reform Judaism is the largest, fastest-growing division of Judaism.

Box 11-3 lists the beliefs and practices that need to be clarified for each patient and nursing interventions that have importance for health care workers in contact with patients who are Jewish.

CHRISTIANITY

Christianity is a 2000-year-old religion based on the belief that **Jesus Christ** was the son of God. Followers of Christianity are called Christians, and a common symbol of this faith is the cross (Figure 11-2).

Box 11-3	Beliefs, Practices, and Nursing Interventions for Jewish Patients

GENERAL
Beliefs and Practices
Jews believe in God but do not have a belief in Jesus Christ.
Nursing Interventions
Avoid references to heaven or Jesus.

OBSERVATION OF SABBATH
Nursing Interventions
If observed, provide time for rest, prayer, and/or study from sunset on Friday until after sunset on Saturday.
If observed, provide yarmulke (skullcap) or prayer shawl. Ask family to provide these items.

OBSERVANCE OF DIETARY RULES (KOSHER DIET)
Beliefs and Practices
If following a kosher diet, meat may be consumed a few minutes after drinking milk, but 6 hours must pass after eating meat before drinking milk.
Some Jews do not eat pork, ham, Canadian bacon, eel, oysters, crab, lobster, shrimp, or eggs with blood spots.
Nursing Interventions
Clarify if patient follows these dietary rules.
If desired by patient, make arrangements for separate utensils for preparing and serving meat and milk dishes. If separate dishes are not available, these foods can be served in the original containers or on paper plates.

DYING JEWISH PATIENT
Beliefs and Practices
Family and friends may want to be with the patient at all times.
Some Jews do not believe in autopsies, embalming, or cremation.
Some Jews may not want the nurse to touch the body of a deceased Jew.
Nursing Interventions
Some Jews may request that the nurse notify the Burial Society for preparation of the body for burial.

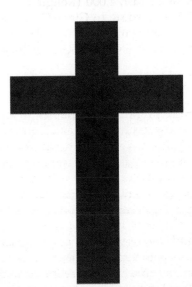

FIGURE 11-2 The cross represents the instrument of the crucifixion of Jesus Christ.

General Beliefs of Christians

The Bible. The Bible is the sacred book of Christians. It contains writings divided into two sections: the Old Testament, which was written before the birth of Jesus, and the New Testament, which was written after his birth. Different Christian groups use different versions of these writings. The numbers and names of the books in the Bible differ in the Catholic and Protestant versions.

Many Christian patients will find comfort in reading or having someone read to them selected passages from the Bible. Treat the patient's Bible with respect. In addition to believing it contains the inspired word of God, some people received their Bibles as gifts commemorating special occasions, such as a wedding, a graduation, Confirmation, Holy Communion, an anniversary, or a jubilee. Some Bibles list passages that can be used in specific patient situations, such as pain, sorrow, and sleeplessness.

Baptism. Baptism is the rite of admission to the Christian community. Christian groups give different meanings to baptism. Some consider this rite a means of salvation, a way of washing away sin, a means of receiving the Holy Spirit (the third person of the Holy Trinity, the belief of some Christians of three persons in one God), an imprinting of character on the soul, or a promise of divine grace. Christian groups differ as to the age (infant, adult) at which a person may be baptized. Although water is used for baptizing, the method differs among groups (pouring, sprinkling, immersion).

If an infant is in danger of death, baptism may be given if the religious beliefs of the parents include infant baptism. If the patient is Protestant and baptism is desired, it is preferable to have a witness. If death is imminent and the patient is Catholic, a witness is not necessary, and anyone with the right intention may baptize. The procedure for baptism can be found in Box 11-4. Baptism beliefs and practices of Catholics and some Protestant denominations are included in Boxes 11-5 and 11-6.

Box 11-4 Procedure for Baptism

If baptism is desired/allowed, the nurse can participate in the baptism as follows.

NURSING INTERVENTIONS

Allow water to flow over and contact the patient's skin while saying the words "Name (if known), I baptize you in the name of the Father, and of the Son, and of the Holy Spirit."

If the patient desires to be Catholic, death is imminent, and it is uncertain whether baptism was received in the past, baptism is administered conditionally. In this situation, the following words are used: "If you are not baptized, I baptize you in the name of the Father, and of the Son, and of the Holy Spirit."

Report the baptism to the chaplain or pastoral care team and the family.

Document the baptism in the patient's record.

Box 11-5 Beliefs, Practices, and Nursing Interventions for Catholic Patients

ROMAN CATHOLIC (WESTERN)

Baptism Beliefs

Necessary for salvation and initiation into the Catholic community. This sacrament removes all sin. Person receives the Holy Spirit. Infant or adult may be baptized, usually by pouring of or immersion in water.

Nursing Interventions

If the patient is a gravely ill infant, a stillbirth, or a fetus, the nurse may baptize without a witness.

If a patient or family member requests baptism and death is imminent, the nurse may baptize before the priest arrives.

Communion Beliefs

Believe that the bread and wine become the body and blood of Jesus Christ.

Nursing Interventions

If sacrament is desired, follow agency privacy policy, developed to carry out HIPAA guidelines, to receive communion. Medicine and water may be taken before Communion.

If the patient's mouth is dry, water may be given after Communion.

SACRAMENTS

Nursing Interventions

If requested, follow agency privacy policy to arrange for the sacrament of Reconciliation and provide privacy when the priest hears the patient's confession.

If desired by patient, follow agency privacy policy for arranging the sacrament of the Anointing of the Sick. (Some

Roman Catholics may refer to this as the Sacrament of the Sick. Older Catholics may refer to this as the Last Rites or the sacrament of Extreme Unction.) This sacrament is for anyone seriously ill or weakened by old age. This sacrament is believed to offer hope, consolation, and peace; assist in physical, mental, and spiritual healing; and provide strength to endure suffering.

If requested, follow agency's privacy policy to make arrangements for the priest to administer this sacrament. Catholics can receive this sacrament more than once, as requested.

Dietary Restrictions

If there are no health restrictions, Roman Catholics 14 years of age and older are to abstain from meat on Ash Wednesday and all Fridays during Lent. Catholics ages 14 to 59 must fast (eat only one full meal, although food that does not add up to a full meal can also be eaten) on Ash Wednesday and Good Friday. Fasting and abstaining are excused during hospitalization. Eastern Rite Catholics may be stricter about fasting.

Nursing Interventions

Clarify practices with patient.

Sexuality

Abortion is not allowed. Natural methods of family planning are strongly promoted.

Dying Catholic Patient

Catholic patients facing death may want to receive the last sacrament of the Christian. In addition to the anointing of the sick, the sacraments of Reconciliation and Viaticum (the last

Box 11-5   Beliefs, Practices, and Nursing Interventions for Catholic Patients—cont'd

Communion that provides food for the journey from this life to the next) are administered.
Nursing Interventions
Follow agency privacy rules to make arrangements for the priest to administer this sacrament. Cremation and organ donation are allowed.

EASTERN ORTHODOX CHURCHES
Baptism Beliefs
Necessary for salvation. Infants are baptized by sprinkling or immersion.
Communion Beliefs
Believe the bread and wine are the body and blood of Jesus Christ.
Follow procedure for Communion as with Catholic patient.
Sacraments
Celebrate seven sacraments.

Nursing Interventions
Follow procedure for Anointing of the Sick as with Catholic patient.
Dietary Restrictions
Abstain from meat and dairy products on Wednesdays and Fridays during Lent.
Ill patients are excused from this requirement.
Sexuality
Birth control and abortion are not allowed.
Dying Eastern Orthodox Patient
The Last Rites are obligatory.
Beliefs and Practices
Autopsy and organ donation are not encouraged. Euthanasia and cremation are discouraged.
Nursing Interventions
Follow agency privacy policy to arrange for priest to administer the Last Rites, preferably while the patient is conscious.

Box 11-6   Beliefs, Practices, and Nursing Interventions for Protestant Patients of 10 Denominations

NURSING CONSIDERATIONS THAT PERTAIN TO ALL PROTESTANT PATIENTS
Nursing Interventions
Because of federal privacy laws, inform patient that if a visit by a personal minister or pastor is desired for Communion, Anointing, and other sacraments, the patient must follow agency policy.
Provide privacy if patient reads the Bible.
Include on data-gathering list:
If patient is an infant and condition is serious, do parents desire baptism if child is not baptized?
If patient is dying, what are family's beliefs about death and dying?

OLD ORDER AMISH (HOUSE AMISH)
Amish are a conservative division of the Mennonites. Old Order Amish worship in private homes. The Amish do not believe in health insurance and Social Security, and they rely on mutual aid in time of need. Patients may believe that sudden fright or blood loss may cause loss of the soul. Female patients may object to cutting their hair because of their belief that Holy Scripture forbids it.
Baptism: Adult baptism.

ASSEMBLY OF GOD
One of several American Pentecostal denominations. May believe in the power of prayer for healing.
Baptism: Receive Jesus Christ as Lord and Savior. Administered by immersion when person understands the meaning of baptism.
Communion: Yes.

BAPTIST
Started in the seventeenth century in the United States. Baptists regard the Bible as a complete, sufficient, and final authority in matters of faith. Interpret the Bible literally. Stress personal relationship with Jesus Christ. Discourage alcohol consumption.
Baptism: No infant baptism. Person needs to understand the meaning of baptism. Adults are baptized by immersion. Baptism not considered a means of salvation.
Communion: Considered a symbol and a remembrance of Jesus Christ's death.

EPISCOPALIAN
Began in the sixteenth century in England. Also called the Anglican Church in England. Service book is Book of Common Prayer. Clergy include bishops, priests, and deacons. Priests may marry. Women may be ordained.
Baptism: Believe baptism is necessary for salvation. Infant baptism is performed by sprinkling.
Communion: Believe that Jesus Christ is present in the bread and wine.

LUTHERAN
There are several Lutheran bodies in the United States. Ministers may marry. Believe in anointing and blessing when ill.
Baptism: Conveys grace. Infants are baptized at 6 to 8 weeks of age by pouring, sprinkling, or immersion. In case of illness, invasive procedures, and emergent situations, infants may be baptized by their pastor, if possible. Baptism by a layperson is acceptable.
Communion: Believe the presence of Jesus Christ is real. Conveys grace.

METHODIST
Methodism started in the eighteenth century. There are several branches of the Methodist Church.
Baptism: An outward and visible sign of an inward and spiritual grace. Infant and adult by sprinkling or immersion.
Communion: Conveys grace. Open to everyone.

PRESBYTERIAN
Began in Scotland and evolved from John Calvin in the sixteenth century. May avoid alcohol.
Baptism: Infant, usually by sprinkling. Signifies the beginning of life in Jesus Christ and not its completion.
Communion: Believe Jesus Christ is present in spirit.

QUAKERS (RELIGIOUS SOCIETY OF FRIENDS)
Beliefs and Practices
Believe they receive Divine Truth from "inner" light supplied by the Holy Spirit. Services called "meetings." Generally regard sacraments as nonessential to Christian life.

Continued

Box 11-6 Beliefs, Practices, and Nursing Interventions for Protestant Patients of 10 Denominations—cont'd

Nursing Interventions

Clarify baptism beliefs with patient. At birth, infant's name recorded in official church book.

SEVENTH-DAY ADVENTIST

Adventists observe the Sabbath from sunset on Friday to sunset on Saturday. Do not pursue their jobs or worldly pleasures during this time. Many Adventists are vegetarians and use soybean products as a protein source. These dietary practices are not mandatory. Adventists generally do not smoke or drink alcoholic beverages. Some Adventist patients may avoid beverages with caffeine. They believe that at death the body rests in the grave until the second coming of Jesus Christ. Organ donation is acceptable.

Nursing Interventions

Clarify diet restrictions.

Baptism: Makes one a church member. Adult by immersion. Opposed to infant baptism.

Communion: May practice washing of the feet in preparation.

UNITED CHURCH OF CHRIST

Formed in 1957 by merger of Congregational and Evangelical and Reformed Churches.

Baptism: Infant by pouring, sprinkling, or immersion. When baptized, become church members.

Communion: Celebrated and open to all.

Holy Communion. Holy Communion (or Holy Eucharist) is partaking of consecrated (blessed) elements of bread and wine. Depending on the group, the bread is leavened (with yeast) or unleavened. Some groups use grape juice instead of wine. Holy Communion has different meanings for different denominations. Examples of these differences include a remembrance of the Last Supper and a remembrance of the death of Jesus Christ. Some groups consider the bread and wine to be only symbols of Jesus Christ, whereas others believe they are the body and blood of Jesus Christ. When caring for a patient of a specific affiliation, question the patient and family regarding specific beliefs and practices regarding Communion. Boxes 11-5 and 11-6 include Communion beliefs and practices of Catholics and some Protestant denominations.

Major Divisions of Christianity

The major divisions of Christianity are Catholicism, Protestantism, and Eastern Orthodoxy.

Catholicism. Catholicism consists of the Western or Roman Catholic Church, including Catholics of the Eastern Rite. Sometimes there is confusion between the Eastern Churches and Roman Catholicism. The Eastern Churches are either Catholics of the Eastern Rite or Eastern Orthodox.

Catholics of the Roman Rite. There are 57,199,000 Catholics in the United States (American Religious Identification Survey, 2009). Catholics trace their faith from Jesus Christ through an unbroken line to the pope. The pope, currently Pope Francis, is considered to be the representative of Jesus Christ on earth and is considered infallible; that is, incapable of being in error when speaking of matters of faith and morals. Beliefs are found in the Bible and tradition. Catholic clergy, called priests, are not allowed to marry because of tradition (custom), not dogma (law). Women cannot be ordained. The administrative hierarchy of the Catholic Church consists of cardinals, archbishops, bishops, priests, and deacons. Buildings of worship for Catholics are called churches and cathedrals. A cathedral is the headquarters of a bishop, archbishop, or cardinal. Celebration of the Mass is the center of worship. Weekly attendance at mass, including receiving the Holy Eucharist, is an expectation. The seven sacraments of the Catholic Church are Baptism, Confirmation, Holy Eucharist, Penance, Anointing of the Sick, Holy Orders, and Matrimony. The Virgin Mary is revered and prayed to, particularly through the Holy Rosary.

Catholics of Eastern Rites. Catholics of Eastern Rites have the same beliefs as the Western or Roman Catholic Church. They recognize the Vatican and the pope. They keep their own canon law, customs, and liturgy. Clergy are priests and bishops, and priests of this Eastern Rite (with the exception of monks) may marry. Bishops are selected from among monks. Examples of Catholics of Eastern Rites include Armenian Catholic, Chaldean Catholic, Maronites, and the Catholics of the Byzantine Rite (e.g., Greek Catholics, Bulgarian Catholics, and Russian Catholics).

Eastern Orthodox Churches. The Eastern Orthodox Church considers itself catholic (that is, universal) but does not recognize the pope. The Roman Catholic Church considers these churches to be in schism because they refuse to submit to the authority of the pope. Beliefs come from the Bible and tradition. Clergy are bishops, priests, and deacons. Priests may marry before ordination. *Matuska,* meaning "Little Mother," is a title given to wives of Orthodox priests. Monks may not marry, and bishops are selected from among monks. These Eastern churches have no central authority. They are self-governed by a board consisting of a bishop and laypersons. Some of these churches are headed by a patriarch. Seven sacraments are celebrated. The Virgin Mary is respected. Liturgies differ among nationalities but have similarities to the Roman Catholic Church, although the services are more elaborate than Roman Catholic liturgies. Examples of Eastern Orthodox Churches are Orthodox of the Byzantine Rite (e.g.,

Greek Orthodox and Russian Orthodox), Armenian Orthodox, and Jacobite churches. Box 11-5 lists beliefs and practices that need to be clarified for each patient and nursing implications for patients who are Catholic (Roman and Eastern). Eastern Orthodox beliefs and practices are also listed.

Protestantism. In the sixteenth century, Germany was part of the Holy Roman Empire and almost entirely Roman Catholic. Protestantism began in 1517 when Martin Luther separated from the Catholic Church in protest because of the many scandals that were taking place in the church. This was the beginning of the Reformation and Lutheranism. As Lutheranism spread throughout Germany, Catholic clergy tried to limit changes affecting the Catholic Church and to retain its authority in all church matters. John of Saxony led a group to a Catholic Church assembly, where they objected to the Catholic Church's plans to limit innovations in doctrine and practices in the Catholic Church. The group then signed a *protestation* and became known as *Protestants* from then on (Gritsch, 2002). Protestants believe that their convictions are closer to New Testament Christianity. The chief characteristic of Protestantism is the acceptance of the Bible as the sole authority in matters of faith. It is believed that Christians are justified in their relationship to God *by faith alone*. Examples of denominations and sects that came from the Reformation include Lutheran, Reformed, and Presbyterian. Depending on the denomination, Protestant clergy are called ministers or pastors. Protestant places of worship are called churches or temples. During the second half of the nineteenth century, opposition to changes in Protestantism resulted in a conservative type of Protestantism called Fundamentalism. Southern Baptists are an ultraconservative form of Protestants. Box 11-6 lists beliefs and practices that need to be clarified for each patient and nursing interventions for patients of 10 Protestant denominations.

ISLAM

The Arabic word *Islam* implies peace, submission, and obedience (Giger, 2013). This contrasts greatly with the extremist members, who often are a reference point for United States citizens. This alone exemplifies why solid knowledge and avoiding stereotyping is important to the delivery of health care.

In the sixth century AD, the prophet Muhammad founded Islam in Arabia. Followers of Islam are called Muslims. There are 1,349,000 Muslims in the United States (American Religious Identification Survey, 2009). Muslims believe in one God: **Allah**. Salvation depends on one's commitment to Allah and his teachings in the Qur'an (Koran). This holy book contains the words of Allah as he spoke to Muhammad. Muslims pray in Arabic and worship in mosques. The imam is the leader of the Muslim congregation (Figure 11-3).

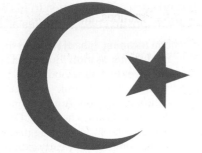

FIGURE 11-3 Crescent moon and star is an internationally recognized symbol of Islam.

Muslims have many beliefs that are similar to Judeo-Christian doctrine; for example, angels and prophets such as Abraham, Moses, and Jesus. Muslims believe in heaven, hell, the last judgment, prayer, fasting, and giving to the poor.

Islam is not one entity but has many interpretations, resulting in diversity in its practice. The two main divisions in Islam are the Sunni and Shi'ite sects. The majority of Muslims worldwide are Sunnis. Because Muhammad did not designate a successor when he died, the Sunni sect chose a successor, who became the political leader of the community. Sunnis believe they must follow the Sunnah, the ethical and religious code from the sayings of Muhammad and vest religious and political authority with the community as guided by Islamic law and consensus of the Qur'an and the leaders. The Shi'ite sect believes that Muhammad designated his cousin and son-in-law, Ali, to be the leader of Islam after his death and vest all authority with the imam (the leader of a Muslim congregation) and ultimately the ayatollah (a high-ranking religious and political leader), and these leaders guide the teachings of Islam (Gellman & Hartman, 2002).

Despite different sects and divisions, the Five Pillars are the essential and obligatory practices all Muslims accept and follow:

1. **The Profession of Faith:** This is a verbal pledge that there is only one God, Allah, and that Muhammad is the messenger of God. (Muslim mothers may whisper this pledge into a newborn's ear.)
2. **Prayer:** Muslims are called to prayer five times a day.
3. **Almsgiving:** This involves an annual payment of a certain percentage of a Muslim's wealth and assets. This money is distributed among the poor.
4. **Fasting:** During Ramadan, the ninth month of the Islamic calendar, adult Muslims abstain from dawn to sunset from food, drink, and sexual activity. Exceptions can be made for the sick and elderly.
5. **Pilgrimage:** Adult Muslims who are physically and financially able are expected to perform the pilgrimage to Mecca (Islam's holiest shrine) at least once in their lifetime.

Jihad, meaning "to strive or struggle" in the way of God, is sometimes referred to as the Sixth Pillar of Islam, although it has no such official status. In his book *Islam: The Straight Path*, Esposito (1998) explains as follows:

> In its most general meaning, [jihad] refers to the obligation incumbent on all Muslims, as individuals and as a community, to exert themselves to realize God's will, to lead virtuous lives, and to extend the Islamic community through preaching, education, and so on. A related meaning is the struggle for or defense of Islam, a holy war. Despite the fact that jihad is not supposed to include aggressive warfare, this has occurred, as exemplified by early extremists like the Kharijites and contemporary groups such as jihad organizations in Lebanon, the Gulf States, and Indonesia.

Male infants are circumcised. Islamic law does not prohibit contraception for married couples. No permanent damage to reproductive organs is allowed. Abortion is permitted if the mother's life is at stake and the fetus is not older than 4 months' gestation. Saving a life is one of the greatest merits and imperatives in Islam. Box 11-7 lists beliefs and practices that need to be clarified, and nursing considerations for Muslim patients.

? Critical Thinking

Avoid Stereotyping Your Patients

How would you avoid stereotyping and making false assumptions about a Muslim patient who is dying? Do the same for a patient of a religious group that is frequently seen in your community.

ADDITIONAL CHRISTIAN AND NONCHRISTIAN RELIGIOUS GROUPS

Box 11-8 lists beliefs and practices that need to be clarified for each patient and nursing interventions for patients of various religious groups.

EASTERN RELIGIONS AND PHILOSOPHIES IN THE UNITED STATES AND CANADA

Because the Western and the Eastern worlds contain different value systems, the two worlds represent different ways of thinking that have molded the culture, including the worldview of two different parts of the world. In the twenty-first century, cultures and religious practices of other countries have become more known to us because of travel, the mass media, and immigration of people from all over the world to the United States and Canada.

The Eastern world (e.g., India, China, Japan, and Korea) emphasizes the following virtues:
- Self-discipline and control
- The inner nature of self
- Moderation in all things
- Nonattachment to worldly things
- Awareness that selfish desire is the cause of much suffering
- Tolerance of other religions and points of view
- Respect for family, elders, and authority
- The principle of not harming any living creature

Box 11-7 Beliefs, Practices, and Nursing Interventions for Muslim Patients

GENERAL BELIEFS
Members of Islam may desire to pray to Allah five times a day (after dawn, at noon, in midafternoon, after sunset, and at night). Friday is a day for communal prayer.

Beliefs and Practices
Rules of cleanliness may include eating with the right hand and cleansing self with the left hand after urinating and defecating.

Nursing Interventions
If patient requests to face Mecca, the holy city of Islam, a bed or chair may be positioned in a southeast direction from the United States.

If a Muslim brings the Koran, the holy book of Islam, to the health care facility, do not touch it or place anything on top of it.

If a Muslim wears writings from the Koran on a black string around the neck, arm, or waist, these writings need to be kept dry and remain on the patient because they are passages from the Koran.

OBSERVATION OF DIETARY RULES
Beliefs and Practices
Some Muslims might not eat *haram* (prohibited food); for example, pork and pork products (ham, bacon), meats from animals that have not been bled to death by a Muslim, and gelatin.

Foods that are permitted are called *halal* (legal).

Some Muslims might not drink alcoholic beverages.

Nursing Interventions
Clarify dietary restrictions.

OBSERVATION OF FEMALE MODESTY
Beliefs and Practices
Some Muslim women prefer to be clothed from head to ankle.

Nursing Interventions
During a physical examination, female Muslims may prefer to undress one body part at a time.

DEATH PRACTICES
Beliefs and Practices
Women may be barred from the room of a dying family member.

The family may pray for the dying family member. The imam usually reads from the Koran for the patient after death. After death:
- Body is turned toward Mecca.
- Body is wrapped in a white cloth for burial.
- Family washes the body, including all orifices, and seals them with cotton.
- Family may not permit organ donation, autopsies, or cremation to keep the body intact so the person may meet God with integrity. These decisions may vary by country of origin.
- Body may not be embalmed or cremated.
- Ideal to bury the body within 24 hours.

Nursing Interventions
The nurse may touch the body only after donning gloves.

Box 11-8 Beliefs, Practices, and Nursing Interventions for Additional Christian and Non-Christian Religious/Spiritual Groups

CHRISTIAN SCIENTIST (CHURCH OF CHRIST, SCIENTIST)

Founded in nineteenth century by Mary Baker Eddy, who wrote *Science and Health with a Key to the Scriptures*.

Beliefs and Practices

Believe sin causes sickness and studying Eddy's book and the Bible will heal them.

Patient may believe that sickness can be overcome through prayer and spiritual understanding that God is good and the only reality.

Healing considered an awakening to this belief.

There are no clergy, but patient may want a Christian Science practitioner to give treatment through prayer.

No baptism.

Consider the Lord's Supper a spiritual communion with God and may sit quietly during this time.

No smoking or drinking alcohol. They do not accept blood transfusions or surgery.

Nursing Interventions

Clarify baptism beliefs with patient.

JEHOVAH'S WITNESSES

Originated at the end of the nineteenth century in the United States. Witnesses base their beliefs on the Bible.

Beliefs and Practices

Believe the Second Coming has begun, Armageddon is imminent, and the millennium will soon follow. At that time, repentant sinners will have a second chance for salvation.

They do not believe in the Trinity. Consider Jesus inferior to God, the Father, Jehovah.

No ordained ministers.

No churches but worship in Kingdom Halls. Publications include Awake and Watch Tower.

Witnesses will refuse to receive whole blood products, including plasma. Receiving such products is viewed as a violation of the law of Jehovah (Genesis 9:3 4; Leviticus 17:14; Acts 15:28-29). They will accept blood transfusion alternatives.

Alcohol and tobacco are discouraged.

Believe the soul dies at death. Autopsy decided by family.

Cremation is acceptable.

Organ transplants are a private decision. Before transplant, organs must be cleansed with a nonblood solution.

Baptism: Necessary for salvation. Considered a symbol of dedication to Jehovah. Adult by immersion. No infant baptism.

Communion: Occurs one time a year.

MORMONS (CHURCH OF JESUS CHRIST OF LATTER DAY SAINTS)

In the nineteenth century, Joseph Smith founded the Mormon Church. The headquarters are in Salt Lake City, Utah.

Beliefs and Practices

Revelation is emphasized to establish doctrine and rituals.

The Book of Mormon contains accounts of ancient peoples in America. This book is considered complementary scripture to the Bible.

Mormons emphasize tithing and community welfare.

Mormons worship in temples and tabernacles.

Mormon adults wear undergarments at all times as a symbolic gesture of the promises made to God.

There is no ordained clergy. High priests are members of the church; they form the Council of Twelve and exert spiritual leadership. Three high priests vested with supreme authority form the first presidency of the church.

A Mormon may be anointed and blessed before planned hospitalization.

Abortion is not allowed unless the mother's life is in danger.

Natural methods of birth control are allowed. Artificial means may be used when the physical or emotional health of the woman is in question.

May avoid tobacco, alcohol, coffee, and tea.

Baptism: Considered necessary for salvation. Causes remission of sins. Allows the person to receive the gifts of the Holy Spirit. Baptism is given at age 8 or older by immersion. Baptism may be given after death by proxy.

Communion: The Lord's Supper with bread and water. Considered a symbol and renewing of covenant with Jesus Christ.

BAHA'I

Founded in the nineteenth century in Persia (now southern Iran).

Beliefs and Practices

Believe in world peace, the unity of all religions and humanity, and the equality of men and women.

There is no clergy.

Members meet in homes. The house of worship in the United States is in Wilmette, Illinois. There is an annual 19-day fast from sunrise to sundown during the last month of the Baha'i calendar. You can find more information at www.bahai.us/welcome/principles-and-practices/bahai-calendar/.

May avoid alcohol.

At death, the soul, the real self, journeys through the spiritual world, which is the timeless, placeless extension of the universe.

No embalming, unless required by state law. Cremation discouraged.

Burial to take place within 1 hour's travel time of death.

There is no baptism or Communion.

Their special book is The *Book of Certitude*.

The Western world (e.g., Europe, Canada, and the United States) emphasizes the following virtues:

- The value of individual worth
- The need to be responsible for one another, which gives rise to many social programs
- A personal relationship with one God that translates into love of neighbor and environment

Because of immigration and acculturation of Eastern peoples and interest in and adoption of Eastern philosophies by Western society, both traditions can be seen in the other. For example, there are a large number of Christians among Eastern peoples. Westerners have adopted meditation, yoga, complementary therapies (including use of herbs and oils), and a focus on inner development.

HINDUISM

Hinduism dates back to prehistoric times. This oldest religion is the third largest religion in the world and is composed of a diverse system of thoughts and beliefs (Figure 11-4). Only 766,000 Hindus live in the United States (American Religious Identification Survey,

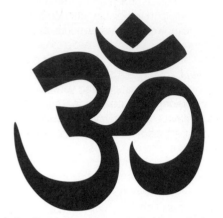

FIGURE 11-4 Om (Aum). This represents Brahman, the impersonal Absolute of Hinduism and the source of all manifest existence.

2009). The essence of Hinduism is based on a vast body of scriptures, including the Vedas and the Bhagavad-Gita. These texts teach the path to the proper way of living through *dharma* (ethics, duties), *karma* (action, deeds), and *bhakti* (devotion and knowledge that God is the ultimate power and exists in many forms). With these in mind, Hinduism is more a way of life than a religion. Hindus believe in **reincarnation**: One is reborn to a higher or lower level of existence based on one's moral behavior in the prior phase of existence. The cycle of birth and death continues until the soul achieves *moksha* (or Nirvana), the self-realization and unification of the soul with the ultimate being.

There is no common creed or doctrine in Hinduism; it is based on the accumulated treasury of spiritual laws discovered by different people in different times. Most Hindus venerate many gods and goddesses, including the Trinity: *Vishnu*, the Protector; *Shiva*, the destroyer; and *Brahma*, the Creator. These gods, along with their equally powerful consorts, are worshipped in their various incarnations and forms. Tables 11-1 and 11-2 present general beliefs and practices of Buddhist and

Table 11-1 General Religious Beliefs/Practices and Nursing Interventions for Buddhist and Hindu Patients	
BELIEFS/PRACTICES	**NURSING INTERVENTIONS**
Not having a central authority or dictated doctrine, the **Buddhists** and **Hindus** in North America exhibit a variety of traditions, beliefs, and practices.	Clarify with the patient his or her preference of practices to be observed.
Buddhists believe pain and suffering result from actions in this or a past life.	Accept the patient's right to this belief; neither agree nor disagree.
Buddhist and **Hindu** patients accept traditional medical treatment. However, to maintain a clear state of mind, **Buddhists** may refuse drugs that alter the state of the mind.	Inform physician of patient's concern. Explain to patient/family the action of all medications before administering them. Report to physician and chart any medications refused and reason for refusal.
Generally, **Buddhists** do not believe in healing through faith. Healing for **Buddhist** patients may be promoted by awakening to the laws of Buddha. After many years of searching, Siddhartha Gautama, the founder of Buddhism, finally found the truth of existence and became the Buddha, the Enlightened One. Many persons since then have become Buddhas by becoming enlightened.	Avoid references to "God" (e.g., "God will help you get through this").
Hindu patients may prefer a light diet in the morning and evening and a heavy meal at noon. Some **Hindu** patients may fast on a specific day of the week or month.	Allow patient/family to select diet for each meal. Encourage patient/family to write in food preferences when not listed. Arrange for visit by dietitian.
Hindus may practice Ayurveda, the traditional Indian science of health that uses herbs to treat disease. Some **Hindus** also practice folk medicine.	As with patients of all cultures and in all settings: Question use of herbs in daily life so possible drug interactions can be avoided. Question use of folk medicine. If practice is not harmful, include practice in plan of care. If practice is harmful, repattern practice. See Chapter 10 for details regarding folk medicine. **Buddhist** patients may use incense, images of Buddha, and/or prayer beads in worship.

Table 11-1	General Religious Beliefs/Practices and Nursing Interventions for Buddhist and Hindu Patients—cont'd

Respect these objects if used by patient. Provide these personal objects if patient asks for them.	
Hindu patients may have a thread on their torso or around their wrist to signify a blessing.	Avoid removing the thread.
Buddhist patients may have a visit from a Buddhist priest, monk, or nun to conduct a religious ceremony. **Hindu** priests generally are not involved with illness care.	Provide privacy for visit of priest, monk, or nun.
Buddhist families may perform traditions with patient.	Arrange the environment to accommodate the family.
Significant others of **Hindu** patients may do the same.	Provide quiet and privacy.
Buddhist patients may chant or meditate to help calm and clear their minds.	Avoid interrupting the patient during meditation or chanting.
Puja, the worship of **Hindu** deities, is preceded by outer purification. **Hindu** patients may request a daily bath.	Provide necessary equipment for bathing for ambulatory patients. If patient requires assistance, assist with bath before meal. If bathing required in bed, add hot water to cold water (Lipson & Dibble, 2006).

Table 11-2	Death Beliefs, Practices, and Nursing Interventions for Buddhist and Hindu Patients

Buddhists believe in many reincarnations until they achieve Enlightenment and are freed from worldly illusion, passions, and suffering. Until this is achieved, death provides the opportunity to improve in the next life. Understanding the Four Noble Truths and the Noble Eightfold Path will allow one to achieve Enlightenment and enter Nirvana (a state, the absence of self, extinguishing of desire and suffering), at which time the cycle of rebirths and deaths ends. Resources within the person to achieve Enlightenment are stressed rather than reliance on ancient gods.	
Hindus believe in the wheel of birth, life, and death (reincarnations) until they break through the illusions of the world and participate in the manifestation of the true self (Atman, the deathless self, the soul). Meditation and grace will help the Hindu believer to realize the Supreme self, which is hidden in the heart. When this occurs, eternal peace or Brahman (the universal soul and source, the Absolute Truth) is the reward.	

BELIEFS/PRACTICES	NURSING INTERVENTIONS
Buddhists and **Hindus** believe in rebirth and death (reincarnation). They do not believe in the concept of an immortal soul.	Accept the patient's right to this belief; avoid agreeing or disagreeing.
Buddhists and **Hindus** believe in karma, the law of cause and effect by which thoughts, words, and deeds of each person create his or her own destiny. One reaps what one sows. Karma is carried over to the next life and determines the form of each new existence. **Buddhists** believe it is the state of one's consciousness at the time of death that usually determines one's rebirth.	For dying patients, make provision for rites and ceremonies by the family and/or spiritual leaders. Avoid interfering with praying, singing, and chanting. **Buddhist Patients** Provide an environment for the dying patient that will allow a clear, calm state of mind and a peaceful death. **Hindu Patients** Allow the family/spiritual leader to place water in the mouth of Hindu patients.
Buddhists and **Hindus** treat the body with respect. Cremation is common for **Buddhists** and **Hindus**. The **Hindu** patient's ashes are saved, to be disposed of in a holy river (e.g., the Ganges). Family may want to wash the body in preparation for cremation.	Inform funeral director of patient's religion. **Hindu Patient** When requested, provide family with equipment to wash the body. Present possibility of organ donation to family in a private environment.
Organ Donations	
Buddhists may allow organ donation if it will help someone pursue enlightenment. **Hindus** allow organ donation.	Follow agency policy for obtaining permission for organ donation.
Autopsies	
Buddhists and **Hindus** permit autopsies.	Follow agency policy for obtaining permission for autopsy.

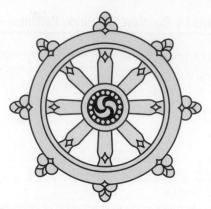

FIGURE 11-5 Buddhist Wheel of Life. The eight spokes symbolize the Noble Eightfold Path. The three swirling segments in the center represent the Buddha, the teachings, and the spiritual community.

Hindu patients and nursing interventions. For more information about Hinduism, access www.religionfacts.com/hinduism/fastfacts.htm.

BUDDHISM

Siddhartha Gautama (**Buddha**) founded Buddhism in the sixth century BC in India. Buddhism can be considered a religion, a philosophy, and a way of life (Figure 11-5). Much of Eastern beliefs have evolved from Buddhism. Well before Christianity, Buddhism originated in India, as did Hinduism. It shares much with Hindu philosophy but also radically departs from it (see Table 11-1). Buddhism spread to China, Japan, Korea, Tibet, Burma, Sri Lanka, Laos, Cambodia, and Vietnam. As Buddhism spread, the core beliefs were adapted to the culture of the host country. The beliefs were shaped and influenced by rituals and the belief system of each country. Two core beliefs of Buddhism that remained constant, however, are the Four Noble Truths and the Noble Eightfold Path leading to Nirvana:

1. Life is suffering.
2. Suffering is caused by desire. Desire is described as the craving or longing for the pleasures of the senses and life itself. Suffering is also caused by ignorance, which is interpreted as not being able to see things as they are.

3. Suffering can be eliminated by eliminating desire (craving or longing for the pleasures of the senses and life itself).
4. To eliminate desire, follow the Noble Eightfold Path:
   a. Right views
   b. Right intention
   c. Right speech
   d. Right action
   e. Right livelihood
   f. Right effort
   g. Right concentration
   h. Right ecstasy

Because of the variation in beliefs and history of Eastern groups, the time interval since immigration, and the degree of socialization, it is difficult to provide clear-cut examples of what a Japanese American or East Indian Hindu American believes and practices. As much diversity exists among Eastern religions and philosophies as exists among Christians.

NURSING INTERVENTIONS FOR EASTERN RELIGIONS

In patient care, the LPN/LVN can come in contact with a Japanese Buddhist, a Korean Buddhist, and a Tibetan Buddhist, among others, as well as American/Canadian patients who have blended Buddhism with their chosen religion. Develop an awareness that not everyone sees the world as you do. Applying the principles from Chapter 10, avoid stereotyping individuals and considering them all the same just because they are Buddhist or Hindu. Table 11-1 presents a comparison of general religious beliefs and practices that *may* be found in Buddhist and Hindu patients, along with appropriate nursing interventions. Table 11-2 presents general death beliefs and practices of Buddhist and Hindu patients and appropriate nursing interventions.

◎ Try This

Learning About Different Belief Systems

Gather information about a religion, philosophy, or group (not discussed in this chapter) other than your own that interests you. Focus on nursing interventions appropriate for the topic you chose to research. Use Chapter 2 as a resource to gather information.

Get Ready for the NCLEX-PN® Examination

Key Points

- The practical/vocational nurse has a responsibility to care for the total person, including physical, emotional, and spiritual needs.
- Spiritual needs of patients arise from their desire to find meaning in life, suffering, and death.
- Gathering data about spiritual needs and providing spiritual care are routine parts of all patients' care, not only in times of crisis.
- To meet the spiritual needs of patients, you need to be aware of the patient's personal spiritual beliefs or the absence of them.
- Members of the health care team who assist the LPN/LVN in providing spiritual care to patients are the minister, priest, rabbi, chaplain, the pastoral care team and other representatives of religions, groups, and philosophies.
- Many patients help to meet their personal spiritual needs by their participation in an organized religion.
- Spirituality can be part of religion, but religion is not necessarily part of spirituality.
- Spiritual distress can occur when patients cannot fulfill the rituals and practices of their religion or when they experience conflict between their spiritual beliefs and their health regimen.
- LPNs/LVNs need to develop an awareness of religious differences and an understanding of the basic beliefs, rituals, and practices of the many religious denominations, groups, and philosophies that exist today.
- Avoid assuming that patients who belong to a specific religion or belief system adopt all of the beliefs and practices of that religion or belief system.
- Clarify personal religious beliefs and practices for all patients.
- Although many patients in the United States are Protestant, Catholic, and Jewish, you will encounter other denominations and groups, such as Muslims and members of Eastern religions and philosophies, as well as persons who have no religious affiliation. By learning more about these groups, you will be able to accommodate their beliefs and practices and focus your care on meeting the goals of the total person.

Additional Learning Resources

evolve Go to your Evolve website (http://evolve.elsevier.com/Knecht/success) for the following FREE learning resources:
- Answers to Critical Thinking Review Scenarios
- Additional learning activities
- Additional Review Questions for the NCLEX-PN® exam
- Helpful phrases for communicating in Spanish and more!

Review Questions for the NCLEX-PN® Examination

1. When providing care to a Muslim patient, the nurse may be requested to facilitate the patient's ability to pray to:
   a. Jesus Christ
   b. Zeus
   c. Allah
   d. Yahweh
2. Select the statement that *best* describes the role of the pastoral care team.
   a. The pastoral care team is the social services department in acute care facilities and extended care.
   b. The pastoral care team works with the nursing staff to help meet the spiritual and religious needs of patients.
   c. Religious care and spiritual support are offered to seriously ill and dying patients by the pastoral care department.
   d. Because of pastoral care, the nursing staff does not have to worry about meeting the spiritual needs of patients.
3. If a Catholic patient requests the Sacrament of the Sick before surgery, the LPN/LVN responds by:
   a. Reassuring the patient that he is not going to die during surgery.
   b. Notifying the patient's family that his condition has changed.
   c. Calling the patient's physician to report the patient's mental state.
   d. Notifying the pastoral care team of the patient's preoperative request.
4. If a patient with a bleeding peptic ulcer is a Jehovah's Witness and refuses to receive an ordered blood transfusion preoperatively, select the priority action of the LPN/LVN.
   a. Notify the nursing supervisor STAT and report the patient's refusal.
   b. Encourage the patient to accept the transfusion as a life-saving measure.
   c. Explain that the transfusion is needed because of severe blood loss.
   d. Alert family members of the crucial need to notify church authorities.

Alternate Format Item

1. A patient of Jewish descent is admitted to the extended care unit on your shift. Which of the following nursing interventions will definitely be applicable? (*Select all that apply.*)
   a. Provide quiet time for prayer on the Sabbath.
   b. Order all meals to be served using kosher preparation.
   c. Arrange for milk to be delivered at least a half hour before meals.
   d. Clarify the patient's Jewish beliefs to determine the best plan of care.
   e. Assist the patient in using the elevator on the Sabbath.

2. Najid, age 76 and a devout Muslim, has died on your shift after an illness with pancreatic cancer. Family wishes and his traditional belief system have been documented. Select the interventions the LPN/LVN would include in Najid's care. *(Select all that apply.)*
   a. Turn Najid's bed in a southeast direction.
   b. Provide the family with bathing supplies.
   c. Obtain permission for an autopsy.
   d. Arrange for Najid's body to be wrapped in a white cloth.
   e. Only touch Najid's body with gloved hands.

Critical Thinking Scenarios

Scenario 1

Amy has an assigned patient who is Muslim. His wife visits daily and always wears a scarf over her head. Amy sees this manner of dress occasionally in her town. She is puzzled about this practice. Help Amy understand the reason for wearing a scarf in this manner if one is a Muslim female.

Scenario 2

An elderly Catholic woman in a long-term care setting appears sad every Sunday morning. Sunday mass is not available at the institution. She quietly sits in her room and refuses to join her friends for Sunday breakfast. Discuss what steps you would initiate.

The Nursing Process: Your Role

chapter 12

Objectives

On completing this chapter, you will be able to do the following:

1. Discuss how the nursing process has evolved from the 1950s to the present.
2. Define your role in the nursing process according to the Nurse Practice Act (NPA) in your state, territory, or country.
3. Describe assisting with four out of the five steps of the nursing process for the practical/vocational nurse.
4. Describe the fifth step, nursing diagnosis, as the exclusive domain of the registered nurse (RN).
5. Explain why the nursing process and critical thinking are part of the practical/vocational nursing program curriculum.
6. Briefly describe how North American Nursing Diagnosis Association International (NANDA-I), Nursing Interventions Classification (NIC), and Nursing Outcomes Classification (NOC) can be used together to plan patient care collaboratively with the RN.

Key Terms

assisting
data collection (DĂT-ă kŏ-LĔK-shŭn)
dependent role (dĕ-PĔN-dĕnt)
desired patient outcome (dĕ-ZĪRD PĂ-shŭnt ŎWT-kŭm)
evaluation (ĕ-VĂL-ū-Ă-shŭn)
goals
implementation (Ĭ-plĕ-mĕn-TĂ-shŭn)
independent role (ĬN-dĕ-PĔN-dĕnt)
interdependent (ĬN-tĕr-dĕ-PĔN-dĕnt)
intervention
North American Nursing Diagnosis Association International (NANDA-I)

Nursing Interventions Classification (NIC)
Nursing Outcomes Classification (NOC)
nursing diagnosis (NŬR-sĭng DĬ-ăg-NŌ-sĭs)
nursing process (NŬR-sĭng PRŎ-sĕs)
objective information (ŏb-JĔK-tĭv)
outcome (ŎWT-kŭm)
planning (plăn-ĭng)
subjective information (sŭb-JĔK-tĭv)
taxonomy (tăks-ŎN-ŭ-me)
validate information (VĂL-ĭ-dāt)

Several students are debating about the licensed practical nurse/licensed vocational nurse (LPN/LVN) role in the nursing process, particularly regarding assessment. CJ states, "Of course the LPN can assess the patient. They could never plan care and evaluate the patient unless they also assessed the patient." However, Stephanie reminds CJ, "The LPN could collaborate with the registered nurse during the assessment and then continue to develop the plan." Susan, overhearing the conversation, states, "Let's be real. I work in a nursing home on the weekend. If the LPN is not able to assess the patient, no one would assess the patient. It is not realistic, given the number of registered nurses working in the nursing homes." Stephanie concludes, "Maybe that is happening; however, the LPN needs to be sure they are working within their scope of practice. Each state nurse practice act has different regulations. Generally, there is some restriction on assessment, particularly the initial assessment. Therefore, the LPN

needs to collaborate with the registered nurse as indicated. This results in safe, high-quality patient care."

As you learn about the nursing process, think of this dialogue. How will you prepare for this issue as a new graduate?

Keep in Mind

The nursing process provides a common strand that unites all nurses in their delivery of relationship-centered care, at the individual, family, and population level. It provides one way nurses communicate with each other to identify what the nurse will do to safely help the patient reach desired outcomes. It provides for continuity of safe, relationship-centered care.

As a student, you will develop nursing care plans. Nursing care plans are learning tools for student practical nurses/student vocational nurses (SPNs/SVNs). Often, they are traditionally used in LPN/LVN nursing programs to help students learn about patient needs and goals. *A critical-thinking exercise is using your role in the* **nursing process** *to devise a care plan as an SPN/SVN in preparation for patient care.* Devising a nursing care plan before patient care is necessary to ensure safe patient care.

Some of the tasks and skills performed by nurses (LPNs and registered nurses [RNs]) can be completed by unlicensed assistive personnel (UAP). It is the nursing process and critical thinking that separate the LPNs/LVNs from the UAP. These distinctions make LPNs/LVNs a strong member of the health care team. The LPN/LVN today uses critical thinking and the nursing process to carefully identify patient needs, health issues, expectations, lifestyle, and risks involved through focused thinking. LPNs/LVNs also use these same skills to identify wellness strategies in the community aimed at improving the community's health. Judgments are based on evidence rather than assumptions and minimal training. The LPN/LVN thinks before acting and collaborates with the RN, who uses the nursing process and critical thinking at a higher skill level based on education and makes final decisions on nursing diagnosis and the creation and application of patient care plans. The LPN/LVN is both a "doer" and, more importantly, a "thinker."

THE NURSING PROCESS: THE 1950S

The nursing process originated in the 1950s to provide structure for thinking in nursing. According to Peseit and Herman (1998), "The nursing process was designed to organize thinking so that the problems encountered by patients could be anticipated and solved quickly." The 1950s four-step process was based on a scientific method that included data collection, planning, implementation, and evaluation. A major difference between the scientific method (problem-solving method) and the nursing process is that the scientific method identifies the problem first and then goes on to gather data and other information. The nursing process gathers data first and then identifies the problem (nursing diagnosis). Initially, nursing did not yet see itself as having something unique to contribute to patient care that was separate from and in addition to its **dependent role** to physicians. Consequently, nursing education programs and textbooks focused on patients' medical problems and associated nursing interventions. To add to the confusion, suggested nursing interventions varied in nursing textbooks and at health care agencies. Although the nursing process had been introduced, it still had a long way to go. The most important **outcome** of the nursing process for nurses was to provide a structure for thinking before acting as well as implementing a communication process.

THE NURSING PROCESS: THE 1970S TO THE 1990S

When the American Nurses Association (ANA) published the standards of nursing practice in 1977, it established a five-step nursing process for the RN: assessment (data collection), nursing diagnosis (a new step for RNs), planning, intervention, and evaluation. The problem-solving format of the original nursing process was replaced with a *reasoning* model. It introduced a way for nurses to identify and respond to patient needs within the scope of nursing. These included the following types of needs:

- Physiological
- Psychologic
- Social
- Spiritual

It also gave nurses an organized, unique way of contributing to patient care that was separate and additional to its dependent role to physicians. It involved the following steps:

- Collecting data (assessment)
- Nursing diagnosis (RN responsibility)
- Planning
- Implementation
- Evaluation of nursing care
- Including the patient in planning
- A way to communicate with other nurses and caregivers

Initially, SPNs/SVNs were not taught the steps of the nursing process or how to think critically. Although nursing diagnosis was, and continues to be, within the RN's legal role, it became clear that LPNs/LVNs have an important role in **assisting** the RN in all the other steps of the nursing process. In addition, the focus is on relationship-centered care today. Thus the patient and their family (significant others) are engaged in planning their care. This is an important focus, particularly in community settings where many LPNs/LVNs work.

◎ Try This

The Nurse Practice Act

Using the Internet, review the Nurse Practice Act (NPA) in your state, territory, or country. Your role in the nursing process is dictated by this law. As you read the law/regulations, discuss with a peer any areas of your state regulation, related to the nursing process, that are not clear. Seek assistance from your instructor as needed. There are variations within the states, territories, and countries. It defines your scope of nursing practice. It is your legal responsibility to know and practice within that scope.

THE NURSING PROCESS: 2000 AND BEYOND

In 2002, the National Council of the State Boards of Nursing (NCSBN) integrated the nursing process into all areas of the National Council Licensure Examination for Licensed Practical Nurses (NCLEX-PN®). By doing so, the council validated the significance of the nursing process and critical thinking for the LPN/LVN as the way to do the work of nursing. The nursing process remains integrated throughout the clients' needs categories and subcategories in the 2014 NCLEX PN detailed test plan. The nursing process, also called the clinical solving process, in the 2014 NCLEX PN detailed test plan is defined as "a scientific approach to client care that includes data collection, planning, implementation and evaluation" (NCSBN, 2014, p. 5). The definition of these terms has remained consistent since 2001 (NCSBN, 2014).

Definitions of the nursing process for the NCLEX-PN® examination (NCSBN, 2001) are as follows:

- **Data collection** (assessment) is a systematic gathering and review of information about the patient, which is communicated to appropriate members of the health team.
- **Planning** involves assisting the RN in the development of nursing diagnosis, **goals**, and interventions for a patient's plan of care while maintaining patient safety.
- **Implementation** is the provision of required nursing care to accomplish established patient goals.
- **Evaluation** compares the actual outcomes of nursing care with the expected outcomes, which are then communicated to members of the health care team.

The LPN/LVN role in the nursing process is governed by state law, through the state nurse practice acts. This is often referred to as regulation or "scope of practice." Corazzini et al. (2013) indicate that there is great variability in how state nurse practice acts include components of the nursing process, particularly assessment, as part of the LPN practice. Thus the LPN/LVN's role in the nursing process and ultimately in developing a patient care plan differs throughout the nation. This can cause confusion and lack of clarity for the LPN/LVN. Knowing your LPN/LVN nurse practice act, specific to the state you will be licensed and work in, is critical to safe practice. A broad discussion follows assisting you in understanding this role and the importance of collaboration with the RN.

WHAT DIFFERENTIATES THE LICENSED PRACTICAL NURSE/LICENSED VOCATIONAL NURSE ROLE FROM THE REGISTERED NURSE ROLE

Because of the depth of the RN's basic education, the RN functions independently in all five steps of the nursing process (including nursing diagnosis). The nursing actions based on nursing diagnosis do not normally require a physician's order. Both RNs and LPN/LVNs share an **interdependent** relationship with other health team members. For example, RNs and LPNs/LVNs both carry out orders for treatments and medication written by a medical doctor or other health care provider with prescriptive authority.

The LPN/LVN acts in a more dependent role when participating in the planning and evaluation phase of the nursing process but acts in a more **independent role** when participating in the data collection and implementation phases of the nursing process. However, LPNs/LVNs at all times work collaboratively with the RN or physician. An LPN/LVN is not an independent practitioner.

RNs are taught in-depth assessment skills as part of their basic education. The skills include patient interview and physical assessment of all body systems. LPNs/LVNs continually gather data about the patient, family, environment, and the community (when indicated). Data collection for the SPN/SVN includes taking vital signs, checking therapeutic responses to medications and treatments, and collecting data on symptoms of health problems, among other functions. While in nursing school, the focus of data collection is based on the current unit of study for the SPN/SVN. With each course, SPNs/SVNs increase their data collection capabilities, achieve competency with basic skills, and expand their knowledge and skill set. Basic assessment skills are taught in the LPN/LVN curriculum. However, the emphasis on assessment skills can vary based on the nurse practice act of the state where the education is delivered. Given the job role of the LPN/LVN, as evidenced by the 2012 NCSBN job analysis, it is evident that the LPN/LVN is involved in the nursing process. According to the NLN vision statement (2014), the LPN/LVN plays a significant role in meeting the needs of the elderly and other vulnerable populations in many diverse settings. Their role in care planning, driven by the nursing process, is essential to advance the health of the nation. However, as mentioned earlier, state nurse practice acts do differ in how they define assessment. Some describe the LPNs/LVNs as collecting data and some describe the LPNs/LVNs as performing a focused assessment. Despite the terminology, you as a student should develop interview, observation, and physical assessment skills. You will use these skills in collaboration with the RN to provide high-quality patient care.

RNs will identify the patient's nursing diagnosis, which provides a basis for the creation of the patient's plan of care. The *International Journal of Nursing Terminologies and Classifications* (2008) defines **nursing diagnosis** as "a clinical judgment about individual, family, or community responses to actual or potential health problems/life processes. A nursing diagnosis provides the basis for selection of nursing interventions to achieve outcomes for which the nurse is accountable." The RN uses an established list of current nursing diagnoses developed by the **North American Nursing Diagnosis Association International (NANDA-I)** (www.nanda.org). NANDA-I was developed as a standardized, orderly, systematic language (**taxonomy**) that would provide a common language for nurses to communicate with one another. RNs are encouraged to use this approved nursing diagnosis list. NANDA-I was updated in 2014. In your LPN/LVN program, you may create patient care plans using a problem list in lieu of the approved nursing diagnosis list. In clinical, your instructor may ask you for your "top five." This is a method to assist you in identifying existing and emerging patient problems throughout your clinical experience. It can also assist you in learning to prioritize. If you do use nursing diagnosis when creating care plans for educational purposes, remember that the nursing diagnosis can only be determined by the RN in a practice setting. Once identified, the LPN/LVN can proceed with the plan of care.

DEVELOPING YOUR PLAN OF CARE FOR ASSIGNED PATIENTS

Patient care for you as a student is a learning experience. It is necessary to plan for patient care assignments. Legally, your NPA will require you to give care at the level of an LPN/LVN. The nursing diagnosis is the problem the patient presented with, and the RN fits this into the categories established by NANDA-I. Because you do not study the NANDA-I diagnostic categories in most LPN/LVN programs, it is helpful (i.e., clearer, more objective, more explanatory, makes more sense to you in the learning situation) if you use the original nursing problem the patient presented with. Turn the nursing diagnosis back to the presenting problem. In this way you clearly understand what you are working with in everyday terms. At this stage you have the benefit of your instructor to help you through the planning process. Planning for patient care becomes easier with each plan. You internalize your role in four steps of the nursing process and are improving your ability to think critically as a practical/vocational nurse.

STEPS OF THE NURSING PROCESS

STEP 1: DATA COLLECTION

Data collection includes many aspects.

Systematic Way of Gathering Data

Data collection begins on admission and continues with each patient encounter. The patient is the primary source of information in data collection. After all, patients know themselves and their body better than anyone else. All patient interview questions should be directed to the patient unless he or she is unable to respond. The RN interviews the patient to obtain the health history and assesses body systems. The LPN/LVN assists in the assessment process by collaborating with the RN.

- **Subjective information** is based on the patient's opinion. Some refer to subjective information as symptoms. This usually includes feelings of physical discomfort, anxiety, and mental stress that are more

difficult to measure. The nurse cannot experience subjective symptoms.

- **Objective information** includes data that the nurse can verify; it is also known as "signs." A physical assessment provides objective data. The terms *check, observe, monitor, weigh, measure,* and *smell, touch, and hear* provide cues that you may be involved in objective data collection. Obtaining initial data, such as vital signs, height, and weight, is often assigned to the LPN/LVN. Objective information helps support or cast doubt on subjective information. For example, a patient's subjective statement about feeling feverish can be verified by measuring his or her temperature (objective).

Verify the Information

Verifying information (validating) is an important step in thinking critically. A nurse should never assume and always validate. As an SPN/SVN, you should seek the assistance of your instructor to discover what resources are available to you for verification of data. Suggestions for verifying information include the following:

- Verify the data and question any information that is not a match to your data collection.
- Differentiate between subjective and objective data. Remember that decisions must be based on evidence, not assumptions. However, the patient's subjective comments are important. Confirm with evidence whenever possible. Patients can express a subjective feeling (i.e., "a feeling of doom") before a change in vital signs. Continue to monitor the patient when subjective comments do not match objective data.
- Compare findings with the RN and other staff involved with the patient.
- Other staff may help verify when a client has mental limitations.
- Patients or family members may be able to validate information you obtained during data collection (family members with patient permission).
- Document all data and sources, especially when they are not congruent.
- Compare the data you collected with the medical records.
- Know that what you do for verification will depend on your skill level, experience, and education.
- As a student, ask your instructor or an RN for guidance on how to verify data and how to determine if there is a relationship between presenting problems.

Communicate Information to Appropriate Health Care Team Members

- **Emergency data** are reported immediately. For example, suppose you learn that the patient with a fracture has diabetes and fell on his way home from a bar, where he goes daily for "just four beers." If he says, "I pace myself," does that reassure you that this is not an immediate issue? Recall that what you have heard is subjective data, but as a student you will not be in a position to verify it further without direction from the RN. Report what you have heard and any objective data, such as vital signs and observations, to the appropriate person.

- **Incomplete toolbox:** Subjective data will be charted as "Patient states . . ." Objective data such as temperature, pulse, and respiration (TPR); blood pressure (BP); weight; and skin color will be charted as what you observe and measure without judging or drawing conclusions. Your involvement in this step depends on your place of employment and your experience and skill level. The LPN/LVN usually has more responsibility in long-term care or community settings, where the patient's condition is more stable. At the conclusion of your LPN/LVN program, you will have acquired strong, although incomplete, data collection skills: "The toolbox is not complete." As a newly licensed practical nurse you will continue to expand your toolbox learning through collaboration with other members of the health care team, particularly the RN. Experienced LPNs can also be great mentors. However, remember that the LPN/LVN must collaborate with the RN or physician when developing a plan of care. The LPN/LVN is a critical member of the team.

Other Aspects of Data Collection

Data collection continues. Data collection starts during the patient's admission. It continues daily at the beginning of the shift for the baseline observations, then periodically during the shift, and right before doing your final documentation and reporting off. The LPN/LVN is always collecting data on therapeutic responses to treatments, interventions, and medications (Box 12-1).

Accuracy in data collection. Florence Nightingale said that if you do not observe your patient, you should not be a nurse (Nightingale, 1993). With each contact the LPN/LVN must see, hear, smell, and touch the patient when necessary, and use all the senses to gather data about the patient and the environment. Data collection is vital; the patient's condition changes throughout the day. This is why accuracy in measuring vital signs; describing vomitus, bleeding, or a skin lesion; and determining level of consciousness, for example, are so important. Has the patient's skin lesion changed since the last time you checked the lesion? How has it changed? How much has it changed? Did you use objective assessment skills (i.e., measuring the lesion)? Every piece of data is important to assist the patient in achieving the best possible health outcome.

| Box **12-1** | Examples of Practical/Vocational Nurse Data Collection |

These examples can apply to acute care, long-term care, or community-based care:

- Observing results of a laxative or enema
- Observing for signs of congestive heart failure for a patient taking furosemide (Lasix) and digoxin (Lanoxin)
- Observing an ulcer on the lower leg of a diabetic (i.e., size [measure it], location, appearance, drainage)
- Observing behavior for signs of disorientation or confusion
- Observing the patient self-administering insulin following a teaching demonstration
- Observing position in bed (acute care)
- Observing gait and posture (community care)
- Observing whether a 76-year-old patient is showing signs of ego integrity or despair (Although the patient should be at ego integrity, he is not capable of being there. Because of his cerebrovascular accident [CVA], he has to be washed, fed, and lifted everywhere. He is incontinent. His needs remind you of those of an infant. You will work at establishing trust in the patient instead of ego integrity.)
- Observing family interactions
- Observing the environment for need for safety factors: spills, bed rails, glasses on table, hearing aids, dentures, and so on
- Observing the urine for color, odor, amount, and other characteristics

Introduce yourself. Data collection, whether partial or total, involves courtesy. Introduce yourself to the patient and explain what you are going to do. Always use a minimum of two identifiers (i.e., name and birth date).

- The patient's first impression of you tends to remain. Address the patient as Mr., Mrs., Miss, Ms., or another title, as appropriate. Avoid using a first name unless you have the patient's permission.
- Remind yourself that this is a *professional*, not a personal, relationship that you are building. The most common complaints by patients include "I don't know which one is the nurse" or "I am treated with disrespect" or "I am not their grandma"; and so on. Familiarity (that is, acting toward a patient as though he or she is a family member or friend) does not give the patient a sense of confidence in your nursing skill. Never address the patient as "honey" or "sweetie."
- Patients often experience fear on being hospitalized or transferred to a new facility.
  - When in the patient's presence, stand or sit where he or she can see you.
  - Confusion or lack of skills on the nurse's part serves to increase that fear.

Asking questions. Avoid asking questions that have been asked before unless you are directed to do so or your observation based on critical thinking alerts you to do so.

- Be sure that you have looked at the record before entering the patient's room.
- Explain why you are asking questions and reassure the patient that he or she has the right to not answer questions that cause discomfort.
- Be a good listener. Encourage confidence, but do not promise to keep secrets.
- Request clarification rather than pretending that you understand: "I am not sure that I understand what you mean by that statement." Check out what you think you understand: "Am I correct in saying that you are worried about the kind of care you will receive here?" Avoid using reassuring promises that you cannot deliver, such as "Don't worry; everything will be just fine."
- Also avoid giving approval; for example, "That's right." This statement may make it difficult for a patient to change his or her mind.
- Nursing responsibility does not involve judging the patient's behaviors, values, or decisions.
- Finally, avoid verbalizing disapproval or belittling the patient with statements such as "You know you shouldn't have done that."
- Chapter 8 elaborates on communication techniques that will assist you in making the best use of the limited time you have to obtain needed data from the patient.

Barriers in Data Collection
You must be alert to several possible barriers to data collection:

- Barriers include insufficient time, cultural differences, poor skills in data collection, and communication failure, such as a comatose patient, a patient who presents a language barrier, the presence of distractions, or a patient who is too sick to speak well.
- A personal bias can be a barrier. You may label the patient before the interview is complete, instead of basing decisions on facts.
- Respectful distancing is necessary if the nurse is to remain objective and use all senses clearly.

STEP 2: PLANNING

Planning includes assisting the RN to develop nursing diagnoses, outcomes, and interventions.

Assisting the Registered Nurse to Develop the Nursing Diagnosis
The LPN/LVN assists the RN to collect and group the data that have been collected in a logical order. Only the RN can develop the nursing diagnoses, goals, interventions, and plans of care. It is unacceptable for the LPN/LVN to write the plan, without collaboration, and for the RN to initial it. The LPN/LVN assists in determining a significant relationship between data

and patient needs or problems. The focus is on patient functions that will benefit from nursing interventions. After the problems are identified and organized, the RN makes the nursing diagnosis. Thus the LPN and the RN collaborate to create the plan of care.

◎ Try This

Assisting During Planning

In the planning phase, the SPN/SVN takes the nursing diagnosis and states it as a nursing problem the patient presented with. SPNs/SVNs state the problem, set outcomes, list interventions, and then list data collection for care plans. This process seems to be the opposite of the RN's, but remember that LPNs/LVNs do not have primary responsibility for data collection (phase 1). The SPN/SVN does not study NANDA-I lists in most nursing programs and relies on the RN for the final nursing diagnosis. To demonstrate understanding of the nursing diagnosis, the LPN/LVN states the nursing diagnosis in objective and specific terms as a nursing problem in the patient's care plan (Table 12-1).

Realistic, useful nursing care plans. For a nursing care plan to be a useful, realistic tool for the nursing staff, priorities must be established:

- A care plan may not include all of the patient's health problems. It is unreasonable to think that nurses will be able to respond to all of the patient's needs and concerns.
- The most important problems, those that are potentially life threatening or most impacting to the patient, must be taken care of immediately.
- Nurses often use Maslow's hierarchy of needs (Chapter 13) to assist in prioritizing patient needs.
- The lowest level of needs, according to Maslow, is the physiologic (survival) level of needs. This means that in prioritizing patient needs, attention is paid first to problems related to food, air, water, temperature, elimination, rest, and pain.
- When working on several problems at the same time, you will often find that a relationship exists between problems.
- Priorities may also change rapidly, depending on the patient's condition. The nurse has to remain flexible and recognize the need to shift priorities according to patient needs.
- Patients will be far more cooperative with the care plan if they and their family (when appropriate) are included in identifying the priorities of care.
- According to Maslow, regression takes place during illness. The amount of regression depends on the circumstances and severity of the illness. As the patient recovers, he or she advances on Maslow's hierarchy.
- Ideally the patient is able to regain the former level of functioning. Cooperation is much more likely when the nurse understands this and respects it.

Table 12-1 Example of a Student Assignment Sheet and Patient Care Plan

Student _____

Patient Initials _____ Room _____ Doctor _____ Allergies _____

Age _____ Marital Status _____ Religion _____ Occupation _____

Admission Date _____

Date of Surgery _____ Diet _____

MedicalDiagnos s _____

Surgical Procedure _____

Meaning in Own Words _____ Meaning in Own Words _____

Primary Nursing Problem _____

CATEGORIES OF HUMAN FUNCTION	DATA COLLECTION	NURSING PROBLEMS	OUTCOMES	NURSING INTERVENTION	EVALUATION
Protective (e.g., personal care and hygiene, environment, surgery)	You will: Check, observe, monitor, weigh, and measure. Collect data (1) at beginning of shift for baseline, (2) periodically during shift, and (3) right before reporting off duty.	What is the problem, in your own words? Be specific and objective. Could use nursing diagnosis, but	The patient will: (Reverse the problem and state positively what patient will do; realistically, measurably, time-referenced).	The nurse will: (Be objective and specific. Care plans in texts rarely are. What the nurse will do to help patient meet outcomes.)	What progress is patient making toward outcomes? Results of data collection in objective terms.
Sensory-perceptual					
Comfort, rest, activity, and mobility (e.g., sleep and rest, body alignment)					
Nutrition					
Growth and development (e.g., identify Erikson developmental stage)					
Fluid-gas transport					
Psychosocial cultural (e.g., emotional support, spiritual support, diversion, and recreation)					
Elimination (e.g., urinary and gastrointestinal elimination)					
Need for community resources					

- Whenever a new problem emerges, LPNs/LVNs collect data about the problem because of their data collection skills.
- They collaborate with the RN, and the RN formulates a new nursing diagnosis.

? Critical Thinking

The Seven Survival Needs

Write an example of a problem for each survival need.
1. Food
2. Air
3. Water
4. Temperature
5. Elimination
6. Rest
7. Pain

POSSIBLE ANSWERS:
1. Not enough or too much food intake
2. Shortness of breath
3. Dehydration, caused by vomiting
4. Temperature above or below normal
5. Diarrhea
6. Sleeping too much or too little
7. Pain that interferes with functioning

Assisting the Registered Nurse to Develop Outcomes

Think back to Step 1, data collection, and ask yourself the following questions: What did the patient say on admission about expectations, wants, or needs while a patient? Did you explore the patient's concerns once they are discharged from this facility? Did you also remember to collect data on the patient's strengths?

Strengths. Strengths are building blocks in developing a realistic plan. Strengths include whatever the patient and family continue to be able to do that will aid patient care. Patient and family are important partners in attaining the goals/outcomes. Building on patient and family strengths provides a sense of contribution and some control for the patient and family. The following are sample questions that may help make the question of strengths patient and family focused:

- What does the patient list as their strengths that will assist them in their recovery?
- Can the patient move from the bed to the chair and back alone?
- Does the patient feed himself or herself? Completely? With some assistance?
- Does the patient eat best if someone is present? Alone? During conversation about family?
- Are there any family members who can be instructed in how to act as partners in meeting patient goals?

- How can the patient and family assist as the patient transitions in care to home? Who will provide the care? What community resources are available?
- Is responsibility for the intervention within the LPN/LVN role? If not, who should the LPN/LVN collaborate with to meet the patient's needs?

Goals and outcomes. Goals state a general intent about what is being accomplished (e.g., "I will learn the medical prefixes, roots, and suffixes by the end of the semester."). Outcome describes a specific result that can be observed at some point (e.g., "I will learn the prefixes, roots, and suffixes well enough by the end of the semester to get an A on the final exam."). The terms are used interchangeably in some agencies, although the ANA prefers the term *outcome*. The focus of the outcome is on the patient, not the nurse. An outcome is thought of as "The patient will . . ." What is agreed on is that well-written outcomes include patient and family input, if at all possible, and must have the following characteristics:

- Realistic (attainable, based on the patient's condition and desire)
- Measurable (tells how you will know that the outcome has been reached)
- Time-referenced (an educated guess on the part of the nurse as to how long it will take to attain the outcome)

It may be easier for an SPN/SVN to use the phrase *desired* (or *observable*) *patient outcome*. This focuses directly on what the patient will accomplish rather than on what the nurse will do. For example, the phrase consists of the following characteristics:

- It uses the word *patient* as the subject of the statement.
- It is realistic for the patient and his or her problem.
- It uses a measurable verb. It is specific for the patient and his or her problem.
- It includes a time frame for patient reevaluation.

To state an outcome as a student, reverse the problem and state it in positive terms.

The statement tells what the patient **will** do to overcome the problem rather than what the patient will **not** do. Here are some examples:

- Observable outcome: The patient will eat 1500 calories of ground foods and liquids during each 24-hour period.
- Unclear statement: The patient will not miss any feedings during a 24-hour period.

Assisting the Registered Nurse to Develop Nursing Interventions

Nursing **interventions** identify specifically what the nurse will do to assist the patient to reach **desired patient outcomes**.

- Sometimes this means encouraging the patient to do certain activities, such as self-feeding. (Think back to the patient strengths that were initially identified and additional strengths you have noted since then.)

- Interventions are also called *nursing approach, nursing action,* or *nursing care.* Interventions focus on the "related to" (R/T) portion of the nursing diagnosis. They tell nursing personnel who, what, where, when, and how much.
- When nursing interventions are clearly written, all nursing staff members, according to their skill level and if within their legal role, will be able to carry out the nursing action. *It needs to be identified on the care plan if the RN, LPN/LVN, or UAP will carry out the intervention.*
- Check the nursing interventions: Are they objective and specific as written? Interventions you will develop in your care plan as an SPN/SVN are based on courses you have taken, additional reading, and finding information from alternate sources.
- Developing interventions requires critical thinking and collaboration. (See Chapter 2 for information on learning resources.)

Table 12-2 takes you through the process the SPN/SVN can use to plan care for an assigned patient:

- The nursing diagnosis, as written by the RN, is shown.
- The nursing diagnosis is turned back into the problem the patient presented with to make it clearer and more specific.
- The SPN/SVN wrote the outcome by reversing the problem statement; it states clearly what the patient will do and what the observable outcome will be.
- The nursing interventions identify what the SPN/SVN will do to assist the patient in attaining the desired outcome.
- After checking the plan with the instructor, the SPN/SVN is prepared to begin patient care.

Care plans vary. Different kinds of care plans are available:

- An individualized written care plan has been demonstrated.
- Some facilities use *standardized care* plans. These plans are based on research of the best possible options for a nursing diagnosis (nursing problem). To individualize a standard plan, cross out interventions that do not apply to the patient and add appropriate interventions that do apply.
- *Computerized care plans* are generally part of the electronic medical record. Individualized plans can be entered into the computer.
- More commonly, standardized care plans are used and then individualized to deal with the nursing problem.
- *Multidisciplinary (collaborative) care plans* work well in settings in which staff from varied professions and disciplines are involved with the patient. This is true in many settings today as interdisciplinary care is an expectation. An example is a long-term care or psychiatric setting. More recently, they are being used in medical-surgical and other units. Plans are developed by a multidisciplinary team and reflect specific interventions used by each discipline (e.g., physical therapist, social worker, nutritionist, nurse, and physician). Maintaining a separate plan for each profession is considered repetitious. The plan is developed with an interdisciplinary focus for each professional involved. The language must be common to each discipline involved. Therefore, the medical diagnosis may be used rather than a nursing diagnosis. A prioritized problem list is developed based on the medical diagnosis, providing a common language for all health team members involved. The plan identifies shared and specific responsibilities for all professions represented.
- Progress is usually documented on a common form or computer to provide easy access for all involved with the plan. A clinical pathway is another type of multidisciplinary plan that schedules clinical interventions over an anticipated time period for a specific type of patient health problem. The clinical pathway is frequently used for high-risk, high-volume, high-cost care. Often, care is documented right onto the clinical pathway.
- A concept map, another type of care plan, is a diagram of a patient's condition and treatments. Concept maps can be used to plan care for patients and are increasingly employed in all types of nursing education programs. It can help the nurse plan

Table 12-2	Nursing Diagnosis, Nursing Problem, Outcome, and Interventions	
NURSING DIAGNOSIS	**NURSING PROBLEM**	**OUTCOME**
Altered nutrition: less than body requirements. Related to (R/T) decreased calorie intake.	Eats only 5% of each meal. R/T loss of appetite and weakness.	The patient will eat 1500 calories of ground foods and drink 2000 mL of liquids during each 24-hour period. (The problem is reversed and stated positively).
INTERVENTIONS		
1. Six small, ground meals at 8 AM, 10 AM, noon, 2 PM, 4 PM, and 6 PM. Patient seated in an easy chair with minimal assistance. Encourage self-feeding. Assist only if needed.		
2. Offer 240 mL of liquids at 6 AM, 9 AM, 11 AM, 1 PM, 3 PM, 5 PM, 7 PM, and 9 PM. Vary choices: likes Jell-O, ice cream, 7-Up, chocolate milk, and pineapple juice. Drinks herbal tea with meals.		

interventions and is also a way to monitor patient progress. From a student perspective it encourages critical thinking and can enhance learning.

Maintaining patient safety. All steps of the nursing process are directed toward patient safety. Do you remember the patient for whom you were collecting admission data? You discovered that he was diabetic, had four beers at the bar, and fell on his way home, which resulted in a fracture. You reported it immediately to the RN, along with a statement about his vital signs. Your critical thinking made you alert the RN to a potentially serious safety issue.

Documenting the care plan. Documenting (charting) the plan of care is essential. Legally, if it was not charted, it was not done. In a lawsuit, a lawyer reviewing the chart or computer charting record may interpret sloppy charting as sloppy nursing care. Where the documentation takes place depends on the facility and the type of care plan used. Almost all institutions use some type of electronic record. However, documentation may be completed longhand in the nurse's notes, on flow sheets, or on the plan itself, especially in the case of a natural disaster or in a remote setting.

STEP 3: IMPLEMENTATION

- The key for all your activity, regardless of your position and the agency involved, is to use the care plan as the basis for your nursing actions and reporting.
- For example, as an SPN/SVN you draw information from the care plan on how to provide individualized patient care.
- While providing care you continue to collect data based on your knowledge of the patient's strengths and disease conditions.
- You chart on flow sheets, nurses' notes, or electronic records, following the priorities indicated by the nursing problem, plus any new observations you have made according to the charting system in the agency.
- You use the care plan as your guideline when reporting to the RN and offer information on any changes you have noted.

Specifically you focus on the nursing interventions outlined in the care plan: Do interventions continue to be appropriate? What patient changes, or lack of changes, have you observed? With this information the RN can update the plan of care and needs only to validate the data. Implementation includes many aspects, which are discussed in the following sections.

Nursing Action

- Follow the established plan of care. Assist the patient in performing activities of daily living. Sit with the patient during meals, encourage eating, and assist minimally, if necessary.
- Review the procedure before preparing the patient. Prepare the patient for the procedure. Ask for help if you are uncertain about what to do.
- Teach the patient and family as indicated, ensuring understanding through return demonstration when appropriate.
- Participate in the patient care conference and offer input. Report specifically on tasks assigned to you, any changes, and progress or lack of progress.

Maintaining Patient Safety

- Use safe and appropriate techniques during patient care. Check the patient's position before lifting up safety rails to be sure arms do not get caught between the bed and the rail. Always survey the room before leaving the patient for safety violations (i.e., bed in high position, call bell out of reach)
- Use precautionary and preventive interventions in providing care to patients. Make sure that wheelchair wheels and bed wheels are locked before moving the patient from the chair to the bed and back again.
- Institute nursing interventions to compensate for adverse responses. If the patient gets weak while standing, assist him or her to lie or sit down and place the patient's head between his or her knees (if not contraindicated by physical condition). Ease the patient to the floor if necessary avoiding injury from a fall.
- Initiate life-saving interventions for emergency situations. For example, if the patient begins to choke on food, perform the Heimlich maneuver.
- Monitor care given by unlicensed personnel. As a charge LPN/LVN, you are responsible for the care provided by the unlicensed personnel.
- Collect data during every patient contact. Be alert to even minor changes in skin color, breathing, respirations, and so on, even though your contact does not occur at a scheduled time (i.e., perhaps you just brought in the lunch tray).

Initiating Teaching That Is Within Your Role and Supports the Registered Nurse's Teaching

- Encourage patients to follow their plan of care and treatment regimen. Be alert to any deviations from the care plan. Know all staff persons' roles so that you have a basis for your observations.
- Assist patients to maintain or enhance optimal functioning. Passive range of motion is done every morning as part of basic care for the bedridden patient who has been assigned to you.
- Provide an environment that is conducive to attaining observable patient outcomes. For example, if the room smells of feces, locate the source and deal with it.

- Reinforce teaching of principles, procedures, and techniques for maintenance and promotion of health. For example, if the patient has been newly diagnosed as having type 2 diabetes, reinforce the steps of foot care the RN taught earlier in the morning and continue to observe for any patient knowledge deficit. Be alert to questions that the patient has, based on lack of understanding, and seek answers to the questions as needed. Demonstrate techniques used by the RN, if requested. Check with the instructor if this is something you have not done before.

Reporting and Documenting

- Collect data during every patient contact. If you observe abnormal symptoms, collect additional data. For example, if the patient is beginning to perspire profusely for no apparent reason, measure their vital signs and obtain their blood sugar.
- Report observations to relevant members of the health team. Report the aforementioned observation immediately to the RN. Report all daily observations before leaving the unit.
- Document the patient's response to nursing intervention, therapy, or teaching. Document all interventions, responses, and changes. Use the care plan as your guide for documentation and reporting.

◎ Try This

Implementing the Plan of Care

As an SPN/SVN, the next phase is *implementing* the plan of care that you have developed with your instructor's supervision. Did you remember to include the patient strengths you identified during your data collection? *Which interventions are within the LPN/LVN role?*

The Difference Between Licensed Practical Nurse/ Licensed Vocational Nurse and Student Practical Nurse/Student Vocational Nurse Responsibility

As a graduate, your responsibility will vary according to the work area in which you are involved and whether you are functioning in a beginning or expanded role. In an acute care setting, your primary responsibility will be to use the established care plan as a guideline for providing direct patient care, continuing data collection, making verbal reports to the RN, and charting. However, it is more likely that you will be working in a long-term care or a community-based setting and functioning in the role of an LPN/LVN charge nurse, responsible for managing patient care, under the supervision of the RN.

STEP 4: EVALUATION

The evaluation phase includes assisting in determining patient progress and communicating the findings.

Table 12-3   Data Collection, Outcome, and Evaluation

DATA COLLECTION LIST	OUTCOME	EVALUATION
Check intake: Amount and type of liquid in milliliters Amount of food taken at each meal	The patient will eat 1500 calories of chopped foods and drink 2000 mL of liquids during each 24-hour period	By day 2 the patient was able to consume 1500 calories in ground meals and 1600 mL of liquids during a 24-hour period

Assist in Determining Patient Progress Toward Meeting Desired Patient Goals/Outcomes

- Collect data during every patient contact. If the patient outcome is written correctly and the data collection list is complete, evaluation will be the result of your daily data collection. The continual data collection helps make daily evaluation part of the natural flow of good nursing care (Table 12-3).
- Compare actual outcomes with desired patient outcomes. If progress is being made toward meeting the outcomes, continue as is.
- Assist in determining the patient's response to nursing care. If the patient is not meeting the outcome, check the way the outcome is written. Is it measurable, realistic, and time-referenced? If you cannot evaluate the outcome, the outcome probably is not measurable or realistic. If necessary, change the portion that needs revision or restate the desired outcome.
- Assist in identifying factors that may interfere with the patient's ability to implement the plan of care. Talk with the patient. He or she may be able to tell you why progress is not being made. Review your daily data collection notes. There may be a pattern that emerges. Have the patient's strengths been considered in the plan of care? Are the stated observable outcomes less than or beyond what the patient can accomplish? Are they realistic? Is the focus on evaluating nursing care, as opposed to evaluating patient progress toward meeting desired outcomes? If necessary, revise nursing interventions that are not working.

Communicate Findings

- Document patient's responses to care, therapy, or teaching.
- Report findings to relevant members of the health care team.

Have you noticed how heavily dependent each step of the care plan is on the others and how the steps are often going on simultaneously? Have you noticed that as desired outcomes are met, other problems emerge?

Recall that according to Maslow's hierarchy, regression occurs with illness. As observable outcomes are achieved at the lower level (patient begins to improve), higher levels of needs begin to emerge. Be aware that the patient may be functioning on more than one level. Continual communication with the patient and their family will identify needs as they emerge and improve overall patient outcomes.

◎ **Try This**

Evaluating Patient Progress

The time-referenced portion of the desired outcome states the approximate date by which the patient will attain an observable outcome. It is an educated guess on the part of the RN, based on education and experience. The SPN/SVN makes an educated guess on the assignment care plan regarding the time it will take the patient to meet his or her outcome. As an SPN/SVN, your daily data collection assists the interdisciplinary team in evaluating how far the patient has progressed and identifying any difficulties. A complete daily data collection list is essential and, as pointed out, is the basis of your data collection during every patient contact. Further assessment and analysis of that data in collaboration with the RN and other members of the interdisciplinary team results in revisions in the plan of care as indicated.

WHERE ARE WE NOW IN THE NURSING PROCESS?

Nursing continues to grow as a profession. Nursing research and health industry focus and policy all drive the change from general to specific nursing interventions and measurement of outcomes. Two such well-researched projects are the **Nursing Interventions Classification (NIC)** and the **Nursing Outcomes Classification (NOC)** taxonomies, recognized by the American Nurses Association (ANA). Visit www.nanda.org/nanda-i-nic-noc.html for more details. As research has continued on NANDA-I, NIC, and NOC, specific ways have been devised to link the three taxonomies to provide a plan of care for patients. As an SPN/SVN, you should recognize the terms *NANDA-I*, *NIC*, and *NOC*, even though you may not be studying these taxonomies during your basic nursing programs. Your place of employment after graduation may have adopted these taxonomies and will expect you to use them in assisting planning for patient care.

NURSING INTERVENTIONS CLASSIFICATION

Nursing Interventions Classification (NIC) focuses on intervention; what the nurse does to enhance patient outcomes. Dochterman and Bulechek (2006) of the University of Iowa head a research team who have worked on developing a language that standardizes, defines, and assists in choosing appropriate nursing interventions. Whereas NANDA-I focuses on the patient concerns, NIC is about nurse behaviors (interventions) to support the patient to attain outcomes the patient desires. NIC interventions are both direct and indirect and can be directed at the patient, family, and community. NIC is useful for nurses, student nurses, other health professionals, administrators, and faculty. It includes interventions in the categories of physical and psychosocial; illness treatment and prevention; health promotion; individual, group, family, and community; indirect and direct care; and independent and collaborative. Some nursing programs are planning their curricula around NIC. For example, during the early classroom and clinical experience, patient care planning interventions chosen are basic and related to the course of study. As the nursing program continues and courses are more advanced, so are the interventions.

NURSING OUTCOMES CLASSIFICATION

Johnson, Mass, and Moorehead (2000), also of the University of Iowa, developed Nursing Outcomes Classification (NOC). This taxonomy standardizes the terminology and criteria for measurable or desirable outcomes as a result of nursing interventions. It identifies desired outcomes for individual patients and family caregivers, as well as family- and community-level outcomes. A 5-point Likert scale is used to measure progress and can be done at any time during use of the chosen intervention(s). The Likert scale is as follows:

1. Never demonstrated
2. Rarely demonstrated
3. Sometimes demonstrated
4. Often demonstrated
5. Consistently demonstrated

This scale helps the nursing (or other) staffs to determine if the intervention is working or if changes in interventions need to be made to attain outcomes desired by the patient.

LINKING NORTH AMERICAN NURSING DIAGNOSIS ASSOCIATION INTERNATIONAL, NURSING INTERVENTIONS CLASSIFICATION, AND NURSING OUTCOMES CLASSIFICATION

NANDA-I is a source that helps the RN to determine nursing diagnosis. NANDA-I identified what concerns the patient. NIC is a source for choosing standardized nursing interventions. NOC identifies desired outcomes as a result of nursing interventions and uses a scale to identify if the intervention(s) are producing the desired outcomes. If linked interventions are used in the health care facility where you are working, you will find the information specific and easy to apply. The RN has the final decision on nursing diagnosis, choice of nursing interventions, and measuring desired patient outcomes (Figure 12-1).

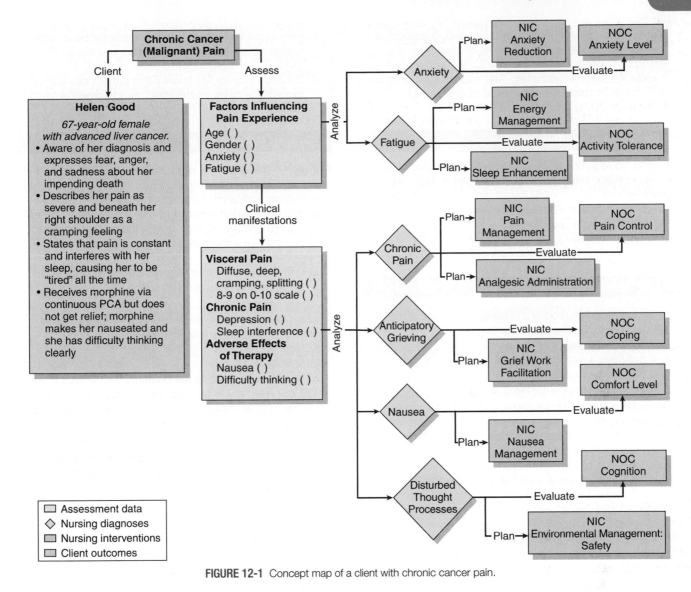

FIGURE 12-1 Concept map of a client with chronic cancer pain.

Get Ready for the NCLEX-PN® Examination

Key Points

- The Nurse Practice Act of your state identifies your legal role in the nursing process as an LPN/LVN. Take time to read it and question what you do not understand.
- The nursing process was originated in the 1950s to provide structure for thinking in nursing. The four-step process included data collection, planning, intervention, and evaluation (problem-solving model).
- The ANA standards of nursing practice, published in 1997, added nursing diagnosis to make a five-step nursing process (reasoning model). Nursing diagnosis is the exclusive responsibility of RNs because of their broad, science-based education.
- In 1996, the nursing process was included in the NCLEX-PN® for the first time. The nursing process and the practical/vocational role became an important part of nursing education for LPNs/LVNs.

- In 2002, the nursing process and critical thinking were integrated throughout the NCLEX-PN®. Four steps of the nursing process for LPNs/LVNs were redefined. The additional step, nursing diagnosis, is considered the exclusive responsibility of the RN.

Step 1: *Data collection* Patient data are gathered and reported to appropriate personnel.

Step 2: *Planning* The LPN/LVN assists the RN to develop the nursing diagnosis, outcomes, and interventions for the patient's plan of care. This includes maintaining patient safety.

Step 3: *Implementation* Nursing interventions in the care plan are put into action.

Step 4: *Evaluation* Actual outcomes of the interventions are compared with desired patient outcomes (emphasis is on patient progress toward meeting outcomes). Results are reported and documented. Critical thinking and nursing process are mandated for SPN/SVN education.

- NANDA-I is a systemized taxonomy used to determine any patient concerns. NIC is a way of identifying standardized nursing interventions. NOC is a system for measuring patient outcomes. Trial implementation in select hospitals has shown the value of combining NANDA-I, NIC, and NOC.

Additional Learning Resources

evolve Go to your Evolve website (http://evolve.elsevier.com/Knecht/success) for the following FREE learning resources:

- Answers to Critical Thinking Scenarios
- Additional learning activities
- Additional Review Questions for the NCLEX-PN® exam
- Helpful phrases for communicating in Spanish and more!

Review Questions for the NCLEX-PN® Examination

1. How did the origination of the nursing process in the 1950s change the course of nursing?
   a. It provided a reasoning model.
   b. It provided a specificity model.
   c. It provided a quality model.
   d. It provided a critical-thinking model.

2. Some RNs and instructors have questioned the value of teaching SPNs/SVNs nursing process and critical thinking. Which statement provides a valid reason for including both in the SPN/SVN curriculum?
   a. Knowledge of the nursing process and critical thinking encourages postgraduate education so that one day the LPN/LVN can be an RN.
   b. LPNs/LVNs and RNs collaborate, assisting the patient to meet their outcomes. A common language and thought process provides an organized way of understanding what is to be done.
   c. Learning the nursing process and critical thinking provides the opportunity to be working on both LPN and RN levels of nursing at the same time.
   d. Learning the nursing process and critical thinking provides a cookbook method of learning and provides time to deal with job stresses.

3. Which request by the RN will you refuse to do because it is beyond the LPN/LVN scope of practice?
   a. "Update Mr. Frederic's plan of care, and we will discuss it as soon I get back from lunch."
   b. "Catheterize Mrs. Jones as soon as you can and report total output to me STAT."
   c. "Check Mr. Neap's pressure sore on his right hip for changes since his admission."
   d. "Assist Sally (RN) by doing an assessment of our new admission on the south wing."

4. Which action is within the LPN/LVN scope of nursing practice when a patient aspirates a piece of meat and you are sitting opposite the patient in the dining room?
   a. Ask someone to get help as you move quickly toward the patient to perform a Heimlich maneuver.
   b. Ask another patient to straighten up the patient while you go to get an RN or other qualified staff member.
   c. Immediately call the patient's doctor for permission to perform the Heimlich and mention you are an SPN/SVN.
   d. Because you do not know if this patient has a do-not-resuscitate order on the chart, send someone to check.

Alternate Format Item

1. Which of the following is an important reason for verifying data? *(Select all that apply.)*
   a. Patient and family account of what happened differ.
   b. You believe that persons of this culture are dishonest.
   c. Patient complains of fever, but the forehead feels cool.
   d. You note that the patient's body language and words match.
   e. Patient indicates that they have no pain but they grimace when you touch their left leg.

2. A new patient has arrived, and the RN has asked you to begin data collection while she finishes taking doctor's orders. *Prioritize the following steps.*
   a. Identify the patient
   b. Measure vital signs.
   c. Introduce yourself to the patient.
   d. Explain what you are planning to do.
   e. Report information to the RN and ask for further instructions.

Critical Thinking Scenarios

Scenario 1

You overhear a conversation among peers stating that the nursing process is a waste of time. Someone states, "Nurses know intuitively what a patient needs because of their love for patients. After all, this is the reason a person becomes a nurse." You have decided to engage in the conversation. What evidence will you share to support why you believe the nursing process is critical to delivering high-quality patient care?

Scenario 2

Amy wants to improve her grades. She learned about using the nursing process during class a couple of days ago. "If it works for planning patient care, why can it not work for me? I am going to give it a try."

Answer the following questions of what Amy can do for each step of the nursing process to improve her grades:

1. How might Amy **gather data** on her study habits?
2. In the **planning** stage, Amy discovered that she periodically fell asleep while studying (maybe because she was studying in her bed). She was surprised to count that she had a total of 30 cell phone calls or text messages during that time. She spent time talking on the cell or texting in response. She did not even finish the chapter she was trying to concentrate on. What changes could she **implement** to ensure future success?
3. How would Amy **evaluate** her success?

Nursing Theory, Research, and Evidence-Based Practice

Objectives

On completing this chapter, you will be able to do the following:

1. Provide one reason for the development of nursing theories.
2. Briefly describe each of the following theories as they relate to the nursing process:
   - Maslow's hierarchy of human needs theory
   - Nightingale's environmental model
   - Rosenstock's health belief model
   - Orem's self-care deficit theory
   - Leininger's culture care theory
   - Peplau's interpersonal relations theory
   - Sister Callista Roy's adaptation model
   - Jean Watson's theory of human care
3. Briefly explain the importance of nursing research.
4. Compare and contrast quantitative and qualitative research studies.
5. Define evidence-based practice (EBP).
6. Explain the three elements of EBP.
7. Briefly describe how best evidence for practice is determined by systematic reviews of research studies.
8. Discuss how your site of clinical experience adopts evidence-based guidelines for nursing interventions.
9. Explain the role of the licensed practical nurse/licensed vocational nurse (LPN/LVN) in nursing research and evidence-based practice.

Key Terms

evidence-based practice (EV-ĭ-dĕns bāsd)
Leininger's culture care theory (KŬL-chŭr KĀR)
Maslow's human needs theory
nursing research
nursing theories
Orem's self-care deficit theory (SĔLF KĀR DEF-ĭ-sĭt)
Peplau's interpersonal relations theory (ĭn-tĕr-PER-sŭn-ăl)

qualitative research study (KWĂL-ĭ-tā-tĭv)
quantitative research study (KWĂN-tĭ-tā-tĭv)
Rosenstock's health belief theory
Sister Callista Roy's adaptation model (ă-dăp-TĀ-shŭn)
spirit of inquiry (SPI-rĭt ĭn-KWĒR-ē)
Watson's theory of human care

Keep in Mind

Becoming acquainted with terminology assists in learning when it becomes necessary in your career.

NURSING THEORIES

RATIONALE FOR THEORIES

Numerous **theories** have been developed for nursing, and some of them are the basis for curriculum development. In addition, these theories provide a basis for research on the effectiveness of nursing care. The following three concepts are important to nursing:

a. *Person* (the recipient of care)
b. *Health* (the goal of nursing)
c. *Environment* (the setting where nursing care takes place)

It is important to discuss nursing theories because if you decide to become a registered nurse (RN), you will encounter name recognition when studying theories used as a framework for nursing education and clinical practice. Practical nurses are sometimes asked to gather data for research being done by Masters/Ph.D. candidates or research staff. Although the licensed practical nurse/licensed vocational nurse (LPN/LVN) does not evaluate the data for the study, recognize that the data gathered will influence the outcome of the research.

FLORENCE NIGHTINGALE: THE FIRST NURSING THEORIST

Florence Nightingale was the first to emphasize the environment: ventilation, warmth, noise, light, and cleanliness. Nightingale is considered the first nursing theorist. She strongly believed that environmental issues influenced the course of illness. She also saw the nursing role as separate from the nurse as a "handmaiden" to the doctor. She was the first to collect data and use evidence to make clinical decisions. Nightingale determined that an environment that was warm, clean, well lit, and with minimal noise resulted in a decreased death rate for soldiers. As a consequence, she instructed her nurses to adhere to these standards and the soldier death rate plummeted.

ABRAHAM MASLOW'S HUMAN NEEDS THEORY

Although Abraham Maslow is a psychologist, his **human needs theory** has been adapted by many professional programs, including some nursing programs, as a framework for education. Here is a general description of the theory:

1. Abraham Maslow's theory states that certain internal, external, physical, and psychological needs are common to all people.
2. Common needs are arranged in a hierarchy.
3. Unmet needs create tension, which motivates the person to react to meet the need.
4. When needs are met, the person is no longer aware of the need, and the need (now met) no longer motivates them.
5. Dominant needs that matter to a person can vary in life.

Figure 13-1 provides examples in identifying patient care priorities and responding to the needs according to the patient level of functioning. Remember that a person may be functioning on more than one level of needs at the same time. Read the list on the lowest level of needs again. Individuals go back to the physiologic level periodically to satisfy basic needs; for example, nutrition.

Applying Maslow's Human Needs Theory to the Nursing Process

The first data collection (assessment) of a patient is the lowest level of needs:

- *Physiologic needs:* Oxygen, food, water, elimination, safety, sleep, activity, mental stimulation, and sexual procreation (e.g., the nurse collects data on whether the patients are eating enough to maintain their strength and health, if they have relief from pain, and if interventions are planned with the

patients to meet the need). Once physiologic needs are met, data can be collected on safety and security needs.

- *Safety needs:* Security, freedom from harm, and protection (e.g., data are collected on real or imagined safety needs; for example, do you need more than one nurse to move the patient safely from the bed to the toilet?). The primary areas that involve hospital nursing care are the first two levels: physiologic and safety needs.

- *Love and belonging needs:* Love, affection, and companionship (e.g., data are collected on whether or not the patient has a support system to assist with care once hospitalization is over). This is a part of discharge planning to be sure that the patient has the support to meet his or her needs posthospitalization. Engaging the patient's family in their care and assisting them in understanding the possible behavior changes that they will experience (i.e., a "flat" affect following a stroke) may assist the patient in feeling loved. The nurse may be involved in doing follow-up care in the home after hospitalization (home health, visiting nurse service, etc.).

- *Esteem needs:* Respect and recognition (e.g., data are collected on what the patient is doing or can do that will assist in earning a positive sense of self). Is the person able to do volunteer work (i.e., Retired Senior Volunteer Program [RSVP]) or join a senior center that has activities, provides an opportunity to help others, and offers meals at a reasonable price)? Once esteem needs are met, the individual may be ready to focus on self-actualization. A parish nurse, caseworker, or other member of the health care team may be providing care at this level.

- *Self-actualization:* This is the highest level of needs, and not everyone attains this level. This involves maximum realization and fulfillment of the individual's potential. People who have reached this level include Mother Teresa and Gandhi. However, you do not have to be famous to achieve self-actualization.

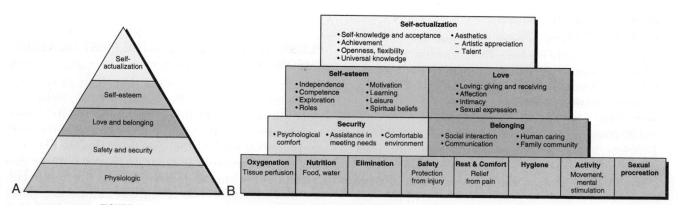

FIGURE 13-1 A. Maslow's hierarchy of human needs. **B.** Evolving hierarchy of needs adapted by nursing.

OREM'S SELF-CARE DEFICIT THEORY

Dorothea **Orem's self-care deficit theory** is a general theory that consists of three subtheories:

1. *Self-care:* This involves a goal that is directed toward a safer environment for life, health, and well-being. (Ideally, individuals learn to respond to health cues in themselves or the environment as a way to maintain personal health.)
2. *Self-care deficit:* Personal care does not meet therapeutic self-care demands. (The individual does not recognize or know what to do in regard to personal health situations.)
3. *Nursing system:* Nurses empower the patient through their interpersonal relationship to help meet their self-care demands. (Nursing responds to the person's care needs totally, partially, or in a supportive role according to the need.)

Orem's theory is concerned with growth and development needs, as well as physiologic and psychosocial needs. Nurses can use the data collection step of the nursing process to identify specific self-care deficits. By working with the patient, nurses can then choose interventions that will have the desired outcomes for the patient. During the last several decades many hospitals, particularly rehabilitation hospitals, used Orem's self-care deficit theory to guide their practice.

MADELINE LEININGER'S CULTURE CARE THEORY

Leininger's interest in cultural care and how nursing responds to people of different cultures began when she was working with children who had special needs. She recognized a link to understanding care based on their cultural background. When developing her **culture care theory,** Leininger identified two kinds of care in every culture: *generic,* meaning home remedies used in care, and *professional,* which is provided by people who are specifically trained to provide care.

Leininger proposed three modes to guide nursing decisions when providing care:

1. *Cultural care preservation or maintenance.* This means assisting persons of particular cultures to maintain care values that help them to maintain health or restore health. As an example, some cultures use periodic "cupping" (bloodletting) as a way to relieve symptoms of hemochromatosis (excess iron deposits throughout the body). A method in other cultures is to periodically give blood at a blood blank to reduce the hematocrit (the percentage of your blood that is made up of red blood cells).
2. *Cultural care accommodation or negotiation.* In some cultures, Vicks VapoRub is placed in the nostrils, which can potentially be aspirated and lead to pneumonia. A cultural care accommodation is described: The home health nurse demonstrated placing the Vicks on the chest and neck and rubbing it in a soothing manner. A warm cloth was placed on the chest for the night. The vapor's fumes relieved the congestion.
3. *Culture care repatterning or restructuring.* Leininger's theory is concerned with respecting cultural differences and yet providing a safe and protective environment (e.g., in some cultures, mud is placed on the infant's umbilicus after delivery). Because of concern for local and systemic infection, the visiting nurse provided clean pads. The nurse demonstrated their use, how to clean the area, and how to leave the area uncovered for a period so the umbilicus could be exposed to the air.

Applying Leininger's three modes when providing nursing care developed a foundation for what we refer to today as providing culturally competent or congruent care.

HILDEGARD PEPLAU'S INTERPERSONAL RELATIONS THEORY

Nurses who work with adult or child psychiatric patients are more likely to use **Peplau's interpersonal relations theory** as a basis for developing a therapeutic relationship with the patient. The relationship that is developed has certain parameters and is the major part of the treatment.

Peplau describes four overlapping phases:

* *Orientation:* The patient seeks assistance because of a felt need. A problem has been identified, and the nurse works with the patient to help him or her recognize the problem. The process is often complex, but personal and social growth can develop during this step.
* *Identification:* During this phase, the patient understands the situation and responds to the nurse who supplies the needed help.
* *Exploitation:* During this phase, the patient begins to depend on the nurse and uses the help offered, exploring all possibilities.
* *Resolution:* The dependent behavior that developed must now be given up as the therapeutic relationship comes to an end. How the nurse handles this phase is crucial because faulty resolution can possibly end with vague physical symptoms.

During the therapeutic relationship, the nurse fulfills the roles of resource person, teacher, leader, surrogate, and counselor.

ROSENSTOCK'S HEALTH BELIEF THEORY

Irwin Rosenstock developed the **health belief theory** that tries to explain why or why not a person will take action to prevent or detect illness. According to this theory:

1. *Perceptions vary and may have no basis in reality.* For example, Marta came to the emergency room because she was no longer able to sit down. Upon examination, it was determined that she had advanced cancer of the vulva. Marta was very shy, and even though she was aware of changes, she just hoped that whatever it was would just go away. Even Marta's sister, with whom she lived, was unaware that there was

any disease process going on. She explained, "We have never seen each other naked." The thought of being examined embarrassed Marta: "No one has ever looked at me down there."

2. *Beliefs are connected to existing barriers* (e.g., may see the preventive or treatment activity as expensive, painful, or inconvenient). If there are fewer perceived negative aspects, the possibility of doing something is higher: If more negative aspects exist, the person is more likely not to act. For example, Cora, age 82, began to have gastrointestinal symptoms and asked her son to make a doctor's appointment for her. He did so and drove 8 hours to take her to the appointment. When he arrived, she refused to go in, explaining, "I've changed my mind. It's nothing." This went on several more times over a period of years before she was so uncomfortable that she finally kept the appointment. Cora was diagnosed with advanced cancer of the colon. Cora explained that she had already had seven surgeries and did not want to put up with another uncomfortable healing process. Because of the pain she was having now, Cora agreed to surgery. The surgery was palliative, which gave her relief from pain, but she was told she probably had only 6 months to live. Financial barriers can also exist. The Affordable Care Act was designed to minimize cost barriers experienced by the underemployed and promote prevention of disease (Koh & Sebelius, 2010).

3. *A cue to action is seen as necessary* (e.g., pain, a news story, a reminder call from the doctor's office). The cue (finally) for Cora was the pain she began to experience.

This theory can be useful when using the nursing process to promote health. It can be used to promote yearly examinations, vaccinations, and wellness classes. It is also helpful to the nurse and patient when developing interventions and outcomes to deal with a disease process or health problem that has been identified.

SISTER CALLISTA ROY'S ADAPTATION MODEL

Sister Roy describes the recipient of care (the patient) as a "holistic adaptive system" in her **adaptation model**. Both internal (from inside the patient) and external (from outside the patient) stimuli affect the system. She identifies the following types of stimuli:

- *Focal*: meaning something direct, such as a patient experiencing pain
- *Contextual*: meaning other factors that affect the focal stimuli, such as being examined in the area of pain
- *Residual*: meaning both internal and external factors that may not always be evident, such as a memory of previous pain and the effect it had on the patient

Coping methods are known as *regulator* and *cognator* subsystems:

- A *regulator* subsystem refers to the internal effects that take place in response to what is happening internally. These include neural, chemical, and endocrine

processes. The body automatically attempts to regulate the system when it is being affected negatively.

- A *cognator* subsystem refers to learning, processing, judging, and emotion that the patient uses to cope with what has happened.

Two adaptive modes are available to help the patient deal with the situation:

1. *Physiologic*, which includes the senses, fluids, electrolytes, neurologic, and endocrine systems
2. *Self-concepts, role functions, and interdependence*
   - Self-concepts are related to psychological and spiritual aspects of the patient.
   - Role functions are related to the patient's role in society.
   - Interdependence is related to love, respect, and values and can include the patient's support system.

The response is either:

- *Adaptation:* The patient reaches his or her goal of recovery.
- *Ineffective:* The patient does not survive or has a poor outcome.

JEAN WATSON'S THEORY OF HUMAN CARE

According to **Watson's theory of human care**, health is harmony between the body, mind, and spirit. It also involves self-perception and how the self is experienced. Illness is a lack of harmony within the self and the soul. The nursing role is a caring process to help the patient regain harmony and health. Through the caring, the patient develops self-knowledge and self-healing. The enabling actions allow the patient to solve problems and grow. Both the patient and the nurse grow through this process.

We have only presented a few classic nursing theories. Countless other theories, such as Pat Benner's theory from novice to expert, are used in nursing practice and nursing education. If you want to learn more about theories, visit www.nursing-theory.org. In addition, most nursing fundamental and foundations texts have a chapter devoted to theories and models.

NURSING RESEARCH

Research in any profession supports existing knowledge and develops new knowledge based on observation and experimentation. Starting with Nightingale's study of soldier morbidity and mortality data during the Crimean War through to today's emphasis on evidence-based practice, **nursing research** has improved existing nursing knowledge and generated new knowledge that influences nursing practice. Research studies in nursing are important because they do the following:

- Identify specific nursing interventions that are proven effective and not merely based on tradition. "That is the way we have always done it . . ."

- Provide evidence that supports the quality and cost-effectiveness of what nurses do.
- Generate knowledge for clinical practice, nursing education, and delivery of nursing services.

Nurses of all educational levels are encouraged to participate in and promote nursing research in varying degrees (Cherry & Jacob, 2011). These are the two main types of research studies done in nursing:

- **Quantitative research study**, which is objective study. A *variable* is the event the researcher is trying to measure. There are two types of variables: One variable is the group receiving the intervention and the other variable is the group that does not receive the intervention. Numeric data are collected and measured using statistics to describe variables, examine relationships among variables, or determine cause-and-effect interactions between variables. A randomized control trial is an example of a quantitative study. An example follows: The study is conducted to determine the effect of a new medication to treat Alzheimer disease on the progression of dementia-like symptoms. One group of patients (experimental) receives the new medication and another group (control) receives the current standard of treatment. The observed effect (identified symptoms) is measured and compared for each group.
- **Qualitative research study**, which is subjective study. Data are gathered by interviews and/or direct observations and the study is a narrative description of the "lived experience" of individuals or possibly groups; for example, living with chronic pain or understanding how nursing students' confidence is increased in the clinical setting. *Phenomenology* is a type of qualitative study. Other types of research such as *grounded theory* studies are implemented to discover theory about a phenomenon of interest. The theory development is not abstract; it is rooted in the observations. All of these research methodologies contribute to the development of the science of nursing and have assisted in establishing nursing as an independent science.

See Evolve for a Quantitative Research Study of Practical Nursing Students and a List of Terms used in Quantitative Research.

EVIDENCE-BASED PRACTICE

BACKGROUND OF THE EVIDENCE-BASED PRACTICE MOVEMENT

- Dr. Archie Cochrane (1901-1988), a British epidemiologist, challenged the public to pay only for medical care that was proven to be effective and advocated the use of randomized, controlled trials (RCTs) as a means of reliably informing health care practices. In 1993, the Cochrane Collaboration, an independent, not-for-profit organization, was established to prepare and promote the accessibility of *Cochrane Reviews*, a collection of evidence-based health care interventions obtained by systematic reviews of research.
- In 1999, the Institute of Medicine (IOM) issued the report *To Err Is Human: Building a Safer Health System*, which discussed the incidence of medical errors in health care and the need for reform.
- In 2001, the IOM issued *Crossing the Quality Chasm: A New Health System for the 21st Century*, calling for consistent, high-quality health care for all people. Included in the 10 rules or general principles issued by the IOM was, "Patients should receive care based on the best available scientific knowledge."
- During the last two decades, insurance companies began to pay for health care practices only if their effectiveness is supported by scientific evidence.
- During the last decade, hospitals are denied payment when complications in a Medicare patient develop if evidence-based guidelines are not followed.
- Patients and families are seeking the latest evidence on websites about the most effective treatment for illnesses and diseases.
- Large national demonstration projects are funded by the federal government and other partners aimed at identifying patient outcomes, grounded in evidence (i.e., The National Council of State Boards of Nursing [NCSBN] study aimed at examining the relationship between clinical simulation in nursing schools and nursing program outcomes; www.ncsbn.org).
- Today, countless sites exist allowing quick easy access to current evidence-based practice guidelines (e.g. , evidence available at NCSBN, National League for Nursing [NLN], IOM, the Joint Commission on Accreditation of Healthcare Organizations [JACHO], and the Joanna Briggs Institute).

HOW BEST EVIDENCE FOR PRACTICE GUIDELINES IS DETERMINED

Best evidence is determined through a complex, rigorous process:

- The clinical question being investigated is formulated in an objective, concise manner.
- Using professional resources, the latest, most relevant research evidence that pertains to the clinical question is located (Box 13-1). Be sure that your Internet source is credible.
- An expert or panel of experts conducts a systematic review, which is a summary of the results of selected studies.
- Guidelines are determined. These are specific practice recommendations derived from the summary of research articles.
- Using critical-thinking skills, the gathered evidence is combined with clinical experience and the patient's preferences and values for use in a specific clinical situation.

Box 13-1   Systematic Reviews Used to Develop Evidence-Based Practice Guidelines

PUBMED (http://pubmed.gov)
The U.S. National Library of Medicine (NLM) database of biomedical citations and abstracts.
- **Medline** is the largest component of PubMed and is freely accessible. (Fact Sheet//www.nlm.nih.gov/pubs/factsheets/dif_med_pub.html).

CUMULATIVE INDEX OF NURSING AND ALLIED HEALTH LITERATURE (CINAHL)
- A source for practical/vocational nurses for evidence-based practice (EBP) interventions.

COCHRANE REVIEWS (www.cochrane.org/cochrane-reviews)
- Each review addresses a clearly formulated question. All of the existing research on a topic that meets certain criteria is searched for and collated and then assessed using stringent guidelines to establish whether or not there is conclusive evidence about a specific treatment. The reviews are updated regularly, ensuring that treatment decisions can be based on the most up-to-date and reliable evidence.

AGENCY FOR HEALTHCARE RESEARCH AND QUALITY (AHRQ) (http://www.ahrq.gov/)
- An agency of the U.S. Department of Health and Human Services.
- The National Guideline Clearinghouse™ (NGC) (http://www.guideline.gov) is an initiative of AHRQ. Provides a comprehensive database of evidence-based clinical practice guidelines and related documents with syntheses and comparisons. It provides Internet users with free online access.

THE JOANNA BRIGGS INSTITUTE (JBI) (http://www.joannabriggs.edu.au/)
- An international not-for-profit membership-based organization in the Faculty of Health Sciences at the University of Adelaide, Australia. The Institute develops methods to appraise and synthesize evidence, conducting systematic reviews and analyses of the research literature to provide the best available evidence to inform clinical decision making.

⦿ Try This

How do agencies where you have clinical rotations obtain their guidelines for evidence-based nursing interventions?

EVIDENCE-BASED PRACTICE IN NURSING

Nursing care that is based on comments such as, "This is how we do that procedure here" or "This is how I was taught to do this nursing intervention 20 years ago" or "We always do things this way" is not sufficient in today's health care environment. Nursing interventions such as cleansing wounds with Betadine or hydrogen peroxide and massaging over bony prominences are examples of common nursing interventions in past years that have been proven through research to be potentially harmful (Ackley et al., 2008). The clinical practice of nurses needs to be based on scientific knowledge with proof that the knowledge is effective. Research provides the foundation for evidence-based nursing practice. Most health care institutions use evidence-based practice to develop or update policy and procedure. Be sure to read and understand all the information provided.

ELEMENTS OF EVIDENCE-BASED PRACTICE

The elements of **evidence-based practice** are like a triangle with the following three areas (Figure 13-2):
- Best research evidence
- Nurse's clinical expertise
- Patient preferences

THE NURSE'S ROLE

In 2010, the National League for Nursing (NLN) established competencies of nursing graduates at all levels. The competency that addresses nursing research and

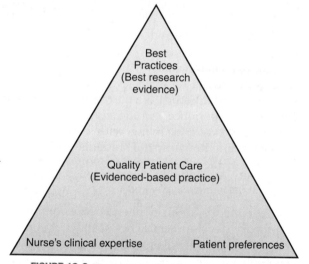

FIGURE 13-2 The triangle of evidence-based practice.

evidence-based practice is **spirit of inquiry**. A nurse with a spirit of inquiry is one who "will raise questions, challenge traditional and existing practices, and seek creative approaches to problems." The following describes what the NLN expects of all levels of nurses in regard to research and evidence-based practice:
- Nurses with a *research doctorate* design and implement research studies and publish findings.
- Nurses with a *practice doctorate* review present research and formulate evidence-based protocols.
- Nurses at the *masters level* formulate research questions and evaluate the effect of evidence-based solutions on nursing problems.
- Nurses with a *bachelor's degree* identify questions needed to be studied, critique published research, and use evidence as solutions to nursing problems.

- *Associate degree/diploma* nurses challenge the status quo, question assumptions, and offer new insights to improve the quality of care.
- *Practical/vocational nurses* question the basis for nursing actions by considering research, evidence, tradition, and patient preference (Outcomes and Competencies for Graduates of Practical/Vocational, Diploma, Associate Degree, Baccalaureate, Masters, Practice Doctorate, and Research Doctorate Programs in Nursing, 2010).

The Licensed Practical Nurse/Licensed Vocational Nurse's Role in Evidence-Based Practice

SPNs/SVNs participate in the nursing research process by reviewing current articles in professional sources as part of their student learning experience and support nursing interventions on care plans and in practice with evidence-based nursing practices. As students and graduates, they need to follow protocols and procedures for nursing interventions of the agency in which they practice. Protocols are the general outlines used to manage a clinical situation; for example, a care plan. Procedures include the detailed steps of nursing interventions for implementing the protocol. Objective data gathering is essential for evaluation of the effectiveness of selected evidence-based practices. The LP/LV nursing program outcome related to the spirit of inquiry states, "By collaborating with health care team members, utilize evidence, tradition, and patient preferences in predictable patient care situations to promote optimal health status (NLN, 2015)."

Get Ready for the NCLEX-PN® Examination

Key Points

- Nursing involves many different theories. Choosing the appropriate theory for a nursing curriculum can be used as a guide to improve the course of study.
- Maslow's human needs theory is based on Maslow's hierarchy of needs, which says that as needs on one level are met, others emerge.
- Rosenstock's health belief theory tries to understand why people do or do not take action to prevent or detect disease.
- Orem's self-care deficit theory looks at why some individuals are goal-oriented toward taking care of their health and well-being, why some do not meet their self-care demands, and how the nurse, through an interpersonal relationship with the patient, can assist the patient with a self-care deficit to meet his or her self-care demands.
- Nursing research is a scientific process that validates and refines existing knowledge and generates new knowledge that influences nursing practice.
- The clinical practice of nurses needs to be based on scientific knowledge with proof that the knowledge is effective.
- Research provides the foundation for evidence-based practice in nursing.
- The elements of evidence-based practice are best research evidence, resources including, nurse's clinical expertise, and patient preferences.
- Spirit of inquiry for an LPN/LVN means a nurse who "will raise questions, challenge traditional and existing practices, and seek creative approaches to problems."
- LPNs/LVNs participate in the nursing research process by reviewing current articles in professional sources; supporting clinical interventions on care plans and in practice with evidence-based nursing practices; collecting data for research studies as requested by the registered nurse; following protocols and procedures of the agency in which they are employed; and providing objective data gathering to evaluate the effectiveness of selected evidence-based practices.

Additional Learning Resources

evolve Go to your Evolve website (http://evolve.elsevier.com/Knecht/success) for the following FREE learning resources:
- Answers to Critical Thinking Scenario
- Additional learning activities
- Additional Review Questions for the NCLEX-PN® exam
- Helpful phrases for communicating in Spanish and more!

Review Questions for the NCLEX-PN® Examination

1. Elements of evidence-based practice in nursing do not include:
   a. Best research evidence
   b. Nurse's clinical expertise
   c. Patient preferences
   d. Tradition in agency

2. An abstract found on a database or at the beginning of a research study is:
   a. Something difficult to understand
   b. Something designed to distract you
   c. A summary of the research performed
   d. A complete account of the research study

3. Which of the following statements is accurate regarding theories useful to nursing?
   a. Orem's interpersonal theory defines roles and steps in developing a therapeutic relationship.
   b. Maslow's culture care theory is concerned with how to meet cultural needs through nursing care.
   c. Rosenstock's needs theory focuses on meeting patient needs that may have no basis in fact.
   d. In Maslow's theory unmet needs create tension, which motivates the person to react to meet the need.

4. Crystal is explaining qualitative research to a classmate. What response indicates a need for clarification regarding qualitative research?
   a. A cause/effect relationship of variables is confirmed.
   b. Interviews are used to gather data.
   c. Lived experiences (for example, pain) are studied.
   d. Problem areas of participants' lives are studied.

Alternate Format Item

1. List in order the steps below that are implemented to identify best practices in nursing.
   a. Find the latest, most relevant research evidence.
   b. Formulate the clinical question being investigated.
   c. Using critical thinking skills, combine the gathered evidence with clinical experience and the patient's preferences and values.
   d. Evaluate the validity, relevance, and how you can apply the evidence to the clinical situation selected.

5. Select the items that describe the LPN/LVN's role in nursing research and evidence-based practice. *(Select all that apply.)*
   a. Collect data for research studies as requested by the registered nurse.
   b. Collaborate to formulate clinical questions that need to be investigated for validity.
   c. Follow protocols and procedures of the agency in which they are employed.
   d. Gather data for evaluation of the effectiveness of evidence-based practices.
   e. Support clinical interventions in practice with evidence-based nursing practices.

Critical Thinking Scenario

Corey, an SPN, has his medical/surgical clinical experience in a hospital that uses evidence-based practice when selecting nursing interventions to implement. During pre-conference, Corey's clinical instructor notes on his care plan that he will instill 5 cc of air into the patient's gastric feeding tube while auscultating over the epigastric area for a "swooshing" sound to ascertain proper tube placement. The patient is receiving an intermittent tube feeding. The instructor questions Corey's source of information, and Corey states that he found the information on the Internet. If you were the instructor, what would you discuss with Corey?

The Interdisciplinary Health Care Team: The Role of the Practical/Vocational Nurse

Objectives

On completing this chapter, you will be able to do the following:

1. Explain in your own words what is the interdisciplinary health care team.
2. List 10 members of the interdisciplinary health care team.
3. Identify the nursing personnel who are part of the interdisciplinary health care team, according to education, role and responsibilities, licensing, and sites of employment.
4. Discuss the different roles and responsibilities between the direct care worker, licensed practical nurse (LPN), registered nurse (RN), and other members of the interdisciplinary health care team.
5. Describe in your own words the following methods used to deliver nursing service: total patient care (also referred to

as case nursing); functional nursing; team nursing; primary nursing; case management.
6. Describe the role of the licensed practical nurse/licensed vocational nurse (LPN/LVN) in the methods used to deliver the nursing services listed in objective number 5.
7. Describe how the philosophy of relationship-centered care impacts nursing care.
8. Discuss how the Affordable Care Act (ACA) and the supply of nurses (LPNs and registered nurses [RNs]) impact jobs for the LPN/LVN.

Key Terms

advanced practice (ăd-VĂNSD PRĂK-tĭs)
associate degree nursing (ă-SŌ-sē-ăt dĕ-GRE)
bachelor's nursing program
case management method (kās MĂN-ăj-mĕnt)
certification (SŬR-tĭ-fĭ-KĀ-shŭn)
clerk receptionist (rĕ-SĔP-shŭ-nĭst)
clinical pathway (care maps) (KLĬN-ĭ-kăl PĂTH-wāy)
diploma program (dĭ-PLŌ-mă)
functional method (FŬNK-shŭn-ăl)
general supervision
independent (ĬN-dĕ-PĕN-dĕnt)
interdependent (ĬN-tĕr-dĕ-PĕN-dĕnt)
nurse manager
nursing assistant (NŬR-sĭng ă-SĬS-tĕnt)

nursing case management
patient-centered care (PĀ-shĕnt SĔN-tĕrd)
practical/vocational nurse (PRĂK-tĭ-kăl/vo-KĀ-shŭn-ăl)
primary care method (PRĬ-măr-ē)
registered nurse (RĔJ-ĭ-stĕrd)
skill mix (skĭl mĭks)
standards of care (STĂN-dĕrds)
student nurse (STOO-dĕnt)
team leader
team method (tēm)
total patient care
unit manager (YOO-nĭt MĂN-ăj-ĕr)
unlicensed assistive personnel (UAP) (ŭn-LĬ-sĕnsd)

Keep in Mind

You cannot identify the players without a structure to your program of health care delivery. This chapter is your program to identify players on the health care team.

WHO IS RESPONSIBLE FOR MRS. BROWN'S DISCHARGE?

Mrs. Amelia Brown, age 75, lives with her daughter on a 200-acre farm in rural Wisconsin. While working in the barn, Mrs. Brown fell and broke her right hip. She required surgery to repair the hip. Under general anesthesia during surgery, Mrs. Brown's blood pressure reached dangerously

high levels, but it quickly stabilized under the anesthesiologist's interventions. Despite this setback, Mrs. Brown was discharged after 3 days in the hospital. She and her family agreed that she was not ready to return home at that point in her recovery, so she was discharged to a sub-acute setting, where she was given physical therapy to learn how to function at home with her restrictions in ambulation. Two weeks later, Mrs. Brown was discharged from the extended-care facility to her home.

This sounds like just another success story for nursing, doesn't it? We will follow Mrs. Brown as she progresses through the health care system and then decide who should get credit for Mrs. Brown's discharge back to the farm.

MRS. BROWN'S EMERGENCY CARE

After Mrs. Brown falls, her daughter calls the emergency squad to transport her mother to the nearest hospital. The hospital is located 20 miles away in a city with a population of 98,000. The three people manning the emergency squad are *emergency medical technicians* (EMTs). Each EMT has taken an approximately 150-hour course in basic life support skills and has been certified as an EMT after passing a national test. The EMTs are currently taking an 18- to 24-month paramedic course, which is preparing them to provide more advanced life support skills. On the way to the hospital, the EMTs monitor Mrs. Brown's blood pressure, pulse, respirations, and level of consciousness. They keep her right leg immobilized. The EMTs maintain contact with the hospital emergency room by means of a two-way radio.

On arriving at the *emergency room* (ER), the EMTs provide the *registered nurse* (RN) with verbal and written reports of Mrs. Brown's status. The emergency room doctor examines Mrs. Brown and orders an x-ray film of her right hip. The *x-ray technician* brings the x-ray equipment to the ER and takes an x-ray film of Mrs. Brown's right hip. This x-ray technician has taken a 2-year program conducted by a hospital or technical college to prepare her to perform diagnostic measures involving radiant energy. The *radiologist* on duty reads the x-ray film of Mrs. Brown's right hip. On the basis of the physical examination and the results of the x-ray, the ER physician diagnoses a fracture of Mrs. Brown's right proximal femur. The ER physician notifies Mrs. Brown's *family physician* and contacts the *orthopedic surgeon* whom Mrs. Brown requests.

The RN receives Mrs. Brown in the ER, assesses her, and provides care until she is admitted to the hospital. The RN is a graduate of a baccalaureate program in nursing (RNs can also be a graduate of an associate degree or diploma in a nursing program). This nurse has passed a national examination, the NCLEX-RN®, to become an RN. RNs who work in the ER participate regularly in continuing education courses at the hospital and at seminars given regionally and nationally for ER nurses and often achieve certification as an emergency nurse practitioner (ENP-BC). Mrs. Brown's RN prepares her for surgery.

To be qualified to be in charge of the medical care of Mrs. Brown, the family physician has attended 4 years of college, 4 years of medical school, 1 year of internship, and approximately a 3-year residency program. Medical school consists of a program that provides the basic knowledge and skills needed to be a medical doctor. Internship involves a program of clinical experiences designed to complete the requirements for licensure as a practicing physician. The residency program prepares physicians for practice in a specialty. The specialty in this situation is family practice. The ER physician, the radiologist, and the orthopedic surgeon have had the same education as the family physician, up to the residency experience. The ER physician has completed a residency program in emergency or trauma medicine. The radiologist has completed a residency program in the reading and interpretation of x-ray films. The orthopedic surgeon has completed a 3- to 5-year residency in performing surgery for problems of bones and joints. Each of these physicians has passed the board examinations, which licenses them as physicians and allows them to practice under the state medical practice act. Each physician in this scenario is board certified in his or her specialty area.

Mrs. Brown also has visits from physician extenders who are working in collaboration with the physicians. These extenders are generally nurse practitioners (NP) or physician assistants (PA). An NP is an advanced practice registered nurse. These nurses have a minimum of a Master of Science degree in Nursing (MSN), obtained in a 1- to 2-year program of study at the graduate level. Organizations such as the American Association of Colleges of Nursing (AACN) recommended NPs be educated at the doctoral level. They are licensed specifically as an NP and have a unique role as defined by the nurse practice act in their state. A PA generally has a minimum of a baccalaureate degree and health care experience. A PA is nationally certified and state licensed as a health care provider. Although still acting as a member of the interdisciplinary team, NPs in some states can function in an autonomous manner. PAs and NPs in other states must work in collaboration with a physician for some activities such as prescribing medication.

Laboratory studies are ordered preoperatively. *Lab personnel* draw blood for these studies. Lab personnel have varied educational backgrounds. Some have on-the-job training to obtain blood samples. A medical lab technician has 2 years of education. A medical technologist (MT) has more than 4 years of education and can be certified by a national examination. Lab personnel are responsible for collecting the specimens needed for lab tests, performing the tests, and reporting the results to physicians and staff.

The family members request that their parish *priest* be contacted to give Mrs. Brown the sacrament of the sick (see Chapter 11). Because surgery is imminent, the pastoral care department is notified. A Roman Catholic priest, a member of the pastoral care team, anoints Mrs. Brown with holy oils, prays with her, and gives her Holy Communion. To be able to meet Mrs. Brown's spiritual needs, the priest has had 4 years of college and 4 years of theological school before being ordained.

Throughout Mrs. Brown's experience in the ER she is cared for by direct care workers. These can be nursing assistants, transport aides, patient-care technicians, or various other support care staff (i.e., admissions representative). These individuals have completed short-term training (2 to 16 weeks), specific to their job role. Training is often provided by the employer but can be achieved through a community-based educational program. These health care workers may need to be listed on a statewide registry.

THE SURGICAL EXPERIENCE

In the ER the nurse *anesthetist* prepares Mrs. Brown and her family for the anesthesia part of the surgical experience. This health care worker is an RN with a Bachelor of Science in Nursing (BSN). This nurse has studied an additional 2 to 3 years in an approved school of anesthesiology after the 4-year BSN program and works collaboratively with an anesthesiologist. The nurse anesthetist provides anesthesia to patients undergoing surgery. Mrs. Brown is transferred to the surgical suite, where she undergoes a right hip pinning procedure under general anesthesia. This type of anesthesia will put Mrs. Brown in a state of unconsciousness. During surgery, the nurse anesthetist monitors Mrs. Brown's vital signs continuously while she is unconscious. The *surgical technician* assists the orthopedic surgeon. The surgical technician sets up the sterile environment in the operating room. This health care worker makes sure the surgeon's instruments and supplies are available when he requests them for the pinning of Mrs. Brown's right hip. The surgical technician is a graduate of a 1-year *diploma program* at a local technical college. The professional nurse, who has a minimum qualification of a BSN, coordinates the overall functioning of the surgical team.

During surgery, the anesthetist notes that Mrs. Brown's blood pressure is rising to a dangerous level. She contacts the anesthesiologist STAT (i.e., immediately!). The *anesthesiologist*, a medical doctor with a residency in anesthesiology, orders antihypertensive drugs (i.e., drugs that lower the blood pressure). The situation is quickly brought under control. Surgery is completed, and Mrs. Brown is sent to the postanesthesia care unit (PACU).

POSTANESTHESIA CARE UNIT

The purpose of the PACU is to monitor the patient's vital signs, level of consciousness, movement, and any special equipment required by patients after surgery. When patients' conditions are stable, they are transferred to their hospital room. The PACU registered nurse, who is a graduate of a diploma (3-year) school of nursing program (also could be from a 2-year or 4-year nursing program), assesses Mrs. Brown. After 1.5 hours, Mrs. Brown is assessed as being ready to leave the PACU. Because of the episode involving high blood pressure during surgery, Mrs. Brown's surgeon orders her to go to the intensive care unit (ICU) overnight for closer observation instead of to the postoperative surgical unit. A *transport aide*, who is trained on the job, and a *staff nurse (RN)* from the PACU take Mrs. Brown to the ICU.

INTENSIVE CARE: A TIME FOR CLOSE OBSERVATION

The ICU is staffed by RNs who went to school for 2 years (associate degree nurses), 3 years (diploma nurses), or 4 years (bachelor's degree nurses). Each nurse has taken the same national examination (NCLEX-RN®) to become an RN. None of these nurses are qualified to work in the ICU immediately after graduation from their nursing programs. Most institutions prepare a nurse for the responsibilities of this unit through inservice classes after a minimum amount of experience or through a postgraduate or continuing education course. Mrs. Brown's nurse, a *2-year graduate (in some regions of the U.S. the hospital employer requires the RN to have a minimum of a BSN)*, is responsible for the care and observation of two patients.

The family is unable to answer some additional questions about Mrs. Brown's medical history. The family physician asks the *clerk receptionist (ward clerk or unit secretary)* to obtain Mrs. Brown's medical records from the medical records department. The clerk receptionist assumes the responsibility for many of the clerical duties that are a necessary part of any patient care area. The clerk receptionist learns these skills by taking a course that varies in length, depending on the area of the country. The course averages approximately one semester of theory and clinical experience. The *medical records department* is staffed by personnel who have attended a Health Information Technology or Health Information Management Program of study at the associates degree or baccalaureate degree level and learned the skills required for indexing, recording, and storing patient electronic records, which are legal documents. Thanks to Mrs. Brown's old records, which are sent to the ICU, the family physician receives answers to his medical questions.

The surgeon writes postoperative orders for Mrs. Brown, including an order for patient-controlled analgesia (PCA) to control postoperative pain. The hospital *pharmacist* has studied for approximately 8 years (doctoral level) to become licensed to prepare, compound, and dispense drugs prescribed by a physician or dentist. The pharmacist fills the order for Mrs. Brown's drugs and intravenous solutions.

The *respiratory therapy department* is contacted to evaluate Mrs. Brown's respiratory status and suggest treatment to prevent respiratory problems. Health care providers in the respiratory therapy department can be certified respiratory therapists (CRTs) or registered respiratory therapists (RRTs) based on their level of educational preparation and performance on the national exams: Therapist Multiple Choice Examination (TMC) and the Clinical Simulation Examination (CSE). Today, respiratory therapists are educated at a minimum of a baccalaureate level, inclusive of course work specific to the specialty area. Within 24 hours of admission to the ICU, Mrs. Brown is judged to be in stable condition. A *transport aide* and an *ICU staff member* transfer her to the surgical unit.

SURGICAL UNIT: AN EYE TO DISCHARGE

The **nurse manager** on the surgical unit at this hospital is an RN who has graduated from a baccalaureate nursing program (4-year) and is enrolled in a Master of Science in Nursing (MSN) program. As manager of the unit, this nurse is responsible for all the care given to patients and the overall functioning of the nursing unit, including budgetary responsibilities. Mrs. Brown's **team leader** is an RN from an Associate Degree in Nursing program (2 year). This nurse is responsible for formulating a plan of care for each of the assigned patients, collaborating with other members of the team to execute the plan, and modifying these plans as needed.

The team leader receives a verbal report and the current care plan for Mrs. Brown from the ICU personnel. The team leader begins assessment of her new admission. The **licensed practical nurse/licensed vocational nurse** (LPN/LVN) assists Mrs. Brown to bed and immediately takes her vital signs. The LPN/LVN is a graduate of a 1-year vocational program in nursing. The LPN/LVN has taken a national examination (NCLEX-PN®) to become licensed. The LPN/LVN is assigned to give Mrs. Brown bedside care and administer her medications. In some states, the nurse practice act limits the LPN/LVN role in intravenous therapy administration and initial assessment of the patient.

A referral is sent to the physical therapy department. The *physical therapist* (PT) assesses the strength of Mrs. Brown's unaffected extremities. The PT sets up a program of exercises and ambulation with no weight bearing on the right extremity. The goal of treatment is to restore function and prevent the development of complications. Physical therapy keeps up the strength of Mrs. Brown's unaffected extremity until she is able to bear weight fully on the right side. The PT is now educated at the doctoral level (5-6 years of college). The *physical therapy assistant* (PTA) has been educated in a 2-year community college or technical school setting. The PTA carries out the plan of care developed by the PT.

You may also have an occupational therapist (OT), working with the patient to rebuild skills needed for everyday activities (e.g., activities of daily living [ADL]). In addition, other health care members may assist in providing care.

Soon after the patient is transferred to the surgical unit, the *social worker* or *case manager, who could be a RN,* visits Mrs. Brown and her family to discuss discharge plans. Although discharge planning begins from the moment the patient is admitted, there will be a focused effort on the transition of care at this point in the patient's recovery. The social worker suggests that Mrs. Brown stay in an extended-care facility for 2 weeks to participate in extensive physical therapy before returning to the farm. In addition, she begins to assess what care and services Mrs. Brown might need following her stay at the extended care facilities and provides for transition in care from the hospital and ultimately, to home. A focus on relationship-centered care is instrumental to successful patient outcomes and avoidance of complications and readmission to the hospital. The financial impact of the care is also discussed. Social workers obtain a bachelor's degree in social work in 4 years and a master's degree in 1 additional year of college. Mrs. Brown's social worker talks to the patient, PT, and the family. All agree that with exercise and skills teaching, the family eventually will be able to care for Mrs. Brown at home.

A direct care worker, often called a *patient care technologist* (PCT) in a hospital setting, is assigned to take Mrs. Brown's vital signs. PCTs perform treatments and skills assigned to them by the RN or the LPN/LVN. PCTs are trained by the hospital for the specific duties they are to perform. Training involves classes (sometimes autotutorial or self-study classes) and a clinical component. The training a PCT receives is short and varies among facilities. The job titles *unlicensed assistive personnel* (UAP), direct care worker, *nurse's aide, nursing assistant,* and *patient care assistant* are used in some facilities. Minimum educational hours and core content is mandated by the federal government if the nursing assistant is employed in a facility receiving Medicare.

Because Mrs. Brown is 50 pounds overweight, her physician orders a weight-reduction diet. The *dietitian* teaches Mrs. Brown and her daughter the elements of weight reduction that will be carried out when Mrs. Brown returns to the farm. A hospital's dietitian is responsible for planning the meals and supplementary feedings for patients and the cafeteria meals for staff. The dietitian also supervises the preparation of food and instructs the patients and their families about nutritional issues and therapeutic diets. This health professional is educated in a 4- to 6-year college program, followed by a year of internship in a health care agency.

The *housekeeper* cleans Mrs. Brown's room and bathroom every day of her stay. Maintaining cleanliness is an effort to maintain medical asepsis (absence of germs) and to provide a pleasant environment. The housekeeper receives training in the needed skills by the employing institution or through a short course in a technical school.

Finally, Mrs. Brown is discharged from the hospital. She leaves by *Medi-Van* and is transported to the extended-care facility.

EXTENDED-CARE UNIT: ON THE ROAD TO REHABILITATION

Mrs. Brown's roommate in the sub-acute facility is an 80-year-old woman who has had a stroke. The roommate is also preparing to go home after additional physical therapy. The *PT* conducts an initial assessment of Mrs. Brown and incorporates the hospital physical therapy plan of care with her findings. The *PTA* helps

Mrs. Brown daily with exercises and ambulation, using a walker, and minimum weight bearing on her right leg. A *nursing assistant* (NA) is assigned to assist Mrs. Brown with her personal care. NAs are educated to give bedside care through courses of a minimum of 75 hours. Successful completion of this course of study makes the NA eligible to be placed on the state registry as a certified nursing assistant (CNA).

A referral is sent to the occupational therapy department. The *occupational therapist* (OT) completes an assessment of Mrs. Brown. The *occupational therapy assistant* (OTA) carries out the plan of care. The goal for Mrs. Brown is to be as *independent* as possible when she returns to the farm, despite her physical limitations. Occupational therapy helps patients restore body function through specific tasks and skills. Educational requirements include a 5- to 6-year occupational therapy program. A 2-year program prepares OTAs for their roles.

Mrs. Brown receives her newly prescribed blood pressure medication from the *LPN/LVN*, who also is functioning in her expanded role as charge nurse in this facility. The *day supervisor*, an RN with a BSN, checks Mrs. Brown daily to monitor her progress. In addition, a nurse practitioner collaborates with the staff to carefully assess for any complications and monitor Mrs. Brown's progress. Ten days later, Mrs. Brown excitedly waits for her family to take her back to the farm. She is pleased with her progress and is confident about going back to her home. She knows that at this time she is unable to gather the eggs each day, but she is anxious to get back in the kitchen.

HOME CARE: SMOOTH TRANSITION TO PREVIOUS FAMILY ROLES

Home care is coordinated, providing physical therapy and occupational therapy. The OT will assess the home for safety hazards and provide recommendations to improve Mrs. Brown's outcomes. These recommendations could include installation of safety devices (i.e., grab bars) and removal of safety hazards (i.e., throw rugs, loose boards on a deck, secure entrance ways) throughout the home. An LPN/LVN or RN may also be a member of the home care team to assist with activities of daily living (ADLs), medication administration/management, treatments, and other supportive services.

? Critical Thinking

Who Is Responsible for Mrs. Brown's Recovery?

Who is responsible for Mrs. Brown's return to the farm? Think about all aspects of Mrs. Brown's care.

INTERDISCIPLINARY HEALTH CARE TEAM

A primary goal of health care is to restore optimal physical, emotional, and spiritual health to patients. This goal is accomplished by promoting health, preventing further illness, and restoring health when illness or accident has occurred. Health care includes a large number of specialized services. It is necessary for these health care workers to work together to integrate care that will provide patients with all the services they need to maintain safe, quality, comprehensive health care. These groups of health care workers are called the interdisciplinary *health care team.*

For Mrs. Brown to be rehabilitated after her fall, it took a minimum of 127 years of education for all the health care workers in this scenario to learn how to perform their respective jobs. The x-ray technician's x-ray film confirmed the presence of a hip fracture. The pharmacist supplied the narcotic pain reliever that relieved pain after the surgical procedure, allowing Mrs. Brown to move more freely and avoid complications. The treatment by the RRT helped prevent pneumonia. The PTs, OTs, and nursing staff all helped restore Mrs. Brown's health and prevent further illness by avoiding complications. The dietitian's expertise allowed Mrs. Brown to receive the basic nutrients she needed to maintain her health, heal her fracture, and lose weight. Teaching about weight-reduction diets promoted health by pointing out the importance of keeping Mrs. Brown's weight within acceptable limits.

As you can see from Mrs. Brown's case, each member of the interdisciplinary health care team, because of his or her specific preparation in a field of study, can increase the quality of health care for a patient. It is impossible for one person to provide the knowledge, expertise, and skills that the health care team as a whole can provide. Everyone needs to work together. It is a team effort. The nurse is an important member of this team, often coordinating patient care.

The members of the interdisciplinary health care team are generally on duty in acute or residential health care organizations 24 hours a day, 7 days a week. Some members of the team may not be scheduled at night or on weekends or holidays, and some of these persons are available on an on-call basis. In the community, health care workers' hours vary depending on the site of employment. Some sites are open Monday through Friday, during day hours only, whereas others also offer services in the evening. Other sites are open 7 days a week and sometimes 24 hours a day.

Each member of the interdisciplinary health care team needs to have good communication skills. Good communication ensures that care is coordinated for the patient's benefit (see Chapter 8). Fragmentation of care can be avoided. Each team member has to be able to anticipate problems and avoid them when possible. This is accomplished by using critical-thinking skills. When problems do occur, the team needs to use problem-solving skills to find solutions in the process of delivering care. In this way the quality of patient care is continuously improved. The team must strive continually to keep its patient care relationship-centered.

The team needs to realize that a cooperative effort is needed to reach patient goals.

WHAT IS *NURSING*?

Virginia Henderson (1966), a nursing theorist, stated, "The unique function of the nurse is to assist the individual, sick or well, in the performance of those activities contributing to health or its recovery (or to peaceful death) that he would perform if he had the necessary strength, will, or knowledge." Henderson refers to nursing's interest in illness and wellness. The direction of LP/LV nursing has been channeled by this definition. For a definition of nursing provided by the American Nurses Association or the International Council of Nurses, visit www.nursingworld.org/EspeciallyForYou/What-is-Nursing or www.icn.ch/who-we-are/icn-definition-of-nursing/.

It is necessary for LPNs/LVNs to understand their role in Mrs. Brown's care. An understanding of the education, licensure, roles, and responsibilities of the varied members of the interdisciplinary health care team is also necessary.

NURSING'S PLACE ON THE HEALTH CARE TEAM

Nursing staff on the interdisciplinary health care team includes *advanced practice nurses, RNs, LPNs/LVNs, student nurses, NAs,* and *cross-trained staff.* Direct care workers assist the nursing staff. Clerk receptionists, although not nurses, are an important part of the unit staff. Most people are unaware of the different types of nurses on the health care team. Sadly, some RNs do not know the educational requirements for LPNs/LVNs, and some LPNs/LVNs do not know what education professional (RN) nursing entails. A common question from the public is "What is the difference between a registered nurse and a licensed practical/vocational nurse?" Members of the health care team generally, and nursing specifically, need to know about one another. For this reason, general information about the education for and the many roles of registered nursing is provided in this section, which describes the members of the nursing team.

DIVERSITY IN EDUCATIONAL PREPARATION OF NURSES

REGISTERED NURSES

Education

Registered nurses (RNs) are the largest group of health care workers in the United States. Approximately 2.9 million RNs were active in the workforce in 2012 (HRSA, 2014). The graduates of the three types of educational programs for professional nurses (2-, 3-, and 4-year programs) currently take the same licensing examination. On successful completion of the NCLEX-RN® examination, all of these graduates hold the title of registered nurse.

Associate degree nursing program

- An **associate degree nursing** (ADN) program is a 2-year educational program (often completed over 3 years) that can be found in community colleges, junior colleges, and technical schools.
- The ADN program includes general education courses (e.g., courses in the biologic, behavioral, and social sciences), nursing courses, and clinical practice.
- On graduation, the graduate receives an associate degree in nursing and is eligible to take the NCLEX-RN® examination to become a registered nurse.

Diploma program

- A **diploma program** is a 3-year educational program conducted by a hospital-based school of nursing.
- The diploma program comprises the same general education courses as 2-year programs, with nursing courses and clinical practice. Diploma programs traditionally have emphasized clinical experience.
- Today, many diploma nursing schools have a University educational partner. The nursing student is likely to be dual enrolled (e.g., enrolled at diploma nursing program and the University).
- On graduation, the nursing graduate receives a diploma in nursing and is eligible to take the NCLEX-RN® examination to become a registered nurse.

Bachelor's nursing program

- A **bachelor's nursing program** is a 4-year nursing program that can be found in public and private colleges and universities.
- The bachelor's program emphasizes course work in the liberal arts, sciences, and nursing theory, including public health. Clinical practice is included.
- On graduation, the nurse receives a BSN and is eligible to take the NCLEX-RN® examination to become a registered nurse.

Role of Registered Nurses

Graduates of all three nursing programs are prepared for entry-level staff nursing in a hospital, long-term care, or community setting. Although you may find 2- and 3-year RNs in supervisory and administrative positions, only bachelor's graduates have been prepared in their nursing education programs for advancement to these positions. Bachelor's graduates are also prepared for beginning positions in public health agencies.

Approximately 55% of RNs in 2010 held a bachelor's degree, representing a 5% increase from 2000 (HRSA, 2013). This education trend is expected to continue as the complexity of patient care increases. Some demographic locations require a bachelor's degree to obtain employment in a hospital setting. This is particularly true for Magnet designated institutions.

All RNs function under the Nurse Practice Act of the state in which they are working. RNs use the nursing process to identify patient problems, formulate nursing diagnoses, and plan and evaluate care. **Standards of care** are used instead of care plans in some acute care agencies. These standards include the priority nursing diagnosis for each patient, with appropriate assessments, nursing interventions, and expected outcomes (goals). Standards provide minimum guidelines for a consistent approach to delivering patient care. The RN uses standards as a reference when individualizing patient care.

Registered nurses assign routine care and the care of stable patients to assistive personnel. This allows RNs to do the following:

1. Plan care.
2. Coordinate all the activities of care, including care from interdisciplinary health care team members.
3. Provide care that requires more specialized knowledge and judgment.
4. Teach patients, families, and other members of the health care team.
5. Act as a patient advocate.

Independent role of the registered nurse. Registered nurses function **independently** in nursing, initiating and carrying out nursing activities. For example, to prevent complications in the respiratory and circulatory systems, RNs assess the patient on bed rest. They identify the need for a turning routine, deep breathing, leg exercises, and range-of-motion exercises. If not contraindicated by the patient's diagnosis and/or treatment, RNs add these nursing interventions to ordered care. Because of their level of education, RNs can identify which patients can and cannot receive these nursing interventions. In the community, RNs will initiate dietitian and social worker referrals. *It is the independent role in decision-making that distinguishes RNs from LPNs/LVNs.* Registered nurses have the ultimate responsibility for the nursing care given to patients.

Interdependent role of the registered nurse. When RNs carry out the legal orders of another health professional (e.g., the physician or physical therapist), they are functioning in an **interdependent** role. RNs function interdependently (collaboratively) when carrying out decisions about patient care that are made jointly by members of the interprofessional health care team. The complexity of care delivery warrants collaboration to maximize high-quality patient outcomes.

Education in Addition to the Basic Nursing Programs for Registered Nurses

The postgraduate educational opportunities available to RNs are presented here to explain the various RNs found on the health care team.

Bachelor of science in nursing completion program
After passing the NCLEX-RN® examination, associate degree and diploma graduates can enroll in a program that will grant a BSN. Programs vary in length, content, and mode of delivery, including online and competency-based programs.

Accelerated bachelor of science in nursing program. Individuals with an undergraduate degree in another discipline can earn a Bachelor of Science degree in Nursing in approximately 15 months. The 15-month program is very intensive, and when completed, the student is eligible to take the NCLEX-RN® examination.

Master of nursing programs. Masters of Science in Nursing programs prepare registered nurses for a specialty area in nursing, such as medical-surgical, pediatrics, management, nursing education, psychiatric/mental health, and geriatrics. The MSN is a requirement for teaching in associate degree programs. Generally, nurses with BSN degrees are the only nursing graduates who may elect to do graduate work in nursing at the masters and doctoral levels. However, MSN programs exist that offer an MSN degree to nurses with an undergraduate degree in an area other than nursing. The MSN then becomes the entry degree into nursing. Various nursing educational pathways exist, encouraging nurses to be life-long learners.

Certification. Passing the NCLEX-RN® examination provides initial licensure in nursing and ensures basic competence for entry into nursing practice. After gaining work experience, RNs can receive **certification** from numerous professional nursing groups. The certificate that is awarded after passing a comprehensive examination indicates that the nurse has demonstrated competence in a select area of practice. The American Nurses Credentialing Center (ANCC), a subsidiary of the American Nurses Association (ANA), makes certification available to all RNs. Often, there is no difference in credentials based on type of RN educational program from which one is a graduate for basic specialty certification. All basic specialty-certified nurses are board certified (AACN Nurse Certification, 2011). The requirement of a Master's degree in nursing remains for certification as an **advanced practice** registered nurse. Because certification needs to be renewed periodically, certification through ANCC allows the registered nurse to demonstrate ongoing competence in a selected area of nursing.

Advanced practice registered nurse. With an additional degree, RNs can pursue expanded roles, called *advanced practice.* These nurses acquire specialized nursing knowledge and skills, and demonstrate a greater depth and breadth of nursing knowledge and an increased complexity of skills and interventions. The term *advanced practice registered nurse* (APRN) identifies the advanced practice roles of a clinical nurse specialist, a nurse practitioner, a nurse anesthetist, and a certified nurse-midwife. Each of these nurses has a minimum of a Master's of Science degree in Nursing (MSN), obtained in a 1- to 2-year program of study. Additional studies can include the Doctor of Nursing Practice (DNP), preparing the APRN for the highest level of clinical practice.

- **Clinical nurse specialist (CNS).** This registered nurse has a minimum of an MSN in a specialty area (e.g., medical-surgical nursing). The CNS is a clinical expert in nursing practice based on the latest research and has certification as a clinical nurse specialist. When employed by health care organizations, the CNS serves as a mentor, role model, and resource person for staff by setting standards for nursing care. The CNS provides direct care in challenging patient situations and shares knowledge, experiences, and resources with staff. The CNS is employed by hospitals, clinics, nursing homes, nursing schools as instructors, and in other community settings. In all sites of employment, the CNS can serve as an educator, consultant, researcher, and administrator.
- **Nurse practitioner (NP).** This registered nurse has a minimum of an MSN and certification by a national body. Additional studies can include the Doctor of Nursing Practice (DNP), preparing the APRN for the highest level of clinical practice. Some states may mandate the doctorate. There are many areas of specialization for nurse practitioners, such as acute, adult, gerotological, pediatric, and psychiatric/mental health. Some NPs provide primary care in the community in physicians' clinics or in their own offices. Others provide acute care services in hospitals and long-term care settings. NPs order and interpret lab and diagnostic tests, develop diagnoses, and prescribe treatments, including drugs, for acute and chronic diseases. Their care differs from medical care because of their interest in and awareness of psychosocial aspects of illness. State regulations differ for NPs regarding prescriptive privileges and other responsibilities. Review your state nurse practice act for details.
- **Certified nurse-midwife (CNM).** This registered nurse has a minimum of an MSN and certification as a nurse-midwife. The CNM provides holistic maternal/family-centered health care in the area of prenatal low-risk pregnancy, childbirth, the postpartum period, care of the newborn, and family planning at home, in hospitals, and birthing centers and in the gynecologic care of women. They diagnose and treat illness, including prescribing drugs.
- **Certified registered nurse anesthetist (CRNA).** This registered nurse has a minimum of an MSN, is a graduate of an accredited nurse anesthesia educational program, and has certification as a nurse anesthetist. CRNAs work in every setting where anesthesia is given: operating rooms, clinics, and outpatient surgical centers. They prepare patients for anesthesia; induce and maintain local, regional, and general anesthesia; provide postanesthesia care, including pain management; and provide emergency resuscitation.
- **Nurse executive/Certified Nurse Educator (CNE).** The American Association of Colleges of Nursing (AACN) offers several types of certifications including a nurse executive certification. In addition, National League for Nursing (NLN) offers a certification for nurse educators called the CNE (www.nln.org).

Doctoral nursing education. The National League for Nursing advocates for advancing the nation's health by positioning the nurse educator, educated at the doctoral level, leading educational reform (2013).

There are two types of doctoral programs in nursing:

- Research-focused: These programs lead to an academic doctorate (PhD) or professional doctorate (DNS or DNSc). Most DNS or DNSc programs have transitioned to PhD programs to better meet the needs of the nursing industry. Graduates are prepared as a scientist and do rigorous investigation into, for example, clinical or educational issues, to help build the science of nursing (NLN, 2010).
- Practice-focused (DNP): These evolving programs graduate nurses who are considered nursing's expert clinicians (nurses working in health care agencies) and most effective practice leaders who will promote and facilitate changes in practice that enhance quality care (NLN, 2010).

Nursing Management, Leadership, and Executive Roles

The twenty-first century health care system requires nursing managers who also possess leadership skills. These nurses possess the ability to develop a shared vision with nursing staff of quality, safety, and cost control that will help improve outcomes in patient care. The typical four levels of nursing management are supervisor, nurse manager, director, and chief nursing officer (CNO) (Box 14-1). The practical/vocational nurse's role as charge nurse is discussed in Chapter 17.

Try This

Get to Know the Nursing Team

During an unhurried moment in the clinical area, ask the RN with whom you are working about the educational requirements to be employed for his or her position. If there are initials behind his or her name, ask for them to be explained. Ask them why and how they achieved the certifications identified by the initials.

Box 14-1	Nursing Management and Executive Roles

Supervisor: BSN preferred; deals with specific problems with nursing personnel; makes rounds to all nursing units on assigned shift to ensure patients' needs are met according to organization's procedures; clinical resource for collaborative decision making

Nurse manager: Middle management position; MSN preferred; leader of a specific clinical department (for example, medical services); responsible for personnel, quality of care, safety, and cost of running department.

Director: Entry level of executive role; MSN or Masters degree in business or health-related field required; coordinates the development and implementation of strategies to initiate new programs and improve current services of several departments.

Chief nursing officer (CNO): Highest-ranking administrative nurse in a health care organization; MSN, Masters in business or health-related field required; doctorate may be required in larger organizations; organizes and coordinates the nursing department; responsible for excellence in nursing that is consistent with the mission, vision, and values of the organization.

Modified from Hader R. (2009). Is being a chief nursing officer in your future? NSNA imprint, www.nsna.org.

LICENSED PRACTICAL NURSE/LICENSED VOCATIONAL NURSES

Background

Approximately 730,000 LPNs were active in the workforce in 2012 (Health Resources and Services Administration [HRSA], 2014), representing the second largest group of licensed health care workers in the United States. The LPN population contributes to the diversity of the nursing profession. The HRSA (2013) report, *The US Nursing Workforce: Trends in Supply and Education,* states, "LPNs are more likely to identify as racial/ethnic minorities when compared with RNs. In particular, the proportion of Black/African Americans is higher among LPNs (23.6 percent in the ACS 2008 to 2010 vs. 9.9 percent for RNs)." LPNs work in a variety of diverse care settings in collaboration with the interprofessional health care team.

Education

The educational program for practical/vocational nurses varies from 12 to 18 months. Part-time study can extend the program a few months longer. The LP/LV nursing program is located in trade, technical, and vocational schools, as well as community colleges. These institutions are usually public institutions. LP/LV nursing programs are also found in private schools.

LPN/LVN education concentrates on clinical care at the bedside, based on fundamentals of biologic sciences. Courses in basic nursing care, the behavioral sciences, and the biologic sciences are included. Basic nursing care includes the administration of medications,

inclusive of intravenous (IV) therapy in some states. Critical thinking is emphasized, and the LPN/LVN's assisting role in the nursing process is included in all phases of the nursing program, as determined by each state's Nurse Practice Act. Clinical experience in acute care facilities, long-term care facilities, and the community is included. On graduation, the LPN/LVN receives a diploma in practical nursing and is eligible to take the NCLEX-PN® examination.

Role of Licensed Practical Nurses/Licensed Vocational Nurses

LPNs/LVNs must be aware of the content of the Nurse Practice Act (NPA) of the state in which they are employed. The LPN/LVN's role and scope of practice is found in this law, and the law differs from state to state. Administrative rules and regulations and interpretations of the state's Board of Nursing provide more *specific* details and clarification. Some NPAs list specifically what LPNs/LVNs can do, but others are written more broadly to allow for changes in the evolving role of the LPN/LVN. This eliminates the need for state legislatures to reopen the act and revise it each time a change is required. However, it also can cause the blurring of professional role boundaries. It is your responsibility to be aware of the law of the state in which you are employed. Generally, the role of the LPN/LVN includes the following:

- Cares for patients within the scope of the state's NPA while upholding clinical standards
- Regardless of the site of employment, provides care in basic and complex patient situations under the **general supervision** of an RN, physician, podiatrist, or dentist, as determined by the state Nurse Practice Act
- Primary responsibility in the care of vulnerable populations with chronic, stable conditions
- Provides safe patient care, serves as a patient advocate, teaches patients, and communicates effectively, all while functioning as a collaborative member of the health care team

Employers expect LPNs/LVNs to think critically and solve problems in patient care situations. LPNs/LVNs function interdependently when they offer input to the RN about the effectiveness of patient care or offer suggestions to improve care. When LPNs/LVNs provide actual care at the bedside in acute care situations, their collection of data while engaged in giving care is valuable in determining whether or not progress is being made to meet patient outcomes.

A major criterion in differentiating between the roles of the registered and practical/vocational nurse is that the LPN/LVN does not function independently. LPNs/LVNs must function safely and are accountable for their actions. They function interdependently (collaboratively) with other members of the health care team, but the LPN/LVN role is basically a dependent role. They should assume responsibility only for nursing actions that are within their legal role and that they feel

| Table 14-1 | Differences Between the Roles of Registered Nurses and Licensed Practical Nurses/Licensed Vocational Nurses |

FIVE NURSING ROLES	ROLES OF RN AND LPN/LVN
Professional	
Registered nurse (RN)	Can join and be involved in American Nurses Association (ANA) at state/local levels.
Licensed practical nurse/licensed vocational nurse (LPN/LVN)	Can join and be involved in National Federation of Licensed Professional Nurses (NFLPN) and/or National Association for Practical Nurse Education and Service (NAPNES) at state/local levels (see Chapter 18).
Provider of Care	
RN	This is an independent and interdependent role. Initiates all phases of nursing process; formulates nursing diagnoses.
LPN/LVN	This is a dependent and interdependent role. Assists with all phases of the nursing process. Works with established nursing diagnoses. Identifies possible new nursing problems and reports same to RN.
Manager of Care	
RN	Controls decisions regarding staff and care of patients.
LPN/LVN	First-line manager in long-term care and other community settings. Responsible to RN nurse manager or physician.
Teacher	
RN	Initiates all health teaching.
LPN/LVN	Initiates health teaching for basic health habits (e.g., nutrition and cleanliness). Reinforces and assists with health teaching as directed by the RN in other areas.
Researcher	
RN	Theory included in 4-year program. All levels interpret and implement evidence-based practice guidelines. Participates in the research process.
LPN/LVN	Assists in implementing evidence-based practice guidelines. Collects data, as instructed, for research studies.

competent in carrying out. Table 14-1 identifies the differences between the LPN/LVN and the RN roles.

? Critical Thinking

The Licensed Practical Nurse/Licensed Vocational Nurse Role in Assisting with the Nursing Process

Identify the major difference between the RN's and LPN/LVN's roles in the nursing process. How is the LPN/LVN's role in the nursing process determined? How does the LPN/LVN contribute to the plan of care?

Expanded Role of Licensed Practical Nurses/Licensed Vocational Nurses

In some settings, LPNs/LVNs are being used in their expanded role. An example of the expanded role of the LPN/LVN is the charge nurse position in long-term care facilities. During implementation of care by the LPN/LVN, the RN is available for collaboration, assisting with decision making when questions arise, either onsite (direct supervision), virtually, or by phone (general supervision). See Chapter 17 for further discussion of the expanded role of the LPN/LVN.

? Critical Thinking

Expanded Role of the Licensed Practical Nurse/Licensed Vocational Nurse

Refer to your state's Nurse Practice Act. Describe care situations when you should be sure to immediately collaborate with the RN or physician.

STUDENT NURSES

Student professional and practical/vocational nurses come to the clinical area under the supervision of clinical instructors. The clinical area is an extension of the classroom. It provides an opportunity to apply theory to practice. When assigned to patients, these **student nurses** have a responsibility to give safe care and function responsibly under the supervision of the instructor. Students are in the clinical area to learn, not to give service. It is possible that a clinical instructor can remove students from the assigned clinical site at any time for additional learning experiences.

Students are members of the interdisciplinary health care team. They are expected to assist other team members in addition to performing their patient assignment.

Examples of such assistance include passing trays, answering call lights in acute care and long-term care situations, and assisting patients and staff in the community. These activities assist students in developing communication and team-building skills.

Student practical nurses/student vocational nurses (SPNs/SVNs) are responsible for giving the same safe nursing care that LPNs/LVNs provide. This is a legal matter. Therefore, the student role demands preparation and supervision.

NURSING ASSISTANTS

Nursing assistants (NAs) are trained for their positions by combining federally mandated classroom instruction with close supervision by RNs while in the clinical area. Vocational and private schools offer programs that last a minimum of 75 hours and are up to 12 weeks in length. These programs combine classroom or autotutorial instruction with clinical practice. At the completion of the course, testing for competence occurs to meet federal Omnibus Budget Reconciliation Act (OBRA) requirements. When test results are satisfactory, the names of NAs are placed in a registry.

NAs function under the direction of RNs or LPNs/LVNs. NAs who work in hospitals, specialty hospitals, sub-acute units and long-term care settings assist in providing personal and comfort needs for stable patients. They are assigned routine tasks, sometimes involving housekeeping chores. A large number of NAs are employed by long-term care settings. The supply of NAs does not meet the demands of employers. According to the Bureau of Labor and Statistics (2013), personal care aides, nursing assistants, and home health aides are expected to be in jobs with the most growth between 2012 and 2022. People in some areas of the country refer to male NAs as orderlies.

Some states offer an advanced NA course that teaches more complex skills. These skills can include tasks that are performed by an LPN/LVN. The demand for home health care workers continues to increase. NAs are allowed to perform a wider variety of skills in the home as home health care workers. Some states offer a postgraduate course for NAs to prepare them for the transition to home care. The comprehensive home care program may also be available to individuals without NA experience.

UNLICENSED ASSISTIVE PERSONNEL

In an effort to use health care workers more efficiently and effectively, health care organizations have added another level of worker to the health care team. **Unlicensed assistive personnel (UAP)** are trained by health care organizations to function in an assistive role to RNs and LPNs/LVNs. Some health care organizations require applicants for UAP positions to be registered as NAs. These workers learn selected skills, sometimes by the autotutorial method or module method, combined with some clinical teaching. Actual skills learned depend on which skills are needed in specific patient care units. UAPs are also known by the terms *patient care technician*, *patient care associate*, *care pair*, *nurse extender*, and *multiskilled worker*.

CLERK RECEPTIONISTS (UNIT SECRETARY)

The job of the **clerk receptionist** is mainly secretarial in nature, but the duties vary from site to site. Given the increase in the use of electronic medical records, the role of this clerk is changing; however, their skills continue to assist nurses and other members of the interdisciplinary health team. Clerk receptionists are trained on the job or in programs of several months' duration in technical schools or community colleges. Clerks prepare, compile, and maintain patient electronic records on a nursing unit. Duties include transcribing physicians' orders; scheduling lab tests, x-ray procedures, and surgeries; scheduling other appointments for services; routing charts on patient transfers or discharges; compiling the patient census; answering the telephone; maintaining established inventories of supplies; distributing mail to patients; and generally ensuring that the unit functions smoothly.

UNIT MANAGERS

Some large health care organizations have **unit managers** to supervise and coordinate management functions for patient units. A college background and supervisory experience are desirable for this position. This job is combined with on-the-job training for specific duties. Responsibilities include budgeting, supervision, assignment, and evaluation of all staff on the unit; coordination with all members of the interdisciplinary health care team; responsibility for patient and unit outcomes, including satisfaction and quality ratings; and clarification of hospital compliance with Medicare requirements. If a health care organization does not have unit managers, the clerk receptionist and the nurse manager assume these duties.

💡 Keep in Mind

Diversity of Age for Coworkers on the Nursing Team

In addition to a diversity of educational preparation, the nursing team needs to contend with four generations of its members. Four generations of personnel on the nursing team can have different goals, priorities, and work preferences (Yoder-Wise, 2011). Awareness and understanding of these differences is necessary for successful communication and working as a team. See Chapter 1 for details.

❓ Critical Thinking

Know Your Health Care Team

When on the clinical area, list the various members of the interdisciplinary health care team with whom you have contact. Draw a concept map describing their role on the team and education required for their job.

DELIVERY OF NURSING CARE IN ACUTE CARE SETTINGS

With the goal of providing optimal care, the nursing team uses different methods to assign patients to staff. The methods evolved as a response to changing needs of the health care system, including staffing. Each of the methods is discussed in its general form as it was intended to function. Health care organizations modify these methods to fit their individual needs.

TOTAL PATIENT CARE (CASE METHOD)

At the turn of the twentieth century, families hired nurses to meet a patient's special needs in the home. By the 1920s, private-duty nursing was popular. This **total patient care** or **case method** of patient care continued in various degrees into the 1960s. Vestiges of the case method, or a one-to-one relationship with a patient, are found today in acute care situations and described as total patient care (comprehensive care). In the case method, one nurse is assigned to one or two patients and is responsible for planning, organizing, and carrying out the care for these patients. Today, total care nursing occurs in intensive care or special care units, as Mrs. Brown experienced in the ICU after she left the PACU. Nursing instructors frequently use the total patient care method when assigning beginning students to the acute care clinical area.

FUNCTIONAL NURSING

During World War II, the **functional method** was a popular method of patient assignment. Registered nurses were in scarce supply because of the war. Hospitals increased the number of LPNs/LVNs and NAs to provide care for patients. The functional method of patient care is task-oriented. The tasks that have to be done for patients are divided among the staff. For example, one person might measure all vital signs, another might do all treatments, and still another might make all the beds. This method's emphasis on efficiency and division of labor is based on the assembly-line-production concept found in industry.

The long-term care facility nearest Mrs. Brown's home schedules resident assignments by the functional method. An NA helped Mrs. Brown with her physical care. An LPN/LVN gave her medications and did her treatments. In addition to assuming responsibility for all care given to residents, the charge nurse, an LPN/LVN would be kept busy with managerial (e.g., staff evaluations) and nonnursing duties (e.g., inventory of supplies).

Functional nursing can easily overlook holistic care, especially in the area of psychosocial needs. This results in fragmentation of care. Although this method is efficient and appears to be less costly to implement, it can discourage patient and staff satisfaction. The functional method, however, may work well in times of critical shortages or need of large numbers of personnel, such as disaster situations and emergencies.

TEAM NURSING

After World War II, the shortage of registered nurses continued. The **team method** of patient care was introduced, aided by the increasing number of LPNs/LVNs and NAs. The team method is based on the belief that goals can be achieved through group action. The patients on a unit are divided into small groups. Small teams are assigned to care for the patients in each group. Assignments are based on the needs of each patient and the skills of the team members. The team leader, the RN, leads the team. The RN continues to have the final responsibility of planning, coordinating, and evaluating the implementation of care for each patient and supervising the personnel giving the care. Although in long-term care settings the LPN can lead a team, collaboration with an RN supervisor is required.

In team nursing the capabilities of each team member are used effectively. This increases the quality of care for the patient and the satisfaction of the team member. An integral part of the team method is the team conference. During this conference, which should be held daily, team members share information about specific patients. Patient problems are identified and solved, and plans of care are developed and revised. The team method is rarely carried out in this manner. When busy, the team leader may administer medications and perform treatments. Team conferences are often postponed. The team method then becomes a functional method of assigning care. Several years ago, the nurses on the medical unit where Mrs. Brown was a patient used the team method, but often the team leader functioned as the medication nurse.

Modular nursing is a method of delivering nursing care that modifies team nursing by arranging the physical layout of units so nurses can stay near the bedside of assigned patients for convenient patient access and record keeping. For consistency, the same group of caregivers is assigned to a specific patient area.

PRIMARY NURSING

The hospital in which Mrs. Brown was a patient adopted the **primary care method** several years ago to replace the team method of assigning care. The intention was to increase the quality of care for patients. This method was instituted in the 1970s as a result of the dissatisfaction of professional nurses with their lack of direct patient contact and the fragmentation of care that resulted from functional and team nursing. In primary nursing, RNs individualize patient care and accept responsibility and accountability for total patient care, generally eliminating the need to delegate to other licensed staff persons. Ideally, staffing for this method requires a nursing staff composed entirely of RNs. Each nurse is assigned a maximum of four to six patients in a hospital setting. It is unlikely to see the primary nursing model used in a long-term care setting. There are no team leaders in this method. Each primary nurse is a bedside nurse, who has received the assignment from and in turn reports to the nurse manager.

The major characteristic of this method is the responsibility and accountability of the primary nurse. The primary nurse is assigned to a patient on admission, develops the nursing diagnoses after the admission interview, develops a plan of care, and is responsible for the care of that patient 24 hours a day until he or she is discharged. When the primary nurse is off duty, an associate RN continues care as planned by the primary nurse. If any changes are contemplated in patient care, the primary nurse must be contacted. LPNs/LVNs are used as assistive nurses in primary care situations.

Primary nursing facilitates continuity of care but has advantages and disadvantages. Positive aspects of the primary method include shorter hospital stays for patients, improved communication among staff, and a more holistic focus of care. The challenge of recruiting a sufficient number of RNs is one negative aspect, but the greatest drawback is the cost of a staff composed entirely of RNs. However, research by nursing experts such as Linda Aiken report that the use of an all BSN prepared nursing staff improves patient outcomes, such as patient mortality rates.

NURSING CASE MANAGEMENT

In acute care, nursing case management focuses on achieving patient outcomes within a specified time frame. **Clinical pathways** or critical paths are used as a tool by all health care workers involved with the patient's care to identify incidents that must occur at specific times to achieve patient outcomes within an appropriate length of stay. These pathways provide a blueprint for care that includes a time frame of significant events that are expected to occur each day a patient with a specific diagnosis is in the hospital.

Nursing case management became popular in the 1980s in response to the increasing complexity of patient care, the need to use scarce nursing resources, and meeting patient needs in a *cost-effective* manner in acute care. Depending on patient needs, this method uses bachelor degree registered nurses, diploma and associate degree registered nurses, licensed practical/ licensed vocational nurses, nursing assistants, and direct care workers in varying ratios to deliver nursing service.

Some institutions use care maps, which are a combination of care plans and critical paths. The case manager keeps an eye on timely discharge and continuity of care in the community by planning, directing, and evaluating care throughout the patient's stay in acute care. The strength of the **case management method** of delivering nursing services is its focus of delivering cost-effective, quality care to patients with complex needs. Quality, service, and cost are timely considerations for health care in the twenty-first century.

SKILL MIX

Skill mix refers to the different levels of educational preparation of members used to staff the nursing team. The skill mix on the nursing team can be varied. Some hospitals are converting to all-RN staffs, and in some regions all baccalaureate-prepared RNs. Some hospitals use LPNs/LVNs and direct care workers to deliver patient care.

Research and data are needed to evaluate the quality of care provided by variously composed teams of RNs, LPNs/LVNs, and NAs in a variety of health care settings. Research does exist supporting the hiring of BSN-prepared RNs (Aiken et al., 2008; Tri-Council for Nursing, 2010). Limited research exists examining the impact of LPN/LVN and direct care worker ratios on patient care outcomes. Plan to investigate the skill mix of nursing staff in health care agencies at which you have clinical experiences and reflect on the skill mix and impact on patient outcomes.

PATIENT-CENTERED–RELATIONSHIP-CENTERED CARE—A PHILOSOPHY

Nursing has always been concerned with total patient care, focusing on the patient's physical and emotional needs, preferences, and values when giving care. The Institute of Medicine (IOM), an independent organization that advises the nation about health care, focuses on safety and quality in health care. You can find information about the IOM and its role in health care at www.iom.edu/About-IOM.aspx.

The IOM defines **patient-centered care** as "providing care that is respectful of and responsive to individual patient preferences, needs, and values and ensuring that patient values guide all clinical decisions" (Mitchell, 2008). The NLN states, "Core to nursing practice, relationship-centered care includes caring; (therapeutic relationships with patients, families and communities; and professional relationships with members of the interprofessional team [NLN, 2010])." The interdisciplinary health care team partners with patients and families to plan care that reflects the patient's needs and preferences and ensures that the patient has the information needed to make health care decisions. All nursing care delivery systems must include these elements of patient and relationship-centered care (see Chapter 13).

THE HIDDEN NURSING SHORTAGE

Hospitals and health care, as well as nursing, have always been considered to be "recession-proof." Nursing jobs in acute care were widely available until the recession of 2008. As people lost jobs nationwide, they also lost health insurance benefits. Many postponed needed and elective health care. Nurses began having difficulty finding jobs in acute care facilities. This situation began to ease in some parts of the country in 2010. Reasons for the sudden downturn in acute care jobs over the last several years include the following:

- A stock market drop in 2008 caused older RNs to delay retiring to allow their retirement funds to recover.
- Some nurses retained their jobs because a spouse was laid off.
- Nurses working part-time switched to full-time employment.
- Hospital services and programs cut during the recession were not restored.
- The Affordable Care Act supports high-quality, low-cost care alternatives. Many of these options are found in community settings. "Transitions in care" is a key theme.

Since World War II, nursing shortages have been common. With the beginning of retirement for Baby Boomers in 2011, a nursing shortage looms, but it has been impacted by the sluggish growth in jobs (Box 14-2). The number of elderly in society and their potential need for increased health care, including long-term care, has resulted in varying projections of the need for nurses in the future. Because of the long-term care

---

Box 14-2   The U.S. Nursing Workforce: Trends in Supply and Education

- The nursing workforce grew in the past decade
  - RNs growing by more than 500,000 (24%)
  - LPNs by more than 90,000 (16%)
- Nurses over 50 entered the workforce during the recent recession (Buerhaus & Auerbach, 2011)

Despite this growth, a shortage is predicted because . . .

- About one-third of the nursing workforce is older than 50 years
- Other trends continue, increasing the demand for nurses:
  - aging population
  - increasing patient acuity
  - hospital staffing and hiring preferences
  - nursing schools cannot admit all qualified applicants because of a shortage of faculty and clinical facilities
  - the average age of nursing faculty is 55 years; they face retirement in about 10 years or less.

Modified from Health Resources and Services Administration (HRSA) (2013). The U.S. Nursing Workforce: Trends in Supply and Education, http://bhpr.hrsa.gov/healthworkforce/supplydemand/nursing/nursingworkforce/

---

needs of an aging society and a future general increase in demand for health care services, employment of LPNs/LVNs and RNs is predicted to increase faster than the average at 25% and 19%, respectively, between 2012 and 2022 (Bureau of Labor Statistics, 2014).

Get Ready for the NCLEX-PN® Examination

Key Points

- Health care organizations include a large number of specialized services and health care workers to provide these services. Patients in the United States have some of the most expensive health care services in the world; however, the United States underperforms compared with other countries on several outcomes.
- Each member of the interprofessional health care team provides a valuable service to the patient. All members of the interprofessional health care team are equal in importance to each other.
- Members of the nursing team are registered nurses (including nursing management), licensed practical/licensed vocational nurses, student nurses, cross-trained staff, unlicensed assistive personnel, and clerk receptionists (support staff).
- To understand where the licensed practical/licensed vocational nurse fits into the interprofessional health care team, be aware of the educational background, role, responsibilities, and possible licensing requirements of all levels of personnel on the team.
- To understand your position on the interprofessional health care team, keep current regarding new levels of health care workers and the method of delivering nursing care in your health care agency.
- Functional, team, and primary nursing are examples of methods used to deliver nursing care in acute care and long-term care facilities.
- Nursing case management focuses on achieving patient outcomes within a specified time frame using clinical pathways.
- The IOM defines patient-centered care as "providing care that is respectful of and responsive to individual patient preferences, needs, and values and ensuring that patient values guide all clinical decisions."
- The NLN states, "Core to nursing practice, relationship-centered care includes caring; (therapeutic relationships with patients, families, and communities; and professional relationships with members of the interprofessional team [NLN, 2010])."
- The increasing number of elderly in society increases demand for health care workers.
  - Although not professional registered nurses, LPNs/LVNs are licensed professionals who share with the entire nursing community a commitment to providing safe, quality, cost-effective care and whose practice behavior is grounded in those shared values (NLN, 2014).

Additional Learning Resources

evolve Go to your Evolve website (http://evolve.elsevier.com/Knecht/success) for the following FREE learning resources:

- Answers to Critical Thinking Scenarios
- Additional learning activities
- Additional Review Questions for the NCLEX-PN® exam
- Helpful phrases for communicating in Spanish and more!

Review Questions for the NCLEX-PN® Examination

1. Which of the following nurses, identified by the initials after their name, is most likely to be the Director of Nursing at a large-size long-term care facility?
   a. RN
   b. RN BSN
   c. LPN
   d. RN MSN

2. Select the statement that indicates an understanding of a major difference between the RN and LPN/LVN.
   a. The LPN/LVN initiates all health teaching for patients.
   b. The registered nurse formulates nursing diagnoses.
   c. By law, the LPN/LVN functions in an independent role.
   d. The LPN/LVN interprets the results of research studies.

3. Which of the following statements best describes team nursing as a method of delivering nursing care?
   a. The method is based on the level of staff skill and patient need.
   b. Task-oriented efficiency is divided among staff across all shifts.
   c. The RN plans and is accountable for total patient care 24 hours a day.
   d. This method uses scarce nursing resources in a cost-effective way.

Alternate Format Item

1. The following describe likely job settings and the job role of an LPN/LVN working as a vital member of the interprofessional team (Select all that apply.)
   a. Community: Team member for a chronically ill pediatric patient in their home
   b. Long-term care: Charge nurse on the evening shift of a skilled care facility
   c. Acute care: Charge nurse on a surgical unit
   d. Community: Team member in a geriatric clinic
   e. Long-term care: Director of Nursing supervising skilled care and personal care units

2. Which of the following statements differentiates the role of the LPN/LVN from the professional nurse? (Select all that apply.)
   a. The LPN/LVN is responsible for formulating all nursing diagnoses.
   b. The LPN/LVN has a collaborative role in health teaching for patients.
   c. The LPN/LVN is not employed in any charge/management positions.
   d. The LPN/LVN is responsible for triaging patients in an urgent care setting.
   e. The LPN/LVN is responsible for all members of the health care team.

3. Which of the following are methods of delivering nursing care in acute care agencies? (Select all that apply.)
   a. Primary care
   b. Case method
   c. Team method
   d. Functional method
   e. Delegation method

Critical Thinking Scenarios

Scenario 1

From the beginning of her PN student year, Amy set her sights on working as an LPN as a charge nurse in a long-term care setting. Amy is hearing through the grapevine that these jobs are highly competitive and often require a minimum of a year of experience as an LPN, before hire. Assist Amy in creating a plan for success in meeting her goal. When should she initiate this plan? Why?

Scenario 2

During Paul's medical-surgical clinical rotation, an assigned patient, Mr. R., is preparing to go home after a 2-day hospitalization. The patient shows Paul a list of health care workers he has come in contact with during his hospitalization and marvels at the number of people involved in his care in only 2 days of hospitalization. Mr. R. asks Paul to explain why there are all types of nurses, RNs, LPNs, and SPNs. What is Paul's explanation?

Objectives

On completing this chapter, you will be able to do the following:

1. Compare public and private health care agencies according to source of funding, services provided, examples of agencies, and possible places of employment for licensed practical/licensed vocational nurses (LPNs/LVNs).
2. Differentiate between official and voluntary agencies.
3. Explain what is meant by private health care agencies as the usual entry into the health care delivery system in the United States.
4. Give an example of: official government public health care agency in your area; official government public health care agency in your state; official government public health care agency at the federal level.
5. Identify the federal health care agency in the United States that is headed by an appointee of the president and advises the president in health matters.
6. List eight agencies that make up the U.S. Public Health Service (USPHS).
7. Describe the responsibility of the World Health Organization (WHO).
8. Explain the difference between for-profit (proprietary) and nonprofit health care agencies.
9. Discuss how primary care relates to family practice physicians.
10. Differentiate between general and specialized hospitals.
11. Explain the purpose of teaching and research hospitals.
12. Discuss the difference between ambulatory and acute care settings.
13. Describe free clinics as a source of primary care.
14. Differentiate among the types of long-term care.

Key Terms

acute care (ă-KŪT)
adult day care center (ă-DŬLT)
ambulatory care facilities (ĂM-bū-lă-tŏr-ē kar fă-sil-i-tēs)
ambulatory surgery centers (ĂM-bū-lă-tŏr-ē SŬR-jĕr-ē SŬN-tĕrs)
assisted care (ă-SĬS-tĕd kār)
board and care homes (bŏrd kār hōms)
community health nursing (kŏm-Ū-nĭ-tē)
continuing care retirement community (CCRC) (kŏn-TĬN-ū-ŭs)
Department of Health and Human Services (HHS)
free clinic (frē KLĬ-nĭc)
freestanding (frē STĂN-dĭng)
general hospitals (JĔN-ĕr-ăl HÔS-pĭ-tăls)
Green House (grēn hŏws)
home health nursing (hōm hĕlth)
hospice care (HÔS-pĭs)
long-term care (LTC) (lŏng tĕrm kār)

official (government) health care agencies (ō-FĬSH-ŭl)
outpatient clinic (ÔWT-pă-shĕnt KLĬ-nĭc)
palliative care (PĂL-ē-ă-tĭv)
primary care (PRĪ-măr-ē kār)
private health care agencies (PRĪ-vĭt)
proprietary hospitals (for profit) (prŏ-PRĪ-ĭ-tĕr-ē)
public health care agencies (PŬB-lĭk)
rehabilitation (rē-hă-bĭl-ĭ-tā-shēŭn)
residential care (rĕz-ĭ-DĔN-shŭl)
skilled nursing facility (SNF) (skĭld)
specialized hospital (SPĔ-shŭl-īzd HÔS-pĭ-tăl)
teaching and research hospital (TĔ-chĭng, RĒ-sĕrch)
United Nations (UN) (ū-NĪ-tĕd NĀ-shŭns)
U.S. Public Health Service (USPHS)
voluntary health care agencies (VÔL-ŭn-tăr-ē)
wellness center (WĔL-nĭs)
World Health Organization (WHO)

Keep in Mind

Over the course of a normal lifetime, most patients will need all levels of care and effective transitions between those levels. Understanding health settings along the continuum of care will assist you in guiding patients to resources and identifying your best "fit" as a new graduate licensed practical nurse/licensed vocational nurse (LPN/LVN). Find your passion and you will love your work!

All health care agencies are not the same. They differ in size, focus, quality of service, and how they are financed. Do some research before making an application for a job so you can make an informed choice about employment after you graduate. Compose questions to ask during an employment interview. Refer to Chapter 18 for ideas.

Critical Thinking

Why is it important for the LPN/LVN to understand the various types of health care settings. How does this assist the patient?

What is your vision for working as a nurse after you complete nursing school? What type of setting do you imagine yourself working at?

PUBLIC VERSUS PRIVATE HEALTH CARE AGENCIES

Health care entities, providing a vast array of services, are owned and operated today by public (government) and private entities, including both profit and non-profit entities. Table 15-1 outlines the major differences between public and **private health care agencies**. As you read about public and private health care agencies, think of them as potential sources of employment for the LPN/LVN. Also consider how the patient accesses these services, when they are needed, and how do patients finance the services provided.

PUBLIC HEALTH CARE AGENCIES

There are two types of **public health care agencies**: official and voluntary. Official (government) health care agencies have the following characteristics:

- Supported by tax money
- Accountable to the taxpayers and the government
- Primary emphasis on the delivery of disease prevention and wellness promotion programs
- Provider of direct health care services

Voluntary health care agencies have these characteristics:

- Supported by voluntary contributions
- Charges a fee for services (sometimes)
- Tuned in to public opinion but are accountable to their supporters
- Activities determined by supporter interest, not legal mandate
- Primary emphasis is on research and education
- May offer direct health services to the patient

Some official and voluntary health care agencies operate at the local, state, federal, and international levels.

EXAMPLES OF PUBLIC HEALTH CARE AGENCIES

Official Government Agencies

Local. The official health agency at the local level is the city or county health department. These agencies have the following characteristics:

- They are funded by local tax money, as well as by subsidies from the state and federal levels of government.
- They carry out state laws (mandated) concerning community health.
- They carry out nonmandated programs, such as health promotion programs.
- In collaboration with other government agencies they respond to community health issues (e.g., outbreak of a contagious disease)

Table 15-1 Comparison of Health Care Agencies in the Public and Private Sectors

	PUBLIC		PRIVATE
	OFFICIAL (GOVERNMENT)	NONOFFICIAL (VOLUNTARY)	
Support	Tax money	Voluntary contributions and fees for service	Fees for service
Primary service	Programs of disease prevention and wellness promotion	Research and education	Curing disease and illness
Additional services	Sometimes direct service of health care	Offer direct health services	Disease prevention and wellness promotion
Accountability	Taxpayers and government	Supporters, boards, and so forth	Owners
How programs determined	Mandated* and nonmandated	Supporter interest	Defined goals of the organization

*Some mandates can apply to all types of settings

State. Each state has a state health department. This official health agency has the following characteristics:

- It is funded by state tax money.
- It sometimes receives money from the federal government.

Federal (National). The official health agency at the federal level in the United States is the U.S. **Department of Health and Human Services (HHS)**.

- A person appointed by the president of the United States is head of the agency. This person advises the president in health matters.
- It is funded by federal taxes.

HHS has 11 operating divisions, including eight agencies in the **U.S. Public Health Services**. Pertinent agencies to your studies include:

- *U.S Food and Drug Administration (FDA).* Ensures that food, human and animal drugs, biological products, and medical devices and electronic products that emit radiation are safe and if applicable, effective.
- *Centers for Disease Control and Prevention (CDC).* Provides leadership in health prevention and promotion programs, and responds to public health emergencies.
- *National Institutes of Health (NIH).* Funds biomedical research in its own laboratories and in universities, hospitals, private research institutions, and private industry. Trains new researchers and promotes collecting and sharing of medical knowledge. The NIH consists of 27 institutes and centers, including the National Institute of Nursing Research (NINR).
- *Health Resources and Services Administration (HRSA).* Improves access to medical care by strengthening the health care workforce, building healthy communities, and achieving health equity.
- *Substance Abuse and Mental Health Services Administration (SAMHSA).* Improves the quality and availability of prevention, treatment, and rehabilitation services for persons who are dealing with addictive and mental disorders, as well as for their families and communities.
- *Agency for Healthcare Research and Quality (AHRQ).* Supports research aimed at improving the quality of care, reducing costs, broadening access, and improving patient outcomes.
- *Agency for Toxic Substance and Disease Registry (ATSDR).* Works to prevent exposure and to minimize adverse health effects associated with exposure to hazardous substances from waste sites, unplanned releases, and other sources of environmental pollution.
- *Indian Health Services (IHS).* Provides comprehensive health services to American Indians and Alaskan Natives.
- *Centers for Medicare and Medicaid Services (CMS).* Provides oversight of the Medicare Medicaid (federal), Children's Health Insurance Programs, the Health Insurance Marketplace, and related quality assurance activities.

The preceding definitions were based on information retrieved from HHS.gov

International. Health activities take place at the international level through the **World Health Organization (WHO)**, an agency of the **United Nations (UN)**. It acts as a coordinating authority on international public health.

- WHO is located in Geneva, Switzerland.
- The major objective of WHO is the highest possible level of health for people all over the world.
- WHO defines *health* as a state of complete physical, mental, and social well-being and not merely as the absence of disease or infirmity.
- WHO is funded through fees paid by member nations of the United Nations.
- Coordinates international efforts to control outbreaks of infections, such as Middle East Respiratory Syndrome (MERS), Sudden Acute Respiratory Syndrome (SARS), malaria, tuberculosis, influenza, and human immunodeficiency virus/acquired immune deficiency syndrome (HIV/AIDS). Also sponsors programs to prevent and treat such diseases.

◎ **Try This**

Local Health Care Agency

Identify an official and voluntary health care agency in your geographic area. What services does each agency provide locally?

VOLUNTARY HEALTH CARE AGENCIES

Voluntary or nonofficial health care agencies (Table 15-2) are so named because they are nonprofit. The health services they provide are complementary to **official (government) health care agencies**. They often meet the needs of persons with specific diseases (e.g., heart disease) and certain segments of the population (e.g., those with disabilities). Although paid personnel work in voluntary health agencies, volunteers support the system. Voluntary organizations are sites for volunteer service and can provide a clinical experience for student practical nurses/student vocational nurses (SPNs/SVNs) and LPNs/LVNs. (Visit the Internet for additional names and numbers of voluntary health care agencies in your region.)

PRIVATE HEALTH CARE AGENCIES

You may be most familiar with private health care agencies:

- Entrance to the health care delivery system in the United States is generally gained through private health care agencies.
- Private health care entities include both profit and nonprofit institutions.
  - Faith-based entities often own health care facilities as a nonprofit entity
  - Corporations often own a chain of health care facilities. This has been increasing in the last

Table 15-2 Examples of Voluntary Agencies

AGENCY	PURPOSE	CONTACT
American Cancer Society (ACS)	Cancer research, public information resource to patients, families, professionals	www.cancer.org
American Diabetes Association (ADA)	Resource for diabetic care and management including nutrition information, resources, and educational programs	www.diabetes.org
American Lung Association (ALA)	Research, professional education, resource for professionals and public	www.lungusa.org
American Heart Association (AHA)	Research and education on heart disease and stroke	www.heart.org
American Stroke Association	Research and education on stroke	www.strokeassociation.org
Alcoholics Anonymous	Rehabilitation help and support to patients and families experiencing difficulty with alcohol addiction	www.aa.org
ALS Society of America	Collects data on persons with amyotrophic lateral sclerosis (Lou Gehrig's disease) for research purposes; resource for public and professionals	www.alsa.org
Easter Seals National Headquarters	Research and rehabilitative services for disabled children and adults	www.easterseals.org
La Leche League	Information and support for breastfeeding mothers; breast milk for infants because of health reasons but lack a source	www.lalecheleague.org
Narcotics Anonymous (NA)	Rehabilitation help and support to patients and families experiencing difficulty with narcotic addiction	www.na.org
United Ostomy Association of America (UOA)	Education, information, and advocacy for patients undergoing intestinal or urinary diversion procedures	www.ostomy.org

decade in an effort to achieve low-cost, high-quality outcomes.

- Small groups of individuals (i.e., physicians, community members) can own a health care facility. This has been decreasing in number because of increasing health care costs.
- Health care systems often exist offering a continuum of health care services (i.e., acute care, subacute, long-term care, home care, and outpatient services).
- Charge a fee for their services. Generally achieved by a payment system consisting of a patient copay and health care insurance or government-based payment (Medicare/Medicaid).
- Primary emphasis in the last decade was to cure disease and illness, however, a strategic shift has occurred focusing on disease prevention and wellness promotion,
- Government mandates, such as the recent Affordable Care Act (ACA), can impact access for patients and payment structures.

Family Practice Physicians

Primary care is the term used to describe the point at which an individual enters the health care system. Family practice physicians are a source of primary care. They provide diagnosis and treatment. The patient is billed a fee for these services. If further diagnostic evaluation is needed, the patient is referred to a specialist. Medical doctors function within the Medical Practice Acts of their respective states. Physician extenders are often used today to meet the needs of patients, particularly in urban and rural areas. Physician extenders include physician assistants and advanced practice registered nurses (APRN).

Private Practice Nurses

Specializing in primary health care, APRNs provide consulting and counseling services to groups or individuals. These nurses practice in all areas of health care. APRNs fill an especially acute need in rural areas where physician services are sometimes difficult to obtain. In addition, the Affordable Care Act has fueled the need for APRNs in all geographic settings. The nurses function within the Nurse Practice Act of their respective states. (See Chapter 7.)

TYPES OF HOSPITALS

According to the American Hospital Association (AHA) 2013 Annual Survey, there are 5686 registered hospitals in the United States. The majority of these hospitals comprise three groups: community hospitals, federal government hospitals, and nonfederal psychiatric hospitals. Both federal government hospitals and community hospitals can be teaching and research hospitals.

COMMUNITY HOSPITALS

AHA defines community as including nonfederal, short term general, and **specialty hospitals**. Most of the registered community hospitals are short-term **general hospitals**, providing a diverse range of medical services. This setting for health care is generally called **acute care**.

For most conditions, a general hospital is able to accommodate a patient's needs. However, a general hospital may not have specialists with expertise for treating serious or unusual medical problems. They also may not have the equipment, laboratory facilities, and other resources necessary to treat a serious or unusual medical condition. The patient may need to be treated in a hospital center that has highly-skilled specialists with advanced knowledge of the condition. Specialty hospitals offer services related to a particular disease or condition (e.g., trauma center, obstetrics and gynecology; eye, ear, nose, and throat; rehabilitation; orthopedic; and other).

Community associations and religious organizations operate nonprofit community hospitals. These nonprofit hospitals provide short-term inpatient care for people with acute illnesses and injuries. **Nonprofit community hospitals** are dependent on gifts and donations to supplement sources of revenue. Ultimate responsibility for the hospital rests with the board of trustees, usually chosen from the community's business and professional people, who serve without pay. The board of trustees appoints a paid administrator to manage the hospital.

For-profit community hospitals, sometimes referred to as **proprietary hospitals**, are operated for the financial benefit of the owner of the hospital and investors. The owner may be an individual, a partnership, or a corporation. With good management techniques, the hospital can be run efficiently, and a profit can be realized.

FEDERAL OR STATE GOVERNMENT HOSPITALS (PUBLIC HOSPITALS)

Public hospitals include Veterans' Health Administration (VHA), state, county, and municipally owned and operated nonprofit hospitals. Hospitals for people with serious mental illness continue to be funded by federal, state, or county funds.

TEACHING AND RESEARCH HOSPITALS

Both community hospitals and federal government hospitals can be **teaching and research hospitals**. These hospitals have a variety of goals, including the following:

- Treating patients, especially those with serious or unusual conditions
- Training sites for physicians, nurses, and other health professionals
- Researching and developing treatments for disease conditions, health promotion and strategies to deliver low-cost, high-quality care.

These hospitals are almost always affiliated with medical schools and have access to highly skilled practitioners.

CRITICAL ACCESS HOSPITALS

HRSA has provided specific Medicare Conditions of Participation for hospitals located in rural settings who meet several criteria. According to HRSA (2015) some of the requirements for critical access hospital (CAH) certification include:

- no more than 25 inpatient beds
- an annual average length of stay of no more than 96 hours for acute inpatient care offering 24-hour, 7-day-a-week emergency care
- located in a rural area, at least 35 miles drive away from any other hospital or CAH.

CAH provides care for common conditions and outpatient care, while stabilizing and referring more complex conditions to larger health systems.

(◎) Try This

Hospitals

What kind of hospitals do you have in your area? Do they currently employ LPNs/LVNs? If so, which nursing units employ LPNs/LVNs?

BEYOND THE HOSPITAL SETTING

In recent years, accelerated by the implementation of the Affordable Care Act, patient care services are being delivered less in an acute care or specialty hospital. Patients are more likely to receive care in a sub-acute or community-based setting, including their home. Care delivered in an ambulatory care-based or community-based setting versus an acute care setting generally results in cost savings for the insurance company. Patients are incentivized to receive care in these settings through lower copays and deductibles.

AMBULATORY SERVICES

The continual rise in cost of inpatient care has resulted in the rapid development of a variety of ambulatory services. As a consequence, the number of inpatient days and the length of stay in acute care facilities have decreased. Ambulatory services offer less expensive care because admission to an acute care facility is avoided. People come to these facilities for assessment, advice, monitoring, teaching, treatment, evaluation, and care coordination.

Private sector ambulatory settings are located in the following places:

- University hospital outpatient departments
- Community hospital outpatient departments
- Physician group practices
- Health maintenance organizations (HMOs)

- Physicians' offices
- Freestanding ambulatory centers
- Urgent care centers
- Nursing care centers

Public sector ambulatory settings include the following:

- Community health clinics
- Indian Health Service
- Community and migrant worker health centers

OUTPATIENT CLINICS

Outpatient clinics provide follow-up care to patients after hospitalization and have the following characteristics:

- Manage disease on an ambulatory basis for those who do not need to be hospitalized.
- Are a part of health care facilities or are **freestanding** (i.e., not attached to a hospital).
- Function by appointment only.
- Include specialty areas, such as diabetes, neurology, allergy, and oncology.
- Number of specialized clinics depends on the population of the area and the medical needs of the population.
- Employ a diverse group of interprofessional health team members.

URGENT CARE CENTERS

Services are available in **ambulatory care facilities** for walk-in patients who do not have an appointment. For some individuals, they replace doctor's offices. These facilities have the following characteristics:

- Make primary health care available as an alternative to care by a family physician or care offered in a more expensive emergency room.
- Used by people who do not have a family physician.
- Used by patients who desire more convenient service outside of regular office hours.
- Names given to ambulatory care services reflect the type of care provided (e.g., convenience clinics, express care, quick care, urgent care).

ONE-DAY SURGICAL CARE CENTERS

One-day surgical care centers (**ambulatory surgery centers**) perform surgery at a scheduled date and time. Patients are discharged when they have recovered from anesthesia and are considered to be in stable condition. These surgery centers have the following characteristics:

- Eliminate the need and monetary charge for being hospitalized overnight.
- Services are also known as outpatient surgery within an established hospital.
- Freestanding outpatient surgery centers provide outpatient surgery as their only service.
- Most types of surgeries can be performed in these settings.
- Complex surgical procedures or a complex patient history may prevent a patient from receiving care at an outpatient surgery center.

⊚ Try This

Ambulatory Care Providers

What are ambulatory health services in your area called? Do any of them employ LPNs/LVNs? If so, what skills will the LPN/LVN perform under registered nurse (RN)/physician supervision?

FREE CLINICS

Some communities have established **free or reduced fee clinics** as an alternative means of providing primary health care. These free clinics have the following characteristics:

- Persons who cannot afford traditional health services or are reluctant to use more traditional services use the clinics. Cost is based on income.
- Generally have an age and/or income limit.
- Generally staffed by one salaried administrator and volunteer physicians and nurses.
- A volunteer board makes policy decisions for the clinic.

ALTERNATIVES TO NURSING HOMES

COMMUNITY BASED CARE

Many older adults live at home accessing services in the home and in the community to assist in meeting their health care needs. Independent and assisted-living facilities can provide some services while allowing the older adult to "age in place".

Home Health Nursing

Home health agencies are public or private agencies that provide home health services, supervised by a licensed health professional in the patient's home, either directly or through arrangements with other agencies. Some examples of home health agencies include the following:

- Public, nonprofit (e.g., visiting nurse association)
- Public, nonprofit, freestanding (e.g., city, county, including county visiting nurse associations, and state health departments)
- Private or nonprofit hospital-based (e.g., hospital home health agency)
- Private, for-profit, freestanding (e.g., home health care owned by person or corporation)

Home health nursing differs from hospital and nursing home care by increased focus on relationship-centered care (i.e., family and the patient's environment). The purpose is to promote, maintain, or restore health or minimize the effects of illness or disability. An important role is to teach the patient and family self-care. Skilled services in home health care include the following:

- Skilled nursing
- Physical therapy
- Speech-language therapy
- Occupational therapy
- Medical-social services

- Homemaker–health aide services
- Other therapy services may be offered (e.g., respiratory, nutritional, podiatry)

Skilled nursing services are provided and directed by RNs. Basic nursing services are provided by LPNs/LVNs under the supervision of an RN. *Depending on state regulations and agency policy,* LPNs/LVNs are able to provide many home health services. The plan of care for all disciplines requires a treatment plan signed off by a physician and recertified according to current regulations. Examples include, but are not limited to, the following:

- Teaching, supervising, administering, or preparing medications for self administration
- Administering injections
- Blood glucose testing
- Assisting in creating a safe environment
- Treatments
  - Ostomy care
  - Wound care and dressings
  - Bowel and bladder retraining
  - Oxygenation and respiratory care

◎ Try This

Community Health Services

Are there community health nursing services or home-care agencies available where you live? What services do they offer? Which of them employ LPNs/LVNs? What skills are the LPNs/LVNs expected to perform under RN supervision?

Community Health Nursing Services

Nurses have always been at the forefront of **community health nursing** activity. The major focus of community health nursing is to improve the health status of communities or groups of people through public education, screen for early detection of disease, and provide services for people who need care outside the acute care setting.

Community health nurses work with many different people and groups on prevention and modification of health issues. Among the many possible roles are advocate, caregiver, case finder, health planner, occupational health nurse, school nurse, and teacher. Community health nursing services may exist as a part of an outpatient clinic service, a service attached to an HMO, or a freestanding private service.

Adult Day Care Centers

Hospital-based and freestanding **adult day care centers** provide services for individuals who need supervision because of physical or safety needs but are not candidates for residing in a nursing home. Patients with families who are able to assist the person during evening hours and on weekends may prefer adult day care centers instead of admission to a nursing home.

The purpose of adult day care is to provide mental stimulation, socialization, assistance with some activities

of daily living (ADL), and basic observation skills and a safe environment. Some typical services include transportation, meals, therapeutic activities, nursing interventions, and rehabilitation activities. The supervisor is often a social worker or RN. Certified nursing assistants (CNAs) and personal care assistants who meet state requirements assist with ADLs. Volunteers play a major role in some of the adult day care centers. Some large adult care centers employ LPNs working in collaboration with the RN.

◎ Try This

Adult Day Care Services

Is adult day care available in your area? Where are the centers located, what services are offered, and who staffs them? Do they employ LPNs/LVNs? If so, what are the LPNs'/LVNs' responsibilities?

Independent Living Facilities

Independent living apartments are not licensed or regulated for health care delivery. People living in these facilities are not there for personal or medical care, but they like to live with seniors who share their interests. Generally, planned activities and trips and bus service for shopping are offered. Aging in place has been a trend in the last several years. The elderly may effectively and safely age in place in an independent living apartment, however an assisted living environment is designed specifically to support "aging in place".

Assisted Living Programs

Assisted living programs (ALPs) provide "a home with services" (**assisted care**) that emphasizes a resident's privacy and choice. Living quarters are used by older adults who want to remain as independent as possible but cannot manage all of their ADLs. Residents typically have private, locking rooms and bathrooms (or apartments), shared only by choice. Living quarters are handicap accessible and are planned to accommodate the changing needs of residents as they age. Help with daily routine is available but not 24-hour basic care. These services can include bathing, dressing, daily activities, and health maintenance. Care management and skilled nursing services, when needed, come from an outside agency. ALPs accept private pay and some accept Medicaid, and Social Security Supplemental Income (SSI) recipients. The facilities are family oriented, provide activities, and assist the resident with travel to outside appointments. The fee for one- or two-bedroom apartments typically include utilities, weekly housecleaning, and linen changes. An additional fee is charged for meals, assistance with medication administration, and assistance with ADLs. Services may be added assisting the individual to "age in place". However, if needed and desired, the resident can be moved into the skilled nursing facility if that level of care becomes necessary. Some institutions offer a full continuum of 55+ living options, including independent living, assisted living, and skilled care, and are generally called continuing care retirement community (CCRC). Dementia care units may also be available.

Continuing Care Retirement Community

A **continuing care retirement community (CCRC)** provides a continuum of living options from independent living, enriched living, assisted living, and skilled nursing home, all on one campus. Residents can move from one level of care to another, accommodating their changing needs. A complete range of housing and health care are offered. Residents generally enter when relatively healthy and transition to care according to need. Short-term skilled care is also often available for residents who have had a surgical procedure or medical complication and require rehabilitation. Financial payment options can be complex and should be evaluated carefully by the patient and the family. Several options exist including a life-care or extended contract, modified contract or fee-for-service contract. The life care contract has a high entrance fee, however it offers unlimited assisted living and skilled care as needs arise. Some applicants can be denied admission because of their health history. The fee-for-service contract requires assisted living and skilled care to be paid for at market rates. Many variations exists and the "fit" is critical from both a financial and quality-of-life aspect. Visit the site aarp.org for more details.

Board and Care Homes

Board and care homes are also known as adult care homes, group homes, or family-type homes. The facilities offer temporary or long-term **residential care**, housekeeping, and personal care for a small number of adults unrelated to the operator. Assistance with ADLs, self-administration of medication, preparation of meals, special diets, and transportation are usually supervised and provided by the owner or manager. The residence may be a single-family home. The residence is licensed as an adult family home or adult group home. The Department of Social Services generally oversees the operation.

INSTITUTIONAL SETTINGS

Nursing Facilities

Nursing facilities specialize in skilled nursing care (SNF), sub-acute care and long-term care (LTC). The care is paid for by:

- Private pay
- Health insurance
- Medicaid
- Medicare. Health care plans will pay for skilled services but not for personal (sometimes referred to as custodial) services unless they are a part of a skilled care service plan of care. See www.longtermcarelink.net/eldercare/long_term_care.htm for more information.

HOW THE OMNIBUS BUDGET RECONCILIATION ACT RELATES TO SKILLED NURSING FACILITIES

The Omnibus Budget Reconciliation Act (OBRA) of 1987 was partially in response to evidence of mistreatment, abuse, and neglect of nursing home residents during the 1970s and 1980s. The Institute of Medicine set out detailed recommendations for improving care, and these recommendations became the basis of OBRA 1987. The CMS implemented the law over a period of years. Rules were not strongly enforced, and by 1998, changes were made in the law. The change omitted language regarding nursing coverage for SNFs and intermediate nursing facilities (ICFs). In 1999, the language for nursing care was reinstated. It mandates that all SNFs and ICFs would be required to have 24-hour licensed nursing services 7 days a week and at least one RN employed 8 hours a day, 7 days a week. Requests for waivers for LPN and RN coverage are reviewed and approved by the CMS.

According to *www.healthaffairs.org*, the following evidence exists of improvement in care:

- Declining use/elimination of physical and chemical restraints
- Lower rates of urinary infections and use of catheters
- Fewer hospitalizations

Areas that have shown limited change include the following:

- Pressure sore rates
- Malnutrition
- Dehydration
- Other feeding problems
- Increase in bowel incontinence cases

TYPES OF CARE

LONG-TERM CARE FACILITIES

Long-term care (LTC) includes a range of medical services designed to help people who have disabilities or chronic care needs. Common reasons for long-term care include cardiovascular disease, mental and cognitive disorders, and endocrine disease (Christensen and Cockcrow, 2011). All long-term facilities focus on promoting independence, maintaining function, and supporting autonomy. Medicare, Medicaid, and the VHA/Veterans Benefit Administration (VBA) will cover the cost of long-term care under certain conditions. If a veteran is at least 70% service-connected disabled, the VHA/VBA will cover the cost of nursing home care indefinitely (see www.longtermcarelink.net/eldercare/long_term_care.htm).

WHAT IS SKILLED NURSING CARE?

Skilled Nursing Facility

In a **skilled nursing facility**, services and supplies can be provided by or under the supervision of skilled or licensed nursing personnel. Skilled care is considered care that is medically necessary to improve the quality of the patient's health or to maintain or slow decompensation of a patient's condition, including palliative treatment. See www.longtermcarelink.net/eldercare/long_term_care.htm for more information.

- RNs and collaborating LPNs/LVNs plan the care of the patient including wound care after major surgery, administering medications, including administering/monitoring intravenous medications for a severe infection or other health issue.
- Physical therapists (PTs) help to correct strength and balance problems that have made it difficult for a patient to walk or get on and off the bed, toilet, or furniture. This also increases safety.
- A speech therapist helps to regain the ability to communicate after a stroke.
- An occupational therapist (OT) may also be needed on a long-term basis if the patient requires adaptive assistance using the upper body. Examples of therapy may include assistance in learning how to dress or feed themselves. In addition, the OT assesses the environment for adaptive equipment or room redesign to enhance safety and independence.

Monitoring vital signs, administering medications, performing wound care, and other procedures are normally associated with skilled care. Delivery of skilled care is based on a written care plan. Residents who meet Medicare requirements and are classified as skilled care receive payment from Medicare and private sources. There are many specific requirements that must be met to access Medicare dollars, including a recent inpatient hospital (acute) admission, of at least three days. An observation admission at an acute care hospital does not qualify. It can appear confusing to the patient whether they were an observation admission or an inpatient admission, as they may reside on the same unit and receive similar care. Be an advocate. Encourage your patients and families to seek understanding regarding their admission status. The impact can be thousands of dollars. See www.medicare.gov/coverage/skilled-nursing-facility-care.html for details.

Innovative elder living models. Various diverse elder living models exist today that are focused on deinstitutionalizing long-term care by eliminating large nursing facilities and creating smaller units which mirror more closely a typical home environment. A relationship between staff, management, residents and families is encouraged including introducing pets, gardens, and children to the nursing home. These models generally are focused on allowing the resident to have more autonomy and choice as they would enjoy living in their own home. Choices could include when to get up in the morning and timing for meals and activities. Social interaction is emphasized and facilitated by the design of the unit and surrounding environment. Defined resident space is coordinated with small collaborative space creating an environment that encourages interaction. Small dining rooms, encouraging a family like atmosphere, are generally found in lieu of a large dining hall. This design can be described as the Greenhouse Model or the Household/Neighborhood model.

Short-term care. Short-term care, also called sub-acute care and previously referred to as transitional care, refers to Medicare nursing home coverage after a three-day hospital stay. It is provided by many long-term care facilities or hospitals. Included are rehabilitation services, specialized care for certain conditions such as stroke and diabetes, postsurgical care, and other services associated with the transition from hospital to home. The goal is to discharge residents to their home or to a lower level of care (see www.longtermcarelink.net/eldercare/long_term_care.htm).

Try This

Long-Term Care Facilities

What long-term care facilities are located in your area? What level of care do they offer? Do they hire LPNs/LVNs? If so, what skills will the LPN/LVN be expected to perform?

PERSONAL CARE

Personal care is when individuals who are neither trained nor licensed can safely and reasonably provide services and supplies. It includes assistance with ADLs such as the following:

- Bathing
- Dressing
- Eating
- Grooming
- Getting in and out of bed
- Walking around
- Toileting (incontinence care)

OTHER TYPES OF FACILITIES/SERVICES

REHABILITATION SERVICES

After a patient has been stabilized following an acute illness or injury, a **rehabilitation** phase, lasting from days to years, may follow. Rehabilitation may take place in the following facilities:

- Rehabilitation centers
- Long-term care facilities
- Outpatient facilities
- Group residential homes
- Patient's home

The focus, regardless of the setting, is the return of function and prevention of further disability.

Try This

Rehabilitation Services

Where are the rehabilitation health services available in your area? What kind of rehabilitation is available? Do they hire LPNs/LVNs? If so, what skills will the LPN/LVN perform with RN supervision?

Wellness Centers

An emphasis on promoting wellness continues to result in a multitude of services being offered in this area of health care. Not only have hospitals developed programs to detect disease in early stages, but they also have developed programs to promote wellness. **Wellness center** programs include nutritional counseling, exercise programs, stress reduction, and weight control. The private sector continues to be active in the wellness area. People have developed an interest in exercise and fitness clubs, weight-reduction programs such as Weight Watchers, smoking cessation classes, stress control, and parenting classes. Wellness programs also exist within a CRCC. LPNs are often employed to work in collaboration with the RN or APRN.

◎ Try This

Wellness Programs

Choose one wellness program in your area. Find out what services it offers and the qualifications of the staff that provide the information. Which programs employ LPNs/LVNs?

HOSPICE CARE

Hospice, or end-of-life, services are available in many areas to persons who have been certified as terminally ill. The philosophy of **hospice care** is to maintain comfort as death approaches. The hospice may be in an institutional setting, such as a hospital or a freestanding agency. Hospice care is offered in the institution, especially if pain and symptom management is necessary, the family caring for the person needs respite, or for terminal care. Hospice home care is also available to those who wish to die in their own home. Because RNs, LPNs/LVNs, home health aides, CNAs, and volunteers all staff hospice, home care can be tailored to the person's needs. **Palliative care** provides comfort care, similar to hospice care. However, palliative care is often initiated at the onset of treatment and can be accessed at any stage of illness, whether terminal or not. While receiving palliative care, the patient may still choose to receive life-saving implementations.

◎ Try This

Develop Your Own Style

Using clustering (concept mapping) as shown in Chapter 2 as your guide, develop your own style/form to summarize the health care settings described in this chapter.

? Critical Thinking

Has My Vision Changed?

Throughout your course of study, you will find that your interest in a particular area of nursing may change or be modified. Based on what you have learned from reading this chapter, what kind of health care setting is most appealing to you at this time?

? Critical Thinking

Patient Care Transitions

Given the diverse array of patient care settings, how will you support the patient to understand the continuum of care that will best meet their needs and achieve the highest level of patient independence?

Get Ready for the NCLEX-PN® Examination

Key Points

- Health care services are delivered in public and private sectors.
- Public health care agencies are classified as official and voluntary.
- Official public health care agencies are supported by taxes.
- Official public health agencies are local, state, and federal agencies.
- The official health agency at the federal level in the United States is the U.S. Department of Health and Human Services (HHS)
- The public health care agency of the United Nations is WHO.
- Voluntary health care agencies are supported by contributions and provide complementary services to official health care agencies.
- Private health care agencies are generally proprietary (for profit).
- The majority of hospitals comprise three groups: community hospitals, federal government hospitals, and nonfederal psychiatric hospitals.
- Primary care describes the point at which people usually enter the health care system.
- General hospitals deal with a full range of medical and surgical conditions.
- Specialized hospitals are limited to patients with specific diseases.
- Teaching and research hospitals offer treatment for serious or unusual conditions and usually are a training site for health professionals.
- Ambulatory health care services are available in both private and public sectors.
- Free clinics provide primary care for persons who cannot afford traditional health care services.
- Short-term care, also known as sub–acute care or transitional care, provides rehabilitation services and specialized care as a transition between hospital and home.
- Long-term care facilities provide a range of services for people with severe disabilities and chronic care needs.
- New elder living models (e.g., Green House) provide an innovative approach different from traditional skilled care and assisted living facilities aimed at improving the resident experience.

- Board and care homes, also known as adult care homes, group homes, or family-type homes, offer housing and personal care.
- Assisted care facilities support "aging in place".
- Continuing care retirement communities provide a continuum of living options as needs change.
- Community health, public health, and home health share many responsibilities. A major difference in home health is providing direct patient care.
- Adult day care centers provide socialization, mental stimulation, and assistance with ADLs, basic observation, and health referrals.
- Wellness centers provide nutritional counseling, exercise programs, stress reduction, weight control, and other services.
- Hospice staff maintain comfort of the person as death approaches.
- Palliative care staff maintain comfort of the person at any point in their disease process.
- Responsibilities of care agencies continue to be modified because of changes in the health care system.

Additional Learning Resources

evolve Go to your Evolve website (http://evolve.elsevier.com/Knecht/success) for the following FREE learning resources:
- Answers to Critical Thinking Review Scenarios
- Additional learning activities
- Additional Review Questions for the NCLEX-PN® exam
- Helpful phrases for communicating in Spanish and more!

Review Questions for the NCLEX-PN® Examination

1. Which of the following health agencies is most likely to be a major resource if you have a measles outbreak at your health care institution?
   a. WHO
   b. CDC
   c. NIH
   d. FDA
2. Which statement best describes how official and voluntary agencies differ?
   a. Official agencies are proprietary.
   b. Voluntary agencies are tax supported.
   c. Official agencies provide primary care.
   d. Voluntary agencies emphasize research.
3. What quality/skill set described below would indicate a need for staff training when working with hospice?
   a. Knowledge of the physiologic process occurring as death approaches.
   b. Ability to sit without the need for dialogue, if desired by the individual.
   c. Feeling the need to tell the individual your beliefs about life after death.
   d. Willingness to honor the person's request for food, conversation, visitors, and so on.

Alternate Format Item

1. Indicate which statements accurately describe differences between community health nursing services and home health agencies. *(Select all that apply.)*
   a. Home health agencies provide direct nursing services to people in their home.
   b. Community health nursing services work on prevention and case finding.
   c. The Visiting Nurse Association and the County Health Department are examples of home health agencies.
   d. Home health agencies have an increased focus on family and the patient's environment.
   e. Home health agencies focus on population health versus individual health.
2. How do new new elder living models differ from traditional nursing homes? *(Select all that apply.)*
   a. Traditional homes provide personal care by assigning an LPN/LVN to give total care to the resident.
   b. New elder living models follow strict schedules for eating, bathing, and so on to provide a sense of security.
   c. In new elder living models, elders have flexibility in when they get up, eat, bathe, go outdoors, and receive visitors.
   d. New elder living models home design could minimize the need for wheel chairs.
   e. Traditional homes establish time frames for meals that meet the needs of the majority of the resident.
3. How will you explain the different levels of long-term health care to someone planning to seek placement for an elderly relative? *(Select all that apply)*
   a. Personal care can provide assistance with basic care needs and supervision to maintain a safe environment.
   b. Assisted care facilities offer 24-hour supervision and support the elderly to "age in place" - providing a flexible menu of services.
   c. Specialty hospitals can provide rehabilitation services following a major neurological event (i.e., stroke).
   d. Skilled care facilities can provide 24-hour supervision and access to many health care services, including dementia care.

Critical Thinking Scenarios

Scenario 1
Joni is graduating soon and is thinking about where she would like to work. While working in a nursing home, she developed an interest in working with elders. How might Joni find information about what is available in her area and what her responsibilities will be in each facility?

Scenario 2
Carman, is a new charge nurse at a skilled care facility. A current resident is being admitted the next morning for elective surgery. The son states, "It will be great to receive some Medicare coverage for Dad's care here when he returns from his surgery." What should you explain to the son regarding Medicare reimbursement for short-term care?

The Health Care System: Financing, Issues, and Trends

Objectives

On completing this chapter, you will be able to do the following:

1. Discuss the provisions of the Affordable Care Act.
2. Describe two general methods of financing health care costs.
3. Explain the different methods of payment options for patients (personal payment, private health insurance, health care exchanges, and public health insurance).
4. Identify sources of funding for public (government) health programs and private health insurance.
5. Discuss how quality, safety, cost, and access affect the direction of health care.
6. Explain how the licensed practical nurse/licensed vocational nurse (LPN/LVN) participates in increasing the quality and safety of health care and decreasing the cost of care.
7. Discuss the effect of the restructuring of the health care system on health care and employment opportunities for LPNs/LVNs.
8. Identify your reaction to change involving your nursing career and personal life.
9. Develop a personal plan to help you adapt to change in your nursing career and personal life.

Key Terms

alliances (ă-LĪ-ăns-ĕs)
capitation (kăp-ĭ-TĀ-sŭn)
coinsurance (KŌ-ĭn-sur-ăns)
continuous quality improvement (CQI) (kŏn-TĬN-ū-ŭs KWĂL-ĭ-tē ĭm-PROOV-mĕnt)
copayment (KŌ-pā-mĕnt)
cost containment (KŎST kŏn-TĀN-mĕnt)
deductibles (dĭ-DŬK-tĭ-bŭlz)
diagnosis-related group (DRG)
entitlement program (ĭn-TĪ-tĕl-mĕnt PRŌ-grăm)
fee-for-service (SĔR-vĭs)
health care provider (hĕlth kăr pră-VĪ-dĕr)
health maintenance organization (HMO)

Institute of Medicine (IOM)
managed care (MĂN-ăgd kăr)
Medicaid (mĕd-ĭ-KĀD)
Medicare (mĕd-ĭ-KĀR)
National Patient Safety Foundation (NPSF)
preferred provider organizations (PPOs) (prĕ-FĔRD)
premium (PRĒ-mē-ŭm)
private pay (PRĪ-vĭt)
prospective payment system (PPS) (pră-SPĔK-tĭv pā-mĕnt)
restructuring (rē-STRŬK-chŭr-ĭng)
"seamless" systems (SĒM-lĕs SĬS-tĕms)
third-party coverage (thĭrd PĂR-tē KŎV-răj)

Keep in Mind

Do you pay federal or state taxes? If you do, then you help pay for health care for others. Do you have health insurance? If you do not, who pays for your health care?

David, Stephanie, and Diane were chatting during lunch regarding health insurance coverage, particularly the Affordable Care Act. David commented, "It is very difficult to assist the patient in understanding their benefits and the possible advantage of the Affordable Care Act. There are so many rules, it's easy to misinterpret something. Most people know some basic principles, such as you cannot be denied coverage related to a preexisting illness. But beyond these basics . . . it is very complicated." Diane states, "I know what you mean. It is scary for the patient if they do not fully understand their benefits. Last

week, I had a patient who was admitted to the hospital for pneumonia for three days. Following this admission, the patient was being transferred to skilled care for reconditioning before returning home. Luckily, the patient realized the day they were being transferred that they had been on observation status instead of admission status and thus would not meet the criteria for Medicare payment for the skilled care (nursing home) facility. They opted for home care instead, to avoid the large out-of-pocket payment." It is an important role of the nurse to assist the patient in understanding their benefits, as well as assisting them to find the correct data is critical. The licensed practical nurse/licensed vocational nurse (LPN/LVN) plays a lead role in assisting the patients in understanding their benefits, particularly in the nursing home setting. *Consider this as you learn the finances of health care.*

THE UNITED STATES HEALTH CARE SYSTEM

The U.S. health care system has been described as a poorly organized and complicated maze of services that lacks preventive care, wastes resources, and is very expensive. Historical trends assist in understanding how this evolution occurred. In the early 1960s, the physician's key role in health care decision making combined with a fee-for-service payment model, contributed to spiraling health care costs and a lack of attention to cost containment (Cherry & Jacob, 2014). Procedures were ordered if they "might help." This process resulted in the unfolding of a very expensive, inefficient health care system. As a result, in the early 1980s, Medicare changed from a fee-for-service payment model to a prospective payment system based on diagnostic-related groups (DRGs). The hospital was paid for the patient based on the DRG. During this time period, the health care team was focused on minimizing the patient length of stay, through what became known as utilization management. In most cases, the shorter the stay, the more apt the hospital would make money. As time evolved, this payment system extended to include physician payment. Private insurers soon followed Medicare's lead and thus the birth of managed care organizations (MCO). MCOs include health maintenance organizations (HMOs), preferred provider organizations (PPOs), point-of-service plans (POS), and open access plans. Despite these changes, only a small overall improvement in health care costs was realized followed by continuing increased costs and inequities in health care **access**. Not all Americans had **access** to healthcare, particularly the underemployed. In addition, the poor often could not access care, despite health care coverage and a lack of preventative care. When people did have access to health care through some type of health insurance plan, problems of quality, service, and cost remained an issue. Many viewed the American health care system as broke and a drain to the overall economy of the nation.

> ### ? Critical Thinking
>
> **Who Deserves Health Care?**
>
> 1. Should all individuals in our society have access to health care?
> 2. Do you think health care is a right or a privilege?

HEALTH CARE REFORM: THE AFFORDABLE CARE ACT

In 2010, the Affordable Care Act (ACA), frequently referred to as "Obamacare," was signed into law by President Obama. As a national health care initiative, it was the first wide-sweeping piece of legislation to address health care reform in the United States since 1965, when Medicare was added to the Social Security Act.

This program was designed to enhance the access and affordability of health care, particularly to all citizens in financial need in the United States. Although controversial, this law has decreased the number of uninsured in the United States. The Agency for Healthcare Research and Quality (AHRQ) concludes that the proportion of uninsured adults under 65 fell from a high of 22% in 2010 to 16% in the second quarter of 2014, after the implementation of "Obamacare."

The ACA established a Health Insurance Marketplace. This is a resource where individuals, families, and small businesses learn about their health coverage options (including cost-effective, competitive health insurance plans), choose a plan, and enroll in coverage. The Marketplace also provides information on programs that help people with low to moderate income and resources pay for coverage.

> ### ◎ Try This
>
> **Health Care Reform: The Affordable Care Act (ACA)**
>
> How well do you understand how this law affects you and your patients? Answer True or False to the following questions about the law.
>
> 1. The law requires all Americans to have health insurance, or they must pay a fine.
> 2. The law allows a government panel to make decisions about end-of-life care for people on Medicare.
> 3. The law cuts benefits that were previously provided to all people on Medicare.
> 4. The law expands the existing Medicaid program and will cover more low-income, uninsured adults regardless of whether they have children.
> 5. The law will provide health insurance to undocumented immigrants.
> 6. The law increases Medicare payroll tax for Americans making more than $200,000/individual and $250,000/couple.
> 7. The law requires employers with more than 50 employees to provide health insurance.
> 8. The law cuts benefits for people receiving Medicare before implementation of the law.
> 9. The law will provide assistance for Americans (up to 400% of poverty) to purchase health care benefits if they are not covered by their employer.
> 10. The law prohibits insurance companies from denying coverage if you have a preexisting condition.
>
> **ANSWERS**
>
> 1 = T and F; 2 = F; 3 = F; 4 = T; 5 = F; 6 = T; 7 = F; 8 = F; 9 = T, 10 = T
>
> Modified from The Henry J. Kaiser Family Foundation (2015). Health Reform Quiz, http://kff.org/quiz/health-reform-quiz/.
> Explanations for the answers in the quiz and additional information that applies to the ACA can be found at http://kff.org/quiz/health-reform-quiz/. A timeline for implication of the ACA can be found at www.healthcare.gov. **Content in italics, contained in this chapter, further explains the ACA.**

Table 16-1 Comparison of Methods of Payment for Health Care Services

	FEE-FOR-SERVICE	CAPITATION
Services covered	Each health care service claimed by the physician (e.g., diagnostic tests, treatments)	Health care services in group contract
Are preventive tests or treatments covered?	Depends on the plan	Wellness practices covered
Cost	Set fee per member of group	Set fee per member of group
How revenue is increased	Increase health care services Increase patient visits	Decrease health care services Increase number of persons served
Advantages	All tests and treatments for illness covered	Wellness encouraged No deductibles and copayments
Disadvantages	Emphasis on illness, although some wellness activities are covered Deductibles and copayments keep patient from reporting illness in early stages	To realize a profit, needed tests may not be ordered facilitating early diagnosis

FINANCING HEALTH CARE COSTS

The two most common ways to finance health care services are **fee-for-service** and **capitation**.

FEE-FOR-SERVICE

The traditional method of paying health care bills is the system called fee-for-service. In this method, physicians are paid a fee for each service they provide.

- Physicians are directly reimbursed for most ordered diagnostic tests and treatments for illness.
- Some insurance companies do not reimburse the tests and treatments that could keep patients healthy or could identify illnesses in their early stages when they are less expensive to treat.
- To improve their margins of profit, insurance companies charge **deductibles**, **copayments**, and **coinsurance**.

CAPITATION

- Capitation is an alternative to the traditional fee-for-service method of payment.
- Capitation involves a set monthly fee charged by the provider of health care services for each member of the insurance group for a specific set of services.
- **Managed care** plans that use the capitation method of payment include **health maintenance organizations (HMOs), preferred provider organizations (PPOs)**, point of service (POS), and open access plans. In each of these plans, patient choice, copays, and deductibles can vary greatly.
- If health care services cost more than the monthly fee, the provider absorbs the cost of those services.
- At the end of the year, if any money is left over, the **health care provider** keeps it as a profit.
- Suddenly, if a provider of health care services can keep a member of the insurance group healthy, that provider will make a profit!

Before continuing, review Table 16-1 for a comparison of the fee-for-service and capitation methods of payment

Box 16-1 Health Insurance Terms

Premium: The monthly fee a person must pay for health care insurance coverage.

Deductible: The yearly amount an insured person must spend out-of-pocket for health care services before a health insurance policy will begin to pay its share.

Copayment: The amount an insured person must pay at the time of an office visit, when picking up a prescription, or before a hospital service.

Coinsurance: Once a deductible is met, the percentage of the total bill the insured person must pay. The insurance company pays the remainder.

Health care provider: A licensed health care person, such as a physician, dentist, or nurse practitioner, whose health care services are covered by a health insurance plan.

for health care services and Box 16-1 for health insurance terms. See Box 16-2 for different types of managed care plans.

HOW PATIENTS PAY FOR HEALTH CARE SERVICES

PERSONAL PAYMENT

Payment directly by the patient (i.e., **private pay**) was the primary method of payment of health care costs before the 1940s. The cost of health care services discourages the millions of people in the United States who do not have health care insurance from making personal payments.

PRIVATE HEALTH INSURANCE

Health insurance, like any insurance, spreads risk. The risk that is spread in health insurance is that the young and the healthy generally subsidize (support financially) the sick and older individuals in the health insurance group. Those who were likely to have high medical bills were denied health coverage before the ACA. *The ACA prohibits discriminating against people with preexisting*

Box 16-2 Managed Care Plans

HEALTH MAINTENANCE ORGANIZATIONS (HMO)
- Are generally located in buildings that are primarily for HMO business, and most physicians working in the HMO are hired specifically for the HMO.
- Receive a prepaid fee to provide comprehensive care to members of the enrolled group.
- Encourage prevention of disease by the practice of preventive medicine.
- Discourage physicians from ordering excessive diagnostic tests and treatments.
- Patients may not have the option of choosing their physician each time treatment is needed. If a physician is chosen outside the HMO network, the cost has to be paid by the patient.
- Depending on the HMO, a member may go outside the HMO to see a desired physician with a point-of-service (POS) option. With the POS option, the member pays an extra fee.

OPEN ACCESS PLANS
- Allow members to see specialist physicians in the network for treatment without need of a referral, as in traditional HMOs. This option may affect the subscriber's coinsurance.

PREFERRED PROVIDER ORGANIZATIONS
- PPOs are an alternative to the strict utilization review system of some managed care plans.
- Fees are paid by fee-for-service, and health insurance companies contract with physicians and hospitals and negotiate discount fees. These members of the network are "preferred" providers.
- Patients may choose to see any general physician or specialist in the network. If a patient chooses a preferred provider, a larger amount of the cost will be covered by the health care plan.
- Family practice physicians may be hired as members of a PPO. These physicians remain in the same office in which their family practice is located and continue to belong to the same physician group. Part of their day is spent treating patients in their own family practice, and part of the day is spent treating patients who are enrolled in the PPO under the rules of the PPO.

conditions; insurance companies are prohibited from refusing coverage to anyone based on their medical history or health status. The ACA also prohibits individual and group health plans from placing lifetime limits on the dollar value of coverage and prohibits insurance companies from rescinding coverage; for example, for a patient on chemotherapy.

Administrative costs of private health insurance can account for greater than 25% of premiums. These costs involve screening of applicants for denial of coverage, reviewing claims for reimbursement, profits to investors, and marketing.

Private Group Health Insurance

Group health insurance is a method of pooling individual contributions for a common group goal: protection from financial disaster as a result of health care bills. One day in the hospital can cost over $4000.00. Health care insurance provides people with the ability to afford health care. Before implementation of the ACA, many Americans could not afford health care insurance. The ACA has improved access. When insured, an individual is said to have **third-party coverage** (a fiscal middleman). This financial middleman pays the individual's health care bills. Employers offer most of the private group insurance in the United States. *The ACA does not require all employers to provide health benefits. However, it imposes penalties on larger employers (those with 50 or more workers) that do not provide insurance to their workers or that provide coverage that is unaffordable. Small businesses that offer health insurance receive a tax credit.*

Blue Cross and Blue Shield, available in 50 states, are examples of private group health insurance. Health insurance protects individuals from bills for unexpected illness.

Private Individual Health Insurance

Many major insurance companies offer health insurance to individuals who are not part of a group. **Premiums** are based on a person's health risk and age.

PUBLIC HEALTH INSURANCE

Veteran's Health Administration (VHA)

The United States has provided comprehensive health care services to all veterans since the 1800s. Today, the Veteran's Health Administration (VHA) continues to meet the health care needs of our Veterans inclusive of hospitals, outpatient clinics, nursing home care units, and domiciliaries. See www.va.gov for details.

Medicare: A Program of Social Security

People of retirement age find themselves ineligible for group insurance plans because they are not employed. This inability to get insurance occurs at the very time when individuals are more likely to encounter medical costs because of chronic disease.

- In 1965, **Medicare** was added to the Social Security Act.
- This federally sponsored **entitlement program** and public health insurance plan helps finance health care for all persons older than age 65 (and their spouses) who have at least a 10-year record in Medicare-covered employment and are a citizen or permanent resident of the United States.
- Coverage is also given to certain younger persons with disabilities and persons with end-stage renal disease.
- No person is denied coverage based on past medical history.

Box 16-3 Medicare Part A Provisions

Medicare Part A helps pay for inpatient hospital care. Part A is available without cost and is funded by a payroll tax; it includes a deductible and a coinsurance fee that starts on day 61 of hospitalization. In 2011, Medicare Part A helped pay for the following types of situations:

- Inpatient hospital care (e.g., a semiprivate room, meals, drugs, supplies, lab tests, radiology, and intensive care units).
- Twenty days' posthospitalization skilled nursing facility care (full cost) for rehabilitation services. The next 80 days are paid after a daily coinsurance.
- Under certain conditions, home health care services with coinsurance charges for medical equipment and hospice care for terminally ill beneficiaries.
- Part A does *not* pay for long-term care custodial services (e.g., patients who need help only with activities of daily living [including feeding]), private rooms, telephones, or televisions provided by hospitals and skilled nursing facilities.

Data from www.medicare.gov.

- In 2012, there were 49,435,610 Medicare Beneficiaries in the United States (Kaiser Family Foundation, 2015)
- Approximately 10,000 Baby Boomers each day become eligible for retirement benefits, placing huge demands on Social Security, including Medicare.
- Visit www.medicare.gov for more details.

Medicare health care plans (www.medicare.gov)
- Medicare Part A (Box 16-3)
  - Referred to as hospital insurance
  - Covers inpatient hospital stays, care in a skilled nursing facility, hospice care, and some home health care
- Medicare Part B (Box 16-4)
  - Referred to as medical insurance
  - Covers certain doctor's services, outpatient care, medical supplies, and preventive services
- Medicare Part C
  - Offered by a private company that contracts with Medicare
  - Can include HMOs, PPOs and fee-for-service plans, special needs plans, and Medicare Medical Savings Account Plans
  - Also offer prescription drug coverage
- Medicare Part D
  - Prescription drug coverage
  - Medicare drug legislation, passed in 2003, provided prescription drug coverage that helps to pay for brand-name drugs at participating pharmacies
  - Offered by insurance companies and other private companies approved by Medicare

Medicare supplement insurance
Medigap Coverage. Because of the items Medicare does not cover, beneficiaries are encouraged to purchase

---

Box 16-4 Medicare Part B Provisions

Medicare Part B is similar to a major medical insurance plan. Part B is funded by monthly premiums that are income related. Most people pay a standard monthly premium. However, if a person's modified adjusted gross income is above a set amount, you may pay an extra premium. In 2012, Medicare Part B helped to pay for medically necessary (needed for diagnosis and treatment of a medical condition) or preventive services, which included the following:

- Physician visits and other medical services
- Outpatient hospital services (including emergency room visits) and outpatient mental health
- Clinical laboratory services and diagnostic tests (x-rays, magnetic resonance imaging [MRI], computed tomography [CT] scans, electrocardiograms [EKGs])
- Ambulance transportation
- Durable medical equipment (wheelchairs, walkers, oxygen, hospital beds)
- Kidney supplies and services
- Some diabetic supplies
- Physical, occupational, and speech therapy in a hospital outpatient department or a patient who resides in a Medicare-certified bed in a rehabilitation agency
- Preventive services: "Welcome to Medicare" physical exam in the first 12 months after enrolling in Plan B and yearly health visits. A diverse array of health screenings and vaccinations are covered.
- Part B does *not* pay for most prescription drugs, routine physicals, services not related to treatment of illness or injury, dental care, dentures, cosmetic surgery, routine foot care, hearing aids, routine eye examinations, or routine glasses.

Data from www.medicare.gov.

---

private supplemental insurance, called Medigap, in addition to Medicare to cover copayments, deductibles, coinsurance, and limited-coverage situations that exist in the federal program. These policies are sold by private insurance companies.

Diagnosis-related groups. Payment for Medicare is a major item in the federal budget. In 2013, Medicare spending totaled $492 billion (Kaiser Family Foundation, 2015). Before 1983, hospitals submitted a bill to the government for the total charges they incurred for Medicare patients and were reimbursed for this amount. This was called a "retrospective payment" system because payment was based on actual costs.

- In 1983, the federal government attempted to stop the skyrocketing cost of health care.
- The former Health Care Financing Administration (now the Centers for Medicare and Medicaid Services [CMS]) adopted a system of paying hospitals a set fee or flat rate for Medicare services.
- Hospitals were told in advance how much they would be reimbursed.
- Because the federal government announces to a hospital in advance what it will pay for health care

costs, this system is called the **prospective payment system (PPS)**.

- Under the **diagnosis-related group (DRG)** system, a math formula is used to arrive at the fee the government will pay for hospitalization. This fee depends on the DRG category (illness) causing the patient's hospitalization.
- Hospitals receive a flat fee for each patient's DRG category regardless of length of stay in the hospital. Hospitals have an incentive to treat patients and discharge them as quickly as possible. If the hospital keeps the patient longer than the government's fee will cover and the patient cannot be reclassified in the DRG system, the hospital has to make up the difference in costs.
- If the acute care facility can treat the Medicare patient for less than the guaranteed reimbursement, the facility can keep the difference as profit.

Because Medicare patients, like all patients, are discharged sooner from hospitals than they were in the past (as a result of the PPS), extended care units are often used to continue convalescence.

Medicaid

The **Medicaid** program (Title XIX) was added to the Social Security Act in 1965. This program provides medical assistance for eligible families and individuals with low incomes and resources.

- Medicaid is a cooperative venture jointly funded by the federal and state governments. Table 16-2 provides a comparison of Medicare and Medicaid.
- The federal government establishes broad, national guidelines for Medicaid.
- Each state establishes its own program services and requirements, including eligibility. For this reason, when eligible for Medicaid in one state, an individual is not automatically eligible in another state.

- *Under the Affordable Care Act, Medicaid improvements continue to take full effect. The CMS continues to work with states to base their Medicaid and Children's Health Insurance Program (CHIP) on modified adjusted gross income (MAGI). See www.medicaid.gov for details. As a result, the ACA creates a uniform Medicaid eligibility level and income definition across all states and eliminates a prohibition that prevented states from providing Medicaid coverage to adults without dependent children. Undocumented immigrants and legal immigrants who have resided in the United States for less than five years are not eligible for Medicaid.*

COST OF HEALTH INSURANCE

The continual rise in health care costs has resulted in annual increases in health insurance premiums for employers. *The ACA requires the federal government to create a process in conjunction with states where insurers have to justify unreasonable premium increases.*

? | **Critical Thinking**

What Services Should Medicare Offer?

1. Should Medicare pay for new technological procedures that are developed to treat common medical problems of the elderly?
2. Should cost-effectiveness enter the picture for treating Medicare patients?

THE UNINSURED

According to the U.S. Census Bureau (2014), the percentage of people in 2013 without health insurance coverage was 13.4%, or 42.0 million.

This includes:

- **Low-wage employees.** This class of people is employed in low-wage jobs that are less likely to offer insurance benefits.

Table 16-2 **Comparison of Medicare and Medicaid**

	MEDICARE	MEDICAID
Purpose of program	Health care for persons 65 years and older who are eligible for Social Security, the disabled, and persons with end-stage renal disease and Lou Gehrig's disease	Medical and health-related services for persons with decreased income and resources that meet eligibility requirements
Source of funding	Federal government (i.e., your tax money) An entitlement health care program. Congress must fund Medicare each year, as opposed to a discretionary program, in which funding must be approved yearly.	An entitlement program jointly financed by the federal and state governments (your tax money). Medicaid is a major expenditure in federal and state budgets.
Who administers the program?	The federal government	Individual states. Variability relative to the Affordable Care Act.
Cost to individual to enroll	Part A: Hospital insurance for inpatient care. No cost for persons who meet eligibility requirements for Social Security. Part B: Medical insurance covering doctors' fees and so on. A premium or monthly fee is taken out of the monthly Social Security check when person registers for program.	No fee. Must meet income eligibility requirements.

- **The middle class.** Some of these workers are unemployed. Those employed may be priced out of the health care insurance market by rapidly rising health insurance premiums.
- *Since 2014, as a result of the ACA, citizens and legal residents must obtain health insurance or pay a penalty.*
  - *Groups exempt from this requirement include those who:*
    - *would have to pay more than 8.05% of their income for health insurance*
    - *have incomes below the threshold required for filing taxes*
    - *were uninsured for no more than two consecutive months of the year*
    - *lived in a state who did not expand its Medicaid program but who would have qualified for it*
    - *qualify for religious exemptions*
    - *are a member of a health care sharing ministry*
    - *are living abroad*
    - *are incarcerated*
    - *are members of American Indian tribes*
    - *are not lawfully present*
- Unemployment and a downturned economy increase the number of uninsured who seek treatment in emergency rooms.
  - Emergency room treatment is expensive and is intended for seriously ill or injured persons and not for less serious illnesses.
- Lack of access to health care prevents individuals from receiving preventive care and seeking treatment when a health problem develops.
  - These individuals may seek treatment during the later stages of illness, usually at greater expense. Cancer is an example of a disease that is best treated and possibly cured when diagnosed in its early stage.
  - Consider the case of a sinus infection. The most cost-effective means of diagnosing and treating a sinus infection is an assessment by a family physician or nurse practitioner. However, this solution is not realistic if you do not have health insurance, your insurance company does not cover this type of visit, or you do not have the money to pay for deductibles, copayments, coinsurance, or a retail clinic visit such as at Walmart. When the sinus infection reaches an acute stage, the individual might seek treatment at the local emergency department. Many people rely on emergency departments for all levels of health care because of lack of insurance.

? Critical Thinking

Who Pays the Health Care Bill?

If a patient does not have health insurance or the ability to pay the emergency room fee, who pays the bill?

QUALITY, SAFETY, AND COST OF HEALTH CARE

According to CMS (2015), the United States spent over $2.9 trillion on health care in 2013. Some reasons for the high cost of health care are the costs of prescription drugs, medical malpractice lawsuits, and continual development and use of medical technology. The United States has the highest health care spending of industrialized countries but has lower life expectancy and higher infant and maternal mortality than many of the industrialized countries of the world. The 2010 National Healthcare Quality and Disparities report states that Americans too often do not receive care that they need or receive care that causes harm. For all the money spent on health care, patients are not experiencing quality and safety in their health care.

The **Institute of Medicine (IOM)** is an independent, nonprofit organization that serves as an advisor to improve the nation's health. The IOM has released the following two reports that address the issue of quality, safety, and cost in health care. These reports have influenced the direction of health care and education of nurses in the twenty-first century.

- *To Err Is Human: Building a Safer Health Care System* (1999): This report found that up to 98,000 people die each year from preventable medical errors and presents a comprehensive strategy to prevent such errors.
- *Crossing the Quality Chasm: A New Health System for the 21st Century* (2009): This report provided six aims for improving the quality and safety of health care in the United States that should be adopted by all personnel providing health care.
- *Future of Nursing: Leading Change, Advancing Health (2010). This report makes recommendations for an action-oriented plan for the future of nursing, recognizing nurses' vital role in realizing the objectives of the ACA and advancing the health of the nation.*

IMPROVING QUALITY IN HEALTH CARE

1. *Continuous Quality Improvement (CQI)*: Quality by inspecting patient incidences of harm or mistakes *after* they had occurred during care. CQI focuses on *preventing* problems or adverse events.
   - Checklists are an example of a method used to ensure quality and safety when giving care. Checklists are a list of items or actions for a task where each item is checked off when completed. This helps the nurse remember parts of a procedure or intervention.
2. *Aims of the IOM for improving quality in health care:* The six aims of the IOM (2001) to increase *quality* in health care are referred to as STEEEP:
   - *Safe:* Avoid injuries to patients from the care that is intended to help them.
   - *Timely:* Reduce waits and sometimes-harmful delays for both those who receive and those who give care.

- *Effective:* Provide services based on scientific knowledge to all who could benefit and refrain from providing services to those not likely to benefit.
- *Efficient:* Avoid waste of equipment, supplies, ideas, and energy.
- *Equitable:* Provide care that does not vary in quality because of personal characteristics such as gender, ethnicity, geographic location, and socioeconomic status.
- *Patient-centered:* Provide care that is respectful of and responsive to individual patient preferences, needs, and values, and ensure that patient values guide all clinical decisions.

[?] Critical Thinking

Increasing Quality in Providing Care

Provide examples of content from your practical/vocational nursing program that help you meet the IOM aims to increase quality in health care.

3. *Continued competency:* An important component of quality health care is that the providers of that care be able to demonstrate competency throughout their careers. Current nursing licensure considers nurses from all levels of educational preparation minimally competent upon receiving the initial license, and continued competence is assumed throughout a career. Patients, lawmakers, employers, and professional organizations question this assumption. As this matter is debated and a method is devised to assure patients that their health care providers are competent and qualified, LPNs/LVNs need to update themselves continually in their area of practice.

IMPROVING QUALITY IN HEALTH CARE; PAYMENT METHODS/PENALTIES

Two payment methods, pay for performance (P4P) and never events, align payment with patient outcomes. P4P rewards hospitals and other entities for meeting and exceeding standards of care for a variety of diseases (e.g., diabetes, myocardial infarction, pneumonia, and heart failure). Never events are serious and highly preventable events. Hospital-acquired infections and injuries from a fall are examples of never events. Hospitals do not receive any reimbursement for never events, encouraging a proactive approach to preventing errors and promoting a safe environment.

A readmission reduction program has been implemented by CMS, resulting in a reduced payment when patients are readmitted to an acute care hospital within thirty days of discharge The applicable diagnosis includes acute myocardial infarction, heart failure, and pneumonia, and will soon be expanded to include chronic obstructive pulmonary disease and total knee and hip arthroplasty. This readmission reduction program triggered a strategic effort to improve transitions in care, inclusive of intensive education and follow-up services. The LPN/LVN has an instrumental role in identifying early complications and immediately intervening, thus preventing a readmission.

[◎] Try This

Licensed practical nurse/licensed vocational nurse role in decreasing hospital readmissions.

Describe how an LPN/LVN in a long-term care setting can effectively decrease a patient's readmission to the hospital.

IMPROVING SAFETY IN HEALTH CARE

1. *The Joint Commission (TJC) National Patient Safety Goals:* Nursing has always promoted safety first with patients: First, do no harm. TJC reviews adverse incidents studies on causes of serious harm and death to patients. The results are startling. For example, the Institute of Medicine's 1999 study estimated that 44,000 to 98,000 Americans die each year as a result of medical errors. High on the errors list is medication error. Improper patient identification is often a problem in giving medication and also in doing wrong-site surgery. Nurses are often involved in patient preparation for surgery and marking the site so no confusion exists during the surgical process. Additional information is available at http://www.jointcommission.org/PatientSafetyGoals. Box 16-5 provides a list of TJC 2015 Patient Safety Goals for hospitals.

2. *National Patient Safety Foundation (NPSF):* Created in 1997, the current vision of the NPSF (2015) is to create a world where patients and those who care

---

Box 16-5   The Joint Commission 2015 National Patient Safety Goals

HOSPITAL
- Improve the accuracy of patient identification (two identifiers)
- Improve the effectiveness of communication among caregivers
- Improve the safety of using medication
- Reduce the harm associated with clinical alarm systems
- Reduce the risks of health care-associated infections
- The hospital identifies safety risks inherent in its patients' population
- Universal protocol for preventing wrong-site, wrong-procedure, and wrong-person surgery

LONG-TERM CARE
- Improve the accuracy of resident identification
- Improve the safety of using medications
- Reduce the risk of health care-associated infection
- Reduce the risk of resident harm resulting from falls
- Prevent health care–associated pressure ulcers

Modified from The Joint Commission (TJC) (2015). *National patient safety goals*, www.jointcommission.org/assets/1/6/2015_hap_npsg_er.pdf, www.jointcommission.org/assets/1/6/2015_LTC2_NPSG_ER.pdf, www.jointcommission.org/assets/1/6/2015_NPSG_LT2.pdf.

for them are free from harm. As a central voice for patient safety, NPSF partners with patients and families, the community, and other stakeholders to improve patient safety by avoiding errors of commission (doing the wrong thing), omission (not doing the right thing), or execution (doing the right thing incorrectly). The NPSF offers a safety-focused certification, annual events, including patient safety awareness week, and a patient safety congress.

3. *Transition to Practice:* Transition to Practice, an initiative of the National Council of State Boards of Nursing, is aimed at improving the quality and safety of health care by improving the new graduates' transition to work. In collaboration with more than 35 nursing organizations, NCSBN developed an evidence-based Transition to Practice model. The model for acute care settings recommends a 9- to 12-month program to aide in the transition to the clinical setting. Details can be found at https://www.ncsbn.org/6889.

> **[?] Critical Thinking**
>
> **Patient Safety Goals**
>
> Discuss how you implemented TJC Patient Safety Goals in your last clinical experience.

IMPROVING THE COST OF HEALTH CARE

A driving force today in health care agencies is **cost containment** (the need to hold costs to within fixed limits) while remaining competitive in the health care **marketplace**. LPNs/LVNs need to remember that health care agencies are interested in improving their agency's "bottom line" by reducing waste and inefficiency. LPNs/LVNs who identify wasteful practices and inefficient routines in their work settings while maintaining quality may in fact be saving their own jobs. The following are the LPNs'/LVNs' roles in containing health care costs in the work setting:

- Follow facility policy for charging patients for all supplies used in their care.
- Follow facility policy for documenting patient care for reimbursement.
- Organize patient care for effective and efficient use of your time.
- Be efficient and effective in delivering patient care. If some aspect of care needs to be "redone," it means you could have done it right the first time.
- Ensure reimbursement, and decrease the patient's length of stay by implementing nursing care to help prevent complications.
- Meet the patients' needs, not yours.
- Provide patient-centered (relationship-centered) care.
- Remember that quality outcomes (pay-for-performance) and never events impact the institution's bottom line. Asks questions and seek guidance to fully understand factors impacting revenue.

Nurses are an essential factor when it comes to addressing quality, safety, and cost in health care. These attributes of health care need to be understood and brought to all clinical situations by all nurses, regardless of educational preparation (Kovner & Spetz, 2011).

> **[👆] Professional Pointer**
>
> Remember to consider quality, safety, and cost in your practice. It is no longer "good enough" to simply provide quality care. High-quality, safe, cost-effective care is the goal.

RESTRUCTURING THE HEALTH CARE SYSTEM

The changes in health care to improve the delivery of health care (*service*), increase the *quality* and *safety* of that care, and decrease the *cost* of care are continual. A major change that continues to take place in health care services today is the **restructuring** of the health care system. This is a response to escalating health care costs.

- Changes in the delivery of health care in the community involve new organization and structure of health care organizations:
- **Alliances** (partnerships) are formed among hospitals, clinics, laboratories, health care systems, and physicians. By joining together, or *networking*, these alliances can coordinate the delivery of care and contain costs among providers of health care services; for example, supplies can be purchased in bulk, and the staff can share a computer. Patient records can be more readily available on referral to another health care provider in the network. For this reason, alliances are called **"seamless" systems**.
- Consolidated systems of health care include hospital systems found nationwide. Any profits realized go to the investors in a for-profit system.
- Mergers and acquisitions have become commonplace in health care as entities struggle to survive financially. A large health care system has greater power to negotiate with the insurance companies for reimbursement, secure capital for strategic initiatives, and share technology and other costly innovations across the organization.

> **[◎] Try This**
>
> **Identify Restructuring of Health Care in Your Area**
>
> 1. Identify health care alliances, networks, or consolidated systems that have formed in your area of the country.
> 2. Do these systems employ practical/vocational nurses?

DEALING WITH CHANGE

If you had no prior experience in health care before entering the student practical/student vocational nursing program, you may not be aware of the changes taking place in the workplace. If you had prior experience in the health care field, some of the changes you now observe in health care services may be obvious, whereas others may be subtler. Even new workers in a health career will see changes as their program of study progresses. How do you react to changes in your life? Whether changes occur in your personal life or career, it is important for you to remember that you have choices. You can be a victim, a survivor, or a navigator of change. When change is in the wind, are you a victim, a survivor, or a navigator?

- **Victims** look at change in a negative way. They fear the worst will happen because of the proposed change and feel helpless in the situation. They do not willingly participate in the change process, allowing change to control them.
- **Survivors** resist change but go along for the ride. They claim the change will never work, and if their prediction comes true, they say, "I told you so!"
- **Navigators** of change feel in control of the situation. They feel confident and excited about the possibility of being part of the solution to a problem. Navigators believe they have some control over change rather than being controlled by the change.

Professional Pointer

Be a self-directed, motivated, problem-solving employee.

In the twenty-first century, LPNs/LVNs need to define their role as more than the list of nursing tasks and duties they perform. Less trained, unlicensed persons on the health care team are also performing these nursing tasks and duties. *LPNs/LVNs need to define their role in light of their assisting role in the nursing process.* LPNs/LVNs are effective in noting new patient problems and collaborating with registered nurses (RNs) in setting patient goals, performing nursing interventions, and evaluating the results of planning. It is these problem-solving and critical-thinking aspects of nursing that make LPNs/LVNs valuable members of the health care team. LPNs need to be viewed as "thinkers" and not just "doers."

LPNs/LVNs need to present themselves in clinical situations as invaluable to the health care agency. Be self-directed, motivated, positive, and a problem solver in your daily work. Avoid being known as the person who always asks what needs to be done next. Identify what needs to be done, prioritize, and do it, collaborating when necessary. Respond flexibly to changes that are presented. Identify tasks or protocols that could be done more efficiently. Use the critical thinking skills that were encouraged in your nursing program to devise innovative suggestions to make these areas more efficient, effective, and safe. Be a role model for practical/vocational nurses. Ensure that your colleagues and community understand the role of the LPN and their unique contribution to advancing the health of the nation by providing high-quality, safe, cost-effective care.

Get Ready for the NCLEX-PN® Examination

Key Points

- The quality, safety, and cost of health care are major concerns in today's health care system.
- Reports of the IOM highlight concern for the quality, safety, and cost of health care.
- Traditional fee-for-service and capitation are the main ways of financing health care.
- Insurance plans, both private and government-sponsored, are the major third-party payment systems in existence today.
- The number of uninsured is a major concern in health care. The ACA is aimed at addressing this issue.
- Continuous quality improvement, aims of the IOM, continued competency, the Joint Commission National Patient Safety Goals, the National Council of State Boards of Nursing's Transition to Practice Model, and the LPN/LVN role in containing health care costs address the issues of quality, service, and cost of health care.
- Changes in health care delivery include patient-centered (relationship-centered) care, HMOs, PPOs, POSs, open access plans, and health care alliances. LPNs/LVNs need to be self-directed, motivated, and positive problem solvers in their areas of employment.
- Changes in health care need to be approached with flexibility and viewed as an opportunity to improve the quality and safety of patient care.
- Practical/vocational nurses need to ensure quality and safety of patient care by keeping updated and current in their areas of employment.

Additional Learning Resources

evolve Go to your Evolve website (http://evolve.elsevier.com/ Knecht/success) for the following FREE learning resources:
- Answers to Critical Thinking Review Scenarios
- Additional learning activities
- Additional Review Questions for the NCLEX-PN® exam
- Helpful phrases for communicating in Spanish and more!

Review Questions for the NCLEX-PN® Examination

1. A driving force in delivering health care today is:
   a. Safety concerns
   b. Patient demands
   c. Technological explosion
   d. Labor negotiations

2. Select the statement that best describes the impact Medicare has as a prospective payment system.
   a. Hospitals have increased revenue as a result of the prospective payment system.
   b. When the patient is discharged, the hospital calculates the bill and sends it to the federal government.
   c. The hospital is paid based on the DRG (diagnostic-related group).
   d. Physician office visits cannot be covered by Medicare funding.

3. A patient tells the LVN about the new HMO that his employer has chosen to cover employees with health care benefits. Select the statement that indicates that the patient understands the coverage of an HMO.
   a. "Each time I go to the doctor, I pay the charges as I leave the office, and I send the bills to the HMO for reimbursement."
   b. "Having an HMO allows me to choose the specialist I prefer to see, based on my colleagues' referrals."
   c. "The doctors hired by the HMO submit their bills to the HMO and receive reimbursement for the services they provided."
   d. "I must carefully choose a specialist from the list provided or I may incur additional costs."

4. Indicate which statement is accurate regarding the Affordable Care Act (ACA).
   a. The ACA was implemented to expand health care insurance coverage to all people in the U.S., irrelevant of their lawful status.
   b. The ACA mandates that all employers provide health insurance to all employees.
   c. The ACA replaces Medicare coverage.
   d. The law prohibits insurance companies from denying coverage if you have a preexisting condition.

Alternate Format Item

1. Capitation plans include all of the following: *(Select all that apply.)*
   a. HMOs
   b. PPOs
   c. POSs
   d. Fee for Service
   e. Joint Purchasing

Critical Thinking Scenario

During break, a group of LVN students are discussing new health reform legislation. Jason is upset because the Affordable Care Act is socialized medicine. Mike tells the group his grandfather told him the new law makes it necessary to have death panels evaluate care for Medicare patients. Mike said he heard that the new law rations care. How would you address these statements?

chapter

17

Collaboration: Leading and Managing

Objectives

On completing this chapter, you will be able to do the following:

1. Discuss the importance of understanding institutional mission and beliefs statements as an employee and as a front-line leader.
2. Discuss how the role (team member, charge nurse) of the newly graduated practical/vocational nurse can vary in a long-term care facility.
3. Explain the difference between leadership and management.
4. Explain the following leadership styles in your own words: autocratic, democratic, laissez-faire, and situational.
5. Explain the four "I"s of transformational leadership: idealized influence, inspirational motivation, individualized consideration, and intellectual stimulation.
6. Discuss how the four "I"s can guide you to develop as a strong team member.
7. Discuss your role as a licensed practical (LP) charge nurse or team member in understanding how the four "I"s of transformational leadership can help build an effective interdisciplinary health care team in a long-term care or community setting, resulting in improved patient outcomes.
8. Identify how to develop core areas of intellectual stimulation essential to be an effective first-line leader.
9. Identify ways to obtain competency in occupational, organizational, and human relationship skills, in which knowledge and skills are needed to be an effective first-line leader.
10. Describe how the Howlett hierarchy of work motivators can help the licensed practical nurse/licensed vocational nurse (LPN/LVN) leader influence direct care workers (DCWs) to motivate themselves.
11. Discuss how you can use the Knecht (2014) job satisfaction puzzle to improve your team's job satisfaction and decrease job dissatisfaction in a long-term care setting.
12. Using the ABCD method of Ellis, identify an irrational thought you have had on the clinical area, and convert it to a rational thought.
13. Focusing on intellectual stimulation, develop a plan for personal growth as a practical/vocational charge nurse.
14. Discuss the role of the LPN/LVN, as written in your state's Nurse Practice Act (NPA) with special focus on the following: the members of the health care interdisciplinary team who can supervise the LPN; the members of the health care interdisciplinary team who the LPN can supervise in collaboration with the registered nurse (RN); any additional requirements in your NPA that must be met to be an LPN charge nurse; the difference between supervising the assigned work of a DCW and delegating an assignment to a DCW.
15. Discuss the key skills necessary to effectively manage a team in a long-term care or community setting.
16. Discuss the assignment of tasks versus the delegation of duties with regard to the following factors: your state's laws regarding the role of the LPN/LVN and the delegation of duties in the charge nurse position; differences between assigning nursing tasks and delegating nursing duties; legal aspects of assigning nursing tasks and delegating nursing duties.

Key Terms

assigning (assignment) (ă-sīn-ĭng)
accountability (ă-KŎWNT-ă-BIL-ĭ-tē)
autocratic leadership (ĂW-tō-kră-tĭk)
Centers for Medicare and Medicaid Services (CMS)
change-of-shift report (chānj)
conflict resolution (KŎN-flĭkt)
continuum (kŏn-TĬN-ū-ŭm)
delegating (DEL-ě-GĀT-ĭng)
goals (outcomes) (gōlz)
Howlett hierarchy (HĪ-ě-RĂR-kē)
irrational thinking (ĭ-RĂ-shŭn-ăl)
leadership (LĒD-ěr-shĭp)
management (MĂN-ĭj-měnt)

mission statement (MĬ-shŭn)
Omnibus Budget Reconciliation Act of 1987 (OBRA) (RĔ-kŏn-SĬL-Ē-Ā-shŭn)
patient outcomes (PĀ-shŭnt ŎWT-kŭms)
performance evaluation (pěr-FŎR-măntz ĭ-văl-ū-Ā-shŭn)
Quality Improvement Organization (QIO) (KWĂL-ĭ-tē ĭm-PROOV-měnt)
scope of practice (skōp, PRĂK-tĭs)
situational leadership (sĭt-u-Ā-shŭn-al LĒD-ěr-shĭp)
stress management (strěs MĂN-ĭj-měnt)
The Joint Commission (jöynt kŏ-MĬ-shŭn)
time management (tīm MĂN-ĭj-měnt)

"The manager does things right. The leader does the right things."

—Warren Bennis, *On Becoming a Leader* (2003)

Grace and Emily, nursing assistants at Quality Care Home, collapsed in their chairs in the lunchroom. "I had forgotten how hectic mornings can be," said Grace. "I am exhausted." This was the first day back on the day shift on the Evergreen Wing for both nursing assistants. Both women had substituted for a week for vacationing nursing assistants; Grace on nights and Emily on the evening shift.

"I don't care how tired I am, I sure am glad to be back with our charge nurse," said Grace. "I missed Sal Sytchuashun's way of running things," she continued. "On nights, being with that LVN Gina Ivanapleze was like working with mass confusion. Anything you wanted to do was fine with her. It seemed the most important thing to her was the happiness of the nursing assistants, not the residents' care. Anything we wanted to do was hunky-dory. Sal listens to my suggestions but also offers input when I need it."

"That sure is different from my experience," said Emily. "Being with RN Priscilla Pittsy taught me the real meaning of her initials: "real nasty." She commanded us to do everything; she never suggested. Never a 'thank you' or 'good job.' We had a task list and a time sequence to follow, and, no matter what cropped up, heaven help us if we didn't stick to it precisely. We couldn't even ask questions about our assignments. The only time I appreciated Priscilla barking her orders was the evening we had a code. I was shaking in my boots, but she knew exactly what to do. And the resident pulled through."

"I'm glad we didn't have a code with Gina in charge," said Grace. "We have so few codes around here. That is a situation in which I would appreciate having some direction."

"I liked the way Sal handled the situation this morning in the lounge when a resident complained of chest pain," Grace added. "Sal gave us each something to do STAT. After the situation was over, we all discussed the emergency as a team. Sal listened to our suggestions on how to make things go more smoothly in the next emergency situation. Sal makes me feel like a real team member and not a slave!"

Grace and Emily finished their lunches. As they went back to Evergreen Wing, they both agreed that LVN Sal had a way about him that gets the job done, makes you feel comfortable about going to him with a concern or question, and makes you want to come back to work for the next shift. You feel good about your contributions to the team. Both agreed he is a good role model for the vocational nurses and nursing assistants.

LICENSED PRACTICAL NURSE/LICENSED VOCATIONAL NURSE AS FIRST-LINE LEADER

Have you ever experienced employment situations similar to the ones just described by Grace and Emily?

Perhaps you received directions as a nursing assistant or in another job capacity and did not like the way you were approached by your supervisor.

Nurses at all levels need to manage patient care. Some nurses will also be leaders. Licensed practical nurses/licensed vocational nurses (LPNs/LVNs) have proved themselves effective as first-line leaders. First-line leaders are responsible for supervising nursing assistants who deliver care in long-term care units or community settings. Such positions are referred to as charge nurse positions. If you are a manager of patient care and a leader, you will be more effective in this expanded role in LP/LV nursing.

LPNs/LVNs need to develop leadership and management skills so they can direct and supervise others in a manner that will effectively meet the goals of the employing agency. In your LP/LV nursing program, you started to build a strong, solid base in these skills. This chapter will help you to continue to develop skills to lead and manage. It focuses on the leadership and management role, and provides interactive and reflective exercises to assist you in becoming an effective charge nurse and emerging as a leader. These roles are critical to both patient and employee satisfaction. As you can see from the story above, the leader's role is critical to patient and employee positive outcomes. In addition, this chapter will be a useful resource if you accept an LP/LV charge nurse position as a recent graduate. Understanding the definition of a mission statement is a good starting point on your journey to being an informal or formal leader.

MISSION STATEMENTS

All organizations have a **mission statement** or vision statement that defines their purpose (goals) and states their values, culture, and norms, thus providing the foundation for collaborative decision making. Core values and/or beliefs can flow from a mission statement and often include topics such as customer service, teamwork, respect, trust, honesty, excellence, patient-centered care, cost-effective, and safe care.

The LP/LV charge nurse needs to be aware of the mission statement of their employer. An example of a mission statement follows: "This non-profit, consumer-oriented institution aims to provide relationship-centered, low-cost, high-quality, safe care in a supportive environment of compassion, trust and respect, resulting in positive patient and institutional outcomes." All staff are required to understand and live the mission statement. It will be your role as a charge nurse to embrace the mission of the institution and ensure all members of the team are committed to the mission.

In a long-term care facility, a unit may focus on specific aspects of the mission statement that require a renewed team approach. For example, if your unit has a decrease in their patient satisfaction surveys, specifically related to compassionate care, the unit may collaboratively develop a goal to improve in this area, thus contributing directly to the overall mission of the institution. As a charge nurse you will be instrumental in creating a climate of the work environment that motivates staff to meet this goal. Types of leadership styles and the four "*I*"s of transformational leadership will be presented in this chapter to assist you in building a solid team ready and willing to meet individual unit and institutional goals. Even if you are not in a formal leadership role as an LVN/LPN, this chapter will assist you in your professional and personal growth.

THE DIVERSE ROLE OF THE NEWLY LICENSED PRACTICAL NURSE/LICENSED VOCATIONAL NURSE

The newly licensed PN/VN job role can differ significantly based on the setting in which you are employed and the acuity level of the patients. In a long-term care setting and in some community settings, the LPN/LVN, even as a new graduate, can be hired as a first-line leader. The organizational chart of an institution is a tool that can assist you in understanding your role in the hierarchy of the organization. The organizational chart is a picture of responsibility in an employment situation. In the traditional organizational chart, individuals who are lower on the organizational chart report to the person directly above them on the chart. Figure 17-1 shows where the LPN/LVN fits into the traditional organizational chart as a first-line leader. In Figure 17-1, the LPN/LVN reports to the nurse manager, who is a registered nurse (RN). Nursing assistants and other DCWs report to the LPN/LVN. To whom does the nurse manager report?

Because of changes in the structure of organizations, organizational charts have become more horizontal than vertical in appearance. Figure 17-2 provides an example of a contemporary organizational chart. This "flattening out" has eliminated some of the middle manager positions in organizations. As a result, the remaining middle managers have taken on more responsibilities and are spread thin. Middle managers in this system have more persons reporting to them than in the past. Middle managers depend on the people who report to them, such as the LP/LV charge nurse, to think critically and problem solve. Middle managers expect to be contacted when you have tried and are unable to solve your own problems. However, always remember that LPNs/LVNs are expected to collaborate with RNs as stated in their Nurse Practice Act (NPA). Always be sure to understand the impact of your NPA when in a leadership role. It is easy to step outside the boundaries in an attempt to "get the job done." This can result in disciplinary action by the state, particularly if an adverse patient event occurs, such as a fall with injury.

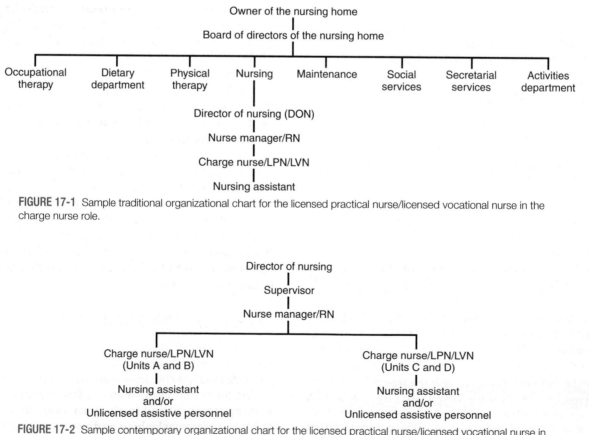

FIGURE 17-1 Sample traditional organizational chart for the licensed practical nurse/licensed vocational nurse in the charge nurse role.

FIGURE 17-2 Sample contemporary organizational chart for the licensed practical nurse/licensed vocational nurse in the charge nurse role.

Examining Organizational Charts

Resources needed:
- Organizational charts from clinical sites used by students in your practical/vocational nursing program
- Organizational charts may differ by region of the United States. Obtain organizational charts of long-term care facilities in your area. Clarify specific levels of responsibility as they apply to the LPN/LVN. Identify whether these charts reflect a traditional or contemporary style of organization.

EXPANDED ROLE OF LICENSED PRACTICAL/ LICENSED VOCATIONAL NURSING

REVIEW THE CURRENT NURSE PRACTICE ACT OF YOUR STATE.

This law legally defines the exact role and boundaries for practical/vocational nurses. Also review the National Association for Practical Nurse Education and Service (NAPNES) standards of practice and educational competencies of graduates of LP/LV nursing programs (www.napnes.org) and the National Federation Licensed Practical Nurse (NFLPN) nursing practice standards for the LPN/LVN (www.nflpn.org). See the Collaborative Care, Leadership Activity: Determining Your State's Requirements to Assume the Position of Licensed Practical/ Licensed Vocational Charge Nurse box.

Determining Your State's Requirements to Assume the Position of Licensed Practical/Licensed Vocational Charge Nurse

Resources needed:
- Your state's Nurse Practice Act

Obtain a current copy of your state's NPA. Identify the part of the act that addresses your state's position on the practical/vocational nurse who is assuming the charge nurse position in the following areas:
1. Requirements before assuming the LP/LV charge nurse position
2. Site of employment
3. Scope of practice

If your state's Nurse Practice Act does not address the issue of charge nurse, how can this information be obtained?

An example of the expanded role of the LPN/LVN is the first-line manager position, also called charge nurse, in a nursing home or long-term care facility. In these situations, the LPN/LVN has the responsibility of supervising the care given by nursing assistants and other DCWs. The LPN/LVN will direct, guide, and supervise these health care workers as they attempt to meet the goals of the resident's plan of care.

The most recent practice analysis of entry-level LPNs/LVNs by the National Council of State Boards of Nursing (NCSBN, 2013) for which data are available occurred in 2012. This survey identified that 43.4% of LPNs/LVNs responding to the survey reported they had administrative responsibilities. This represented two primary settings: long-term care (32.4%) and community-based (7.3%) settings. In addition, 62.2% of these respondents performed these administrative duties as their primary position. To succeed as a first-line manager/charge nurse role effectively, you will need the abilities found in both a leader *and* a manager. The 2012 LPN/LVN practice analysis can be obtained at www.ncsbn.org.

PREPARING FOR A LEADERSHIP AND MANAGEMENT ROLE

The topic of leadership and management for the LPN/ LVN is a vast one. All LPNs/LVNs are already managers in the sense that they consistently need to direct, handle, and organize care for assigned patients. It is worthwhile for you to review the ways in which your LP/LV nursing program helps prepare you for a management position. The LP/LV nursing program encourages development of the following skills, which are necessary for functioning successfully as a first-line manager:
1. Basic nursing skills, including the nursing process
2. Time-management techniques for home and clinical time
3. How to learn new information, including using evidence for learning and decision-making
4. The power of positive self-talk and thinking
5. Rules for assertiveness
6. Communication skills
7. Ethical aspects of health care
8. Legal aspects of health care
9. Problem solving and critical thinking
10. Stress management
11. Participation in clinical evaluation

Learning leadership and management involves much more than taking one course or reading one chapter about becoming a leader. Learning leadership is a process (continual development) that includes many skills and is something that evolves over time. This chapter encourages you to think specifically of a leadership role, and it provides leadership hints that practical/vocational nurses need.

DIFFERENCE BETWEEN MANAGEMENT AND LEADERSHIP

Management is the organization of all care required of patients in a health care setting for a specific period.
- The focus of management is planning and directing to meet patient and institutional outcomes.
- The manager asks how and when, and has her eye on the bottom line (day-to-day operation).

- Managers often value control.
- Management is a formal role given to a person by the employer.
- Managers are appointed by their employers.
- The tools needed for management could be written in a step-by-step manner and given to you to follow.
- Following the directions for using the management skills would possibly get the job done in an efficient manner.

Leadership is how a person empowers and develops a team to meet and exceed patient and institutional outcomes.

- The focus of leadership is to produce changes in the workplace that will meet the goals of the employing agency.
- The leader asks what and why and keeps her eye on the future.
- Leaders inspire trust.
- Leadership is an informal role that is given to a person by a group of workers. You become a leader when your team members decide to follow you.
- Leaders, if appointed, will fail quickly if no one follows.
- The leader needs to influence others in the work setting to want to implement desired change.
- Directions for leadership skills can also be learned, but it is through experience that leadership skills are truly developed.

The LPN/LVN who has the skills of both management and leadership will get the job done in the most efficient and effective manner, and the LPN/LVN manager and coworkers will experience greater job satisfaction. A manager is not automatically an effective leader, and a leader is not automatically an effective manager. Your goal will be to develop skills of leadership *and* management.

WHAT KIND OF LEADER ARE YOU?

You can lead in several different ways. What is your predominant leadership style? Each of the statements given in the Collaborative Care, Leadership Activity: Discovering Your Personal Leadership Style box is an extreme. The responses are not positive or negative. One answer does not have value over another answer. They just are.

Collaborative Care
Leadership Activity

Discovering Your Personal Leadership Style

Put a checkmark next to the statement that *best* describes the way you *might* be at work, not how you *want* to be.

A Short Test of Leadership Style

1. My primary goal at work is to:
   a. Get the job done.
   b. Get along with the people with whom I work.
   c. Do the job correctly.
   d. Hope the work I do is noticed.

2. My clinical coworkers would say I am:
   a. Domineering in my relationships.
   b. Friendly and personable in my relationships.
   c. Likely to attend to details of the resident care plan.
   d. Creative and energetic in giving care.
3. At work, I feel like I have to be:
   a. In control of the resident situation.
   b. Liked by my coworkers.
   c. Correct in giving care.
   d. Recognized and praised for my care.
4. When I communicate on the nursing unit:
   a. I am usually direct and to the point.
   b. I am more considerate of the person to whom I am talking rather than strongly getting my point across.
   c. I usually give detailed information.
   d. I usually elaborate on the point at hand.
5. My coworkers would say I am a person who:
   a. Gets the job done regardless of what shift I work.
   b. Is very likable and patient.
   c. Is precise and accurate in giving nursing care.
   d. Is optimistic and has good verbal skills.
6. My charge nurse might describe my behavior while on my shift by saying that:
   a. Sometimes I alienate people.
   b. Sometimes I waste time and fall for excuses others may give.
   c. Sometimes I can be stubborn with coworkers.
   d. Sometimes I appear flaky to my coworkers.
7. I react to a stressful incident on the nursing unit:
   a. By being rude, blaming other departments, and yelling at coworkers.
   b. By being accommodating to the person in charge and by passive behavior.
   c. By becoming silent and withdrawing from the situation.
   d. By talking faster and louder.
8. When I deal with my coworkers on the nursing unit regarding patient matters, I like them to:
   a. Get to the point and be businesslike in their behavior.
   b. Be casual and sincere in their behavior.
   c. Use the facts of the matter and go step-by-step when explaining a resident-care situation.
   d. Be enthusiastic about the situation and use demonstrations to explain their points.

Add up your "a" and "c" answers. These answers are more characteristic of a task-oriented person. In leadership terms, this person is called an *autocratic* leader. Add up your "b" and "d" responses. These are more characteristic of a people-oriented person. In leadership terms, this person is called a *laissez-faire* leader. Your score can give you a rough estimate of the tendency of your leadership style.

LEADERSHIP STYLES

The literature abounds with examples of leadership styles. Figure 17-3 illustrates a **continuum** (a line with extreme opposites at each end) of leadership styles. Box 17-1 compares and contrasts the leadership styles found on this continuum.

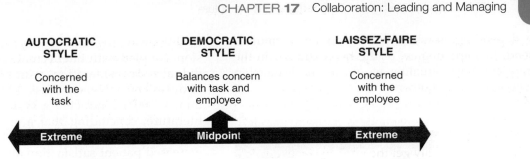

FIGURE 17-3 Extremes of leadership styles on a continuum.

| Box 17-1 | Comparing Autocratic, Democratic, and Laissez-Faire Styles of Leadership |

GENERAL DESCRIPTION

Autocratic: Does not share responsibility and authority with employees

Democratic: Shares responsibility and authority with employees

Laissez-faire: Gives away responsibility and authority to employees

IMPORTANCE OF AGENCY'S POLICIES

Autocratic: Emphasis is on policies

Democratic: Enforces policies but with concern for employees

Laissez-faire: Puts employees before policies

HOW LEADER GETS THE JOB DONE

Autocratic: Tells employees what tasks to do; does not seek input from employees

Democratic: Seeks input from employees and encourages problem solving

Laissez-faire: Tries to please everyone

WHAT GETS DONE

Autocratic: May reach goals

Democratic: Because of involvement of employees, goals may be achieved with positive staff feelings

Laissez-faire: Maybe nothing, but at least staff feels good

WHEN STYLE CAN BE USED

Autocratic: Crisis situations, code situations, emergencies

Democratic: Daily nursing care situations, meetings, committees, review of care plans

Laissez-faire: When agency goals/policies are not a consideration

BENEFITS AND DISADVANTAGES OF LEADERSHIP STYLES

A purely task-centered leadership style (called **autocratic leadership**) thrives on power. It involves telling someone what to do, with little regard for the employee as a person who may have ideas about how to improve resident care or reach the goals of the employer. Adopting the autocratic or laissez-faire style in Box 17-1 to use consistently as a leadership style is unrealistic. Its consistent use could be disastrous. However, there are opportunities when an autocratic leadership style is

necessary; for example, in times of emergency. On the following lines, list two additional examples of situations that might require the autocratic style of leadership.

1. _____

2. _____

A purely people-oriented style (laissez-faire) focuses on people's feelings but ignores the task at hand. It allows employees to act without any direction. The goals of the employer will be compromised when the laissez-faire leadership style is used. At times, persons in leadership roles may feel the need to be liked by all team members and use this leadership style, but the task of accomplishing goals will be compromised.

Focusing on both the task and the employee is characteristic of the democratic style of leadership. In this style the LP/LV charge nurse displays concern for the work that needs to be done, as well as for the team performing the work. When using this leadership style, the LP/LV charge nurse encourages supervised nursing assistants to discuss resident care, make decisions, and problem solve improvements in care. It may take longer than the autocratic style for work to be accomplished, but patient goals (outcomes) will be achieved, with staff having positive feelings about their supervisor and the experience. Examples of situations in which the democratic style of leadership is useful include daily nursing care situations, unit meetings, and reviews of patient care plans.

Situational Leadership

A popular system of leadership for the twenty-first century is called situational leadership. **Situational leadership** involves varying your leadership style to meet the demands of the situation in the work environment. According to this system, the LPN/LVN needs to use a leadership style that fits the work situation at hand.

USING THE LEADERSHIP CONTINUUM AS A GUIDE

The value of a continuum, as shown in Figure 17-3, is that as you move along the continuum from each extreme toward the center or midpoint, the two extremes begin to blend together. You have some of each style, depending on where you are on the continuum. A blend, to some degree, of the two extremes in the appropriate work situation would be the leadership style needed at the moment.

Collaborative Care

Leadership Activity

Plotting My Leadership Style Score

Using your leadership style score from the Discovering Your Personal Leadership Style box, place an "X" on the continuum in Figure 17-3 to indicate where you are at this point in general leadership style tendencies.

Do the exercise in the Collaborative Care, Leadership Activity: Plotting My Leadership Style Score box. Remember, this score is your tendency. If your "X" is far to the left or right, it will benefit you to be aware of this tendency and to avoid using this style consistently. Remember the continuum and the need to be flexible in your style. Balance task and people orientation as needed. Knowing what your predominant style of leadership is will be helpful in your evaluation of work situations and the style needed at that time. Some situations require a supportive style, whereas others require a more directive approach.

CORE KNOWLEDGE AND SKILLS NEEDED FOR LEADERSHIP

To function well in your expanded role as LP/LV charge nurse, you will strive to be a good leader. The scenario at the beginning of this chapter provides examples of what not to do as a nurse leader. Much research in learning about the business of leading others and theories, such as transformational leadership, is available in the literature (Bass, 1985). *Core knowledge and skills lay the foundation for leadership.* They will help you develop other necessary knowledge and skills for your leadership role. We identify five core areas of knowledge and skills that are necessary for the practical/vocational charge nurse to be an effective leader. These core areas include the ability to do the following:

1. Motivate team members to accomplish team goals.
2. Communicate assertively.
3. Problem solve effectively.
4. Build a team of cooperative workers.
5. Manage stress effectively.

THE FOUR "*I*"S OF TRANSFORMATIONAL LEADERSHIP CAN HELP LEAD THE WAY

Transformational leaders are viewed as motivating their followers without a focus on their own personal power, elevating their team's needs through effective mentoring/coaching, and providing a clear vision to lead the way. Together as a team, this collective mission, coupled with intellectual stimulation and individualized consideration, results in heightened levels of overall effectiveness (Bass, 1985). Wong and Cummings (2007) conducted a systematic review of the literature, concluding that a significant association exists between transformational leadership style and increased patient satisfaction and decreased adverse patient events. Thus strong evidence supports the use of transformational leadership in health care settings. Bass (1985) identified four key behaviors of transformational leadership, commonly referred to as the four "*I*"s: idealized influence, inspirational motivation, intellectual stimulation, and individualized consideration.

An in-depth understanding of each of these key behaviors will assist in the journey of the LPN/LVN in becoming a highly effective leader. The information below describes how the leader exemplifies each of these key characteristics, and Box 17-2 provides examples of LPN/LVN behaviors based on the four "*I*"s of transformational leadership that will improve the work environment resulting in improved patient outcomes.

Idealized Influence	The leader acts as a charismatic role model, promoting desirable behavior and establishing trust and respect of the team
Inspirational Motivation	The leader establishes a clear, focused vision and creates collective pursuit of this vision
Intellectual Stimulation	The leader encourages creative thinking and problem solving and is supportive of taking risks based on knowledge
Individualized Consideration	The leader communicates genuine concern for all followers, providing personal attention and individualized coaching and mentoring, supporting the development of followers

Adapted from Knecht, P., & Sosik, J. J. (2012). Transformational leadership of nurses in long-term care contexts: Propositions and implications for research and practice. Proceedings of the Institute of Behavioral and Applied Management, Nashville, TN.

Keep in Mind

When transformational leaders display individualized consideration and inspirational motivation, they create a democratic and participative climate to enhance followers' performance (Bass, 2008; Sosik & Jung, 2010).

UNDERSTANDING MOTIVATION AND HUMAN NEEDS

As a leader, you will have the task of getting your team members to meet goals set by your employer. Getting people to do what needs to be done is a complex task.

Box 17-2	Licensed Practical Nurse/Licensed Vocational Charge Nurse Behaviors/Actions That Use the Four "I"s of Transformational Leadership (Bass, 1985) to Improve the Work Environment

IDEALIZED INFLUENCE
- Model a high level of ethical and moral conduct
- Act confident and optimistic
- Lead by example
- Share and explain risks taken by the institution
- Avoid using power for personal gain
- Use teamwork language, such as "we" and "us." Convey the attitude "We have common goals, and together we will meet them"

INSPIRATIONAL MOTIVATION
- Review the mission statement of the facility and unit with your team
- Assist the team to see the value of their work
- Model and set high standards of care visible by the team
- Be optimistic and enthusiastic in the clinical area modeling this behavior for others on the team
- Highlight and reward positive outcomes
- Highlight the benefits of change

INDIVIDUALIZED CONSIDERATION
- Encourage politeness, cooperation, trust, and respect among nursing assistants
- Encourage honest feedback among nursing assistants
- Model active listening
- Be open to hear valid concerns and collaboratively identify solutions
- Provide an opportunity for sharing of ideas among nursing assistants

- Ask nursing assistants for ideas on how to do unit tasks more effectively
- Provide individual and group words of acknowledgment, praise and thanks
- Be fair regarding who gets acknowledgment and thanks based on commitment and contribution as an individual and as a team
- Treat nursing assistants on your team as you would like to be treated
- Advocate for your entire team
- Provide occasions for the team to spend time together

INTELLECTUAL STIMULATION
- Provide opportunities for your direct care workers (DCW) team to participate in training
- Provide opportunities for your DCW team to contribute to the patient's plan of care
- Discuss how their job role impacts the patient's, unit's, and institution's outcomes
- Encourage all to challenge the "status quo"
- Provide evidence for decision-making
- Empower the entire team to offer ideas to improve patient care, before providing input
- Mentor DCW to advance in their job and the nursing profession
- Ensure fair workload distribution

What motivates one person does not necessarily motivate another. Understanding motivation and human needs coupled with the four "I"s of transformational leadership will assist you in becoming an effective leader.

Motivation

Motivation is a drive that causes individuals to set personal goals and behave in a way that will allow them to reach those goals. The motivation drive comes from within an individual and is intrinsic. Herzberg's two factor theory (1959) states that intrinsic factors (also known as motivating factors or satisfiers) improve job satisfaction and extrinsic factors (also known as maintenance factors or dissatisfiers) decrease job dissatisfaction. Satisfiers (motivator factors) contribute to personal or psychological growth, increase job satisfaction, and arrive from intrinsic conditions of the job itself. Satisfiers include: achievement, recognition, the value of the work itself, potential for growth and advancement, and responsibility (Herzberg, 1959). All of these intrinsic factors have to do with the job itself. In contrast, dissatisfiers are extrinsic to the work itself and include company policy and administration, supervision, salary, interpersonal relations, and work conditions (Herzberg, 1959). A

good leader will address both intrinsic and extrinsic motivators in their workplace. Herzberg's theory (1959) parallels Maslow's theory of needs hierarchy, relevant to the human's need to engage in higher order work.

Human Needs

All individuals have needs that must be filled to meet goals. Individuals are internally motivated to engage in various activities to meet these needs. The activity they engage in is called behavior and can be observed. Here are some facts about needs:
- Abraham Maslow, a psychologist, presented a pyramid of human needs that ranks those needs and can assist the learner in understanding self and others (see Figure 13-1, A).
- Meeting needs on one level of the pyramid acts as a motivator for meeting the needs on the next level.
- Progression through these levels is not clear-cut. In reality, as most of your needs are met on one level, you are already beginning to check out the next level.
- When faced with overwhelming difficulties, physical or emotional, some regression takes place; for example, physiologic needs become a priority if you have lost your job or housing.

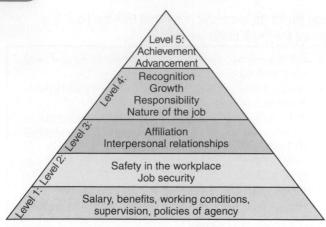

FIGURE 17-4 Howlett hierarchy of work motivators. (From Hill, S.S., Howett, H.S. [2013]. *Success in practical/vocational nursing* [ed. 7]. St. Louis: Elsevier.)

- Safety and security needs become a major issue if you are facing a serious illness, move into an unsafe neighborhood, or are facing a divorce.
- Once these issues have been dealt with or resolved, higher needs will reemerge.

Motivating Nursing Assistants

Maslow's hierarchy of needs can be adapted to help the first-line LPN/LVN leader understand motivation of team members in a health care setting based on needs (Figure 17-4). Remember all behavior is internally motivated. Herzberg, like Maslow, noted that feelings of self-actualization and growth are true motivators. As an LPN/LVN manager, you can influence what nursing assistants might be motivated to do. If nursing assistants see that doing a good job helps them meet personal needs, they will also be meeting the goals of their employer. Providing for growth opportunities will further enhance their motivation.

All levels of the pyramid in Figure 17-4 are considered to be needs of employees in an employment situation. As you go up the **Howlett hierarchy**, strategies could be used to encourage meeting needs of nursing assistants at each level. The opportunity to meet these needs can be encouraged or discouraged by the employer and/or the work environment, including the charge nurse (extrinsic motivators). If these needs are met, the person can proceed to the next highest level of the pyramid. If these needs are not met, a person may become dissatisfied with the work situation. Strategies for levels 3 and 4 can play an important role in motivation for team members at any level of the Howlett hierarchy. Praise, recognition, and rewards are extremely important tools for leaders.

What Motivates You as an Employee?

List what motivates you specifically in clinical situations to get your assignment completed.

Motivating Nursing Assistants

Resources needed:
- Readings on motivation, the Howlett hierarchy, and your creativity to find ways to meet the needs of nursing assistants.

This exercise inspires the charge nurse to be creative in finding ways to encourage motivation in nursing assistants. Examples of behaviors that encourage meeting needs at each level of the hierarchy are given; the person responsible for the behavior is listed in parentheses. Space is provided for you to fill in additional suggested behaviors at each level to encourage motivation of nursing assistants. Identify whether the employer needs to initiate the strategy or whether the strategy could be initiated by the first-line LP/LV nursing leader.

LEVEL 1 SALARY, BENEFITS, WORKING CONDITIONS, SUPERVISION, AND POLICIES OF AGENCY
Examples
- Explanation of policies that affect employees (employer)
- Cafeteria-style benefits; pick and choose benefits (employer)

LEVEL 2 SAFETY IN THE WORKPLACE AND JOB SECURITY
Examples
- Provision of adequate equipment to carry out standard precautions (employer and first-line LPN/LVN leader)
- Establish policy for hostile patients (employer and first-line LPN/LVN leader) and visitors

LEVEL 3 AFFILIATION AND INTERPERSONAL RELATIONSHIPS
Examples
- Plan monthly potluck dinners, pizza lunches, get-togethers (first-line LPN/LVN leader)

LEVEL 4 RECOGNITION, GROWTH, RESPONSIBILITY, AND NATURE OF THE JOB
Examples
- Encourage attendance at continuing education seminars, inservice training, and so on (employer and first-line LPN/LVN leader)
- Recognize employees when working short-staffed (employer and first-line LPN/LVN leader)

LEVEL 5 ACHIEVEMENT AND ADVANCEMENT
Examples
- Recognition of successful completion of class or seminar (employer and first-line LPN/LVN leader)
- Provide objective examples of how you can implement each of your suggested behaviors. For example, level 5 could be implemented by the following examples: A written account in the facility's newsletter
- Posting an announcement on a special section of the bulletin board
- A personal note of congratulations from the charge nurse

APPLYING COMMUNICATION SKILLS AS A LICENSED PRACTICAL NURSE/LICENSED VOCATIONAL NURSE LEADER

One of the LPN/LVN leader's most productive tools is the effective use of verbal and nonverbal communication. The principles of communication in Chapters 8 and 9 are building blocks for the communication skills you will need as an LP/LV charge nurse. See the Collaborative Care, Leadership Hint: Communication of the Licensed Practical/Licensed Vocational Charge Nurse box and the Collaborative Care, Leadership Hint: Encouraging Verbal Communication from Nursing Assistants box.

Collaborative Care

Leadership Hint

Communication of the Licensed Practical/Licensed Vocational Charge Nurse

VERBAL

1. When talking to nursing assistants, deliver your message with clear, specific language. Spell out objectively what has to be done for residents. If you work with nursing assistants who do not speak English as a first language, determine their proficiency with English. Verify that intended messages were received.
2. As an LP/LV charge nurse, you are a role model for nursing assistants. Discourage profanity, personal criticisms, gossip, and rumors.
3. Use *I* instead of *you* messages. *I* messages indicate you take the responsibility for the message; for example, "I saw you tie the patient's wrist restraint to the side rail. This could cause injury to the patient when the side rail is lowered. I suggest you review the videotape on application of restraints. Also review the policy this facility has about the danger of restraint application." *You* messages imply that you are blaming the person to whom you are speaking; for example, "You did a poor job applying that wrist restraint." Take responsibility for your messages.
4. When talking with your supervisor, be valued for your input. Avoid being known as someone who just brings up problems. After objectively stating the problem, offer solutions.

NONVERBAL

1. Be sure your body language and message are consistent and professional. For example, avoid smiling when you are delivering a needed reprimand. Face the person to whom you are speaking.
2. When delivering your message, appear sure of yourself. Have an attentive posture.

WRITTEN

1. Use language that all staff will understand.
2. Review your written messages before posting them to be sure the intent of the message is clear.
3. Provide written work assignments that do not require the nursing assistant to make judgments.
4. Provide written reports of all meetings. If information is not restricted, a report from a meeting with management can dispel/prevent rumors about what "they" are planning now. The reports can be placed in a loose-leaf binder in an area that is accessible for nursing assistants.

TELEPHONE

1. Gather your thoughts before you make a call. This includes the purpose for the call.
2. With a smile in your voice, greet the person by name, identify yourself, and offer a brief inquiry as to his or her well-being, if you know the person you called. For example, say, "Hello, Mrs. Kylie, this is Tricia Zak from the nursing home. How are things going?"
3. State the reason for the call: "I need to order a DVD and wanted to know if you had any specific needs."
4. You initiated the conversation. Terminate it when your business is completed. The exception is when the person you called brings up a work-related question.
5. Avoid long conversations about nonwork-related topics. This is what is considered allowing the telephone to extend into your time.
6. Arrange to have incoming calls answered quickly, by the second or third ring.
7. When you answer, identify the facility and give your name and title: "The nursing home, Tricia Zak, charge nurse."
8. Speak clearly in a moderate tone of voice. Most people talk too loudly on the phone.
9. Callers are "customers." Treat the caller respectfully and cordially.
10. If it is necessary to put the person on hold, ask permission to do so.
11. If it is necessary to put the person on hold, try to get back to her or him within 30 seconds. If you are still delayed, ask for a number so you can call back.
12. Provide the information requested.

Collaborative Care

Leadership Hint

Encouraging Verbal Communication from Nursing Assistants

1. Actively listen to nursing assistants. Avoid distraction and inattention.
2. Stay focused on what the nursing assistant is saying.
3. Avoid forming a response while the nursing assistant is speaking.
4. Avoid judging the message or the nursing assistant.
5. Rephrase the message when the nursing assistant is done to verify that you understand the message.
6. Encourage comments. Your goal is to have the nursing assistant go back to the team and say, "That charge nurse really listened to me!"
7. Encourage constructive evaluation. Create an environment in which nursing assistants are encouraged to give their input, whether positive or negative.
8. Respect all opinions. Nursing assistants need to feel safe to speak up, ask questions, identify problems, and suggest solutions to those problems.

APPLYING PROBLEM SOLVING AS A LICENSED PRACTICAL NURSE/LICENSED VOCATIONAL NURSE LEADER

The basic hint for successful problem solving is to *identify the real issue and solve it*. What is the problem? Avoid spending precious time on finding solutions for what is not really the problem. Chapter 12 introduced you to the nursing process, an excellent problem-solving process. You have been using this problem-solving method throughout your student practical/vocational nursing program. For problem solving, the nursing process can

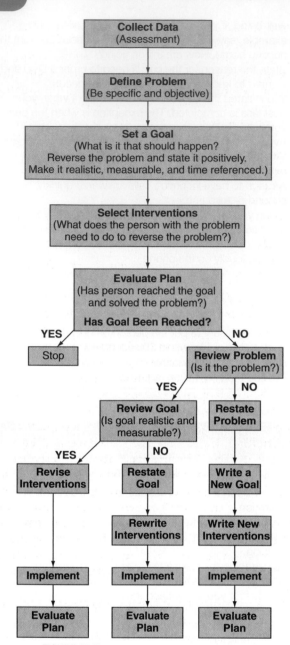

FIGURE 17-5   Decision tree for problem solving.

be used to solve resident problems as well as staff problems. The nursing process also works at home, as well as in the clinical area (Figure 17-5).

Scenario: Late for Assigned Shift

Penny, a nursing assistant, is assigned to the day shift in a long-term care facility. Her shift begins at 6:45 AM with a verbal report from the day LP/LV charge nurse for her wing. All nursing assistants are expected to attend this report and receive their assignments at this time.

Data Collection. On May 8, 10, 15, 16, 23, and 24, Penny came to work either during the charge nurse report or after the charge nurse had finished. When questioned about this behavior, she states she has problems getting her teenagers up and ready for school.

Problem. A record of Penny's tardiness indicates this is a recurring problem and not an isolated incident. A pattern has been established in being late for report.

Goal. Starting immediately, Penny will be on time for the day charge nurse's report and will hear the entire report.

Intervention. As the charge nurse, it is your responsibility to talk to Penny about this tardiness. This includes the times and days of her tardiness. Select a private location for your discussion. Encourage Penny to think through why this behavior is inconvenient for the staff and residents. Review the long-term care unit's policy on punctuality. Encourage Penny to come up with ideas that will allow her to be on time. Set limits with Penny. Identify that she needs to be on time for her assigned shifts. Plan to meet with her in 1 week to discuss her performance. At that time, if she has not improved her performance, a written reprimand will be given and included in her personal file. At the end of the meeting, compliment Penny on an area of her work that has been going well.

Evaluation. During the next week, continue to document Penny's arrival for her assigned shifts. If she complies, note and praise her change in performance.* If she continues to be late for her shift, issue a written reprimand. Place a copy in her file, give a copy to your supervisor, and keep a copy in your file. Be sure the warning contains objective information, such as the following:
1. Days and times late for shift
2. Date of oral warning
3. Seriousness of situation
4. Consequences

TEAM BUILDING

STRESS MANAGEMENT

Stress is a part of all work environments. The long-term care area has its fair share because of increased workloads (especially when a nursing assistant calls in sick) and conflicts with nursing assistants, physicians, families, and residents. Stress and anxiety in the clinical area can result in dysfunctional behavior on the job. Examples of dysfunctional job behaviors include the following:
1. Decreased performance of nursing assistants
2. Negative interactions with nursing assistants
3. Ineffective communication
4. Inappropriate body cues, such as sharp tone of voice
5. High staff turnover
6. Unhappy residents, families, physicians, and nursing assistants

---

*In the next week, Penny actually arrived a few minutes before the other nursing assistants. The LP/LV charge nurse allowed her to choose her break and lunch times. Penny had never experienced this before and was very pleased.

As an LP/LV charge nurse, you have the responsibility to be a stress manager and role model for the team. Your goal will be to do the following:

1. Display the ability to cope with stress as it affects you.
2. Create a work environment with decreased stress levels.
3. Guide and support nursing assistants when they experience stress.

The LP/LV charge nurse needs to learn how to detect stress in the clinical environment. A good place to start is to be aware of your own stress level. See the Collaborative Care, Leadership Hint: Life Skills That Help Control Stress box and the Collaborative Care, Leadership Hint: Creating a Less Stressful Work Environment box.

Collaborative Care
Leadership Hint

Life Skills That Help Control Stress

1. The actual stress reduction/relaxation technique you choose is personal. Whatever works for you is the skill to choose.
2. Massage.
3. Daily exercise: Walking is the easiest and least expensive form of exercise. No special equipment is required, except good walking shoes.
4. Apply the principles you learned in nutrition.
5. Get the amount of rest you need to function at your best.
6. Take your breaks when at work. You will be reenergized and increase your productivity.
7. Develop leisure activities you enjoy (or rediscover activities you put on the back burner during nursing school).

Collaborative Care
Leadership Hint

Creating a Less Stressful Work Environment

1. Your ability to organize your shift will help prevent some stressful situations.
2. Have available the equipment that nursing assistants need to get their job done.
3. Encourage nursing assistants to take breaks as scheduled.
4. Create a calm environment.
5. Treat nursing assistants with respect. Remember your communication skills, especially "please," "thank you," and "I sure appreciate _____."

Collaborative Care
Leadership Activity

Identifying Signs of Stress

Resources needed:
- Any textbook identifying physical and emotional signs of stress

The next time you feel yourself getting stressed, identify how you are feeling and what you are thinking. List the physical and emotional symptoms you experience.

Stress Control Skills for the Licensed Practical/ Licensed Vocational Charge Nurse

Controlling Stress by Altering How You Think. Stress is the body's reaction to the mind's analysis of a situation. It is not the situation, but your reaction to the situation, that creates stress. You have the only **stress management** tool you will ever need right inside your head. If you learn to manage how you think about the many interactions you have daily with nursing assistants, residents, and family members, you can control your reaction and therefore your stress level.

Thinking Before "Irrational Thinking" Class

Nursing assistant (on telephone): "I cannot come in today. I have a headache."

LP/LV charge nurse (*thinking*): *"I'll just bet she has a headache. She probably spent half the night partying."*

The LPN/LVN becomes abrupt with the nursing assistant and hangs up. She feels angry and allows the incident to ruin her entire day. Nursing assistants can sense that the charge nurse is upset and will try to avoid any contact with her.

Ellis (1994) discusses rational versus **irrational thinking**. When we are in a situation, we engage in self-talk about what is happening. This self-talk is often irrational because it is based on judgments we make about the situation. Judgments are subjective and have no bearing on facts. The irrational thinking then causes negative emotions, and stress often results. Ellis offers the ABCD way of increasing awareness of irrational thinking and changing how we think to a more rational way. In learning to do so, we control our emotions and thus the stress that results. The following are examples of how Ellis's ABCD method of controlling irrational thinking applies to the practical/vocational charge nurse.

A—Activating event: The nursing assistant called in sick with a headache.

B—Belief (self-talk) about the situation: The charge nurse thinks the nursing assistant must have been out partying.

C—Consequences: The LPN/LVN manager was abrupt with the nursing assistant on the telephone. She allowed herself to feel angry about the absence. She allowed it to ruin her whole day. Nursing assistants avoided her like the plague.

D—Dispute irrational thoughts: Choose a more rational, assertive response to the situation. Focus on the objective facts (nursing assistant has a headache). Avoid the subjective judgments that your beliefs (self-talk) call up (the nursing assistant was partying). You will avoid the anger over this incident and its effect on nursing assistants. Stress is avoided for all.

Thinking After "Irrational Thinking" Class

Nursing assistant (on telephone): "I cannot come in today. I have a headache."

LP/LV charge nurse (tempted to use irrational thinking but remembers Ellis's ABCD instead): "I'm sorry to hear that. I hope you feel better after you get some rest."

See the Collaborative Care, Leadership Hint: Avoiding Irrational Thinking box.

Collaborative Care

Leadership Hint

Avoiding Irrational Thinking

1. Be aware that beliefs about the situation are self-talk. Self-talk sometimes makes judgments. These judgments, if negative, can cause an emotional reaction. The emotional reaction leads to stress.
2. See situations objectively. Rational thinking is based on facts. Objective facts do not cause emotion. The situation "just is."
3. Avoid thinking that nursing assistants *should*, *must*, or *always* do something. This is another example of irrational thinking and can lead to anger. When you use these words for yourself, they can lead to anxiety and guilt.
4. We do not have the power to make nursing assistants do anything. We can encourage, prefer, or expect that nursing assistants do something.
5. For yourself and team members, use the words *want*, *choose*, and *prefer* in your thinking.

SPECIFIC KNOWLEDGE AND SKILLS NEEDED FOR LEADERSHIP

To be a leader in long-term care, it is necessary to use the aforementioned core areas of knowledge as a base and to develop the following skills in three specific areas:

1. *Occupational (clinical) skills:* The knowledge and skills of nursing.
2. *Organizational skills:* Skills necessary to function in the organization that delivers health care.
3. *Human relationship skills:* The ability to get along with and relate to people.

OCCUPATIONAL SKILLS FOR FIRST-LINE LICENSED PRACTICAL NURSE/LICENSED VOCATIONAL NURSE LEADERS

Nursing (Clinical) Skills, Including the Nursing Process

Solid clinical skills are a must to be a good nursing leader. Visible expertise in clinical skills is a plus with the nursing assistants and also gives you an informal power base. See the resident situation for yourself, assist in providing care, and demonstrate nursing skills to nursing assistants as needed. This conveys the attitude that resident care comes first. This action demonstrates that the facility mission statement and unit goals are not just a written exercise. It communicates that practical/vocational charge nurses are there to support their staff.

Knowledge of your role in the nursing process is an important part of organizational skills. Your practical/vocational nursing program has started your skill development in this area. You will need to keep this area current and fresh. Refer to Chapters 9 and 12 for more about your role in the nursing process.

Documentation

Use the guidelines in nursing fundamentals for your charting. LP/LV charge nurses need to be aware of the documentation requirements of federal and state laws and accrediting agencies. Specific, objective documentation demonstrates whether or not the standard of care has been met. Effective nursing documentation is the basis for payment of resident fees or denial of payment by Medicare, insurance, and/or the state. This is especially important when these agencies mandate patient outcomes. Incomplete or questionable documentation could also result in a citation for the facility. It cannot be emphasized often enough that you must make sure all your charting is specific, objective, and complete. Avoid subjective comments and personal judgments in your charting. Students sometimes find this area of charting difficult, especially if they see examples of general and subjective entries on charts by licensed staff in the clinical area.

Legal Aspects

The nursing assistants and you, the LP/LV charge nurse, are the people who have direct contact with residents and their families on a daily basis. You have the ability to ensure resident and family satisfaction with care. You are also a vehicle to voice concerns. This in turn will decrease the need for legal action to resolve disputes. Chapter 7 provides you with information for being legally sound in your nursing career.

Be aware of your state's NPA, health care facility policies and procedures, state and federal regulations, and published standards of your nursing organizations and codes of conduct. These standards and codes are guidelines to evaluate safe practice. It is your responsibility as a licensed nurse to keep current and informed.

Federal regulations. Your facility must be in compliance with federal, state, and local laws. The impact of federal regulations in your facility is affected by the **Omnibus Budget Reconciliation Act of 1987 (OBRA)** and the **Centers for Medicare and Medicaid Services (CMS)**.

The Omnibus Budget Reconciliation Act of 1987. OBRA contains the Nursing Home Reform Act. The basic objective of the Nursing Home Reform Act is to ensure that residents of nursing homes receive quality care that will result in their achieving or maintaining their "highest practicable" (reasonable) physical, mental, and psychosocial well-being. The act also established a Resident's Bill of Rights. A copy of one state's Resident's Bill of Rights can be found at http://www.health.state.mn.us/divs/fpc/consumerinfo. OBRA regulations will be reviewed with you at the time of your orientation. See the Collaborative Care, Leadership Hint: OBRA Provisions That Deal Specifically with Nursing Assistants box.

Collaborative Care
Leadership Hint

Omnibus Budget Reconciliation Act Provisions That Deal Specifically with Nursing Assistants

1. Nursing assistants require a minimum of 75 hours of instruction before taking a state-approved written and skills competency evaluation. This establishes a baseline proficiency and competence of nursing assistants.
2. Each state must have a nursing assistant registry. This registry is an official list of individuals who have successfully completed nursing assistant training and competency evaluation. To be listed in a state directory, the history of the nursing assistant must be free of incidents of abuse, neglect, or dishonest use of property.
3. Your state's registry must be notified by the employer before employment of nursing assistants. The registry of some states is available online.
4. Nursing assistants' work must be evaluated "regularly."
5. Nursing assistants must complete inservice training hours per year. Number of hours can vary based on the state of registry.
6. If an extended period of time has passed without a person being employed as a nursing assistant, training and competency evaluation will need to be repeated.

Centers for Medicare and Medicaid Services. This agency was formerly called the Health Care Financing Administration (HCFA). CMS, a federal agency of the Department of Health and Human Services (HHS), certifies nursing homes for Medicare and Medicaid reimbursement. To receive payment, facilities are required to meet conditions of participation. The long-term care unit will have the conditions of participation in its policies. **Current** CMS regulations will be presented during your orientation.

Your state's regulations. Long-term care units and nursing homes are licensed by the state in which they are located. Each state sets regulations that must be met to be licensed. Periodically, inspectors will visit the facility to determine whether the facility has any deficiencies. Being cited for deficiencies can affect licensing. Your state's regulations will be reviewed at orientation.

The Joint Commission (TJC) is an independent, not-for-profit organization. The purpose of this organization is to improve quality of care by creating a safe environment for patients through the accreditation process. TJC reviews organizations such as hospitals, long-term care facilities, and home health agencies. Accreditation is a voluntary activity. If your facility participates in TJC accreditation, its requirements will be explained to you at your orientation. Detailed

information about TJC and long-term care can be obtained at www.jointcommission.org.

ORGANIZATIONAL SKILLS FOR FIRST-LINE LICENSED PRACTICAL NURSE/LICENSED VOCATIONAL NURSE LEADERS

Organizational skills are an essential ingredient for leaders as well as team members. The emphasis on the personal and vocational issues/concepts course in your student practical/vocational nursing program has given you the opportunity to learn and apply the principles of time management (see Chapter 2). Continuous quality improvement (see Chapter 19) and conflict management (see Chapter 8) are also necessary skills for the development of any nursing leader in today's health care organizations, including long-term care.

Time Management

Whether your dominance is on the left or right side of the brain, you have been given the opportunity this year to develop **time management** skills by applying the content of Chapters 1 and 2. Your school year has certainly provided the need to use your time effectively (doing the right thing) and efficiently (doing it right the first time, and in the appropriate amount of time) for class, clinical, and home. The step-by-step procedures learned in the nursing skills lab helped you prioritize your care for efficiency and the safety and comfort of the patient. You have experience organizing work for one or two patients in the clinical area. As an LP/LV charge nurse, you will direct the care of approximately 30 residents and supervise a team of possibly three to four nursing assistants.

Time management is more about management and less about time. Your ability to manage time will help you organize tasks and allow you to be successful as a charge nurse. Once again, the nursing process will be the tool to help you get organized. See the Collaborative Care, Leadership Hint: Applying the Nursing Process to Organize Your Shift box.

Collaborative Care
Leadership Hint

Applying the Nursing Process to Organize Your Shift

ASSESSMENT (DATA COLLECTION) OF TASKS

1. Make a *to-do* list that reflects unit routines and schedules. When new to the job, listing unit routines and schedules is helpful until you experience the actual routine. This list includes break times, staff meal times, resident meals and nourishments, scheduled physician rounds, and routine times for vital signs, blood glucose testing, medicine administration, and treatments.
2. Develop a *worksheet* to use during report. Use a style you are comfortable with. Some charge nurses develop a list according to a sequence of room numbers. Others list residents that need special assessments. Others list treatments, vital signs, and so on by time.

Continued

Collaborative Care

Leadership Hint—cont'd

3. *Prioritize* the list. Use Maslow's hierarchy of needs to set priorities for residents. Remember physiologic needs must be met before other needs are considered. "As" are most important needs and must be done. They could be life-threatening or urgent resident needs. "Bs" must be done, but there is more leeway in the exact time they are accomplished. Some "Cs" are necessary but not of urgent status. Some of the "Bs" and "Cs" can be assigned to unlicensed assistive personnel (UAPs) or postponed if appropriate. Some "Cs" might not need to be listed at all. Here are some examples:

TASKS	EXAMPLES	COMMENTS
"A" tasks	STAT med, PRN med, q2h neuro check after resident's fall on prior shift	New "A" tasks always surface during the shift, requiring modification of the *to-do* list. These needs are unpredictable and cannot be planned in advance.
"B" tasks	Routine medicine administration, dressing changes, routine resident personal care, ambulation, activities, routine treatments, nourishments, meals	These needs are recurring and predictable but can have specific timelines.
"C" tasks	Mail and flower delivery, chitchat with family	Important but can be delayed.

PRN, pro re nata (as needed); *q2h*, quaque secunda hora (every 2 hours); *STAT*, statim (immediately).

PLANNING USE OF TIME (GOAL SETTING)

1. Plan tasks within a time frame of 2 to 3 hours. Arrange blocks of time according to unit routine. Planning allows you to have the feeling you are in control of the situation. Take resident preferences into consideration when you are planning. For example, one resident prefers to eat breakfast at 6 AM, but breakfast is served at 8 AM. Arrangements could be made for coffee and crackers at 6 AM, if diet allows.

2. Use the same guidelines for setting goals for planning time as with care plans or personal goals. Focus on goals as outcomes (the results expected after a given period). Using action verbs, make sure goals are realistic and measurable. A measurable goal states specifically and objectively what results are expected after a specified period. Set minigoals for timed tasks to keep you on task.

3. Planning involves having the equipment and supplies that the team needs for the shift and the shift that follows. As you collect data about residents when first starting your shift, check rooms and treatment closets for needed supplies. This includes linen, a well-stocked floor refrigerator, supplies for treatments, and supplies for medicine administration kept on a medication cart.

4. Make sure you have your personal tools for the shift: your watch (working), a pen that writes, bandage scissors, a stethoscope, and a small notebook. Use the notebook to quickly jot down the equipment that is needed and the results of data collection.

IMPLEMENTING YOUR PLAN

1. Remember your plan is written in soft margarine, not hard marble. Be flexible.

2. As you carry out your plan for the shift, expect interruptions of your planned activities. You know they will occur but not when. These include telephone calls, changes in residents' conditions, transfer of a resident, and staff injury.

3. When unexpected events occur, planning assists you to rearrange tasks. If you have a plan, you can return to the plan after interruptions. You can continue or revise the plan as needed.

EVALUATING YOUR USE OF TIME

1. As nursing assistants give you reports for their assigned residents, seek input from them about the effectiveness and efficiency of the shift.

2. Ask for suggestions to improve staff and your use of time at the next shift you work.

3. Keep a log of your shift activities. Look for a pattern of inefficient use of time. Examples of time wasters are putting things off, allowing unnecessary interruptions, socializing with staff, inability to say "no," and allowing telephone calls to exceed needed time for business.

4. At the end of your shift, take a few minutes to plan for the next day. This will allow you to leave work-related activities at work, and allow you to enjoy your much-needed leisure time.

Continuous Quality Improvement

Continuous quality improvement (CQI) is a program found in all health care facilities. The principles of CQI found in health care are borrowed from those of the business world. The focus of CQI is quality of care. Quality is indicated by patient outcomes. **Patient outcomes** are observable, measurable results of nursing activities. The CQI program involves all departments of health care facilities, including long-term care. You will receive information about the CQI program during orientation at your facility. See the Collaborative Care, Leadership Hint: Continuous Quality Improvement Components That the Licensed Practical/Licensed Vocational Charge Nurse Needs to Incorporate into the Leadership Role box.

The CMS is involved with quality improvement in nursing homes and long-term care facilities. The **Quality Improvement Organization (QIO)** program consists of a national network of experts, clinicians, and consumers working together to improve care to Medicare recipients. The core functions of QIO include the following (www.cms.gov):

• Improve quality of care for beneficiaries.
• Protect integrity of Medicare Trust Fund.
• Protect beneficiaries by expeditiously addressing individual complaints, notices, and appeals, such as noncoverage.

Continuous Quality Improvement Components That the Licensed Practical/Licensed Vocational Charge Nurse Needs to Incorporate into the Leadership Role

1. Review job descriptions with your nursing assistants. Emphasize the role they have in achieving quality and safety in care and resident service for a reasonable price (do it right the first time).
2. Remember that CQI is a continuous, daily part of your unit.
3. Encourage nursing assistants to report safety issues in resident care and the work environment.
4. Encourage nursing assistants to offer suggestions to solve safety issues in number 3 of this list.
5. When safety issues are noted, initiate a plan for improvement.
6. Consider volunteering for a CQI committee. Policies and nursing procedures are revised based on the input you and your nursing assistants provide regarding resident care and the functioning of the unit. It is personally rewarding to be included in policy and procedure revision because revisions improve resident care.
7. Document resident information in an objective and specific manner. Your documentation will be used to measure the effectiveness of CQI efforts.

Conflict Resolution

Conflict can occur whenever two or more persons interact. In long-term care, conflicts can arise with nursing assistants, staff, residents, families, and physicians. Conflict is not always a bad thing; sometimes it is an opportunity for growth and learning. Other times the presence of conflict can point out the need for change in an organization. When conflicts are out in the open, the opportunity exists to settle issues. This is preferable to leaving conflicts unsettled. Unsettled conflicts can act like cancer, slowly growing into something much larger that may be more difficult or impossible to resolve. Tools to reduce conflicts include clear communication and the ability to work well as a team. **Conflict resolution** involves people settling their differences. Resolution of the conflict is an exercise in problem solving. See the Collaborative Care, Leadership Hint: Applying the Nursing Process for Conflict Resolution box.

Applying the Nursing Process for Conflict Resolution

DATA COLLECTION: OBTAIN ALL THE FACTS

1. When a conflict arises, avoid pursuing it on the spot. Arrange for the involved parties to meet in an area that will provide privacy. First meet with each separately.
2. Separate the person from the problem. Attack the problem, not one another.
3. Each party has its own perception and strong emotions about what happened. Unclear communication may result. Clarify subjective statements and generalizations. You need to obtain objective and specific facts. For example, clarify what is meant by "she always does that" and "they."
4. Actively listen to the person presenting "the facts."
5. Avoid formulating your response while the other party is giving "the facts."

STATE THE PROBLEM: IDENTIFY THE SPECIFIC ISSUE

1. After hearing all sides, state in your own words what you understand to be the conflict. Use *I* messages when presenting your perspective. For example, say, "Emma, I heard you say that Hannah always leaves the utility room in disarray and does not offer to help the other nursing assistants when she has completed her work and they are swamped."
2. Ask parties for feedback as to the accuracy of your understanding of the conflict: "Emma, am I clear about the nature of your complaint? Is there anything you would like to add or correct?" and "Hannah, is there anything you would like to add or correct about the situation?"

INTERVENTIONS (PLANNING)

1. Convey the attitude of working side by side to settle the conflict. For example, sit side by side to work on the problem.
2. Involve all parties in identifying and discussing possible solutions to the conflict. The more alternatives, the better. The goal is a solution that will be agreeable to everyone's interests.
3. *Avoid* bargaining over *positions* (*what you want*). Egos are identified with positions. The parties involved will focus on defending their positions. In the end, all parties need to save face.
4. *Focus* on *interests* (*why something is wanted*). Behind a *position* is a *motivating interest*. Behind opposite *positions* lie shared and compatible *interests*. *Compromise* involves giving up aspects of an issue that are important to one of the parties involved. This is not a good intervention. *Collaborate* for a win/win solution that focuses on shared or compatible interests.

IMPLEMENTATION: IMPLEMENT THE SELECTED SOLUTION

On a sunny, cool day in the fall, two residents are sitting in the sunroom of a long-term care facility. Resident A's *position* is that he wants a window open, and Resident B's *position* is that he wants the windows shut. The LP/LV charge nurse asks Resident A why he wants a window open. He replies, "So I can get some fresh air." The charge nurse asks Resident B why he wants the windows closed. He replies, "So it won't be drafty."

A solution built on *collaboration* would involve the charge nurse wrapping Resident B in a blanket and moving his wheelchair to the north end of the sunroom. She would move Resident A to the south end of the sunroom and open a window near him. This is a win/win solution. A solution built on *compromise* would involve the LP/LV charge nurse returning one of the residents to his room and accommodating the other in the sunroom. This is an "I win/you lose" solution.

EVALUATION: EVALUATE THE EFFECTIVENESS OF INTERVENTIONS IN MEETING THE GOAL

In the preceding situation, the LP/LV charge nurse returns 30 minutes later and finds both residents peacefully asleep in their wheelchairs.

Human relationship skills for first-line licensed practical nurse/licensed vocational nurse leaders

LP/LV charge nurses can have excellent clinical skills, use the nursing process expertly, and document to the letter of the law. The LP/LV charge nurse can have a good understanding of federal and state laws and requirements of accrediting agencies. Charge nurses can get the job done efficiently, but perhaps human relationship skills are the most important skills for an LPN/LVN leader to have. Leaders with human relationship skills will get the job done with style and tact, without sacrificing quality. Nursing assistants will value their leader's style a whole lot more and be more effective in reaching the goals of the unit. Because success depends on what is accomplished through others, the ability to relate well to others is crucial.

Professional Pointer

Human relationship skills are important skills for an LPN/LVN to have in any clinical setting.

LPNs/LVNs are well versed in clinical skills. They risk bringing *clinical* problem-solving skills to the practical/vocational charge nurse role when leadership/management skills, in the area of human relationship skills, are needed in this position.

Anger Management

Besides providing money on which to live, work provides people with the opportunity to be recognized for what they do, to belong to a group, and to display their competence. (Review the Howlett hierarchy of work motivators.) When any of these needs is threatened in the course of the workday, or when you feel like a victim in a workplace with lack of control, you may get angry. Anger is not automatically bad; it gives you a cue that something is wrong. If your anger is justified, it can help you get your needs met by stimulating you to action. Harassment and discrimination are examples of situations in which anger is justified. If your anger is unjustified, or displayed inappropriately, it can get you and others in trouble. It is always important to remember that all behavior must be professional. See the Collaborative Care, Leadership Hint: Preventing Anger in Nursing Assistants box, the Collaborative Care, Leadership Hint: Personal Anger Management Techniques for the Practical/Vocational Charge Nurse box, and the Collaborative Care, Leadership Hint: Prevention of Workplace Violence box.

Collaborative Care
Leadership Hint

Preventing Anger in Nursing Assistants

1. Meet the needs above level 2 (e.g., belonging, affiliation, and recognition) on the Maslow and Howlett hierarchies.
2. Use assertive communication, especially I messages. This will prevent the LP/LV charge nurse from being perceived as a threat. In your I messages, remember to include what you observed, the possible result of that observation, and your recommendations.
3. Actively listen, using direct eye contact and alert body posture, to convey to nursing assistants that you are interested in understanding their point of view.
4. Successful team building helps nursing assistants feel like part of the group.
5. Seek input of nursing assistants to find solutions for unit problems. This provides a sense of control over one's work environment.
6. Use win/win strategies in conflict resolution to provide a feeling of having control over situations and being treated with respect.
7. Encourage nursing assistants to participate in objective evaluation of their clinical performance to maintain self-esteem, and give nursing assistants some control over what happens to them.
8. Encouraging self-evaluation also helps tone down an important but potentially volatile area, especially when areas for improvement are noted.
9. Attempt to help nursing assistants become self-confident, reach their full potential, and achieve the higher levels of the Maslow and Howlett hierarchies. When needs are met at these higher levels, nursing assistants are more satisfied in their work environment.

Collaborative Care
Leadership Hint

Personal Anger Management Techniques for the Licensed Practical/Licensed Vocational Charge Nurse

1. Learn your personal signs that communicate you are becoming angry. Pay attention to what you are thinking and feeling.
2. How you appraise events causes the anger response. Change irrational thoughts to rational thoughts.
3. If your heart is pounding, take deep breaths.
4. If you feel tension in a body area, rub the area for a few seconds.
5. When angry, speak slowly and in a lower tone of voice, acknowledge how you feel, and take a time-out.
6. View a stimulus to anger as a problem. Use the problem-solving process to arrive at a solution.

Collaborative Care
Leadership Hint

Prevention of Workplace Violence

1. Suggest inservice education in anger management for all employees.
2. Create a work environment that is respectful and fun.
3. As an LP/LV charge nurse, be a positive role model for anger management.
4. Take conflicts in the work environment seriously.
5. Refer to/use your facility's employee assistance program (EAP).
6. If your facility does not have an EAP program, suggest that such a program be developed.

Performance Evaluation of Nursing Assistants

The thought of **performance evaluation** can send shivers up the spine of the person doing the evaluating, as well as of the person being evaluated. Perhaps this goes back to bad evaluation experiences in prior situations. Perhaps it even goes as far back as grade school. Perhaps you and the nursing assistants have learned to associate evaluation with constructive criticism and weaknesses. Keep sight of the main purpose of evaluation, which is to encourage personal and career growth. Constructive evaluation gives you and your team members a profile of strong behaviors and behaviors for improvement, along with a plan to improve. Evaluation encourages the development of employees who will meet the facility's objectives and fulfill the mission statement. See the Collaborative Care, Leadership Hint: Providing Feedback to Nursing Assistants box.

Collaborative Care
Leadership Hint

Providing Feedback to Nursing Assistants

POSITIVE FEEDBACK IDENTIFIES STRONG BEHAVIORS TO BE ENCOURAGED

1. Most nursing assistants know what it is like to be caught doing something "wrong." Catch them doing something "right." This encourages them to repeat the behavior.
2. Let nursing assistants know you notice their efforts, believe in them, and feel good about their contributions to the long-term care facility.
3. Praise people in measurable terms (specific and objective) so that the behavior can be repeated. For example, say, "When you disinfected the shower, I noticed that you paid special attention to the corners and the shower chair. Great job!"

NEGATIVE FEEDBACK IDENTIFIES BEHAVIORS THAT NEED IMPROVEMENT

1. Provide verbal feedback as close to the event as possible. The purpose of constructive feedback is to point out behaviors that need to be modified. Focus on the behavior as one needing improvement. Avoid addressing the behavior as a criticism.
2. Without emotion, objectively point out what is wrong with the behavior and its consequences. You want the nursing assistant to remember the message, not the manner in which it was delivered. You also want the team member to know it is performance that is being evaluated.
3. Negative feedback needs to be accompanied by suggestions to correct the behavior. These suggestions need to be so specific that the nursing assistant will be able to correct the behavior by following them. For example, you might say, "I noticed that the ties of your isolation gown were untied while you were in the room with the patient who has tuberculosis. Once you remove the gown, you risk spreading the bacteria to other patients, staff, and your family because the back of your uniform was not protected. When getting into an isolation gown, be sure to cover the back of your uniform and tie the gown at the waist."
4. Mention behaviors that need improvement first. Offer praise at the end of a reprimand. The message will be heard more clearly. The impact of the praising will not be ruined.

As an LP/LV charge nurse, your responsibilities in evaluating nursing assistants include the following:
1. Observing skill performance and attitudes of nursing assistants
2. Providing daily oral/written feedback, including suggestions for improvement
3. Documenting observations
4. Presenting a final evaluation form

Review the evaluation process and form for your facility. What you are evaluating is not subject to your personal judgment. You will be objectively evaluating the skills and attitudes of nursing assistants. These work-related activities are expected of nursing assistants and are found in their job description and the facility's policy manual. If a checklist format is used for daily observations, be sure you understand the scale used by the long-term care facility. In observing nursing skills, you will be evaluating the application of nursing assistant knowledge of a skill to actual skill performance. Attitudes are more difficult to evaluate. They are stated as observable behaviors and usually involve areas such as dress and grooming, attendance, functioning as a team member, and interpersonal skills. Concerns regarding attitudes should be discussed with your supervisor to facilitate a positive outcome.

The performance evaluation is written documentation of what you have been discussing and documenting throughout the period before the formal process of evaluation. Documentation is a time-consuming task. When you are used to the system for the long-term care facility, you will find it can be completed more quickly.

OBRA mandates regular evaluations for nursing assistants. In addition to scheduled performance evaluations, you will be giving spontaneous feedback to nursing assistants. Evaluation is the responsibility of the LP/LV charge nurse and the nursing assistant. No one needs to "give" another person an evaluation. Evaluation needs to be a joint process. Evaluation is not a secret that you surprise team members with at the end of the evaluation period. It is a tool for personal and career growth. A team member has the right to be able to correct areas for improvement as time goes by. It is unfair to have your discrepancies unloaded (i.e., dumped) on you during the final evaluation interview. See the Collaborative Care, Leadership Hint: Encouraging Nursing Assistants to Participate in the Evaluation Process box and the Collaborative Care, Leadership Hint: Meeting for the Final Evaluation Interview box.

Collaborative Care
Leadership Hint

Encouraging Nursing Assistants to Participate in the Evaluation Process

1. Provide nursing assistants with their own copy of the evaluation form at the beginning of the evaluation experience. Tell them it contains the elements you will be evaluating. Encourage them to read it.

Continued

Collaborative Care

Leadership Hint—cont'd

2. Encourage nursing assistants to evaluate themselves daily/weekly and record their evaluation on their copy of the form. This also gives them the opportunity to become familiar with the form.
3. Remind them to include their strong areas. People are good at identifying areas for improvement but sometimes need reminders to acknowledge their strong points. Dispel the myth that doing so is egotistical or boastful. It is merely stating what is.
4. Encourage nursing assistants to include a plan on the evaluation form for improving areas that need improvement.

Collaborative Care

Leadership Hint

Meeting for the Final Evaluation Interview

1. Remember that the goal of evaluation is to encourage personal and professional growth. In preparation for the evaluation, summarize strong behaviors of the nursing assistant and behaviors that need improvement on your copy of the evaluation form. Develop a suggested plan for improvement. Attach this summary to the front of the evaluation. Remind nursing assistants to do the same and to bring their copy of the completed evaluation form to the meeting.
2. Schedule the interview at a private location.
3. Allow 15 to 20 minutes for the interview.
4. Conduct the interview in a neutral manner. Be careful of both your verbal and nonverbal messages.
5. Use I messages when discussing the summary sheet. For example, say, "The following are the behaviors that I observed when you were working with residents and staff . . . ."
6. Use the information on the 4 I's of Transformational Leadership learned in this chapter to guide your interaction.
7. Start with strong behaviors and compare them with the nursing assistant's list. This creates a good mood.
8. Compare behaviors for improvement.
   a. Similar behaviors appearing on both evaluation forms can indicate insight into the problem. Both the nursing assistant and the LP/LV charge nurse have noted similar behaviors in the clinical area.
   b. When the nursing assistant includes behaviors not noted by the LP/LV charge nurse, this can indicate the value of self-evaluation. The charge nurse cannot observe everything.
   c. If the LP/LV charge nurse includes behaviors not included by the nursing assistant, this can indicate lack of self-evaluation by the nursing assistant.
9. Finish the evaluation interview with the plan for improvement for any behaviors that need to be modified. The nursing assistant's plan is especially valuable because it indicates personal thinking through of interventions needed for improvement and strengths to build upon.

10. Check feedback throughout the interview to ensure clear communication. Have the nursing assistant rephrase feedback to see whether or not your intended message was heard. Some people may distort the message. Clarify messages given by the nursing assistant for information not understood. Encourage questions about any areas on the evaluation that are not understood. For example, say, "What did you understand me to say regarding your areas of strength that I have identified?"
11. Have the nursing assistant sign and date both evaluations. You do the same. The signature indicates that the forms were discussed and all questions were answered.

Your nonthreatening, objective approach to constructive evaluation will result in positive evaluation experiences for you and the nursing assistants on your team. Occasionally you may experience a situation in which a nursing assistant feels threatened and becomes defensive during evaluation. If the defensiveness begins to escalate or the person displays anger, terminate the meeting. Set a new time for another meeting. Have your supervisor present at this time. Such experiences are the exception, not the rule.

Empowering Team Members and Encouraging Personal Growth and Development of Confidence

It is rewarding to see the nursing assistants on your team increase their self-confidence and display career and personal growth. You can encourage personal growth in nursing assistants by demonstrating the leadership skills you have developed in your position as an LP/LV charge nurse. The nursing assistant must do the actual work to achieve confidence and grow. See the Collaborative Care, Leadership Hint: Strategies to Increase Self-Confidence in Nursing Assistants box and the Collaborative Care, Leadership Hint: Strategies to Encourage Personal Growth in Nursing Assistants box.

Collaborative Care

Leadership Hint

Strategies to Increase Self-Confidence in Nursing Assistants

1. Provide opportunities to be successful in new situations.
2. Praise beginning successes in new situations.
3. On clinical evaluation forms, include positive statements as well as negative statements.
4. With administration's support, plan educational opportunities for nursing assistants (e.g., seminars and inservice programs).
5. Include nursing assistants in planning meetings and inservice ideas.
6. Stand up for and support nursing assistants' contributions to the facility.
7. Actively listen to problems involving the clinical area.
8. Coach/mentor nursing assistants on a new skill and/or how to improve an old one.
9. Provide challenging assignments that stimulate thinking.

👥 Collaborative Care
Leadership Hint

Strategies to Encourage Personal Growth in Nursing Assistants

1. Display a balanced interest in the personal problems of nursing assistants.
2. Encourage nursing assistants to solve their own problems.
3. Suggest referral when nursing assistants are unable to solve personal problems. Follow facility policies.
4. Remember nursing assistants are individuals. Clip and give pertinent articles and information.
5. Be a mentor/coach.
6. Be a role model. Display a positive work ethic; demonstrate good clinical skills; get out from behind the desk and see what is going on with residents; display good grooming; give objective, specific feedback; address the problem, not people; and actively listen.

ADDITIONAL RESOURCES FOR THE LICENSED PRACTICAL NURSE/LICENSED VOCATIONAL NURSE TO DEVELOP ORGANIZATIONAL, OCCUPATIONAL, AND HUMAN RELATIONSHIP SKILLS

There are many ways to add occupational, organizational, and human relationship skills for survival in the workplace. Some of the following suggestions for additional learning for the practical/vocational charge nurse offer continuing education credits. See the Collaborative Care, Leadership Hint: Sources of Learning Skills for the Practical/Vocational Charge Nurse Position box.

👥 Collaborative Care
Leadership Hint

Sources of Learning Skills for the Licensed Practical/Licensed Vocational Charge Nurse Position

1. Check with your local vocational/technical school for an LP/LV nursing leadership course.
2. Ask your boss to consider inservice programs on leadership techniques, including transformational leadership strategies, as well as updates on nursing skills. Suggest cosponsoring such inservices with the local technical college and making them available to a wide geographical area.
3. Form a network with other persons who fill first-line leadership positions. Be sure to go outside your institution, as well as the discipline of nursing. You will find that the leaders have similar problems regardless of the discipline.
4. Attend seminars relating to leadership topics as well as nursing topics.
5. Read books and articles that offer hints for leaders. Be sure your personal nursing library is up to date.
6. Enroll for certification courses to enhance your knowledge and skills. See Chapter 18 for additional information.

💡 Keep in Mind

"Effective leadership is putting first things first. Effective management is discipline, carrying it out."

-Stephen R. Covey

Tricia was always a "saver," as her several well-constructed scrapbooks and boxes of books and papers from nursing school verified. Tricia looked at the carefully clipped classified ad she had saved from 5 years ago, when she had applied for her current nursing position. Five years ago, her husband was transferred to the neighboring state of Ohio. After 3 years' experience as an LVN in a nursing home, postgraduate courses in leadership at the local technical college, seminars, inservice programs, personal reading, and workshops, Tricia thought that she was qualified for a charge nurse position.

Tricia smiled as she pictured herself going in for the interview. That navy blue blazer sure paid off! And all her preparation for the interview served her well. What a sage Mrs. Kelly had been in her Transitions to Practice class to recommend that a job applicant read the facility's mission statement before the interview. Although she did not have LP/LV charge nurse experience, she was sure her knowledge of the facility's emphasis on and pride in providing quality care was a big plus in landing the job. And this was in addition to the enthusiasm and positive attitude she displayed to the interviewer about her willingness to learn and her confidence that she would be able to do the job. Also, following the textbook suggestion to obtain the respective state's Nurse Practice Act before employment gave her the opportunity to learn how an LPN/LVN could delegate in the respective state and helped her to think of some supervision/delegation-related questions to ask at the interview.

Five years had passed since she had secured the job as LP/LV charge nurse. Tricia loved her job and smiled as she remembered many of the challenges she had faced early in her job as charge nurse. She began to page through that old eighth edition of her textbook . . .

Licensed Practical Nurse/Licensed Vocational Nurse

Full-time position available for an experienced LPN/LVN to join our long-term care facility as a charge nurse on the evening shift. Must have excellent communication and customer service skills, needs to be team-oriented, and must have current state of Ohio license. We offer a competitive salary and full benefits package. If you qualify, submit resume and cover letter to: cradant

Before continuing with Tricia's story, review the Collaborative Care, Leadership Activity: Determining Your State's Requirements to Assume the Position of Licensed Practical/Licensed Vocational Charge Nurse box in this chapter.

Tricia looked at the job description the director of nurses gave her during her job interview. It all seems such a routine and comfortable part of her job, but Tricia remembers how overwhelming it was to read through the 12 areas of responsibility, along with the 15 duties of the charge nurse.

WHERE TO BEGIN? JOB DESCRIPTION FOR CHARGE NURSE

Read the Collaborative Care, Management Tool: Reviewing Licensed Practical/Licensed Vocational Charge Nurse Job Descriptions box. The charge nurse job description might seem overwhelming at first, but it illustrates the reason some state laws require that LP/LV charge nurses have education, training, or experience beyond the basic LP/LV nursing curriculum and documentation of such. It is difficult to prepare health care workers in 1 year or less to be able to function in this position immediately after graduation. After additional education, training, and experience, many LPNs/LVNs become charge nurses, also called first-line managers, in long-term care units and nursing homes. They are doing an excellent job in that role. The NCSBN (2013) 2012 job analysis survey identified that 43.4% of LPNs/LVNs responding to the survey reported they had administrative responsibilities.

Collaborative Care
Management Tool

Reviewing Licensed Practical Nurse/Licensed Vocational Nurse Charge Nurse Job Descriptions

Resources needed:
- Review LP/LV charge nurse job descriptions of long-term care facilities at sites at which you affiliate during your student year.

HOW LONG WILL IT TAKE ME TO PREPARE TO BE A CHARGE NURSE?

You are probably thinking, "How long will it take for me to get to this point in my practical/vocational nursing career?" The answer is individual to the person asking it. The law of some states specifically dictates that the LPN/LVN charge nurse functions in a nursing home and under the direct supervision of a registered nurse. Also, the LPN/LVN could not function under

---

Quality Care Licensed Practical/Licensed Vocational Charge Nurse: Job Description

QUALIFICATIONS
Licensed practical/licensed vocational nurse with a current license to practice in State XYZ. One-year experience as a charge nurse in a long-term care facility.

STANDARDS
The job of the LP/LV charge nurse is to ensure that residents receive high-quality, low-cost nursing care that has been ordered by their health care provider. The LP/LV charge nurse shall do the following:
- Collaborate with the RN to provide resident care services (e.g., physicians, dietitian, activity director, physical therapist, and social worker).
- Assist the Director of Nurses in the orientation of new employees.
- Evaluate work performance of nursing assistants.

RESPONSIBLE FOR (COLLABORATING WITH THE RN)
- Knowledge of residents' conditions at all times.
- Assigning actual nursing care tasks to nursing assistants.
- Providing nursing care according to physicians' orders and in agreement with recognized nursing techniques and procedures, established standards of care as described in state statutes, and administrative policies of this long-term care facility.
- Recognizing symptoms: reporting residents' conditions, including changes, and assisting with remedial measures for adverse developments.
- Assisting physician in diagnostic and therapeutic measures.
- Administering medications and treatments as prescribed.
- Maintaining accurate and complete records of nursing data collection and interventions, including documentation on the electronic medical record (EMR) and Kardex.
- Efficiency in completing workload, including neatness and orderliness.
- Delegating duties, as appropriate, to nursing assistants.

- Maintaining a safe and hazard-free environment.
- Ensuring the residents' right to privacy.
- Maintaining the dignity of residents.

DUTIES (IN COLLABORATION WITH THE RN)
- Observes and reports symptoms and conditions of residents.
- Administers medications safely and as prescribed by physicians. Gathers data about therapeutic response and side effects of medications.
- Takes and records vital signs accurately when appropriate. Maintains charts and Kardexes, including residents' conditions and medications and treatments received.
- Notifies physician when necessary. Records phone/fax orders.
- Contacts pharmacist for prescription drugs as needed.
- Assists in maintaining a physical, social, and psychological environment for residents that is conducive to their best interests and welfare.
- Receives report at beginning of shift from personnel on previous shift and assigns tasks to nursing assistants under the LP/LV charge nurse's supervision.
- Supervises, assists with, and evaluates delegated duties to nursing assistants.
- Evaluates the completion of nursing assistant assignments in a safe and timely manner.
- Provides report to oncoming shift.
- Evaluates nursing assistants in the performance of their job description and reports same to Director of Nursing.
- Attends patient care meetings and supervisory staff meetings.
- Interprets state and federal guidelines to employees. Uses authority as LP/LV charge nurse to "follow code."
- Participates in orientation of all new employees assigned to LP/LV charge nurse.

general supervision until after passing the NCLEX-PN® examination. *Be sure to check your state's Nurse Practice Act.* Some LP/LV nursing programs offer a postgraduate course that prepares graduates for an expanded role. The answer to the question, "How long will it take for me to get to this point in my LP/LV nursing career?" depends on your state's Nurse Practice Act, additional education, your motivation to learn the manager role, your ability to be a risk taker, how you use your nursing experience and the policy and procedures of the employing institution.

HOW THIS TEXT CAN HELP YOU TO PREPARE FOR A FUTURE CHARGE NURSE POSITION

This text is unable to provide you with a concise recipe of how to function in the role of charge nurse as an LPN/LVN. This chapter begins with a discussion of areas of responsibilities, problems, and concerns that affect the LP/LV charge nurse in a long-term care unit or nursing home. Through active learning and an interactive format, this chapter presents both management and leadership tools. These tools involve you with the many areas that need to be considered, understood, and investigated when assuming an LP/LV charge nurse position. In addition, critical-thinking exercises present the opportunity to apply learning in the area of assignment and delegation.

Scenarios for three residents are interspersed throughout the nursing process guide for *leading*, *assigning*, and *delegating*. You will be expected to be self-directed, to problem solve, and to think critically as you apply the information in this chapter. These are the very attributes employers expect of you as an LP/LV charge nurse. References to specific resources that you will need to work through the leadership and management tools are provided. You are encouraged to use the information from the entire text, your other classes, and your learning resource center. Your instructor is a valuable resource. Remember, also, the usefulness of peer group discussion.

At times we will flash back to Tricia as she reminisces about her early days in the LP/LV charge nurse position. Her initial experiences and adjustment to the charge nurse role will show you the challenges and opportunities the LP/LV charge nurse role provides.

Tricia thought back to the orientation phase of her job. It seemed so overwhelming at the time. The thought of going through those thick manuals of policies, regulations, and routines was enough to give her a headache. However, they sure did contain valuable information. Mrs. Kelly gave the class the following sample checklist as a guide when reviewing these manuals.

A CHECKLIST OF POLICIES, REGULATIONS, AND ROUTINES FOR THE LICENSED PRACTICAL/ LICENSED VOCATIONAL CHARGE NURSE

Not all the areas included in this checklist are the responsibility of the LP/LV charge nurse in a nursing

home/long-term care facility. However, LP/LV charge nurses need to have information for all the areas included so they can carry out their management duties. Because the LP/LV charge nurse has the responsibility to supervise nursing assistants, these personnel also need information about policies and routines. Orientation to your facility needs to include these items.

FACILITY ORGANIZATION/LEGAL ASPECTS

- Mission statement
- Organizational chart
- State statutes for all licensed persons on health care team
- Skills checklists for LPNs/LVNs and nursing assistants
- Skills checklists for all cross-trained personnel
- Job descriptions and duties of RNs and LPNs/ LVNs
- Job descriptions and duties of unlicensed personnel and cross-trained personnel

FEDERAL, STATE, AND PRIVATE AGENCY REGULATIONS

- Inspection protocols/standards
- Current federal (including Health Insurance Portability and Accountability Act [HIPAA] regulations) and state regulations
- Regulations of the Omnibus Budget Reconciliation Act of 1987 (OBRA)
- Regulations of the Centers for Medicare and Medicaid Services (CMS)
- Regulations of The Joint Commission (if facility seeks TJC accreditation)
- National Patient Safety Standards
- Other related accreditation standards

PERSONNEL POLICIES

- Employee manual
- Time sheets: location and interpretation
- Vacation, holiday, sick leave policy
- Special request for time off, leave of absence
- Communication, reporting: on and off duty, sickness, absence, memos, bulletin board
- Meal and coffee break
- Smoking regulations
- Use of facility telephones, personal cell phones, and other electronic devices
- Uniform regulations
- Computer related systems

RECORDS AND UNIT ROUTINES

- General shift routine for days, evenings, and nights
- Duties of each of the three shifts
- Methods of reporting
- Procedure manual
- Facility policy manual
- Procedures specific to each division of the facility

- Nursing care plan system
- Nursing Kardex and Pyxis systems
- Electronic Medical Record (EMR)
- Routine for care planning conferences
- Routine for physicians' visits
- System of transcribing physicians' orders
- Location of reference books

UNIT ADMINISTRATION

- Admission, placement, transfer, and discharge of residents
- Care of clothing and valuables, including personal property list
- Procedure for caring for seriously ill residents
- Procedure for caring for a resident who has died
- Autopsy permit
- Authorization procedure and forms for diagnostic tests and surgery
- Visiting hours
- Notary public

SAFETY POLICIES

- Side rails
- Restraints and bed alarms
- Fire regulations: reporting, evacuation plan, fire exits, location and correct use of fire extinguishers, fire alarms, preventive measures, fire drill procedure
- Use of oxygen
- Transportation of residents by cart, wheelchair
- Body mechanics and back safety policy
- Door alarms
- Standard precautions
- Security policies
- Smoking policy

HOUSEKEEPING, MAINTENANCE, AND SUPPLIES

- Linen: how supplied, extra linen
- Care of contaminated linens and dressings
- Unit cleaning procedure and responsibilities
- How to obtain supplies: drugs, sterile supplies, personal care items, kitchen items
- Maintenance and repairs requests
- Conservation of supplies, linen, and equipment

EQUIPMENT: HOW TO USE IT AND WHERE TO OBTAIN IT

- Oxygen
- Suction equipment
- Therapeutic beds
- Respiratory therapy equipment and services

FOOD SERVICE FOR RESIDENTS

- Ordering diets/diet changes
- Tray service
- Unit food stock items
- Special nourishments
- Policy for feeding residents
- Policy for dining room
- Policy for family trays

NURSING CARE PROCEDURES/ASSISTING PHYSICIAN

- Morning and evening care
- Bathing/showering, bed bath
- Mouth care
- Bed making
- Temperature (devices used), pulse, and respiration
- Blood pressure
- Catheterization
- Enemas
- Suppositories: rectal
- Recording intake and output
- Systems used for pressure ulcer care
- Collecting, delivering, and labeling specimens
- Assisting podiatrist with foot care
- Policies for sterile technique procedures
- Blood glucose monitoring
- Colostomy care
- Nasogastric and gastrostomy tubes: flushing, feeding, administration of medication
- Standard precautions
- Postmortem procedures

MEDICATIONS

- Medication system
- Policy for reordering
- Unit stock
- Ordering from pharmacy
- Review of metric system, proportions
- Drug errors: reporting, incident reports
- Narcotics count
- Sources of drug administration

DOCUMENTATION

- Method of documenting
- Electronic Medical Record
- Specific forms used
- Flow sheets used
- Policy for phone/fax/Email orders
- Incident reports
- Lists for wanderers, hearing aid use, and so on
- Federal and state chart forms and requirements

SPECIAL AREAS

- Emergency supplies
- Central supply area
- Physical therapy
- Occupational therapy
- Laundry
- Maintenance
- Break room
- Dining room
- Kitchen
- Business offices
- Social services

- Director of nurses
- Chaplain services/chapel area
- Staff educator
- Administrator of facility
- Conference rooms
- Recreational areas
- Activity department

MISCELLANEOUS

- Paging system
- Call light system
- Disaster plan
- Procedure for residents who desire cardiopulmonary resuscitation
- Volunteer services
- On-call schedule
- Handling of wanderers
- Procedure for signing resident in and out of facility
- Hair care services
- Podiatrist and dentist list
- Staff break room

See the Collaborative Care, Management Tool: Reviewing Policies and Routines box.

▦ Collaborative Care

Management Tool

Reviewing Policies and Routines

Resources needed:

- Aforementioned checklist of policies, regulations, and routines for the LPN/LVN
- Your opinion and reasons (rationale)

All policies, regulations, and routines of a health care facility are important. After reading the checklist, complete the following:

1. List the five items from records and unit routines that you think are most necessary for effective running of the resident wings of the long-term care unit. Provide the reason (rationale) for your choices.

ITEM	RATIONALE
a.	
b.	
c.	
d.	
e.	

2. List the five items from unit administration that you think are most necessary for effective running of the resident wings of the long-term care unit. Provide your reason (rationale) for your choices.

ITEM	RATIONALE
a.	
b.	
c.	
d.	
e.	

Tricia came across a data list. Mrs. Kelly had stressed the importance of the LPN/LVN's assisting role in collecting data. Mrs. Kelly always said that what the LPN/LVN did with those data really separated the licensed nurse from unlicensed personnel. Mrs. Kelly had provided a helpful list of signs and symptoms to be aware of in various patient situations. She stressed it would not be a complete list but would be something to get us started. It had been some time since Tricia updated that list.

COLLECTING DATA AS A CHARGE NURSE

As LP/LV charge nurse, the *change-of-shift report* when coming on duty provides data for dividing the work of the shift among team members. Baseline data of residents for whom you are in charge also must be obtained. This involves a quick visit of each resident to compare the status of residents with the status reported at change of shift. You will also collect data periodically during your shift. The frequency of data collecting depends on patient condition. Following is a list of signs and symptoms that may indicate illness, exacerbation of a previous disease condition, injury, or decline in prior functioning.

Be observant with each resident interaction. When nursing assistants report that "something does not seem right," visit the resident to collect your own data. After collecting the data, record it on the proper form and report all abnormal observations according to agency policy. The actual data-collecting parameters given here are guidelines. Follow specific parameters given for the resident. Collaborate with the RN or physician as needed.

SIGNS AND SYMPTOMS

1. **Weight:** Increase or decrease of 5 to 10 lb in 1 week.
2. **Temperature:** Elevation over 100° F orally or 100.6° F rectally; temperature under 96.6° F orally.
3. **Upper respiratory:** Head congestion, headache, sore throat, ear pain, runny nose, postnasal drip.
4. **Lower respiratory:** Acute onset or worsening of shortness of breath, dyspnea with exertion, orthopnea, cough (productive or nonproductive), wheezing or other abnormal sounds on inhalation or exhalation.
5. **Cardiac:** Blood pressure over 135/85 (new symptom); blood pressure below 80/50; irregular pulse (new symptom); chest, neck, shoulder, or arm pain; fatigue; increased frequency of angina; shortness of breath; orthopnea; peripheral edema; sacral edema or distended neck veins.
6. **Breast:** Lump found on palpation, discharge from nipple.
7. **Abdomen:** Localized or generalized pain, especially of acute onset; epigastric burning or discomfort; constipation; diarrhea; nausea; vomiting; bloody or tarry stools; loss of appetite.
8. **Musculoskeletal:** Swollen and tender joints, loss of strength in limbs, pain, loss of motion, ecchymosis, edema.

9. **Reproductive system:** Vaginal discharge, abnormal vaginal bleeding.

10. **Genitourinary:** Urgency, frequency, dysuria, nocturia, hematuria, incontinence. Male: Dribbling, inability to start or stop stream.

11. **Sleep and rest patterns:** Changes from normal routine, requirement of medication for sleep, nightmares or dreams.

12. **Appearance of skin:** Changes in color, turgor, contusions, abrasions, lacerations, rashes, lesions.

13. **Mobility and exercise:** Need for support in ambulation, changes in posture, weakness of extremities, changes in coordination, vertigo.

14. **Hygiene status:**
    a. *Mouth:* Condition of mucous membranes, gums, teeth, tongue, mouth odor.
    b. *Body:* Cleanliness, odor, especially of body creases and genital area.
    c. *Hair:* Grooming, distribution, scalp scaling, lesions.
    d. *Nails:* Color, texture, and grooming of fingernails and toenails.

15. **Communication:** Verbal, nonverbal, and affective, aphasia, level of understanding.

16. **Sensory-perceptual:** Ability to hear, and condition of hearing aid; ability to see, and condition of glasses; ability to feel in all extremities; ability to discriminate odors; ability to distinguish tastes.

17. **Cultural/religious:** Food preferences, wellness/illness beliefs, religious practices (e.g., rosary, prayer beads, Bible, Koran, Torah, religious readings, medals, icons, communion, clergy visits, confession, sacrament of the sick).

18. **Psychological status:** Level of consciousness, disorientation, intelligence, attention span, vocabulary level, interests, memory, affect.

Tricia remembered how Mrs. Kelly stressed the importance of getting to a room and personally collecting patient data, especially when there was a change of condition. Tricia found the example Mrs. Kelly gave so that members of the class could avoid the same situation.

THE REPORT THAT WASN'T

A nursing assistant (NA) reported to the LPN/LVN charge nurse (CN) that Mr. Jones "doesn't look too good to me." The charge nurse immediately called the physician.

Doctor Grimm: What seems to be the trouble?
CN to NA: What seems to be the trouble?
NA to CN: I don't know. He just doesn't look right.
CN to doctor: He just doesn't look right.
Doctor: How long has he looked like this?
CN: I don't know. We just noticed.
Doctor: What's his temperature?
CN: Just a minute. I'll find out.
CN to NA: Take Mr. Jones's temperature.
Doctor: What are his other vital signs?

CN: I don't know. The nursing assistant is going to check them.
Doctor: How much fluid has he had?
CN: Just a minute. (She puts the telephone down and goes to check Mr. Jones's intravenous [IV] line.)
CN: He's getting an IV now.
Doctor (with sarcasm in his voice): Is he breathing? Never mind, don't send anyone to check. I will be over to check him myself. (The doctor hangs up abruptly.)
CN to NA: I don't know why he gets so upset every time I call him. What am I supposed to do?

See the Collaborative Care, Management Tool: Reporting Change of Condition to the Physician box.

Collaborative Care

Management Tool

Reporting Change of Condition to the Physician

Resources needed:
- A checklist of signs and symptoms (earlier in this chapter)
- SBAR (situation, background, assessment and recommendation) information from Chapter 8
- A medical-surgical textbook or electronic access to evidence
  List the data you would collect and any other pertinent information you would gather before notifying the physician of a "change of condition" in the following residents:
- Resident has history of compensated, left-sided congestive heart failure.
- Resident has cancer of the esophagus and uses a Duragesic patch for pain control.

Tricia began to think of the "people problems" she continually experiences in her job as LV charge nurse. With each day that passes, handling these problems becomes easier and easier. Mrs. Kelly's basic advice to "treat people as you would like to be treated" has saved the day on many occasions. That was good advice even for reporting change of condition to the doctor: "What information would I need if I was the physician and my patient had a change of condition?" As for dealing with doctors, residents, staff, and families, I sure remember situations that arose as clearly as if they happened yesterday.

Professional Pointer

Treat others as you would like to be treated.

COMMON PROBLEMS OF LICENSED PRACTICAL/ LICENSED VOCATIONAL CHARGE NURSE

Tricia recalled one morning during the second week of work after orientation to the charge nurse position. The nursing assistants were all tied up in knots. The babysitter for the three young children of Margarita, one of the nursing assistants, had quit the evening before, and when Margarita got up the next morning for work, her car would not start. All the nursing assistants were talking about Margarita's problems from the time they hung up their coats, straight through lunch, and beyond. It was only the week before that Margarita found out she was overdrawn at the bank because she wrote checks before her paycheck was deposited by Quality Care Home and cleared by the bank. It seemed as though "things always happened to Margarita, and she was such a nice person. It just was not right." All the nursing assistants were feeling bad because all these problems happened to Margarita. Everyone was involved with how to get Margarita out of her current mess. Several of the nursing assistants forgot to do some of their tasks/duties, and Margarita needed a lot of assistance to get her assignment completed. As Tricia remembered that particular time, a picture flew through her mind. It was Mrs. Kelly standing in the front of the class with a stuffed toy monkey on her back.

WHEN NURSING ASSISTANTS BRING PROBLEMS FROM HOME

As an LP/LV charge nurse, it is important that you do not fall into the "monkey trap," as described by Blanchard, Oncken, and Burrows in *The One-Minute Manager Meets the Monkey* (1991). You fall into the trap each time you take on a responsibility (monkey) that belongs to an employee. Once monkeys are adopted, they take a lot of time in their care and upkeep. LP/LV charge nurses can help nursing assistants become aware of this trap and be a role model for avoiding it. Remember this thought, "This is not my monkey...this is not my circus."

Realize that you do not own any problems that nursing assistants experience. The nursing assistant owns the problem. Avoid feeling bad because you cannot solve the problems of team members. Be supportive and express genuine concern and empathy (individual consideration), but realize that you do not have a license to counsel nursing assistants. Team members need to solve their own problems. Follow facility policies when personal problems interfere with work performance. Report the situation to your supervisor. Professional counseling in the community may be necessary. See the Collaborative Care, Management Tool: When Nursing Assistants Bring Problems from Home box.

Collaborative Care
Management Tool

When Nursing Assistants Bring Problems from Home

Resources needed:
- Reading: The section in this chapter "When Nursing Assistants Bring Problems from Home"
- Creative thinking

Pretend you are the LP/LV charge nurse the morning Margarita comes to work with her problems. Identify a way to handle the situation.

Tricia remembered Betty, a nursing assistant who had been employed at Quality Care Home for 6 months when she told Kay, a nursing assistant on her wing, that she did not know how to use the new patient-lifting device. Kay stated she did not really have time, but Betty coaxed her to take the time to get the resident out of bed for her. Tricia had suggested to Kay a way of handling the situation that she had learned in class, a tip that would help Betty be more accountable.

ENCOURAGING PERSONAL RESPONSIBILITY IN NURSING ASSISTANTS

When nursing assistants cannot do something that is in their job description (for example, transferring a resident by a lifting device) it is their problem. Staff persons need to avoid assuming it is a staff problem. Be sure to follow the policy of the facility. For safety reasons, encourage nursing assistants to report to the charge nurse when they are having problems carrying out their assignment. This gives the charge nurse the opportunity to determine what staff member is skilled and available to assist in the situation. Encourage the nursing assistant to offer suggestions for learning to do the part of their job that they do not know how to do. Praise them for coming up with a plan, and add to the plan, if necessary. Write a note to your supervisor explaining the situation objectively and how you proceeded to remedy the situation. If necessary, request additional training for the nursing assistant. Learning who owns problems will help you control a large part of the stress you experience as an LPN/LVN charge nurse and help ensure the safety of resident care. See the Collaborative Care, Management Tool: Encouraging Nursing Assistants to Be Accountable for Learning Skills box.

Collaborative Care
Management Tool

Encouraging Nursing Assistants to Be Accountable for Learning Skills

Resources needed:
- Reading: The section in this chapter "Encouraging Personal Responsibilities in Nursing Assistants"

Develop a plan to encourage Betty to approach the lifting-device situation in a more accountable manner.

Tricia remembered instances in her student days and throughout her career when families had complained about care given to their relatives. These complaints troubled Tricia, who had high standards and prided herself on the quality of her nursing care. She would take the complaints seriously and investigate each criticism thoroughly. Sometimes nothing could be found out of order, and sometimes she began doubting her ability to self-evaluate. Once again, Mrs. Kelly offered insight into this common problem, which Tricia still uses today.

DEALING WITH DEMANDING/COMPLAINING FAMILIES

A common problem in the nursing home is dealing with complaints of family members regarding care of their relatives. A common complaint involves physical care. Sometimes the family members become verbally aggressive, express concerns in an angry manner, and are very critical of the charge nurse. Others will be nonassertive and sarcastic. Remember the problem-solving process. First, collect data to determine the real problem. If there is a problem with physical care, identify and correct it. Be honest and apologize as appropriate. Sometimes when the problem is identified and solved, the complaints continue. Sometimes when no problem with physical care is identified, the family may continue the attack.

It is necessary to consider the situation in which the family finds itself. They are in a position of seeing their loved one progressively aging and decompensating. This is a time of loss for the family. They may feel guilty about placing a relative in a long-term care facility or about not being able to continue caregiving. They may have grieving issues to contend with. Lashing out may be their attempt at relief. To avoid personal issues, family members may unconsciously project blame onto nursing assistants and other members of the nursing staff. It is similar to looking at skeletons in other people's closets so you do not have to look at those in your own closet. This behavior may make a family feel better. It is important for staff to understand these issues to avoid hurt feelings. Avoid personalizing the situation. Suggested interventions to deal with the demanding or complaining family are included in the Collaborative Care, Management Tool: Interventions to Use for the Demanding/Complaining Family box. When family complaints surface, investigate them, but remember to keep broad shoulders. The exercise in the Critical Thinking: Dealing with the Demanding/Complaining Family box can help you to practice dealing with the demanding and complaining family.

![] Collaborative Care
Management Tool

Interventions to Use for the Demanding/Complaining Family

- Develop a sincere, nonpunitive relationship with the resident's family.
- Encourage the family to vent feelings about the resident's placement in a nursing home, aging, and behavior.
- Apologize if a mistake has been made or if care has not been of high quality as expected.
- Be specific regarding steps taken to remedy the adverse situation.
- Try to identify the unconscious issue (possible hidden bias) and address it.
- Determine the needs the family is trying to fulfill through their demands, criticism, and complaints.
- Spend time with the family when demands or complaints are not being made.

- Establish rapport with the family to provide emotional support during this difficult time.
- Explain the resident's disease and expected behavior.
- Assess the family's understanding of the patient's condition. Clarify any misperceptions.
- Suggest joining a support group. These groups offer explanations for specific diseases, as well as a place to share feelings and frustrations.
- Encourage the family to stay involved with the resident and continue caregiving and visiting.

？ Critical Thinking
Dealing with the Demanding/Complaining Family

Resources needed:

- Reading: Review the Decision-Making Tree for Problem Solving.

Mrs. Duffy, age 82, was admitted 2 weeks ago to Quality Care Home. You are an LP/LV charge nurse on her wing on the evening shift. Mrs. Duffy has osteoarthritis, short-term memory loss, and Parkinson disease. In the past few days her family has been complaining about her hair care, mouth care, appearance, and missing items in her laundry.

- Develop a plan with specific interventions to investigate and alleviate these complaints.
- Despite modifications in Mrs. Duffy's care plan, the complaints continue. Plan specific interventions to handle the continuing specific complaints.
- Inform and engage all members of the interdisciplinary care team.

ASSIGNMENT AND DELEGATION

Tricia stopped at the topic of "Assigning Tasks and Delegating Duties to Nursing Assistants." She remembered well the confusion she experienced in class in trying to understand the difference between "assigning" and "delegating" to nursing assistants. Like most of the students in her class, she thought assigning and delegating meant the same thing. They sure sounded the same. The fact that she went to school in a state that did not allow her to delegate to nursing assistants compounded her confusion in understanding these concepts. Mrs. Kelly, as usual, had the situation well under control. She said that although assigning and delegating had many similarities, there were differences that had legal consequences. The best place to start was to lay down the boundaries of what we were talking about, define and describe the terms, and then go on from there. In case the students thought assigning and delegating were new concepts, Mrs. Kelly read the following quote:

To be "in charge" is certainly not only to carry out the proper measures yourself, but to see that everyone else does, too. It is neither to do everything yourself nor to appoint a number of people to each duty, but to ensure that each does that duty to which he is appointed.

Florence Nightingale
Notes on Nursing, 1859

CHECKING YOUR NURSE PRACTICE ACT

At this time, not every state in the United States allows LPNs/LVNs to delegate in their charge nurse positions. It is crucial that you check your state's NPA to determine whether or not you may delegate as an LP/LV charge nurse in your state. If you cannot clearly find an answer, contact your state's Board of Nursing (BON). Click on your state at the National Council of the State Boards of Nursing website (https://www.ncsbn.org/contactbon.htm) for contact information. Unfortunately, some states are silent regarding delegation. This means that you will be unable to identify any clear direction. In this case, carefully follow the policy and procedure of your employer. See the Collaborative Care, Management Tool: Reviewing Your Nurse Practice Act for Authority to Delegate box.

🖥 Collaborative Care
Management Tool

Reviewing Your Nurse Practice Act for Authority to Delegate

Resources needed:
- Your state's Nurse Practice Act
  - Locate the section of your state's Nurse Practice Act that discusses your ability to delegate nursing duties as an LP/LV charge nurse.
  - In your own words, write that position.

If your state's Nurse Practice Act allows LP/LV charge nurses to delegate duties, you will have the authority to delegate duties to nursing assistants (unlicensed assistive personnel). States may differ in their interpretation of "delegation." This is one reason you need to check with the BON in your state for its interpretation. In addition to your state's NPA, be sure to review the following:

1. Rules and regulations of your state's BON
2. Interpretations, guidelines, and memorandums developed by your state's board of nursing regarding delegation

A state's NPA usually presents information in a general manner. Rules and regulations and interpretations of your BON are more specific statements. They make clearer the intent of the NPA and provide more specific details that describe your nursing practice.

Your state may give you permission to delegate as an LPN/LVN, but to delegate in your place of employment, *your facility must also give permission for that function by including it in its written policies.* For this reason, check facility policy regarding delegation of nursing duties by the LP/LV charge nurse.

The standards of nursing organizations are not legal statements, but they provide support to the legal decisions of your state. Be sure to review the standards of your nursing organizations that apply to delegation by the LPN/LVN. See the Collaborative Care, Management Tool: Locating Positions of Nursing Groups and Employer on Delegation Function of Licensed Practical/Licensed Vocational Charge Nurse box.

🖥 Collaborative Care
Management Tool

Locating Positions of Nursing Groups and Employer on Delegation Function of Licensed Practical/Licensed Vocational Charge Nurses

Resources needed:
- Rules, regulations, interpretations, guidelines, and memorandums regarding delegation of your state's board of nursing
- NAPNES Standards of Practice and Educational Competencies of Graduates of Practical/Vocational Nursing Programs
- NFLPN Nursing Practice Standards for the LPN/LVN
- Policies on delegation of employer
  Review the policies/rules and regulations/interpretations/guidelines/standards of the following agencies in regard to delegation:
- Board of Nursing
- National Association for Practical Nurse Education and Service, Inc.
- National Federation of Licensed Practical Nurses
- National League for Nursing
- Health care facility

GENERAL CONSIDERATIONS

Assignment and *delegation* are terms used in reference to allocating patient care activities to team members. Both terms refer to nursing actions or activities, but the terms do not have the same meaning. Think about and use *assignment* and *delegation* in the way they are legally intended. **To help increase your understanding and decrease confusion, the terms *assignment* (assigning) and *delegation* (delegating) are used in this chapter in the following way.**

- When discussing **assignment**, this topic will be used in reference to **"tasks."** Tasks are activities that are carried out by nursing assistants. Nursing assistants learn "how to" perform a task in their nursing assistant training, and these tasks are listed in their job description.
- When discussing **delegation**, this topic will be used in reference to **"duties."** Tasks are functions that are performed by LPN/LVNs because they successfully passed a licensing exam. The duties are included in the state's Nurse Practice Act. The duties are their *scope of practice.* The LPN/LVN learns "why" a duty is performed and "what" could go wrong during performance of a "duty."

Resident circumstances can change a "task" for a nursing assistant into a "duty" requiring the LPN/LVN to use the nursing process.

Whenever the title "charge nurse" is used, it will be in the context of the LPN/LVN.

DIFFERENCES BETWEEN ASSIGNING AND DELEGATING

Assigning

Assigning is the way that work is distributed among team members for the shift. Assigning is a skill that every LPN/LVN needs to develop if their state allows them to assume a charge nurse position. Distributing the workload by assignment is a routine part of the LP/LV charge nurse's job. Assignment occurs at the beginning of every shift and as the need arises during the shift.

When LPNs/LVNs give assignments to nursing assistants, they are **allotting tasks that are in the job description of these health care workers.** The assigned tasks are tasks that nursing assistants are trained, hired, and paid to perform. The tasks are in *their* job description. These unlicensed personnel have the responsibility to complete the assignment in a safe and timely manner. The LP/LV charge nurse shares responsibility with unlicensed personnel for the quality of the care delivered. In assigning situations, the LP/LV charge nurse needs to monitor the performance of the task and evaluate the quality and effectiveness of the care that was assigned. See the Collaborative Care, Management Hint: Assigning Tasks box for help in understanding assigning tasks.

▣ Collaborative Care

Management Hint

Assigning Tasks

- The need to assign can occur at any time during the shift but *always* occurs at the beginning of the shift.
- The assigning of tasks is part of the LP/LV charge nurse's job.
- The LP/LV charge nurse assigns tasks to nursing assistants that are in *their* job description.
- *Nursing tasks* are tasks that nursing assistants are trained, hired, and paid to perform. Refer to the subsection "Specific Tasks for Nursing Assistant Assignment" for more details.

- Because assignments involve allocating the tasks that are to be done by nursing assistants in *their* job description, these team members cannot refuse the assignment unless they do not feel qualified to perform the task.
- Nursing assistants assume responsibility for completing assigned tasks safely and in a timely manner.

Delegating

LPNs/LVNs receive the authority to provide nursing care from the nursing license they receive after successfully passing the National Council Licensure Examination for Licensed Practical Nurses (NCLEX-PN®) examination. When allowed by your state's NPA and facility policies, **delegating** duties in the long-term care unit involves **transferring the authority to perform nursing duties that are in the job description of the LP/LV charge nurse (the person doing the delegating)** to competent nursing assistants (unlicensed personnel, known as the delegate) in selected situations. These nursing duties are in *your* job description and "emerge" from your nursing license. These duties are in your scope of practice. **Based on your scope of practice, one of the most important duties of LPNs/LVNs is their role in the nursing process.** Table 17-1 presents a comparison of assigning tasks and delegating duties.

Delegating is a complex skill requiring sophisticated clinical judgment. Delegation information, including scenarios, might be included in theory classes in your LP/LV nursing program, but opportunities to apply the information on clinical may be limited. To be effective, delegation is a skill that needs to be developed with a licensed nurse as a mentor after graduation (Grumet, 2005; NCSBN, 2005).

Delegating duties and assigning tasks are written in the job description of the LP/LV charge nurse at Quality Care Home. When allowed by your state's NPA and your facility, **delegating is a voluntary function.** You do not *have* to delegate because the facility allows it. The Collaborative Care, Management Hint: Delegating Duties box contains helpful information for delegating duties.

Table 17-1	Assigning Versus Delegating by the Licensed Practical/Licensed Vocational Charge Nurse	
	ASSIGNING TASKS	**DELEGATING DUTIES**
To whom may tasks or duties be assigned or delegated?	Nursing assistants and other unlicensed personnel	Nursing assistants and other unlicensed personnel
Are tasks or duties in nursing assistant's job description?	Yes	No. The duties delegated are in the job description of the licensed practical nurse/licensed vocational nurse (LPN/LVN). Specific duties are not listed. Delegated duties depend on the situation.
May nursing assistant refuse nursing task/duty?	No, unless nursing assistant thinks he or she is unqualified for the assignment.	Yes. In addition, the nursing assistant must voluntarily accept delegation function.
Who has accountability for nursing task/duty?	The nursing assistant is responsible for completing the task and in a safe manner.	The LPN/LVN is accountable for delegating the right duty to the right person.

Collaborative Care
Management Hint
Delegating Duties

- When delegating duties, you are asking nursing assistants (unlicensed personnel) to do part of *your* job.
- Delegation involves the ability to share power with nursing assistants.
- Delegation is *not* asking nursing assistants to do duties that the LPN/LVN dislikes doing.
- As LP/LV charge nurse, you are asking nursing assistants to help you perform some of *your* job description so that you may perform other responsibilities, with the ultimate goal of improving resident care and meeting resident goals (outcomes).
- Because you are delegating part of *your* job as charge nurse, nursing assistants must give approval to the assignment. Nursing assistants must voluntarily accept the delegation; they cannot be forced to accept the delegated duty.
- When delegating duties, the LP/LV charge nurse needs to provide the nursing assistant with the necessary information, assistance, and equipment to safely carry out the delegated duty.
- Employers may suggest that certain duties be delegated, but the LP/LV is ultimately responsible for the following:
  - Deciding *to* delegate a duty
  - Deciding *what* duty to delegate
  - Deciding *to whom* to delegate a duty
  - Deciding *under what circumstances* to delegate a duty
  - Retaining the ultimate responsibility for the delegated duty.

WHY DELEGATING IS IMPORTANT

When allowed by your NPA and facility policies, learning to delegate some of the duties in your job description to nursing assistants can have many advantages. Delegating can do the following:

- Increase your effectiveness and efficiency as an LP/LV charge nurse
- Be instrumental in realizing patient goals (outcomes) in a cost-effective manner
- May help nursing assistants increase and improve their job skills

LEGAL ASPECTS OF DELEGATING

In the long-term care facility, the LP/LV charge nurse, who is under the *general* supervision of an RN, is managing and directing the activities of nursing assistants. The RN might be in the building on days and evenings. On the night shift the RN might be at the other end of a cell phone. When the RN delegates a duty to the LP/LV charge nurse and the charge nurse then delegates to a nursing assistant, the registered nurse is *ultimately* responsible for the supervision of nursing assistants. But the LP/LV charge nurse assists in the supervision of these health care workers, collaborating with the RN, and shares **accountability** with the RN for their actions.

Scope of Practice for the Licensed Practical Nurse/Licensed Vocational Nurse

Never delegate what is in your legal **scope of practice**. Legal scope of practice is what you are able to do

because you are an LPN/LVN. Your scope of practice includes the assisting role in the nursing process. The LP/LV charge nurse can delegate to nursing assistants the duty of checking a resident's IV site for intactness and dryness of dressing. However, nursing assistants are not trained in the basics of collecting data. If the resident complained of being cold at the site of the IV, nursing assistants might provide the patient with another blanket, turn up the heat, or turn down the air conditioning. They may not automatically check to see if the infusion device had come out of the resident's vein and was infusing fluid onto the bed sheets.

Although unlicensed assistive personnel obtain data while caring for residents, they do not have the nursing education to make a judgment about or interpret those data. Therefore nursing judgment cannot be delegated to or expected of nursing assistants. The LP/LV charge nurse needs to use his or her knowledge and experience to interpret data gathered by these members of the team.

Your license is at stake in the matter of delegating nursing duties. To be legally sound when delegating duties, see the suggestions in the Collaborative Care, Management Hint: Suggestions for Legal Soundness When Delegating box.

Collaborative Care
Management Hint
Suggestions for Legal Soundness When Delegating

- Delegate only if allowed by your state's NPA and facility policies.
- Determine stability of the patient's condition.
- Delegate duties for which nursing assistants have demonstrated ability.
- Provide specific, objective, clear-cut directions to nursing assistants for delegated duties.
- Provide assistance and instruction to nursing assistants when you delegate a duty.
- Monitor the activities of nursing assistants when they carry out delegated duties. Depending on the nursing assistant and the situation, this monitoring can mean anything from being "right there" to a periodic check.
- Intervene if correction is needed to maintain safety.
- On completion of the delegated duty, evaluate the safety and effectiveness of duties delegated to nursing assistants.
- If you delegated improperly and a resident was harmed, you are liable. This could result in a disciplinary action against your license and/or a civil suit (see Chapter 7).
- If you delegated properly, including monitoring, and the patient was injured, the nursing assistant is also liable.
- Delegation should always occur in collaboration with an RN.
- According to the American Nurses Association/National Council of States Board of Nursing, the RN should follow the five rights of delegation: the right task, under the right circumstances, to the right person, with the right directions and communication, and under the right supervision and evaluation.

Tricia continued paging through her textbook and notes. What memories they brought back! All those shifts of taking report and focusing on important aspects of each patient or resident on the clinical area had a purpose. Tricia remembered the first time she had taken report as an LP/LV charge nurse. Her new position of responsibility gave her a heightened sense of awareness of the data being given. Based on the data she received in report, she had to decide what to assign and what to delegate to nursing assistants for the shift.

USING THE NURSING PROCESS AS A GUIDE FOR ASSIGNING TASKS AND DELEGATING DUTIES

The nursing process will be used as the device to cover the various aspects that need to be understood and used when assigning or delegating.

- *Collecting data:* Oncoming report, assessment of residents
- *Planning:* Establishing goals (outcomes) for the shift, setting priorities, and assigning/delegating
- *Implementing:* Monitoring, assisting, being available, and intervening
- *Evaluating:* Two-way feedback

COLLECTING DATA

Oncoming Report
National Patient Safety Goals require a standardized approach to communications (for example, change-of-shift report, which is sometimes called "handoff"), including an opportunity to ask and respond to questions during reports. If your facility has TJC accreditation, there may be a standardized form to use when receiving report. The National Patient Safety Goals of TJC are in Chapter 16 and can also be accessed at www.jointcommission.org.

Change-of-shift report allows the LP/LV charge nurse to collect data to determine how the work of the shift will be divided. **Always keeping in mind patient goals (outcomes) for shift report helps guarantee continuity in resident care.**

Report When Starting Your Shift
Reports in long-term care units and nursing homes, as in other health care facilities, are a way to pass pertinent data to the oncoming shift. The report you receive when you are starting your shift will be your basis for collecting data about resident needs. This is legally necessary so you can safely distribute the work of the shift to nursing assistants to provide care for specific residents by keeping in mind patient goals (outcomes). Report may be taped or oral, depending on TJC accreditation or agency policy.

When report is taped, offgoing personnel usually are still on duty. They answer call lights and attend to residents' needs while the oncoming shift listens to report. This enables the charge nurse to question unclear information after report. If facilities do not have a standardized report form, nurses develop personal ways of gathering data when they are taking report, including the use of symbols and abbreviations. See the Collaborative Care, Management Tool: Developing Your Personal Form for Collecting Data During Report box.

Collaborative Care

Management Tool

Developing Your Personal Form for Collecting Data During Report

Resources needed:
- Method of gathering data during report that you have developed during the clinical year
- Sample of forms/method to gather information for report used by clinical sites where you have worked this year
- Your creativity and organizational skills

Develop a form that will help you gather the pertinent information needed to assume responsibility of taking charge of the residents on your wing(s). Include format, symbols, and abbreviations you find helpful and that will allow you to quickly and accurately gather the information. Compare your form with forms of classmates.

Assessment of Patients
Assignment/delegation of patients is usually done after report. Ideally, the LP/LV charge nurse makes rounds to personally assess each resident before making assignments. This baseline assessment allows the charge nurse to note any changes in condition of residents or discrepancies that may have occurred since report. If distribution of work for the shift is done before rounds and a change in assignment/delegation is required, the nursing assistant needs to be notified. In some states an initial assessment of patients can be completed by the LPN/LVN independently. Refer to your respective NPA for details.

PLANNING

"We may be very busy, we may be very efficient, but we will also be truly effective only when we begin with the end in mind."

-Stephen R. Covey

Planning involves deciding goals (outcomes) for the shift, setting priorities of care, and then using specific directions, assigning the appropriate task/duty to the nursing assistant who can safely and effectively complete the assignment.

Before Assigning Tasks/Delegating Duties to Nursing Assistants
Distributing the work to be done among nursing assistants follows change-of-shift report. Encourage nursing assistants to take notes and ask questions

regarding the directions you give for assigned tasks/delegated duties. Resist the urge to think of work only as tasks to be completed and to just divide the work equally among team members. In other words, just because there are 32 patients and 4 nursing assistants, it does not mean that each assistant automatically gets 8 patients. Take time to plan how work will be distributed. At first this part may seem tedious and time consuming, but planning becomes easier with practice and experience. Level of patient acuity and education and experience of team members should be considered when creating an assignment. This part of the nursing process is a good reason why the charge nurse position, by some state laws, can require experience beyond a new graduate.

Hansten and Jackson (2008) state, "Fail to plan. Plan to fail." When nurses must decide what to assign/delegate, they should identify resident goals (outcomes) and set priorities.

Identifying resident goals. To be more effective when assigning/delegating and to make these functions more understandable, think in terms of resident **goals (outcomes)**. Goals are desired results in resident progress after nursing intervention. What should happen after nursing intervention by the nursing assistant? Why is the nursing activity being done? What is the goal (outcome) for each resident for the shift?

? Critical Thinking

Formulating Goals/Outcome for Residents

Formulate a goal (outcome) to be met at the end of the shift for each of the following residents:

- **Harold,** an active 90-year-old with osteoarthritis, had a right total hip replacement and is completing his rehabilitation at Quality Care Home, with the goal to go back to his apartment in assisted living. He is to walk x2 with stand-by assist and have one dry clean dressing change daily. His temp went to 100.4° F last evening, but he is not displaying respiratory symptoms.
- **Goal (outcome) for Harold for day shift:** Harold will maintain hip abduction when turning and getting out of bed to prevent hip dislocation. Harold will have causes of his elevated temp investigated.
- **Adelia,** age 76, and a 2-year resident of Quality Care Home, has type 1 diabetes and receives an intermediate-acting insulin injection each morning and capillary blood glucose monitoring ½ hour before meals with sliding scale short-acting insulin coverage. Adelia can be up ad lib, and today is her shower day, which Adelia is looking forward to. The PM shift had trouble getting a blood sample and had to do *two* fingersticks to obtain a blood sample for testing.
- **Goal (outcome) for Adelia for day shift:** Adelia will have blood glucose monitoring done x2 with only one fingerstick required for each test. Blood sugar will be monitored as ordered.

- **Blake,** age 82, has resided at Quality Care Home for 3 years. He has arteriosclerotic heart disease (ASHD). He recently was hospitalized with a cerebral vascular accident (CVA) and is back at Quality Care Home. Blake has weakness on the right side of his body, is allowed up with the assistance of one person, and uses a walker. He has dysphagia (difficulty swallowing).
- **Goal (outcome) for Blake for day shift:** Blake will eat breakfast and lunch without signs of aspirating.

Setting priorities. Set priorities among the goals (outcomes) for the shift. The priority (most important) care to be done can be evaluated according to the following criteria:

1. *Life-threatening situations: real or potential*
   a. A resident who has unrelieved back pain that started on the last shift. (Goal/outcome: Resident will be painfree at end of shift or pain level will be decreased from the previous shift.)
   b. A resident who is dying. (Goal/outcome: Because of comfort measures provided and presence of family, resident will have a peaceful look on his face and lie still in bed without thrashing and picking at sheets.)
   c. A resident who is showing untoward effects to a newly ordered drug. (Goal/outcome: Resident will have stable blood pressure and respirations of 22 to 26 per minute. This requires frequent monitoring and reporting PRN [as needed] to physician.)
   d. A resident attempted to flee the building several times on the last shift. (Goal/outcome: Resident will be present in the building at the end of the shift, secondary to constant supervision.)
2. *Essential to safety.* This criterion pertains to residents and the nursing team.
   a. Which residents, because of their weight, require two persons to turn and position?
   b. Which residents, because of poor balance, need assistance to get out of bed and/or ambulate?
   c. Who is going to check special equipment (e.g., the stock of supplies used in emergencies) for shift?
   d. Does a resident require standard precautions that infrequently need to be used in the facility? Instruction may need to be given to nursing assistants.
3. *Essential to the medical/nursing plan of care.* Criteria include ordered treatments, facility routines for care, and interventions listed on the nursing plan of care; for example, dressing changes, administration of drugs, measuring vital signs, turning, transferring, ambulating, feeding and encouraging fluids, and monitoring of capillary blood glucose levels.

Criteria for Assigning/Delegating to Nursing Assistants

In 2006, the NCSBN and the American Nurses Association (ANA) issued a joint statement on delegation

Table 17-2 Delegation Decision-Making Tree for the Licensed Practical/Vocational Nurse

Starting with question 1, if you answer "no" to a question, do not delegate. If you answer "yes," proceed to the next question.			
1. Does your Nurse Practice Act give the licensed practical nurse/licensed vocational nurse (LPN/LVN) permission to delegate?	No	Do not delegate	Yes
2. Does the employing agency give the LPN/LVN permission to delegate?	No	Do not delegate	Yes
3. Is the duty to be delegated within the scope of practice of the LPN/LVN?	No	Do not delegate	Yes
4. Does the LPN/LVN have the education necessary to delegate nursing duties?	No	Do not delegate	Yes
5. Has the LPN/LVN collected data of the patient's needs and condition?	No	Collect data and continue	Yes
6. Is the nursing assistant to whom a duty is being delegated competent to accept the delegation? (See later in chapter for suggestions to determine competency.)	No	Do not delegate	Yes
7. Is the delegated duty performed according to a sequence of steps?	No	Do not delegate	Yes
8. Does the delegated duty occur repeatedly in the daily care of patients?	No	Do not delegate	Yes
9. Does the delegated duty involve little or no modification from one patient situation to another?	No	Do not delegate	Yes
10. Can the delegated duty be performed with a predictable outcome?	No	Do not delegate	Yes
11. Is there danger of affecting the patient's life or well-being if the nursing duty is carried out?	No	Do not delegate	Yes
12. Is the delegated duty in the nursing assistant's job description?	No	Do not delegate	Yes
13. Does the nursing assistant accept the delegated duty?	No	Do not delegate	Yes
14. Does the nursing assistant have the knowledge, skills, and abilities to accept the delegated duty?	No	Do not delegate	Yes
15. Does the nursing assistant's ability match the patient's needs?	No	Do not delegate	Yes
16. Can the delegated nursing duty be performed without requiring nursing judgment?	No	Do not delegate	Yes
17. Are the results of the delegated duty reasonably predictable?	No	Do not delegate	Yes
18. Can the delegated duty be safely performed according to exact, unchanging directions?	No	Do not delegate	Yes
19. Can the delegated duty be safely performed without constant data collection, interpretation of that data, and the need for decisions based on that data?	No	Do not delegate	Yes
20. Does the agency have a written policy, procedure, and/or protocol for the delegated duty?	No	Do not delegate	Yes
21. Is the LPN/LVN who delegated the duty available for monitoring the nursing assistant?	No	Do not delegate	Yes → May delegate

Adapted from National Council of State Boards of Nursing *Decision Tree for Delegation to Nursing Assistive Personnel*, App. B of *2006 Joint Statement on Delegation*, American Nurses Association (ANA), and the National Council of State Boards of Nursing (NCSBN). https://www.ncsbn.org/Delegation_joint_statement_NCSBN-ANA.pdf

to assist licensed nurses to delegate safely and effectively in clinical settings. Table 17-2 adapts the NCSBN's decision tree for delegation to nursing assistive personnel. The joint statement and additional materials about delegation can be accessed online at www.ncsbn.org (type "delegation" in the search box).

The joint statement provides a list of five areas to assist RNs (LPN is working in collaboration with the RN) in making decisions about delegation. When discussing delegation, the joint statement uses the term "task." Remember, to help differentiate and understand assigning versus delegating, we use "task" to apply to assigning and "duty" to apply to delegating those functions that require the knowledge and judgment of your nursing license and experience.

1. Right task (duty)
2. Right circumstance
3. Right person
4. Right directions and communication
5. Right supervision and evaluation (Some states use the term *monitor* instead of *supervision* when the LPN/LVN performs this function.)

Right task. A crucial legal consideration in dividing work among nursing assistants is nursing judgment.

The LPN/LVN charge nurse needs to avoid real and potential harm to residents when allocating workload to nursing assistants. You are *legally liable* for improper assigning/delegating. **Change-of-shift report** and rounds for beginning of shift resident data collection gave you the opportunity, as LP/LV charge nurse, to collect data about the specific nursing needs of the residents for your shift and the complexity of those needs. Actual tasks/duties allocated depend on the following criteria:

- Laws in your state
- Policies of the long-term care facility
- Needs and condition of the residents on your unit
- Training of nursing assistants

Assigning tasks. Assigning tasks involves dividing work that is in the job description of nursing assistants. The Collaborative Care, Management Hint: Specific Tasks for Nursing Assistant Assignment box lists specific tasks that could be assigned to nursing assistants.

Collaborative Care
Management Hint

Specific Tasks for Nursing Assistant Assignment

Routine:
- Personal care, including hygiene, dressing, toileting, grooming, and skin care
- Feeding and hydration
- *Basic restorative skills,* including transfer, positioning, ambulation, and maintaining range of motion
- Measuring and recording vital signs, height and weight, and intake and output
- Assistance with elimination, including catheter care and enemas
- Maintaining safety factors, including fall prevention, application of heat and cold, and infection prevention
- Collecting specimens of urine and stool
- Nursing assistants who have displayed an excellent work ethic, job performance, and skills may be offered additional, specialized training to become restorative aides. Additional training occurs for positioning, transferring, performing range of motion, using assistive devices, and preventing pressure ulcers.

Delegating duties. Remember, delegating involves transferring the authority (the right) to perform a selected nursing duty (a duty your license gives you the right to do after attending a practical/vocational nursing program and passing a licensing exam given nationally). Delegation generally involves selected activities in patient care. A nursing assistant can receive an assignment, and within that assignment might be activities that need to be delegated. *Avoid assuming that simpler duties may be automatically delegated.* The Collaborative Care, Management Tool: Criteria for Delegating Duties box lists criteria for delegating duties to nursing assistants.

Collaborative Care
Management Tool

Criteria for Delegating Duties

The following are criteria for nursing duties that can be delegated for residents whose conditions are stable:
- The delegated duty must apply to an unchanging situation. (If there is a chance for a change in the patient during a procedure, do not delegate.)
- The results of the delegated duty must be predictable.
- The potential for risk during performance of the delegated duty must be minimal (e.g., the patient with difficulty swallowing is a risk).
- The delegated duty should be necessary and routine in daily care.
- The delegated duty should not require nursing judgment (e.g., "I think the blood glucose level is normal").
- The delegated duty should not require frequent, repeated collection of data during performance of the duty.

The following suggestions include information to help decide what duty can be delegated.

- A question that can help the LPN/LVN make a decision as to what to delegate is "What is the intended outcome (goal/desired result) of the nursing care in question?" In their article, "Delegating to UAPs— Making It Work," Hansten and Washburn (2001) use a bath given for several different reasons (goals/outcomes) as an example.
  - If the bath of a patient in long-term care who is recuperating from total hip replacement is being used as a teaching situation for family members to learn how to observe for signs of skin breakdown, then a licensed nurse needs to be part of the procedure.
  - If a resident who is recuperating from a stroke has a mobility issue, then a physical therapy assistant may be involved with range-of-motion training for the family during the bath.
  - The aforementioned two baths could be given as a team, with the nursing assistant bathing the resident, while the licensed nurse points out pressure points susceptible to skin breakdown or the physical therapy assistant gives range-of-motion training.
  - If the desired goal of a bath is to have a long-term care resident bathed before being discharged, then the nursing assistant would be assigned.
- Given *specific* directions, nursing assistants can assist to collect, report, and document simple data, but not interpret that data. All this occurs in collaboration with the LPN and RN.
- More complex skills to delegate depend on the following:
  - What is allowed by law in your state
  - Resident needs of your unit
  - Further training of nursing assistants; for example, electronic blood glucose monitoring

A concise, across-the-board list of what nursing duties to delegate and what not to delegate does not exist. The

Collaborative Care, Management Hint: Why Lists of Duties to Delegate Do Not Exist box contains the drawbacks of such lists.

Collaborative Care
Management Hint

Why Lists of Duties to Delegate Do Not Exist

- A duty list for nursing assistants eliminates the need for collecting data of the needs of each patient.
- A duty could be on a list of acceptable duties to delegate to a nursing assistant, but the patient situation might indicate the duty would be dangerous or inappropriate for a nursing assistant; for example, feeding a patient with dysphagia (difficulty swallowing).
- The board of nursing has the responsibility to protect the patient. Licensed nursing personnel carry out this responsibility.
- A duty list for nursing assistants puts the control of nursing care into the hands of unlicensed persons who have had minimal training for patient care.
- The exact duties delegated to nursing assistants are interpreted by each state's board of nursing and by each patient situation.

It is somewhat easier to list what duties of the LPN/LVN/RN should *not* be delegated to unlicensed staff. The Collaborative Care, Management Hint: Examples of Duties Not to Delegate box contains examples.

Collaborative Care
Management Hint

Examples of Duties Not to Delegate

- Sterile technique procedures: Nursing assistants do not have training in sterile technique.
- Crisis situations (you must be there): An example of a crisis situation is a resident who develops chest pain.
- Initial patient education by an RN: In most states, LPNs/LVNs may reinforce initial patient teaching given by the RN.
- Although nursing assistants can collect simple data, they have not been trained to make decisions about or interpret those data. For example, nursing assistants cannot evaluate results of capillary blood glucose monitoring or determine when vital signs need to be rechecked.
- Duties that are part of *your* legal scope of practice may *never* be delegated. Your legal scope of practice is your assisting role in the nursing process.

? Critical Thinking
Delegating Duties

You practice in a health care facility that allows the LP/LV charge nurse to delegate nursing duties to nursing assistants. List two additional items to consider before actually delegating:
1.
2.

Right circumstance. NCSBN emphasizes that the setting and patient situation must be considered when delegating. The same criteria must be considered when assigning tasks. Assignment/delegation of duties would not occur if the following is true:

- Resident is unstable. For example, the LPN/LVN would probably work as part of "pair caring" with the nursing assistant when a patient has difficulty swallowing, needs to be fed, and has a history of choking. The LPN/LVN would feed the resident and could use the situation as an opportunity to teach the nursing assistant techniques to use to avoid choking.
- The unit does not have equipment or supplies needed to safely carry out the procedure. The procedure would not be attempted until equipment and supplies were obtained.
- There are safety issues for the nursing assistant, including infection control issues.
- The staffing level is so limited that:
  - Supervision (monitoring) of assigned/delegated duties would not be adequate.
  - Assistance from the LPN/LVN/RN might not be available when needed; for example, assistance when the nursing assistant has questions or needs directions.

Right person. The National Council's guidelines describe delegation as transferring the authority to perform a "selected nursing task" to a *competent* person. These guidelines also apply to assigning tasks to nursing assistants. According to NCSBN interpretation (Working with Others, 2005), a *competent* nursing assistant should be capable of the following in addition to basic care:

- Communicate effectively
- Collect basic subjective and objective data
- Perform noncomplex nursing activities safely, accurately, and according to standard procedures
- Seek guidance and direction when appropriate

The following suggestions will help you determine competence of nursing assistants.

Review job descriptions. Legally, you need to know the job descriptions of nursing assistants to whom you assign tasks. Check these job descriptions of the facility in which you are employed or on clinical affiliation as a student. See the Collaborative Care, Management Tool: Reviewing Nursing Assistant Job Descriptions box.

Collaborative Care
Management Tool

Reviewing Nursing Assistant Job Descriptions

Resources needed:
- Job descriptions of nursing assistants
- Make a list of the tasks nursing assistants can perform in various health care facilities.

Know level of competence. Know the level of clinical competence of nursing assistants you supervise. The following questions can help you determine the competency of nursing assistants on your team:

- Is the nursing assistant certified?
- How much nursing assistant training have they had?
- What skills are taught in their nursing assistant program?
- What is the nursing assistant's job description?
- Does the facility conduct yearly skills list updates? (Some LPNs/LVNs keep a laminated copy of nursing assistant job descriptions and skills lists on their clipboards.)
- What clinical strengths have you observed?
- Have the nursing assistants demonstrated previous competency when performing the activity?
- What clinical weaknesses have you observed?
- Is orientation to your unit completed?
- What activities do nursing assistants say they feel qualified doing?
- What activities do nursing assistants feel unsure doing?
- Ask nursing assistants to describe what they would do in a specific situation; for example, "Tell me how you would get this resident with a total hip replacement out of bed." If the nursing assistant hesitates or looks baffled, suggest that you will assist the nursing assistant when she gets the patient out of bed for the first time and use it as a teaching situation.
- Ask what the nursing assistant would do if a deviation from the normal procedure should develop. For example, you might say, "While getting this resident to stand up, what would you do if he got dizzy when attempting to stand?"
- Ask if the nursing assistant has done the procedure before. If nursing assistants misrepresent themselves by saying they know how to perform a nursing activity when they do not know how to perform the activity, they could be liable in a court of law. For example, if a nursing assistant tells you that he or she can do a fingerstick test and then does it incorrectly, causing injury to the resident, he or she could be liable. The LPN/LVN/RN can still be named in the suit.

Refusing assignment. If a nursing assistant does not feel qualified to safely perform an *assigned task* and refuses the assignment, the team member is then reassigned. It is a fine art distinguishing between "I don't want to" and "I don't know how to." If there is a training problem, follow the suggestion in the Collaborative Care, Management Tool: Reviewing Nursing Assistant Job Descriptions box. Make arrangements with the staff educator of your facility for this team member to receive the training necessary to safely perform the task(s). Also see the Collaborative Care, Management Tool: Handling Refusal of Assignment by Nursing Assistants box.

Collaborative Care

Management Tool

Handling Refusal of Assignment by Nursing Assistants

Resource needed:
- Reading: The "Refusing Assignment" section in this chapter.

A nursing assistant on the team has refused your assignment to give a resident a whirlpool bath because he does not feel qualified to do the job safely. Write a brief note to the staff educator of the facility regarding this situation. (In a real situation, also send a copy of the note to your supervisor.)

Once you work consistently with nursing assistants, they will prove their dependability and ability to pursue assigned tasks. Nursing assistants have the right to refuse a delegated duty. The LP/LV charge nurse, collaborating with the RN, then uses questioning to determine if the team member feels unqualified or simply does not want to do the activity. Feeling unqualified is a training problem; not wanting to do an activity is an attitude problem. Problems in attitude can interfere with a nursing assistant's growth as a member of the health care team.

Tricia chuckled as she thought about the time she asked a nursing assistant to force fluids for a resident with an elevated temperature. When the nursing assistant was approached during the shift, she kept reporting that she was forcing fluids. At the end of the shift, when asked for the volume of fluid taken by the resident during the shift, the nursing assistant replied that although she had forced fluids every hour, the resident took only 80 cc for the entire shift. Tricia, upon self-reflection, realized that she had not adequately discussed with the nursing assistant the patient expectations for fluid intake and what parameters required an immediate report to the LPN/LVN.

Right directions and communication. Using effective communication techniques is an excellent example of the leadership skills that are needed by LP/LV charge nurses. The LP/LV charge nurse's ability to communicate assignments effectively to nursing assistants for reaching patient goals depends on these skills.

As with all communication, assigning/delegating is a two-way process. The communication skills of LPNs/LVNs and their management styles are crucial for establishing a positive working relationship between charge nurse and nursing assistant. It is not only *what* you say as LP/LV charge nurse but also *how* you say it. *Inadequate communication is the most common reason assigned/delegated duties are not completed as required.* The communication guidelines for delegating duties also apply to communication for assigning tasks. Communication skills need to be learned by studying and using the techniques. Review Chapter 8 regarding straightforward communication.

Do not just tell a nursing assistant what to do. Be sure to give the rationale for duties assigned or delegated. Explain *why* an assigned or delegated duty must be done first or at a specific time. Explain why you need the results at a specific time. Nursing assistants become frustrated and feel unsafe when expected to complete an activity when too little information is given. Most importantly, be sure you are available to collaborate as needed. See the Collaborative Care, Management Hint: Communication/Direction Responsibilities of the LPN/LVN Charge Nurse When Assigning or Delegating box for communication guidelines that apply to assigning *and* delegating.

Collaborative Care
Management Hint

Communication/Direction Responsibilities of the Licensed Practical/Licensed Vocational Charge Nurse When Assigning or Delegating

When assigning tasks or delegating duties, be sure to provide nursing assistants with the following information:

- Give objective, detailed, clear-cut verbal and written directions. Get to the point!
- Consider writing assignments in a concise, objective manner on a master assignment sheet.
- Clarify if the nursing assistant has performed delegated duty in the past.
- Explain what is expected at the nursing assistant's level of understanding.
- Be specific about the results you are expecting and when to report. Do not ask nursing assistants to "find out how the patient is." Instead, ask a patient who has been itching because of a rash if the rash still itches.
- Provide guidelines for reporting after the delegated duty is completed. Provide the time you expect to be informed and why.
- Make sure your directions are specific and complete. Provide all the necessary information, including time, to get the task or duty done correctly and safely. For example, say, "Please report the numbers immediately after you measure Mr. Smith's blood pressure, pulse, and respirations. I need to know the numbers before his 9:00 AM blood pressure medicine can be given."
- Given specific directions, nursing assistants can collect, report, and document simple data. However, they are unable to make judgments based on those data. For example, say, "Please report the results of Mr. Ettle's fingerstick immediately after you perform it so I can determine if he needs insulin."
- Instruct nursing assistants when to consult with the charge nurse during the performance of an assigned/delegated duty. For example, say, "Let me know immediately if you are having trouble getting the specimen."
- Clarify all messages by asking nursing assistants to tell you what it is you expect them to do and when to report.
- A "please" and "thank you" are in order as part of common courtesy.

Inform nursing assistants when you expect a report/rundown on activities. A suggested "routine" for reporting back to the charge nurse is before and after breaks and meals and before going off duty. The exact number of reports depends on your familiarity with how the nursing assistant functions, the condition of the residents, and the nature of the assigned/delegated duty. Examples of delegated duties that need priority or more frequent reporting are blood pressure numbers when the resident is to receive blood pressure medicine and blood glucose monitoring with sliding scale insulin coverage. State when you expect to be informed and why you need to be informed.

⁇ Critical Thinking
Identifying Resident Goals/Outcomes

Using the information in the "Identifying Resident Goals/Outcomes" section, the "Signs and Symptoms" list and a medical/surgical text, write the following activities/observations to be assigned/delegated to nursing assistants in specific, objective, clear-cut terms. The directions need to be realistic, measurable, and time referenced.

1. Be sure to clean up Mr. Collar.
2. Make sure Mrs. Thren drinks today.
3. Mrs. Wall must get up today.
4. If Mr. Jones does not pass any urine, let me know.
5. Have Mrs. Neidert ready for her doctor's appointment.

⁇ Critical Thinking Exercise
Communicating Objectively to Nursing Assistants

This is your first month as charge nurse at Quality Care Home. Provide specific, objective, clear-cut data for the nursing assistant to be aware of while giving care in the following resident situations:

1. Resident has compensated right-sided congestive heart failure.
2. Resident is a poorly controlled diabetic who receives an intermediate-acting insulin each morning.
3. Resident has lost 5 pounds in the past 2 weeks.
4. Resident has an order for a catheterized urine for residual.

Remember. When delegating, clarify that the nursing assistant has accepted the delegation. The nursing assistant's responsibility in delegation includes accepting the delegated duty, as well as safe performance in carrying out the duty.

Tricia Makes Assignments for the Nursing Assistants

See the resident goals on p. 283.

- **Harold:** Tricia has worked with Margarita, certified nursing assistant (CNA), for several years and assigns Margarita to Harold for personal care and assistance with ambulation because Margarita has had training as a restorative aid. Margarita verbally explains that she will make sure Harold gets up from the right side of the bed, does not cross his legs, and does not lean forward while getting up or sitting in the chair. Tricia assigns Margarita to care for Harold and set up for his dressing change. Although Margarita is allowed to change clean dressings, she is to notify Tricia before she starts so Tricia can observe the surgical site because of Harold's temperature.

- **Adelia:** Lenore, CNA, has had training for capillary blood testing. Tricia has worked with Lenore for several months and thinks she has demonstrated proficiency in safely and accurately obtaining samples for glucose testing. Tricia assigns Lenore to Adelia and delegates capillary blood testing. When given information of the need for two fingersticks on the evening shift, Lenore explains she will identify the finger to be used for the fingerstick, warm Adelia's finger under warm water at the sink in the bathroom, and keep that hand down after Adelia sits before attempting to get the sample. Tricia reminds Lenore that she needs the sample at 6:30 AM before breakfast and 11:30 AM before lunch trays so she can determine if she needs to administer Adelia's sliding scale insulin coverage ½ hour before meals.
- **Blake:** Sergio is a nursing assistant with 7 years' experience, but he is new to Quality Care Home. Sergio has had restorative nursing training and does well with ROM, positioning, and transfers. Sergio has generally been doing well feeding residents. However, last week Tricia saw a resident almost choke on a grapefruit segment while being fed by Sergio. Tricia assigns Sergio for the following care of Blake: Assist with AM care in bed, range of motion, positioning, and assist with transfer from bed to chair. Tricia decides to be with Sergio and "care pair" for meals. Tricia will feed Blake and use this as an opportunity to review with Sergio hints and safety techniques for feeding residents with dysphagia.

IMPLEMENTATION

Right Supervision, Feedback, and Evaluation

The National Council (1995) defines *supervision* as "the provision of guidance or direction, evaluation, and follow-up by the licensed nurse for accomplishment of a nursing task delegated to unlicensed assistive personnel." This definition is interpreted to include appropriate monitoring, intervention, and evaluation of the nursing assistant, as needed, while providing the delegated duty and feedback after the delegated duty is completed. The following suggestions also apply to assigning tasks. To comply with the National Council's guidelines, the LP/LV charge nurse needs to carry out the suggestions found in the Collaborative Care, Management Hint: Supervision and Feedback box for nursing assistants regarding assigned tasks/delegated duties.

Collaborative Care
Management Hint

Supervision and Feedback

- How often or closely the charge nurse monitors the nursing assistant carrying out the assigned task or delegated duty depends on the resident condition and status and the nursing assistant.

- The LPN/LVN/RN needs to make himself or herself available for questions or concerns as they arise and to provide guidance and assistance when needed. Ask the nursing assistant if assistance is needed.
- Determine if the assigned tasks or delegated duties are being completed. If not, determine the reason for this (e.g., change of condition).
- If necessary, intervene in the situation to ensure carrying out the assigned task or delegated duty safely.

If you fail to supervise adequately and the resident is harmed, the situation could result in a civil suit in a court of law or disciplinary action against your license. See Chapter 7 for information about nursing and the law.

Assessment of residents and functioning of the team by the LP/LV charge nurse occurs periodically during the shift. Although clear communication with nursing assistants during assignment helps ensure that helpful information about residents will be collected during the shift, nothing can replace the charge nurse's contact with residents and judgment based on knowledge and experience.

Collaborative Care
Management Hint

Tricia Supervises the Nursing Assistants

At 7:30 AM and 11:30 AM, Lenore reports, without reminder, Adelia's blood glucose levels. Lenore states she had no trouble getting the samples with one fingerstick. Tricia interprets that no sliding scale insulin is required.

Tricia sees Margarita and Harold as they walk to the dining room for breakfast, and Margarita reports that Harold is very careful about getting up. Harold informed Margarita that "I need to keep that new hip in its socket" so he always gets up on the right side of the bed and never crosses his legs. Margarita notified Tricia after she set up for the clean dressing change, and Tricia assessed the incisional line. There was no redness or edema at the area. The wound was well approximated. Harold's lung sounds are clear, and he denies coughing or congestion. Tricia asks Margarita to check Harold's temperature again at noon.

Sergio sets up Blake for breakfast and notifies Tricia when his tray arrives. When Tricia enters Blake's room, she notes that Blake is sitting up in bed. Tricia suggests that they have Blake sit in the chair for meals. When seated, Tricia reminds Blake to keep his head straight, slightly flexed forward, and not tilt it back while swallowing. Tricia turns Blake's head to the left (the unaffected side) and starts with a couple of spoonfuls of thickened liquids and explains this will moisten the membranes of Blake's mouth and throat to make swallowing easier. Tricia feeds one-third of a teaspoon at a time of Cream of Wheat and scrambled eggs. Sergio is attentive as Tricia continues with thickened liquids periodically. When done, Tricia arranges with Sergio to be present while he sets Blake up and feeds him his lunch.

EVALUATION

You discovered in this chapter that clinical evaluation is a two-way process. The information applies to this part of the assignment/delegation process. See the Collaborative Care, Management Hint: Evaluation and Feedback box.

Collaborative Care
Management Hint
Evaluation and Feedback

EVALUATION

- Check the completed duty that was assigned/delegated. Was the task/duty completed? Was the task/duty performed safely and correctly?
- Legally, the LP/LV charge nurse may not delegate a duty without checking the outcome of that delegation. Have resident goals (outcomes) been met?
- Has something unusual, undesirable, or unexpected occurred? Does the nursing assistant have suggestions to improve carrying out the delegated duty? What went well and what was challenging?
- Did the nursing assistant report as requested?
- Has the nursing assistant documented the activity?

FEEDBACK

- Encourage the nursing assistant to offer input about the assignment/delegation. For example, you might say, "Harper, what problems did you have while assisting Mr. Paul with his shower?" or "Carlos, what suggestions do you have that would make things flow more smoothly during the shift?"
- The LPN's/LVN's leadership skills again come into importance during evaluation and feedback. Provide feedback as needed by the nursing assistant.
- Review communication strategies important for performance evaluation from Chapter 8.
- Did the LPN/LVN thank the nursing assistants for their cooperation during the shift?

Tricia's Evaluation of and Feedback from Nursing Assistants

Tricia thanks Margarita, Lenore, and Sergio for their help and for getting back to her with information and notifying her as quickly as they did. She asks each aide how he or she thought the day went. Margarita and Lenore say the day went fine and that Tricia was available when they needed to report. Sergio says the hints for feeding Blake, especially getting him up to eat and giving thickened liquids first to moisten membranes, were very helpful. All three say they hope to get the same assignment tomorrow, and Lenore asks to watch Sergio feed Blake so she can pick up some hints to use with patients with dysphagia.

PUTTING IT ALL TOGETHER

See the exercise in the Critical Thinking: Assigning Residents in Long-Term Care box.

? Critical Thinking
Assigning Residents in Long-Term Care

Resource needed:
- As LP/LV charge nurse and with available staff, make assignments for the day shift for wing 1 of the nursing home. Include the rationale (reason) for your assignment decisions. Assign and delegate as you feel is appropriate.

STAFF AVAILABLE FOR THE TEAM

- Two student practical/vocational nurses who have completed half of their nursing program. Instructor makes assignments and is present on the clinical area.
- One nursing assistant who has worked at the facility for 10 years (on state registry). One nursing assistant who has 7 years' experience and has worked at your facility for 6 months (on state registry).
- One nursing assistant who was sent from a temporary agency to fill the position of a nursing assistant who has the flu. She completed a nursing assistant advanced course 2 months ago (on state registry).

TASKS FOR DAY SHIFT OF WING 1

- *Four showers*. Each of these residents transfers with the help of two nursing assistants. Each of these residents needs to be weighed, have blood pressure checked, and have a complete linen change on shower day. One resident scheduled for a shower says she feels dizzy and has a congested-sounding cough.
- *Sixteen AM cares*. Ten residents are able to wash their own face and hands when set up. Of the remaining six, one has developed a rash over his entire body, one needs electronic glucose monitoring ½ hour before breakfast and lunch on day shift, and four are confused and incontinent of urine and feces. Each of these residents needs one assistant to transfer and ambulate.
- *One complex dressing change for a resident on a Clinitron bed*. (This resident is transferred by a patient-lifting device and requires total care.)
- *One percutaneous endoscopic gastrostomy (PEG) tube intermittent feeding with commercial tube feeding formula and drug administration at 8:00 AM and 12:00 noon on day shift*. (This resident is confused and requires two persons to ambulate.)

You have just completed assigning team members, when one of the nursing assistants states that she feels warm and then faints. As it turns out, she has a temperature of 102.2° F and will not be able to engage in resident care. Reassign the residents on wing 1.

? Critical Thinking
Delegating to Nursing Assistants

Resources needed:
- Descriptions of recent clinical assignments for students in your clinical group
- Critical thinking

If your state allows LPNs/LVNs to delegate, use Table 17-2 and the nursing process format in this chapter to practice assigning/delegating recent clinical duties for your clinical group to nursing assistants.

REPORTING AT THE END OF YOUR SHIFT

Giving report at the end of your shift requires planning. As the LP/LV charge nurse, you need reports from the nursing assistants before you can tape or give report. This is where the concise, clear directions that you gave to these team members during assignment/delegation will pay off. You will need to set priorities in deciding pertinent information to give to the next shift. Be sure to personally assess residents who have the following:

- Changes in condition
- Current ongoing problems
- New orders (and resident response to new orders)
- Suspected side effects to medications

Use the same sequence of data for each resident. This will make it easier for the oncoming charge nurse to take notes from your report. An example of a suggested sequence of data for reporting to oncoming shift for residents in a long-term care unit can be found in the Collaborative Care, Management Hint: Reporting to Oncoming Shift box.

Collaborative Care

Management Hint

Reporting to Oncoming Shift

THINGS TO REPORT

Resident name, room number, and physician
1. New problems/concerns
2. Contact with physician and new orders
3. Progress of current, established problems
4. PRN medication: name of drug, time given, and reason for PRN medication; time follow-up is required

5. *Briefly* describe resident's behavior during shift; include any changes in resident's physical and mental status
6. Resident's voiding, bowel movement (continent versus incontinent), intake/output
7. Follow up with residents, family, or team members still needed
8. Highlight and update key patient goals

THINGS TO AVOID DURING REPORT
1. Meaningless chatter that has nothing to do with residents' nursing care and goals/outcomes
2. Routine nursing care, unless it has a bearing on current nursing problems
3. Personal opinions about residents' conditions
4. Value judgments, gossip about residents' lifestyles, behavior, or families

---

Tricia was very tired and began to put away her textbooks and scrapbook. The review of delegation in her old text proved demanding for Tricia, but it also had been very pleasant reminiscing about her school days and early years as an LVN. She felt good with how far she had come since feeling insecure in those beginning days. At least, she now knew what to question and where to find the answers. It felt good to have a grasp of her LP/LV charge nurse position, especially the fine points of assignment and delegation of duties. Later, as Tricia was relaxing, a big smile came over her face. Tomorrow would be a big day in her life. Mrs. Kelly had strongly recommended membership in professional organizations. Tricia had been a member of the National Federation of Licensed Practical Nurses at the national, state, and local levels since graduation. Over the years, she had assumed various committee assignments and officer positions at the local level of the organization. Tomorrow she would be installed as the first president of the organization at the state level from her local district! Tricia was proud to be of service to her career and looked forward to promoting and having a say in the direction practical/vocational nursing would take in the twenty-first century.

Get Ready for the NCLEX-PN® Examination!

Key Points

- When the state's Nurse Practice Act allows, LPNs/LVNs are used as first-line leaders and or managers (charge nurse) in the nursing home/long-term care unit.
- The basic student practical/vocational nursing program offers students the opportunity to develop skills in nursing procedures, the nursing process, critical thinking, communication, time management, assertiveness, and stress control. These are skills needed for everyday practice, as well as leadership and management positions.
- Development of a leadership style is important in guiding nursing assistants to meet the goals of the long-term care facility.
- Established leadership styles range from the extreme of autocratic, with a pure emphasis on the task, to laissez-faire, which emphasizes concern with the employee.

- Situational leadership adapts a leadership style to the environment and situation at hand. It is the suggested way of leading in the twenty-first century.
- No one chapter or course can teach you how to become a leader. The development of leadership skills is a process and evolves over time.
- Understanding and applying the four "I"s of transformational leadership (idealized influence, inspirational motivation, individualized consideration, and intellectual stimulation) can assist the LPN/LVN in becoming a successful leader.
- The five core skills of leadership involve the ability to (1) motivate team members, (2) communicate assertively, (3) problem solve effectively, (4) build a team of cooperative workers, and (5) manage stress effectively. These core skills lay the foundation for the development of other specific skills for leadership.

- Specific skill areas for nursing leadership include occupational skills, organizational skills, and human relationship skills.
- In addition to training given by the institution, first-line practical/vocational nursing leaders need to educate and update themselves continually in the five core and three specific skill areas noted.
- Herzberg's two-factor theory indicates that managers/leaders should implement strategies to support intrinsic and extrinsic motivators in the work setting, thereby increasing job satisfaction and decreasing job dissatisfaction.
- Common charge nurse challenges include nursing assistants who bring personal problems to work, the need for nursing assistants to be accountable for learning new job skills, and dealing with the residents and family members' concerns.
- Oncoming shift report gives the charge nurse the opportunity to collect data about resident needs, identify resident goals (outcomes) for the shift, and assign nursing tasks to nursing assistants for resident care from *their* job description.
- Assessment of each resident after assignment/delegation identifies changes in condition/circumstances that may require a change in assignment/delegation.
- The charge nurse shares responsibility with nursing assistants for the quality of care that is given.
- LP/LV charge nurses routinely assign care to nursing assistants.
- Charge nurses, as part of their jobs, evaluate the thoroughness and safety of all tasks they assign.
- *If allowed in your state's Nurse Practice Act,* and included in facility policies, the LP/LV charge nurse may elect to delegate duties from the LPN/LVN job description to nursing assistants.
- Delegation gives the charge nurse time to focus on duties that cannot be delegated.
- Duties can be delegated, but the accountability that goes with those duties remains with the registered nurse, with whom the charge nurse functions under general supervision. The LPN/LVN shares accountability and collaborates in these situations.
- The charge nurse position is a complex role for LPNs/LVNs. With additional education and experience, many practical/vocational nurses are doing an excellent job in this expanded role position.

Additional Learning Resources

evolve Go to your Evolve website (http://evolve.elsevier.com/Knecht/success) for the following FREE learning resources:
- Answers to Critical Thinking and Scenario
- Additional learning activities
- Additional Review Questions for the NCLEX-PN® exam
- Helpful phrases for communicating in Spanish and more!

Review Questions for the NCLEX-PN® Examination

1. Select the defense mechanism that may be present in a family member who continually finds fault and criticizes the care given to a relative by nursing assistants.
   a. Projection
   b. Validation
   c. Introversion
   d. Conversion

2. Select the statement that indicates the best understanding of delegation.
   a. Nursing assistants cannot refuse a duty delegated to them by the practical/vocational nurse for any reason.
   b. Delegating duties depends on state law, facility policies, resident condition, and the need of the LPNs/LVNs to delegate based on the situation.
   c. Any LPN/LVN may delegate his or her role to a qualified, dependable nursing assistant.
   d. LPNs/LVNs delegate duties routinely to nursing assistants that are in the facility job description of the nursing assistant.

3. Cindy, LPN, is charge nurse on the evening shift at a nursing home. Select the priority action she will use in making assignments to nursing assistants.
   a. Cindy obtains feedback from the nursing assistants as to the type of procedures for which they feel competent.
   b. Cindy distributes the nursing tasks to be completed on the evening shift equally among the nursing assistants on the team.
   c. Cindy checks job descriptions and skills for nursing assistants to clarify who is competent to perform selected duties.
   d. After report when coming on duty, Cindy establishes patient outcomes for residents for the shift and sets priorities for care.

4. Laura, a nursing assistant, has been absent four times this month, each absence occurring on the weekend. Which of the following practical/vocational charge nurses is using problem solving to handle this situation?
   a. Focuses feedback on Laura's frequent absences and explains the related discipline measures according to policy.
   b. Downplays the importance of absences to make Laura feel better.
   c. Provides Laura with all the suggestions needed to correct the problem.
   d. Assumes being present for assigned shift is something Laura cannot do.

5. A nursing assistant, with a history of minimal absences, is attending a practical nursing program. Before the staffing schedule being posted, she requests to be off the night before two final exams. As the LPN/LVN who has the responsibility for the scheduling process you comply. This is an example of:
   a. Individualized consideration
   b. Intellectual stimulation
   c. Idealized influence
   d. Inspirational motivation

Alternate Format Item

1. Select from the following sources where authorization for the LPN/LVN to delegate in long-term care can be found. *(Select all that apply.)*
   a. BON
   b. NCSBN
   c. NFLPN
   d. FACILITY
   e. NAPNES

2. Which of the following LP/LV charge nurses in long-term care facilities are assigning in a legally sound manner? *(Select all that apply.)*
   a. Lilly assigns patients based on geographic location to enhance timeliness of the response to patient inquiries.
   b. Ada clarifies skill levels of nursing assistants by asking the RN to whom she reports to show her where to locate CNA skill lists.
   c. Aiden makes rounds after report to gather data on actual resident conditions so he can develop shift outcomes for residents before making assignments.
   d. Alexander provides specific, concrete information for what nursing assistants should do while engaging in resident care and follows up appropriately.
   e. Michael asks the CNAs which patients they prefer to care for and assigns accordingly.

3. A work-related conflict has surfaced between two nursing assistants on their shift at the long-term care facility, where a licensed practical/vocational nurse is charge nurse. Which of the following intervention strategies does the charge nurse use to resolve the conflict? *(Select all that apply.)*
   a. Develop a collaborative solution to solve the conflict so the two parties are satisfied with the solution.
   b. Limit the number of possible solutions offered to solve the conflict, thus saving time.
   c. Instead of focusing on what solution each assistant wants, focus on why they want that specific solution.
   d. Actively listen while each nursing assistant presents his or her side of the conflict and solutions.
   e. Request that the nursing assistants stay away from each other for 72 hours to encourage time for self-reflection.

Critical Thinking Scenarios

Scenario 1

Sasha, a nursing assistant, has accepted a delegated duty to complete for several evenings. There have been three new admissions to the unit in the last 24 hours. This evening, the LP/LV charge nurse says she will do the duty that has been delegated on prior shifts. Sasha complains to the other nursing assistants that the charge nurse doesn't trust her. Comment about this situation.

Scenario 2

Jill, an LPN, is the new charge nurse on the evening shift at the local nursing home. The nursing assistants on the evening shift are complaining to the nursing assistants on the day shift about the way Jill gives them directions about their assignments. They indicate that she micromanages them and does not respect them for the knowledge that they have regarding the patients. They also never have an opportunity to leave the floor for continuing education. Jill always states that their unit is too busy to attend. As a result, recently they were unable to be certified in dementia care. Provide advice for Jill based on the four "I"s of transformational leadership.

Workforce Trends: How to Find a First Job You Will Love

Objectives

On completing this chapter, you will be able to do the following:

1. Discuss the current and projected workforce trends for licensed practical nurses/licensed vocational nurses (LPNs/LVNs) in your local area, state, and nation.
2. Based on workforce trends, list employment opportunities available to LPNs/LVNs.
3. Discuss professional growth opportunities for LPNs/LVNs that can increase your marketability.
4. Based on your program outcomes, self-confidence, values, and professional expectations, identify job options that will be a good fit for your first job.
5. Discuss how to use your personal and professional network to identify job opportunities.
6. Determine interpersonal styles and how to use them to improve your interview skills.
7. Effectively participate in an informational interview.
8. Effectively role-play an interview, preparing for complex interview questions.
9. Develop a resume, including a cover letter that will result in an interview.
10. Use verbal and nonverbal messaging effectively during an interview.
11. Describe the diverse social media sources to assist with your job search.
12. Discuss the importance of employer follow up both at the time of application and after the interview.
13. Investigate if Transition to Practice or residency programs are available for you at local sites of employment when you graduate.
14. Discuss how Transition to Practice or residency programs can decrease reality shock during your first year of employment as a LPN/LVN.
14. Write an effective resignation letter.
15. Discuss three advantages of belonging to professional organizations.
16. Describe your postgraduate career goals. (Review your answer periodically.)

Key Terms

Certification in Managed Care Nursing (CMCN)
conditional job offer (kŏn-dǐ-shŭn-ăl)
follow-up illusion (ĭl-oo-shŭn)
hidden job market
illegal questions (ĭl-ē-gŭl)
informational interviews (ĭn-fŏr-mā-shŭn-ŭl ĭn-tĕr-vūz)
interpersonal styles (ĭn-tĕr-pĕr-sŭn-ăl)
Long-Term Care Certification (CLTC)
mobility program (mō-BĬL-ĭ-tē)
National Association for Practical Nurse Education and Service, Inc. (NAPNES)
National Certification in Gerontology (jĕ-rŏn-TŎL-ō-jē)
National Certification in IV Therapy

National Federation of Licensed Practical Nurses (NFLPN)
National League for Nursing (NLN)
networking (net-wŭrk-ĭng)
Pharmacology Certification (NCP) (făr-mă-KŎL-ō-jē)
podcast (POD-kast)
preceptor
reference hierarchy (hī-ĕr-ăr-kē)
residency
resignation courtesy (rĕz-ĭg-nā-shŭn)
resume (rĕz-ŭh-mā)
silence (sī-lĭns)
Transition to Practice Model (trăn-zĭ-shŭn)
voice control (vŏys kŏn-trŏl)

💡 Keep in Mind

You've decided what you want to be when you grow up; now get out there and do it!

David and Kamy, students at the Success Practical Nursing Program, are chatting as they leave their clinical experience on Monday afternoon. They had a great day, learned immensely, and felt like an integral part of the health care

team. David had interacted with a wellness nurse in a continuing care facility and Kamy had participated in a pediatric home care experience. During the clinical day, the mom stated to Kamy, "You are going to be a great nurse. My son really connected with you today and performed all his exercises well. It is often a struggle. You have a gift." In addition, they are excited about their upcoming graduation in four weeks. Despite this positive clinical experience, fellow student Diane enters the conversation, sensing frustration as the conversation tone changes. David and Kamy are sharing comments made by friends and community members at a holiday event this past weekend. They were asked by two different people the following question, "Why are you wasting your time in LPN school? I hear there are no jobs available for LPNs; all nurses must soon be an RN who graduated from a University." They share that they felt at a loss for words. David recalls becoming quiet and Kamy changed the topic of conversation. Kamy states to Diane, "I know in my heart this has been a great step on the nursing career pathway for me, but I just did not know what to say . . . and to be honest it makes me worry a bit. I hope this is not true." Diane, unsure of what to say, stated, "Well, you know that it is not true," and walked away frustrated.

As you read through this chapter, write down ideas that could have been a great response. Remember, often the public is misinformed. LPNs/LVNs and all nurses need to be their own advocates ensuring the public knows the facts. In the future, if you were in a situation similar to Diane, how could you help ease you peers' anxiety and spread the word about a great career as an LPN/LVN? Likewise, if you were David or Kamy, how could you communicate effectively the strong and diverse job market for LPNs/LVNs? As you read the chapter, you will see LPNs/LVNs are important members of the health care team and the job opportunities are countless.

LICENSED PRACTICAL NURSE/LICENSED VOCATIONAL NURSE DEMOGRAPHICS

The LPN/LVN workforce trends play a lead role in diversifying the nursing workforce. According to the National Council of State Boards of Nursing (NCSBN) 2012 LPN practice analysis, 87.9% of the LPNs were female, similar to 2009 but lower than 2006. Thus overall the male population is slowly increasing. In addition, they are ethnically diverse with 57.9% reporting being white but not of Hispanic origin. The second largest racial group represented was African American at 18.6% (NCSBN, 2013). This mirrors an overall trend of all LPNs/LVNs. Health Resources and Services Administration (HRSA, 2013) reports that approximately one-quarter (23.6%) of the LPN/LVN workforce is African American as compared with 9.9% of the registered nurse (RN) workforce. The number of Hispanic/Latino nurses in the LPN/LVN workforce is almost double that of the RN workforce (7.5% versus 4.8%). As you can see, the LPN/LVN is important to building a diverse health care workforce. According to the National League for Nursing (NLN, 2014) statement, *A Vision for Recognition of the Role of the Licensed Practical/Vocational Nurses in Advancing the Nation's Health*, LPN/LVN graduates are a critical pipeline to building a diverse nursing workforce, playing a vital role in the delivery of culturally sensitive health care in a variety of settings to vulnerable populations (NLN, 2014).

NURSING: THE LICENSED PRACTICAL NURSE/LICENSED VOCATIONAL NURSE AS A DOOR TO MANY WORKFORCE OPTIONS AND LIFE-LONG LEARNING

Nursing opens the door to an entirely different world, with countless opportunities. Not only will you have access to a financially secure job, you will also experience many intrinsic rewards. Every day, you enter and touch the lives of many individuals and families. Patients trust you without having to prove yourself. They feel safe in the knowledge that you have pledged to do your best in providing care without passing judgment. Some patients and families will let you know their appreciation for your skill in providing nursing care, but some will never tell you how deeply you touched their life and the lives of their loved ones.

Unfortunately, approximately one-third of those who enter a nursing program do not complete the program for any number of reasons. A major reason is that the course of study demands a great deal of personal discipline, time management, and prioritization of needs (knowing the difference between "I want to" and "I need to"). Nursing changes you: You see and hear more in a short period than you ever imagined. Because of confidentiality, most of what you see and hear cannot be shared with anyone out of the immediate setting. Nursing is a maturing experience, often beyond your years. Both self-confidence and the ability to say, "I don't know, but I will find out," grow as your professional honesty is tested. Nursing opens doors for you in traditional and atypical careers and provides a lifelong career pathway. Be proud of choosing nursing as a career, become an advocate for nurses, particularly LPNs/LVNs. Seize opportunities to educate colleagues and community members regarding the critical role of the LPN/LVN.

Nursing challenges you throughout your career. As a student, you are expected to learn and use an entirely new language and yet always explain to a patient what you are doing in terms he or she can understand. The challenge continues when you graduate because you have only scratched the surface of knowledge in nursing. Every day will provide at least one answer to your question, "What did I learn today?" In addition, all of you will continue your education. This may be through inservices, workshops, and collaboration with other health care providers. In many states, you will be required to achieve a minimum number of continuing education units when renewing your license. In addition, some of you will pursue a formal education route resulting in achievement of various certifications and/or the pursuit of a registered nurse (RN). According to the NCSBN 2012 LPN practice analysis, approximately 23.4% of responders reported enrollment in an RN educational program broken down as follows: 82.6% were in associate degree programs, 12.5% were in baccalaureate programs, and 3.1% were in diploma programs.

In response to the Institute of Medicine (IOM) report to increase baccalaureate prepared nurses to 80% of the workforce by 2020 and magnet hospital standards, the trend for baccalaureate-prepared RNs is increasing in specific geographic areas of the country. It is anticipated that the percentage of LPNs enrolled in baccalaureate RN programs will also increase. Being a life-long learner is a strong quality and contributes to job satisfaction and financial security in the United States.

Given the predicted nursing shortage, fueled by the aging nursing workforce, and aging Baby Boomers, your selection of a career in nursing and particularly a career as an LPN/LVN is a great one! Projected job growth for RNs and LPNs is predicted to be 16%, which is greater than the average rate for all occupations (Bureau of Labor Statistics Occupational Outlook Handbook, 2016). In addition, the average age of LPNs/LVNs was 43.2 years, exceeding the median average of all United States workers in 2011 (Bureau of Labor Statistics, Current Population Survey, 2012). This increased age of the LPN workforce coupled with predominance of the LPN as the licensed nurse working in long-term care settings and the prediction by Medicare that 12 million older Americans will need long-term care by 2020, intensifies the predicted shortage of LPNs. Recruitment and retention of LPNs/LVNs will remain a focus for the future. Meeting the job satisfaction needs of LPNs/LVNs will be critical to maintain a robust workforce.

The U.S. workforce consists of 2.8 million RNs and 690,000 million LPNs working in the field of nursing or seeking employment in 2008 to 2010 (HRSA, 2013). National entities support the role of the LPN as noted in the National League for Nursing, *Recognizing the Vital Contributions of Licensed Practical/Licensed Vocational Nurse* (2011) report and the IOM reports, *Retooling for an Aging America: Building the Health Care Workforce* (2008) and *Future of Nursing* (2010). The IOM (2010) report recognizes the unique contribution of LPNs in long-term care, including supervision of direct care workers (DCWs) and other non-licensed individuals and encourages increased education for nurses at all levels. The report states, "Licensed practical/vocational nurses (LPN/LVN) are especially important because of their contributions to care in long-term care facilities and nursing homes (p. E3)."

According to the NCSBN LPN/LVN 2012 practice analysis, newly licensed LPNs employed in long-term care soared from 44.5% to 54.2% from 2003 to 2012 (NCSBN, 2013). Also, 43.4% of newly licensed LPNs indicated that they have administrative duties and LPNs working in long-term care facilities were more likely to have administrative responsibilities than LPNs working in a hospital (32.4% versus 0.8%, respectively) (NCSBN, 2013). In addition, approximately 70% of licensed nursing care is provided by LPNs rather than RNs (American Health Care Association, 2011).

However, geriatrics is not the only setting for LPNs/LVNs. The NCSBN survey also indicates that LPNs/LVNs work with a diverse array of patients in need of chronic care in the community. This includes caring for the chronic pediatric patient who is ventilator dependent, caring for patients with mental health and dependency issues, and providing care in correctional settings, clinic, and urgent care settings.

There have been several workforce trends noted in the newly graduated LPN/LVN workforce, representing a shift from acute care to long-term care and/or community-based care. See the NCSBN 2012 LPN practice analysis for specific details: www.ncsbn.org/3978.htm. This aligns with changes in patient access to health care fueled by the Affordable Care Act, positioning the LPN/LVN for a continued strong presence as a member of the health care workforce team. What does this mean to you? A strong future for continued stable employment despite swings in the economy. The LPN/LVN is a low-cost, high-quality health care team member.

◎ Try This

Consider the following questions:

1. What type of environment do I want to work in: direct health care, state/federal government, private duty, insurance-related, sales, industry, or other?

2. What population (i.e., type of client) do I find most rewarding to work with?

3. What kinds of nursing skills do I find most challenging and rewarding? What new areas would I like to be involved in? How can I become immersed in these areas?

4. What workforce trends impact positively on my practice setting preferences for employment?

COUNTLESS WORKFORCE SETTINGS EXIST: FINDING THE RIGHT FIT IS A REWARDING CHALLENGE

While you are in your educational program, carefully evaluate each unique clinical or volunteer experience. Be proactive, introducing yourself to staff and the human resource department. Be sure to communicate directly if you are interested in a particular specialty area or practice setting. Then, note whether your area of interest is reported as a likely employment setting for new nursing graduates in the LPN/LVN practice analysis. Seriously consider taking additional coursework or obtaining certifications to enhance your employability in the areas of basic life support, intravenous therapy, phlebotomy, advanced cardiac life support, behavioral management, and rehabilitation as available. See the NCSBN 2012 LPN practice analysis for specific details (www.ncsbn.org/3978.htm). Lastly, focus on increasing your knowledge of the diverse health care settings where LPNs/LVNs are employed. Identify your passion, understand the usual role of the LPN/LVN in this setting, and evaluate the future LPN/LVN workforce trend for this setting. The information below provides details of many possible workplace settings for LPNs/LVNs to inform you.

LONG-TERM CARE FACILITIES (INCLUDING SUB-ACUTE UNITS)

Every day 10,000 Americans cross over the threshold of age 65, creating an increased demand on the health care system (Barry, 2011). This has a positive impact on the job demand for LPNs/LVNs. The long-term care population is made up of residents who are:

1. In need of transitional care upon discharge from the acute care hospital, allowing time to recover from surgery or trauma before returning home.
2. Elderly people who are unable to care for themselves because of medical or psychological impairment.
3. Young to middle-aged people with chronic debilitating disease or injuries from accidents.
4. Young, chronically mentally ill persons who need continual supervision and are not candidates for independent living or group homes.

LPNs/LVNs who are hired for direct care measure vital signs, collect data, provide physical care and comfort measures, and administer medications. LPNs/LVNs often have administrative responsibilities in long-term care settings. Some state nurse practice acts permit more extensive use of LPN/LVN skills in nursing homes. Other state regulations are more restrictive.

There are some inconsistencies in the nurse practice acts for LPNs and RNs. Some inconsistencies are noted on course names (e.g., "mental health nursing" instead of "psychiatric nursing") or terms like *assessment*, *delegation*, and *decision-making*. The difference in the terms *assessment* and *data collection* (the preferred term for LPNs/LVNS) is difficult to define. Because critical thinking has been incorporated into the National Council Licensure Examination for Practical Nurses (NCLEX-PN®), critical thinking is now taught as a part of practical nursing programs. As noted in the 2012 Practice Analysis, 43% of the LPNs/LVNs work as charge nurses, primarily in long-term care facilities; some work as team leaders. Critical thinking is a necessary component of their job. The LPN/LVN may no longer just collect the data but also may need to determine what data are most important and how they apply to the patient's plan of care.

Many states and organizations offer postgraduate courses and certifications. The National Association for Practical Nurse Education and Service (NAPNES) offers certification programs in pharmacology, intravenous (IV) therapy, and long-term care (www.napnes.org). The National Federation of Licensed Practical Nurses (NFLPN) offers certifications in IV therapy and gerontology (www.nflpn.org). The American Board of Managed Care Nursing (www.abmcn.org) offers certification in managed care nursing. Other certifications such as wound care, dementia care and end of life care should be obtained as an LPN/LVN. These certifications are valuable assets in a long-term care setting. In addition, some vocational and technical colleges offer postgraduate courses in management and leadership. Some states recognize postgraduate courses and certifications and permit the LPN/LVN to use the skills they have learned in providing care. A major benefit of postgraduate information is knowledge gained for more effective patient care and job satisfaction.

Long-term care as an employment option may be available to you if you possess the following characteristics:

- Use solid nursing process skills in gathering data and use the care plan as a guide.
- Use critical thinking throughout the shift.
- Use therapeutic communication skills; differentiate between therapeutic and personal.
- Enjoy longer-term contact with people. (High turnover rates of staff have been associated with lower quality of care in some extended care facilities.)
- Provide quality nursing care with collaboration but without immediate supervision of an RN or physician.
- Seek assistance or additional instruction as needed to provide safe, quality, cost effective care.
- Apply information about growth and development changes during illness.
- Willingly seek to learn new skills through continuing education and certification courses needed to take care of a diverse population and age group.
- Listen to patients regarding what they see as their needs for care.
- Treat patients of all ages and levels of growth and development with respect.

Other special qualities needed include the following:

- Patience
- Ability to see below the exterior of a person
- Willingness to listen
- Maturity
- Understand the significance of the work you are doing
- Ability to determine priorities
- Ability to set limits
- Interest in working with people with disabilities
- Willingness to collaborate and problem solve with other health care givers, residents, significant others, and family members
- A sense of security in regard to your personal value system
- The ability or willingness to learn to manage and lead a team effectively

Prior experience on a medical/surgical unit, including clinical student rotations, is helpful before working in a long-term care facility.

LPNs/LVNs who work in long-term care are challenged to assist in providing a homelike atmosphere while dealing with chronic, long-term, and terminal health problems of the residents. The level of responsibility in long-term care is great. The LPN/LVN often works in a charge nurse role, and although supervision must be available from an RN or physician, during some periods of the day supervision may be virtual (i.e., at the other end of a cell phone). Consequently, solid knowledge and skills are essential to understanding when to seek help and from whom. The nursing process and critical thinking provide the basis for skilled, compassionate care.

The charge nurse role also means that the LPN/LVN is responsible for managing care given by other LPNs/LVNs, certified nursing assistants, and other DCWs. (Refer to Chapter 17 for more specific details on leadership and charge nurse skills.)

Working as an LPN/LVN in a long-term care facility, much of your work ultimately relates to assisting the residents to achieve their highest level of health and independence possible. Through your efforts, residents who are recuperating from surgery or trauma will realize their goal for recovery and discharge. For other residents, your role includes supporting them through the final step of the growth process: a dignified death.

ASSISTED LIVING FACILITY

Although adults who live in assisted living facilities do not need 24-hour skilled nursing care, they benefit from an LPN/LVN with good nursing process and critical-thinking skills. The LPN/LVN is constantly gathering data on the medical and psychological condition of the client. A skilled LPN/LVN, for example, will note early signs of exacerbations of chronic conditions or an impending acute issue, such as an early cough before it progresses to pneumonia. Assisted living facilities are often a part of a continuing care retirement community (CCRC). The RN in charge evaluates the needs of the resident at the time of admission and assigns specific duties to the LPN/LVN. The RN also identifies the chain of command for the LPN/LVN should there be an emergency. If you like the human connection and you function well with less supervision, this may be an area to consider. The LPN/LVN is generally in a supervisory position.

INDEPENDENT LIVING FACILITY

As the geriatric population continues to grow, the practical nurse continues to excel in various settings. Some independent living centers are using LPNs/LVNs to provide wellness services and health teaching to the residents, in collaboration with the RN.

SCHOOL RELATED POSITIONS

Although the LPN cannot be certified as a school nurse (Post RN Bachelor of Science in Nursing [BSN] certificate required), they are increasingly being hired as part of the school nurse team in school districts. This has been a cost-effective and successful implementation for many school districts. In addition, LPNs are often hired to meet the needs of students with special needs attending regular education or special education classes, Lastly, LPNs are also finding employment in specialty day care centers.

HOME HEALTH NURSING

According to the U.S. Bureau of Labor Statistics, faster-than-average growth is expected in home health services. This is in response to the number of older persons with functional disabilities, preference for home care, implementation of the Affordable Care Act, and technological advances that make it possible to do more complicated treatments/care in the home.

Because of shorter hospital stays, patients are receiving an increased amount of care in the home. The actual care given is under the supervision of an RN, who uses nursing process steps as a guideline to finalize a plan of care approved by the patient. Data from the LPN/LVN involved with care are essential to complete the care plan. Postdischarge (subacute) care fits in well with LPN/LVN basic education, thereby making LPNs/LVNs invaluable in implementing the plan of care. LPN/LVNs' observations of physical and mental changes allow additions to the continuing data collection and evaluation of the plan of care. Because of difficulty in receiving payment from non-private sources, some home health agencies use LPNs/LVNs for private-pay patients only. However, the increase in home health care needs has improved the employment of LPNs/LVNs in home care. According to the NCSBN 2012 LPN job analysis, home health care has increased between 2006 and 2012. In recent years, LPNs have been obtaining positions caring for stable, chronic, complex pediatric patients at home. In addition, they may travel to a school setting with them.

Helpful Qualities for Home Health Nurses

- **Flexibility:** You will have to improvise in the home, yet practice sound nursing principles. For example, this may include improvising when equipment is not readily available, determining how to clean the equipment, and using it to attain desired results. Flexibility is also needed when the patient assignment changes because of the patient's needs.
- **Communication skills:** You are working in the patient's domain. You have to understand the patient's expression of needs and also make sure that you express yourself clearly and tactfully. For example, you may find yourself having to use words in the patient's vocabulary to be understood.
- **Self-confidence:** An air of insecurity or uncertainty will be picked up by the patient, resulting in lack of confidence in the LPN/LVN. This does not imply that you should fake confidence. Have the knowledge and nursing skills that enable you to perform tasks efficiently. Do not ask for unnecessary reassurance from the patient when performing basic skills. Ask

questions away from the patient, unless an emergency exists. For example, you may be tempted to tell the patient, "This is only the second time I have changed a dressing on a foot, and I'm kind of nervous about it." Do not make a comment like this. It will worry the patient. Be adequately prepared at all times. It may be difficult to find the reference needed once in the patient's home.

- **Sensitivity to physical and emotional changes:** Once the initial assessment is completed by the RN, it will be up to you to note any changes in patient status and alert the RN. The RN must be able to depend on your observational skills to assist the patient in meeting their health outcomes, while providing a safe environment. For example, be tuned in to the person's affective communication as well as the verbal and nonverbal. Perhaps the individual is beginning to show signs of agitation that will need to be diffused before continuing the other work you have been assigned.
- **Ability to deal with emergencies:** Staying calm and following agency protocol are essential. For example, the patient may start to bleed from the wound you are dressing. Remembering what you learned to do in basic nursing and during first aid class is more effective than panicking and yelling for a family member to call 911. Initiate emergency help (911) as needed but in a calm and effective manner. In an emergency, your motto is, "Function now, and shake later."
- **Nonjudgmental attitude:** This is a must because you work in the patient's home. You are providing a service. If you are comfortable with your own values, different values are not personally threatening. For example, the home may not be up to your standards in cleanliness, but is a safe environment for the patient. Also, be aware of your hidden biases and reflect often to avoid stereotyping of patients.

MENTAL HEALTH NURSING

Mental health nursing facilities include psychiatric hospitals, community mental health centers, day treatment centers, and group homes for the recovering mentally ill. Many community mental health centers and group homes are staffed primarily with LPNs/LVNs and nursing assistants, with RNs in a supervisory role. The LPN/LVN may also function in a supervisory role collaborating with the RN. The workforce trend has remained relatively constant over the last decade.

In mental health nursing, LPNs/LVNs are involved in the following:
- Performing treatments
- Administering medications
- Tending to activities of daily living
- Observing patients
- Assisting with group meetings and activities

Furthermore, LPNs/LVNs perform a significant role in developing a therapeutic relationship with the patient and following through with the appropriate interventions, according to the patient's care plan. Mental health facilities practice a team concept in which everyone is expected to contribute to the patient's care plan, know the therapeutic guidelines in a patient care plan, and carry out the plan. A solid knowledge of mental health concepts and nursing process is essential.

Specific beneficial qualities for working in a mental health unit include the following:

> **Professional Pointer**
>
> **Desirable Qualities in a Mental Health Setting**
> - Basic knowledge of dealing with psychiatric behaviors
> - Keen observational skills regarding behavioral change
> - Calm and able to make quick decisions
> - Empathetic rather than sympathetic
> - Therapeutic communication skills
> - Separates personal and professional life
> - Nonjudgmental and respectful
> - Sound mental health
> - Excellent nursing process and critical-thinking skills
> - Sets patient-centered limits assertively
> - Knowledge of basic self-defense
> - Does not take unnecessary risks with a patient who is acting out and knows when to seek assistance
> - Experience with medical/surgical patients before working in a mental health unit

MILITARY SERVICES

As an LPN/LVN, you will take basic training if you volunteer for military service in the reserves or for active duty. Contact recruiters for all branches of the military services, including the National Guard. Compare the differences in available nursing careers to determine which branch best fits your needs. The U.S. Army, for example, cross-trains LPNs/LVNs to be able to work in any area of the hospital. The benefits of military service also provide the financial means to continue education, and some LPNs/LVNs have taken advantage of this benefit to become an RN and an officer. Others have gone on to get advanced degrees in nursing.

> **Professional Pointer**
>
> **Desirable Qualities in Military Service Nursing**
> - Interest in teamwork
> - Strong ego
> - Ability to cope with changing situations
> - Emotional stability
> - Good communication skills
> - Self-directed
> - Desire for adventure
> - Flexible and adaptable
> - Empathetic (rather than sympathetic) with patients
> - Self-directed, but knows when to seek help
> - Healthy personal stress-relieving habits
> - A desire for a challenging career and an ability to adjust quickly to new situations

HOSPITAL NURSING

The acute care experience in most practical/vocational nursing programs is found in the medical and surgical units of hospitals. The percentage of LPNs/LVNs working on medical surgical units has trended negatively in the last decade as the acuity of patients increased and the length of stay decreased. However, there have been some positive trends noted as health care systems are hiring LPNs/LVNs to work in their specialty and medical surgical clinics. In some cases, the LPN/LVN is underused in the hospital setting because the RN is not familiar with what the LPN/LVN is permitted to do legally. Your responsibility is to know what your nurse practice act (scope of practice) is in your state. Make this information, plus information on continuing education (including certifications you have earned), known to your RN supervisor. Some RNs do not trust LPNs/LVNs primarily because they have never worked with them. Do your nursing care with skillful professionalism and help pave the way for other LPNs/LVNs to be a collaborative care partner in this important hospital nursing role.

If you consider working in a specialty area, it is helpful to have both theory class and clinical experience, or additional education. Areas with complex nursing duties mean that additional postgraduate education such as inservice, workshops, or courses related specifically to the area are required. Previous nursing experience may also be listed as a requirement. Refer to your state's Nurse Practice Act (NPA) to see how performance of nursing acts beyond basic nursing care is handled. These acts are referred to as the expanded role of the practical/vocational nurse or performance of acts in complex patient situations.

Professional Pointer

Desirable Qualities in Hospital Nursing

- Strong technical skills
- Organizational skills
- Nursing process and critical-thinking skills
- Strong ego
- Copes well during emergencies
- Teamwork: knows own and others' scope of practice
- Knows own limits and asks for help as needed

OUTPATIENT CLINICS, DOCTORS' OFFICES, URGENT CARE CENTERS AND CHIROPRACTIC OFFICES

Outpatient clinics and doctors' offices continue to provide jobs for many LPNs/LVNs. Most clinics and offices are open Monday to Friday, although extended and weekend hours are quickly becoming the norm. Assigned work varies, but it generally includes the following:
- Measuring vital signs
- Weighing patients
- Venipuncture
- Treatments
- Data collection
- Preparing the patient for an examination
- Assisting the doctor or nurse practitioner with the examination
- Performing additional duties delegated by the physician
- Maintaining and ordering supplies
- Data entry and insurance processing
- Managing patient flow and team communication
- Office tasks and management

Cross-training (learning to do jobs other than nursing) is expected in some of these facilities. For example, you might be expected to do basic lab tests, assist with x-rays and other diagnostic tests, and clerical work, including answering telephones and making appointments.

If you are working as a private nurse for a physician, you can also expect to assist with examinations and treatments as needed. When patients remain with the same physician, these nurses develop rapport with the patients, which is an asset to both the patient and the physician.

Professional Pointer

Desirable Qualities in Outpatient Nursing and Doctors' Offices

- Has good communication skills
- Pays attention to details
- Enjoys routine
- Has excellent organizational skills
- Applies nursing process and critical-thinking skills
- Adapts and is self-directed when patient load is small
- Treats all patients and their families with respect and empathy
- Practices confidentiality and is respectful of patient's right to privacy
- Uses a well-modulated voice throughout the work period
- Is flexible and willing to learn

Previous work experience in a medical-surgical unit is advised to prepare you for data collection, administering medications, doing select treatments as assigned by the physician, and keeping records, as required.

OPERATING ROOM NURSING

LPNs/LVNs who have worked in the operating room (OR) for years describe their work as assisting the surgeon with instruments and equipment, collecting data, doing preoperative and postoperative patient care, and supporting postoperative education. They strongly urge that if you are interested in this line of work, stress your education and clinical skills as an LPN/LVN to your future employer.

Overall, the employment options as an LPN/LVN in the OR are limited. In some states, LPNs/LVNs can become trained to become an operating room technician. There is the combined value of being an LPN/LVN and operating room technician. If the operating room is your passion, it may be worth researching the possibility.

VETERANS HEALTH ADMINSTRATION MEDICAL CAREERS

Working with the nation's veterans in Veteran Health Administration (VHA) hospitals or veterans in a long-term care setting or community-based facilities are additional options for LPNs/LVNs. You do not have to be a veteran to apply for employment. More LPNs/LVNs are hired in veteran's nursing homes and community settings than in acute care veteran's facilities.

Facilities generally provide new nurses an extensive orientation during duty hours regardless of the shift you are assigned. Veteran's care includes medicine, surgery, spinal cord injury, alcohol/drug treatment, psychiatry, intensive care, hemodialysis, ambulatory care, and long-term care. Minimum qualifications include U.S. citizenship, graduation, or pending graduation from an accredited nursing school, and English language proficiency. Benefits are normally generous and are based on civil service grades. If interested, go to the "Job Search" section of the VA Careers website at www.mycareeratva.va.gov/careers/career/062000

HOSPICE AND PALLIATIVE CARE

Hospice care is for terminally ill patients of any age, whether in institutional settings or their homes. The same qualities that are important in a long-term care facility are important in a hospice setting. The nurse's role is to maximize patient comfort through pain relief and addressing the patient's physical, psychosocial, and spiritual needs. Palliative care focuses on providing relief from pain and physical, mental, and spiritual stress for any type of disease or illness. It can be provided with a curative approach.

[?] Critical Thinking

Pain Medication for the Terminally Ill Patient

Think about the statement, "You should withhold pain medication from a terminally ill patient so he or she does not become addicted." Does that statement make sense to you? Explain your response.

OTHER JOB OPPORTUNITIES

Private Duty Nursing

LPNs/LVNs have been employed for years as private duty nurses. This is frequently a long-term commitment on the part of an LPN/LVN. The most common responsibility is for ill, elderly individuals who wish to be cared for in their home rather than in an institution. Some private duty nurses accompany the person on extended trips. Private duty nursing can also involve a child or adult with a long-term chronic illness. The LPN/LVN may be part of an around-the-clock care

system with RNs on opposing shifts. Responsibilities vary according to the shift involved and include basic nursing skills. The LPN/LVN works under the general supervision of the patient's physician, collaborating with the RN.

Health Insurance Companies

Health insurance companies provide in-depth orientation for the work required. This work generally includes less direct care, although it can include venipuncture and data collection related to a physical exam. In addition, LPNs/LVNs work in the role of a wellness nurse or health coach. Workman's compensation cases can also be a focus of their work.

Travel Nursing

There are a variety of ways to inquire about travel nursing as a career. Many health care related websites include information. Another option is to make your search selective. Use any search engine available to you on the computer and type in "travel nurse," or "travel nursing career," Placing the words in quotes makes the search more selective. Travel nursing can be an exciting way to experience many different types of care settings in various geographic locations. The cost of the nurse's lodging is generally provided.

Veterinary Clinics and Hospitals

For some LPNs/LVNs, this is an opportunity to combine a love of nursing with a love of animals. In some states you may work as an assistant to the veterinarian in the care and treatment of animals. Other states, such as California, require a special training program and a passing grade in a state test to assist veterinarians.

Pharmaceutical/Medical Equipment Sales

Some pharmaceutical and medical device companies may select LPNs/LVNs to staff this particular area, although it is more likely a job role for a BSN-prepared RN.

Coroner's Office

A former student practical nurse working with a coroner commented, "I never saw myself as doing this, but it is so interesting. I've learned a lot about people, pain, compassion, and myself. The doctor I work with is a born teacher and is always respectful of the person on whom he is doing the autopsy. He has helped me accept the life cycle."

Parish Nursing

Some church parishes employ their own nurse to take care of the basic health needs of the congregation. The work includes basic nursing skills such as measuring blood pressure, temperature, pulse, and respirations, medication education, and contacting a physician as needed. Health education and making healthy choices is also a focus. The LPN can work collaboratively with the RN or nurse practitioner in this role.

Temporary Help Agency

Temporary help agencies are listed under a variety of names. They supply nurses when requested by a health facility. Some provide temporary help exclusively for certain kinds of health facilities (e.g., long-term care). The need for help may be related to a shortage of nurses, lack of availability in the area, and need for temporary coverage. Assignments are intended to be short term, though sometimes the facility decides to hire the temporary nurse. Nurses who work for temporary agencies must be ready to "hit the floor running." Consequently, the temporary agency rarely hires a newly licensed nurse. They prefer a nurse with at least 1 year of experience in a clinical setting. The nurse must be competent in doing the required procedures. The temporary agency handles the contract for the health facility and for the nurse. Because of the immediate need for a nurse, the temporary agency usually pays the nurse at a higher salary than usual. A former student used this method of nursing employment to pay for continuing education to become an RN. The ability to grasp information quickly, good nursing process skills, and good critical-thinking skills are essential. Some temporary help agencies hire nurses for other countries and states.

Countless other possibilities for LPN/LVN employment exist. Consider the following:

- Residential treatment centers
- Medical management companies
- State, federal, or private correctional systems
- Corporate short-term or long-term disability benefit administration case manager
- Day care centers for adults and children
- Weight loss clinics
- Social service agencies
- Entertainment complexes (i.e., amusement park)
- Ambulance and emergency medicine staff
- Dentist office
- Blood bank
- Substance abuse clinics
- Adult day care
- Welfare and religious organization
- Specialized mobile units (e.g., bloodmobile)
- Fitness centers
- VISTA (Volunteers In Service To America) or the Peace Corps
- School nurse
- Industrial/occupational health
- Your own other areas of interest. Dare to apply!

◎ Try This

Area Job Opportunities

Investigate nursing job opportunities in your area. Add ideas to the listed job choices.

HELPFUL PERSONAL ATTRIBUTES

LPNs/LVNs must be caring, have an empathetic (not sympathetic) nature, and have a genuine concern for the welfare of their patients. Emotional stability is essential because work with sick and injured patients can be stressful. LPNs/LVNs need keen observational, critical-thinking, and decision-making skills and be able to communicate at a patient's level to be understood. A comfort level in doing basic nursing skills is absolute. If the LPN has been taught advanced skills that are within the state board's scope of practice for LPNs, then these skills need to be perfected. The condition of a patient may quickly change from stable to acute, and the nurse will have to respond to the situation without panic.

- LPNs/LVNs work as part of a team and will be expected to follow orders and work under close supervision of an RN or physician.
- Assertiveness and patient advocacy are other important attributes.
- Because the LPN/LVN will often hear or see things that cannot be discussed with someone outside of the immediate area, confidentiality is a must.
- The LPN/LVN must also find healthy ways to relieve stress at the end of the shift that will not contribute to his or her personal health problems.

◎ Try This

Personal Skills and Characteristics

Name some additional nursing skills and personal characteristics you have that enhance your ability to work in an area that currently appeals to you.

USING INTERPERSONAL STYLES TO YOUR BENEFIT

Tony Beshara (2008) suggested that by recognizing your personality type and that of your interviewer, it may be easier to answer questions as well as pose your own. With that, it was noted that in 370 BC, Hippocrates defined four basic personality types:

1. The *analytical* type is highly detail oriented, can make difficult decisions without all the facts, is perceptive, and may tend to be pessimistic.
2. The *driver* type tends to be blunt, is objective focused, is a hard worker, makes quick decisions, is independent, and is considered a can-do person. There is a tendency to be assertive, distrusting, impatient, high energy, and motivated by external recognition.
3. The *amiable* type likes to be liked, is easygoing, and is not a big risk taker. He or she likes to blend in, is highly sensitive, has difficulty making firm decisions, and can be quiet and soft-spoken.
4. The *expressive* type is a natural salesperson and storyteller. He or she is gregarious, a good motivator, tends to exaggerate, leaves out facts and details, and is relationship-oriented.

| Box 18-1 | Responding to Individuals Through the Four Major Interpersonal Styles |

Analytical type: Tell me how the patient is. (Speak rapidly and to the point about the patient's status.)

Driver type: How is your day going? (Speak slowly and deliberately, hitting the highlights of the shift.)

Amiable type: How are we doing today? (Start off with small talk, such as, "The day has been going good," and then go on to highlights of the shift. If there is a problem, present it to them with a solution and ask if they are in agreement.)

Expressive type: Did Mr. Jones get his dinner yet? (Start off with small talk, and leave an opening in the conversation for her to fill, such as, "Yeah, but I don't think he was too happy about the peas on his plate.")

An easier way to remember the four types is to associate them with characters from Charles Schultz's *Peanuts* comic strip: Linus, who is the analytical type; Lucy, who is the driver type; Charlie Brown, who is the amiable type; and Snoopy, who is the expressive type (Personality Types, 2011).

Being able to recognize different personality types around you is a plus. It is recommended that you practice this identification skill with other students and friends, so that recognizing personality type comes quickly to you. Some examples of conversation responses to individuals with these types of **interpersonal styles** can be found in Box 18-1.

POTENTIAL REFERENCES

Take a moment to consider who has seen you work and might be willing to confirm in writing and verbally that you are someone employers should hire. Instructors, unit managers, supervisors, team leaders, staff RNs, and LPNs/LVNs are potential sources of references and job openings. With respect to references, ask them in person for permission to use their name as a reference. Do not assume an instructor or anyone will give you a positive reference. Specifically ask, "May I list your name for a positive reference?" If yes, write down the nurse's name (spelled correctly), job title, work address, and work telephone number. Also, take the initiative and ask for a letter of recommendation. Be sure to acknowledge their busy schedule and ask if they'd prefer you to draft a possible letter for their use (Boxes 18-2 and 18-3). Also consider using managers and employees with whom you have worked as a volunteer or health care worker. Lastly, patients and families can also serve as references, especially if you were a consistent caregiver.

| Box 18-2 | Sample Letter to Reference Writer |

May 12, 2014

Ms. Valerie George
Surgical Care Charge Nurse
Veterans Hospital
1000 Veterans Lane
Minneapolis, MN 55402

Dear Ms. George,

Thank you again for agreeing to be a work reference. My experiences on the medical-surgical unit were both challenging and rewarding. I am pleased to have the opportunity to use the skills you taught me.

I am actively seeking employment in medical-surgical units at hospitals within the metro area. A letter of recommendation from you is definitely an asset to my job search.

Knowing your busy schedule, I have enclosed a draft letter of recommendation for your review, edit, and signature. However, if you prefer to write your own letter, you may wish to mention my ability to work under pressure, ability to administer medication on time, communication skills with staff and patients, computer proficiency, and willingness to take on new assignments.

Your assistance in helping me secure employment is greatly appreciated. I plan to give you a call next week to let you know how my job search is going and answer any questions you may have regarding the letter. I look forward to talking with you soon.

Cordially,
Katelyn Bieser

2001 Putt Drive
Cottage Grove, MN 55016
612-555-2728 or ktbieser@star.com

ENC: Reference letter

| Box 18-3 | Sample Letter for Reference Writer to Complete and Place on Facility Letterhead |

Dear Employer:

Please accept this as a letter of recommendation for Ms. Katelyn Bieser, whom I supervised during her medical-surgical rotation. Katelyn was enjoyable to work with and displayed a high degree of skill as a student practical nurse.

Specifically, she learned new tasks quickly, measured patient vital signs accurately, was proficient in computer charting, provided nutritional care, and administered medication safely and promptly. Ms. Bieser was able to follow both physician orders and RN instructions and had a keen sense of knowing when to ask for help.

I believe that Katelyn will make a positive contribution as an employee. Should you have further questions about Katelyn's skills and abilities as a nursing professional, please feel free to contact me.

Cordially,
Valerie George, RN
Surgical Care Charge Nurse

NETWORKING YOUR WAY TO SUCCESS

Smart **networking** of influential people can lead to finding new jobs, better pay, faster promotions, and greater job satisfaction.

- **Placement personnel** are good sources of job opportunities. Register with the school's career service center and local or state Career/Job Workforce Centers. Go to the school's placement office frequently, with a smile on your face. This will make them smile as well and store you in their memory job bank. Also, plan to attend job fairs or professional association conferences. Talk to the recruiters, learn about job opportunities, provide your resume, and obtain their business cards. Visit your local employment center and use free services such as job seeking workshop series and access to job postings. This can augment services received at your school and strengthen your ability to secure a first job. Many of the states in the nation have an Internet site that provides real-time job postings for the entire site accessible by specific county or city location. For an example, visit: www.paworkstats.state.pa.us.
- **Family and friends with nursing contacts.** Ask them for job leads and names of contacts, and follow up with them every 2 weeks until you get the job. And remember to thank these people for all their help once you get it! You never know if you might need their help again in the future.
- **Social media sites.** Your presence on social media sites creates your own personal brand. For example: What passion/interest do you pursue? Who do you chat with? What groups do you join? Social media is now an essential job-seeking tool.
  - LinkedIn (www.linkedin.com) is a professional social media site that can help you find mentors, stay in touch with favorite teachers, and find hiring managers and recruiters in your chosen career. Some people refer to LinkedIn as Facebook with a tie. The advantage of LinkedIn is that it allows you to look at others' networks and reach out to them for suggestions and recommendations. The goal is to make the second connection in hopes that this may be a person with hiring authority. LinkedIn has more than 350 million members (LinkedIn, 2015) from 200 countries, has a makeup of 56% male and 44% female, and is considered the must-have tool for ambitious professionals, whether looking for a job now or possibly in the future. There are several strategies to increase the number of views of your LinkedIn profile. For example, your profile is 11 times more likely to be viewed if you have a picture of yourself. That said, LPNs/LVNs should consider LinkedIn as an investment site like a 401(k) retirement plan. What you do to invest in the plan now (i.e., making sure your profile is 100% complete; adding LPNs/LVNs, nurse managers, recruiters, short- and long-term disability case managers, and

any contacts made through active networking with health care and insurance company staff) will help you later in your career when you are looking for new, higher-paying opportunities. You will also find recent graduates who are looking for jobs and may be contacted by recruiters who use LinkedIn as part of their regular scouting for candidates. Reach out to alumni, creating a common bond and a new network.
- Job boards: Countless job boards exist today. Typing in "LPN" "LVN" "licensed nurse" or "case manager" will yield some jobs through search engines such as Simply Hired (www.simplyhired.com) or Indeed (www.indeed.com). Today, hospitals, facilities, and government agencies are advertising more through these job boards and this is expected to increase in the future. According to Jobvite (2013), 74% of companies made a hire through social media in 2013. Try typing in "LPN," "LVN," or "nurse." As you search through the links, you will find recruiters, companies, and other health care professionals you can contact about employment. General Internet career search sites should be explored to seek job opportunities. Box 18-4 lists several Internet sites for careers that will prove useful.
- Twitter (twitter.com), Facebook (www.facebook.com) can be used to expand your job search network. For a Twitter profile, you should list only the basics about who you are because your online "biography" is limited to 160 characters. Twitter will load your address book and show you which of your contacts are already using the site. And, with that, Twitter will give you the option of inviting people in your address book who are not yet registered to join Twitter. Facebook can be used to access the job sites Simply Hired (www.simplyhired.com) and CareerBuilder (www.careerbuilder.com) to search for job openings. Additionally, it can be used for those who want to post their own ads on a daily basis or on specified dates at a nominal rate.

Box 18-4 **Internet Sites for Careers**

Career site suggestions include typing "practical nurse jobs" into your Internet search engine or visiting the following job boards: Indeed.com; careerbuilder.com; jobcentral.com; monster.com; and simplyhired.com. Other sites such as glassdoor.com can provide employment data such as average wage and information regarding employee satisfaction. This is important for salary negotiation, if you are offered the job.

Also, for a quick reference on the median wage in the state you are looking at, go to www.bls.gov/oes/current/oessrcst.htm. Find the blue map of the United Stated titled "Annual Median Wage," and then highlight the state you are interested in. If looking at opportunities in Canada, check out careerowl.com.

Here are some tips whether you are using professional or social media sites:

1. Do not add your current employer/supervisor to your network of contacts.
2. Be selective about adding coworkers.
3. Do not add someone to your "friends list" unless you know who they are.
4. Never post opinions about any of your employers.
5. Do not post any nonmainstream beliefs, hobbies, or recreational activities.
6. Never let anyone post items on your "wall."
7. Never announce your intention to leave your current employer because this may lead to a rapid termination. *It is not unusual for potential or current employers to browse social medical sites to see if there is a hit and learn what that person's site reveals about them.*
8. Be careful about extra costs: For example, using LinkedIn's "InMail" system to contact people who are not part of your network can cost you money. Try contacting these individuals via Facebook because you can do that free of charge.

Preparation is essential in job seeking even before the interview. Visit company websites to find current job openings, the facility's mission statement, any specialties, and locations. You can also Google the name of a nursing home, clinic, and assisted-living facility to get their URL. When using the Internet, it often takes a while to locate job and career opportunity links. After entering the career/job area, try using the "search box" and type in "licensed nurse" or "vocational nurse" as a possible shortcut. The beauty of the Internet is that you can search your local area by individual state and in different countries.

Skype Webcam (www.skype.com) consists of free computer software used in conjunction with a webcam (cameras are relatively cheap) in which families and businesses may communicate with one another via voice or video anywhere in the world. It is also a useful tool for interviewing when travel or associated costs are not practical to meet with the employer. Create a Skype account so you are prepared if this type of interview is used. Because the Internet is essentially free, this is a tool used often in the first round of interviews to save time and money for all participants. In addition to the computer, Skype can be used on a smartphone, an iPod Touch, or an iPad.

Another good way to find employment is to attend professional conferences or training sessions and *"work the room."* To do this, introduce yourself to someone you don't know or a group of people, learn something about them in 5 to 10 minutes of time, and then move on to the next new person or group. With this in mind, understand that although these are not formal interview situations, the people you are meeting for the first time are "sizing you up," just as you are doing to them. As such, it is recommended that you wear the same type of clothes that you would to an interview. Remember to ask for their card and send a follow-up email thanking them for the conversation and requesting that they keep you in mind for future job opportunities. Your email may arrive just

as they have received two resignations and a medical leave of absence. Great timing can result in a quick hire!

Professional Pointer

First impressions count, and you may be talking with the person who does the hiring, has the boss's ear, or knows of job openings.

Here are some more tips for job hunting:

- Don't bring your "significant other" to the conference. Conscientiously or not, he or she will impose on your time during and after the session. You want to be able to focus on the people you are talking to.
- Plan to arrive early, obtain your name badge, and ask the registration people to point out the key representatives who are conducting the conference. It is likely these individuals know who may be hiring.
- Strike up conversations with the key representatives. If they are not available, look for individuals who are professionally dressed. A good way to start a conversation is saying, "Hi, I am ___ (your first name). Are you part of the conference?" and/or "What part of the session did you come for?" Then, as people sit down for the conference, ask if you might join them.
- Don't sit at a table with other students. They can't offer you a job and don't have the networking connections you're seeking.
- After sitting down with the professional, you might ask, "What are your thoughts about _____ (speaker's topic) and best practices?" Whenever possible, use open-ended questions because they will lead to additional conversation and relationship building. Questions that only require yes or no answers can quickly shut down a discussion.
- At the conclusion of the session, tell the professional that it was a pleasure to have met him or her. Request his/her business card, and if none is available, ask where he/she works. If you are feeling brave, ask, "Is it a good place to work, and why or why not?" Then be prepared to listen. Finally, ask, "Would it be okay to call you at work to check on openings?" If yes, ask for the phone number and the best time to call.

Try This

Networking Your Way to Success

Who are potential individuals I haven't yet contacted? List them in the spaces provided.

NAME	TELEPHONE

Networking should be a never-ending process whether you are happily employed or looking for another job. The successful person makes a point of meeting someone new each day, knowing there will be openings if they lose their job to downsizing or are looking for an opportunity to increase earnings, advance their position, or develop professionally. From your network, mentors are often identified. In your professional and personal lives you can have countless mentors all with a unique skill set, which they share. Seek out mentors and willingly mentor others. When doing so, focus on the following:

- Display a positive affect with everyone you meet (i.e., facility staff, patients and their families, technical vendors, professionals at conferences, etc.).
- Seek the input of your supervisor and other experienced LPNs/LVNs and RNs on how to build your career and ask them to be your mentor.
- Try to build relationships with key people where you work.
- Be willing to lend a hand **without** being asked and mentor others.
- Ask about facility committees you might be able to participate in.
- Join professional organizations; members often know about job openings before they are posted.

INFORMATIONAL INTERVIEWS TO CREATE FUTURE EXPECTATIONS

Chances are, sometime during your educational program you will be asked to visit community health facilities. Your instructor will provide objectives to help make the experience worthwhile. Focus your objectives or questions on the following areas:

- Purpose
- Hours or shifts
- Staffing patterns
- Facility specialty
- The identities of the training staff and their expertise
- Newest technologies being used

Viewing this assignment as an **informational interview** allows you to find out how the facility works firsthand, assists you in determining whether you would want to work there, and allows you to meet the employer before you actually seek a job.

To obtain an informational interview with an employer, practice with another individual before making that telephone call. It may be tempting to use the example script without practicing in advance, but if you do, remember that this is exactly how you will sound: as though you are reading a script! The following is an example of a telephone request:

1. "Hello, my name is _____ (first and last name)."
2. "Who is the manager for the _____ (specialty floor or area you are interested in)?" (Emphasis is on first learning the name of the right person. Do *not* begin by asking, "May I speak to the manager for _____?") You can also try to bypass human resources and talk directly to the decision maker (i.e., cardiac floor nurse manager).
3. "Please connect me with Mr./Ms. _____."
4. "Hello, Mr./Ms. _____. My name is _____ (first and last name)."

5. "I am a student practical/vocational nurse at (school's name)."
6. "As a part of my learning experience, I would like to visit your facility and meet with you."
7. "Would it be possible to set up an informational interview tomorrow at 9:00 AM or perhaps the following day at 2:00 PM?"
    - *If the answer is yes:* "Great! I'll see you on _____ (day). Thank you!"
    - *If the answer is no:* "Is there someone else you can recommend that I contact there?"

Voice control is important as you will be judged on how you sound to others on the telephone and at the interview. It is important to understand that spoken English is broken down into five areas:

- *Low-pitched:* Sounds more mature and truthful
- *Nasal:* Grates on the listener's ears
- *Monotone:* Sounds boring and puts people to sleep
- *Loud:* Viewed as dynamic but shifty
- *Whiny:* Implies a lack of self-confidence—a turnoff

Your friends can help you gain control over your voice by modulating with you, or you can find voice self-help books and/or companies that can help you to speak more clearly and pleasantly.

◉ Try This

Practicing and Getting a Critique of Mock Interviews

With a peer, make a digital recording of you making informational interview requests, using the telephone script in this chapter. Ask them to play the part of the employer on the other end of the telephone line. Then, debrief with your peer. Evaluate the ease with which you present yourself, how your voice sounds, and the pitch and fluency of your speech. Listen to the recording while they give you feedback. Continue to practice with them until your voice sounds right with minimal effort on your part.

You should not encounter any difficulties when you speak directly to senior nursing management to request an informational interview. Management wants to "get the word out" about their facility and will often give tours and let you meet the training staff. However, do not make the mistake of turning this into a job interview. No one likes to be tricked and management tends to have a long memory about such things. Respect that they are extremely busy people and be very flexible with your time and understanding if they need to cancel. Reschedule as soon as possible.

Arrive looking sharp! This is not a T-shirt, shorts, jeans, and sandals casual meeting. Wearing your uniform is acceptable if you are coming directly from a clinical rotation. However, share this information immediately. Consider the interview as an opportunity to get insider information about what employers are looking for in potential employees. Keep a copy of the information you obtained with the name, address, and phone number in a safe place (ask for their business card) for the time when your job search begins. Creating a file on your computer or smartphone will ensure you can retrieve this information easily in the near future. Follow up the informational interview with a thank you letter, and mention the staff you met by name. Employers will sometimes share letters like this with their staff, which will bring a smile to their face. Who knows; this may gain you allies should you apply for a job there (Box 18-5).

SEARCHING FOR EMPLOYMENT OPENINGS

If you expect to work shortly after graduation, apply for employment approximately 2 months before that date. Obtain a telephone answering machine, use a telephone "voice mailbox" service, or use your cell phone so you do not miss any calls from potential employers. Be sure your voice mail is not full and is able to accept messages. Record a professional-sounding message, such as the following:

> *"Hi, this is _____ (first name), and I am not available right now. Please leave your name, telephone number, and the reason for your call. I will return your call as soon as possible." (Be sure you have caller ID enabled on your phone.)*

LPN/LVN employers are often familiar with the unusual graduating times of PN programs; however, it can become confusing to them. Share this information

frequently, during casual conversation throughout the last level/semester of your classes. Employers have immediate unexpected needs and also are planning staffing patterns for the new year. Be responsive to both situations.

You need to do some homework in preparation for seeking employment. Find out all you can about the facility where you would like to work. Facilities often provide websites or give out free pamphlets as part of their advertising. An easy way to locate company websites is to use search engines like Google, Yahoo, or MSN and type in the company name. Look for the facility's "mission statement"; determine the number of people they employ and annual profits earned.

Use the Internet to search for news stories/releases so you can work current events into your interview and talk about how your skills relate. A good site is www.healthcarefinancenews.com, which addresses health care business issues that are of interest to employers. Or if considering a move to another community, check into www.abyznewslinks.com, which enables you to visit hometown newspapers for local stories throughout the world. If applying to a specialty health care setting, visit related associations websites on the Internet (Google the key words).

It is generally accepted that 75% to 85% of all available jobs are not advertised. Do not wait for an ad to appear before seeking employment. Here are some ways to tap the "**hidden job market**":

- Get assistance from family and friends.
- Get employee/staff recommendations from your school's clinical site(s).
- Submit direct applications to employers.
- Do internal job searches. For example, depending on your skills, you could obtain less skilled employment with a health care provider in a different job that would allow you to post for jobs internally before they are released to the public. Jobs might include sterile service technician (process/package surgical instruments), certified nursing assistant, and health care coder (ICD-10). Search company websites, using terms such as "careers," "employment," and "jobs."
- Use State Job Service/Workforce Centers.
- Use Internet job sites (i.e., Careerbuilder.com, Indeed.com).
- Find out about your school's social alumni network sites, or if they don't have one, try Twitter.com to see who may be alumni and then throw out an icebreaker to get the conversation rolling (i.e., "What dorm did you live in the first year?" or "Was instructor _____ there when you were there, and what did you think about her class?").
- Use private employment or recruiter companies (i.e., type "practical nurse recruiters" into your search engine).
- Search state or federal government websites.
- Read school placement office postings/e-newsletters.

Box 18-5 | **Follow-Up Letter After Informational Interview**

January 22, 2016

Ms. Elizabeth Ekholm
Director of Nursing
Lyngblomsten Health Care Facilities
1415 Almond Avenue
St. Paul, MN 55118

Re: Informational Interview

Dear Ms. Ekholm:

Thank you so much for meeting with me yesterday. The information you provided was both valuable and interesting. I found that the variety of programs offered was progressive and individualized to meet the needs of the resident and their families. The tour that followed supported your comments about the positive interactions between staff and patients. I was pleased to have the opportunity to meet staff trainers Ms. Abbinante and Ms. Wexler, who certainly inspire confidence.

Your suggestions about strategies to improve my competitiveness through certification were appreciated. I have already registered for an applicable preparation course. Thanks for your time. This visit confirmed my hope to be fortunate enough to work at such a center after my graduation this June.

Sincerely yours,
Katelyn Bieser

2001 Putt Drive
Cottage Grove, MN 55016
612-555-2728 or ktbieser@star.com

- Do volunteer work, and read professional association newsletters.
- Contact the state's nurses' union and ask about employers who are hiring.
- Use recruiting services. The three types of staffing services are temporary or contract, in which employees work for a specified period of time; temp-to-hire, which allows employees to work with an employer on a trial basis, and if it is a "good fit," they may be offered a permanent job; and direct hire, where the employee is recruited by a staffing service and then hired by the client. Determine which service will best meet your needs.
- Job fairs are typically advertised 2 to 3 weeks before the event, so visit the companies' websites and find out all you can about the companies. You can forward your resume to the fair producers both before and after the event. The producers frequently forward resumes to participating employers at no cost to you. If you attend a job fair, go prepared with a high-energy, *30-second pitch or elevator speech* that covers your key skills, your passion for that type of work, and how it's related to the needs and goals of the recruiter's company. Because most applicants don't have a prepared speech, your presentation will make you stand out.
- Participate in virtual job fairs, such as through http://www.employmentguide.com/job-fairs/. Beware of scam job ads. Since 2006, phony job ads have increased by 345%. With such a tough job market, people's eagerness to find any job until the right one comes along sometimes overrules their common sense. If you see jobs that include home money transfers (convinces the person to open a bank account as a payment representative and then promises a percentage of the money that comes in), an unidentified employer (only willing to discuss the job in an individual or group presentation), requests for personal information via telephone or website, such as a Social Security number, address, and driver's license, to "run a background check" before the interview, or promises of high salaries for "simple" work, it is best to avoid them. At worst, you may become a victim of identity theft (Pyrtle, 2009).

It is standard practice to apply directly to employers using website job applications, emails, or cover letters and **resumes**. Often, a traditional brief, to-the-point cover letter, accompanied by a resume addressed to the director of nursing or nursing recruiter at the facility is best. Box 18-6 provides an example cover letter. Do not include a personal reference list or a photograph of yourself with it. Retain the reference list for your interview and provide it only on request.

It is best to use Sundays and Mondays to research job opportunities and then contact employers from Tuesday forward. The best time to call employers to schedule interviews or make follow-up contacts is after 9 AM. As a rule, most employers don't have the luxury

---

Box 18-6   **Sample Cover Letter for Employment**

April 14, 2016

Ms. Cheryl Krutchen
Human Resources Director
Columbus Hospital & Clinics
2031 Lakeside Drive
Columbus, MN 55025

Re: LPN Staff Nurse Position

Dear Ms. Krutchen:

I will graduate from the Rainy Lakes Technical College practical nursing program this June. While completing a medical nursing rotation at your hospital, I was impressed by the quality of client care, staff professionalism, and learning opportunities.

In addition to this rotation, my work experiences have included a focus on electronic patient documentation, care coordination using a multidisciplinary approach, follow-through on individualized patient/family plans, working with a diverse population, patient advocacy, and participation in the evaluation process toward achievement of patient and institutional outcomes.

I am interested in obtaining employment at your hospital and being able to work with your staff again. I will contact you on Tuesday, April 21, to see whether you have received my resume and to determine when we might arrange an interview. Should you wish to contact me before then, I can be reached weekdays after 3:30 PM. I look forward to speaking with you.

Cordially,
Katelyn Bieser

2001 Putt Drive
Cottage Grove, MN 55016
612-555-2728 or ktbieser@star.com

---

of contacting every prospective job candidate, owing to time constraints and demands of their own jobs. Candidates who are waiting to hear from employers should not hold their breath or be disappointed when employers do not call.

Once you identify an applicable job posting, follow the directions provided which can include e-mailing or uploading a cover letter and resume, completing an on-line application, reporting to an open interview session or calling for an interview. Don't forget that many other people are also reading the job posting. *The candidate who hesitates is lost.* If you call the employer, your conversation needs to reflect the following example:

1. "Hello, my name is _____ (first and last name)."
2. "Can you share the name of the person in charge of hiring?"
3. "May I please speak with Ms. _____?"
4. "Hello, Ms. _____. My name is _____ (first and last name)."

5. "Do you have any practical/vocational nursing positions open now or projected in the near future?"

   a. *If hiring:* "Would it be possible to set up an interview on . . . (give a choice of two upcoming dates and time) [pause for a moment]" *If no:* "What would be a better time and date? [Offered time and date.] Great! I will see you then."

   b. If they are not hiring or are under a hiring freeze, catch your breath and don't be put off. An acceptable reply then would be:

- "Oh, I hadn't heard that. Your facility sounds like a great place to work. Would it be possible to meet with you anyway? I would like to be the first person you consider when an opening occurs or the freeze ends." *If yes,* see 5a. *If no:* "Do you know of anyone who might be hiring?"
- *If yes:* "Would you also know the contact person and/or have a telephone number?"
- *If no:* "I appreciate your time. Thank you." Or if *no:* "Thank you for trying. Would it be possible for me to come in for an informational interview?" *If yes,* see 5a. *If no:* "Well, thank you again. Good-bye."

Deflect the employer's interview type of questions until the actual interview. Often when employers do not have an opening, they feel it is kinder to applicants to ask some questions and then tell the applicant that he/she is not what they are looking for. Also, you do not want to be "washed out" by a telephone conversation if the employer does have a job.

If the employer begins to ask you questions about your background, education, or work experience, you might respond, "I have completed an accredited practical/vocational nursing program, passed the NCLEX-PN® examination, obtained my license, and have the necessary work experience. I would like the opportunity to discuss my qualifications during our interview." The tone of your voice can make a significant difference on the telephone. If you smile while you are talking, you will project a positive tone. Practice the preceding format several times in advance with a friend so there are no hesitations in your presentation and you're prepared for the challenging questions.

Leaving a Voice Mail Message

At some point you may have to leave a phone message for the employer. Here is a script you can practice beforehand:

"Ms./Mr. _____, my name is _____, and I am calling about a licensed practical nurse position. I have strong clinical and interpersonal skills and am willing to work all shifts. I would like to meet with you and can be reached at _____ (phone number). Again, this is _____ (name) at _____ (phone number). I look forward to talking with you."

REFERENCES: A TIMELESS TREASURE

Prospective employers will be more interested in certain types of work references than others. There is a reference hierarchy of individuals who act as references. Ranging from most to least important are current or former nursing instructors, clinical staff from your clinical rotations, and supervisors from past nursing-related work or volunteer experiences; past employers or supervisors from non–nursing-related jobs; and personal references or friends. (Employers rarely contact personal references because their opinions are likely to be biased.)

◎ Try This

Pick Your References

List the people in your reference hierarchy, including the person's name, job title, work address, and telephone number. Most employers request three references. Pick and choose from your list of resources for maximum impression.

The statement "References available on request" does not need to be placed on your resume. Letters of recommendation (preferred) or a reference list should be given to the interviewer if requested, so bring them to the interview. References, however, are a "treasure." Avoid requesting references unless you are interested in a job. People's time is a valuable commodity. Do not abuse their willingness to help and/or mentor you.

RESUMES: THE CONTRIBUTIONS YOU WILL MAKE

Developing two versions of your resume is a must! First is the traditional *design-focused* document you mail and bring with you to the interview. The second is a scannable or *text-focused* resume, which is good for Internet applications and pasting onto email.

Your resume is a painting of your life. Remember that a painting generally uses broad strokes to create an impression. This is your goal. Resumes are not a confession or "tell-all" script, nor should they include reasons for leaving past jobs, salary requirements, or personal photographs. Additionally, listing personal data, such as marital status, race, religion, height, weight, number or age of children and other demographic/personal characteristics is discouraged. Resumes can look different based on the professional discipline. A nursing resume looks very different than graphic designer's resume.

A list of objectives at the top of a resume went out of fashion more than 20 years ago. Resumes should now include a "Summary" or "Profile" (keyword focus) section. Also, statements on "personal goals" or "health" are a waste of both time and valuable space on your resume.

Many traditional resumes are never read because they are too cluttered, too wordy, or contain the aforementioned problems. Use short, bulleted sentences of no more than two to four words, which allow employers to compare resume key words to their job description. Remember that "white space" is your friend.

An employer makes a decision whether to interview in the first few minutes of reading a resume. Plan to modify your resume to contain the keywords from the ads you apply to. This will enhance your chances of being contacted for an interview.

Essentially, all resumes have a format of heading, profile/summary, work and military experience, education, and licenses/professional memberships. With respect to the heading, list your email address so employers can reach you any time of the day or night. Some job searchers, as a time saver or depending on the amount of email traffic they receive, will set up a separate free email account. This can usually be done if your server has a free second email line available or by using free email services such as Gmail or Windows Live Hotmail.

It is recommended that you stop and think about what specific classes or jobs you have performed and record them in your resume. Spell out the job tasks, and do not assume an employer will understand a statement like "Performed nursing duties." It is recommended that

military/work experience be listed in years. Do not list more than 10 years of work history, outdated training (i.e., 2007 CPR certification), or old versions of computer programs (i.e., Windows 2003). In addition, avoid listing job tasks that are very routine for the position. For example: If you were a nursing assistant, do not include a task such as bathing the patient but do include if you were responsible for obtaining vital signs or you mentored new staff.

Remember that your resume must be truthful. Human resource departments will look for inconsistencies such as work experiences that are too good to be true or resumes that appear purposely vague. Keep your resume consistent and well balanced. Communicate in your accompanying cover letter why there are gaps in employment, particularly when there is a logical explanation (i.e., child rearing or training).

The initial impression made by the resume is very important. Box 18-7 lists some basic factors to consider for scannable/personal and traditional resumes. Figures 18-1A and 18-1B show sample resumes.

Box 18-7 Basic Resume Factors

SCANNABLE/ELECTRONIC/EMAIL RESUME FACTORS

For a scannable resume, you want no visual distractions to confuse the OCR (optical character recognition) scanner that reads the resume. As noted previously, a text-focused format is required when completing/submitting online applications or faxing your resume:

- **Length:** Two pages maximum; one page is preferred.
- **Paper:** *Quality bond*. Use colors such as white or off-white only (no designs, textures, or recycled paper). Use matching paper for the cover letter and envelope.
- **Type:** Arial or Times New Roman typeface (10- to 14-point type) is preferred; underlining, italics, or graphics should generally be omitted. Bolding is permitted. Avoid multiple columns, newspaper-style layouts, landscape printing, and designer fonts. Always place your name at the top of the page because scanners assume that whatever is at the top of the page is your name. As such, if your resume has a second page, place your name and a "page 2" designation at the top.
- **Spellcheck:** Use the computer's spellcheck feature, and then proofread the resume from the bottom up so there are no extra marks or spelling or grammatical errors.
- **Printing:** If you don't have a computer, borrow a friend's or go to the library. Type the resume and save it onto a thumb drive, which is inexpensive and fits in your pocket. For printing, use a laser printer, which is less likely to smudge, or take your thumb drive to a quick print shop. Avoid standard copy machines because they often provide poor-quality copies.
- **Faxes:** Avoid faxing your resume unless it's specifically requested because faxing degrades the text.
- **Emails:** If asked to email your resume as a nonattachment, use the scannable resume. Simply copy and paste it into an email to the employer. However, before sending it to the employer, send a copy to yourself first to see what the recipient will see and then decide if you can use

it or need to go with another option of getting the resume to the employer.

- **Balanced space:** An uncluttered, balanced design is desirable so the resume is easy to read. Also, because most managers don't have time to read, a "bulleted" style is recommended when listing your job skills and past duties.
- **Emphasis:** Whether you have a strong or limited work history, keep in mind that your use of keywords will help answer the employer's question "What can you do for me?"

TRADITIONAL RESUME FACTORS

- **Length:** Two pages maximum; one page is preferred.
- **Paper:** *Quality bond*. Use colors such as white or off-white only (no designs, textures, or recycled paper). Use matching paper for the cover letter and envelope.
- **Type:** Arial or Times New Roman typeface (10- to 14-point type) is preferred. Underlining, italics, graphics, and bolding can be used to draw the reader's eyes to points being made. Different resume formats may be used, with conservative design recommended. Multiple columns and newspaper-style layouts are permitted. Make a practice of using your computer's spellcheck feature, and then proofread the resume from the bottom up so there are no extra marks or spelling or grammatical errors. For printing, use a laser printer, or take your thumb drive to a quick print shop. Avoid standard copy machines because they provide poor-quality copies.
- **Faxes:** If specifically requested to fax your resume, use the scannable one.
- **Emails:** Use a scannable resume instead, or send your traditional resume via U.S. mail (snail mail).
- **Balanced space:** Use an uncluttered, balanced design with a "bulleted" list of job skills.
- **Emphasis:** Whether you have a strong or limited work history, keywords are important.

COVER LETTERS: TAILORED TO FIT THE JOB YOU WANT

◉ Try This

Cover Letters

Why do cover letters need to be sent in with resumes?

Include a cover letter with each resume, whether submitted by email, fax, snail mail, or dropped off with an employer's application. Cover letters directly respond to the job's requirements and refer to any prior telephone conversation with the employer, including "dropping the name" of the person who referred you. If the employer is located out of town or out of the country, it is also a means to discuss your plans to move there with a request to interview for the job via Skype because of the distance involved. Also, for cover letters, neatness, correct spelling, and proper grammar are mandatory. Each letter should be one page, should be an original (never photocopied), should contain no errors or white correction ink, and should be typed in block letter format. If an employer asks for specific experience, be sure to list this in the cover letter, even if the experiences are not listed on the resume. The cover letter should provide additional information or highlight critical information from your resume. It should not be repetitive of your resume. Remember that each cover letter is unique to the individual job posting. Use key words from the job posting in your cover letter to highlight how you align with the job requirements.

You may use the same cover letter you send out by post for your electronic mail. It is recommended that you "paste" your resume to the end of the electronic cover letter and send this out as a whole unit rather than as an attachment. This will help you to avoid running into an employer's computer that can't open your attachment and subsequently lose the opportunity. Boxes 18-8A and

---

Katelyn Bieser
2012 Putt Drive
Cottage Grove, MN 55301
Phone: (651) 555-2728
Email: ktbieser@star.com

SUMMARY OF QUALIFICATIONS

Cardiac-oriented Licensed Practical Nurse with rudimentary Spanish who is patient oriented, has working knowledge of sterile techniques, possesses strong clinical judgment, available night shift, and hardworking.

EXPERIENCE

St. Michael Hospital – Minneapolis, MN
Cardiac Unit – Practical Nurse School Rotation   (Spring 2016)
- Worked with interdisciplinary health care team including patients, physicians, nursing staff, patient families, and social workers.
- Performed basic data collection, utilized time management, and infection control.
- Medication administration, measured vital signs, quality assurance, and charting.
- Patient/family education, positive attitude, and positive learning attitude.

Forest View Nursing Home – Hastings, MN
Certified Nursing Assistant   (2014 – present)
- Served on memory unit, health care intervention, and provided direct patient care.
- Promoted daily living skills, resident feeding/hygiene, and room sanitizing.
- Measured/charted vital signs, worked with staff of 10, monitored patients with confusion.
- Positive family interactions, assisted with patient turning/lifting, and duties as assigned.

The Small Town Café – Bloomington, MN
Waitress   (2012 – 2014)
- Strong focus on customer service, promotion of specials, and cashiering.
- Grew café customer base by 20%, participated in marketing strategies, and assisted with food preparation so food served hot.
- Worked full time, including holidays, and welcomed customers by name.

LICENSE/CERTIFICATION

State of Minnesota Board of Nursing – LPN License   (2016 to present)
American Red Cross - CPR Certification   (2011 to present)
Hmong Cultural Awareness Class – School District 916   (Spring 2014)

EDUCATION

Rainy Lakes Technical College – Practical Nursing Diploma

A

FIGURE 18-1 A, Sample typed resume scannable/electronic plain text/fax.

Continued

Katelyn Bieser
2012 Putt Drive, Cottage Grove, MN 55301   (651) 555-2728 • ktbieser@star.com

PROFESSIONAL SUMMARY

Key Strengths

- Cardiac-oriented LPN
- Sterile Tech knowledge
- Willing to move

- Rudimentary Spanish
- Strong clinical judgment
- Quality assurance

- Patient oriented
- Available night shift
- Hardworking

PROFESSIONAL EXPERIENCE

St. Michael Hospital, Minneapolis, MN
Spring 2016
PN School Rotation; Cardiac Unit
- Interdisciplinary H.C. Team
- Time management
- Medication administration
- Quality assurance
- Charted data
- Solicited Sup. feedback

- Basic data collection
- Facilitated Sterile Tech's
- Vital sign measurement
- Patient/family education
- Positive attitude
- Assisted staff as needed

Forest View Nursing Home, Hastings, MN   June 2012 – present
Certified Nursing Assistant; Memory Unit
- Health care intervention
- Resident feeding/hygiene
- Charted vital signs
- Coordinated with 10 staff
- Positive communications
- Duties as assigned

- Direct patient care
- Promoted ADLs
- Room sanitization
- Monitored patient activity
- Patient turning/lifting, etc.

The Small Town Café, Bloomington, MN   May 2010 – May 2012
Waitress; Full Time
- Active customer service
- 20% Sales increase
- Time mgmt./memory dev.
- Worked holidays, etc.
- Duties as assigned

- Promotion of specials
- Cashiering/Inventory
- Assisted food preparation
- Cleaned restaurant

LICENSE/CERTIFICATION

State of Minnesota Board of Nursing, St. Paul, MN   2014 to present
Practical Nursing
License (LPN)

American Red Cross, St. Paul, MN   2011 to present
Cardiopulmonary Resuscitation
Certification

School District 916, White Bear Lake, MN   Spring 2014
Hmong Cultural Awareness Class

EDUCATION

Rainy Lakes Technical College, International Falls, MN   Diploma
Practical Nursing   2014

B

FIGURE 18-1, cont'd B, Sample typed traditional resume.

18-8B show sample cover letters to employers through an unsolicited telephone call and Internet advertisement.

⊚ Try This

Résumé

Develop a resume, and include a cover letter.

Access resources on the Internet and Microsoft word to assist you in writing a resume.

Microsoft word has a template that can be used found by clicking on file, new from template and resume (May vary based on your version of Microsoft word). A simple or block resume is appropriate.

Helpful Internet resources: www.resumehelp.com/home-1?utm_source=bing%20&utm_medium=cpc&utm_keyword=%2Bresume%20%2Btemplates; www.resumetemplates.org/

Purdue Owl: https://owl.english.purdue.edu/owl/resource/719/1/

Box 18-8A	**Sample Cover Letter: Unsolicited Telephone Call**

August 12, 2016

Ms. Jana Williams, RN
Director of Nursing
St. Helen General Hospital
8354 177th Lane
St. Paul, MN 55084

Re: LPN Staff Nurse Position

Dear Ms. Williams:

Thank you for taking the time to speak with me about the Practical Nurse position. As we discussed, I believe that my clinical work experiences and skills are a good match for the job.

In addition to two-plus years of Nursing Assistant experience, my education, job skills, and abilities also include direct patient care, electronic charting of observations, verbal/written communications, strong interpersonal skills, being safety oriented, advocating patient/family rights, and the ability to perform efficiently and effectively during emergencies.

I will contact you on Tuesday, August 18, to see if you have had an opportunity to review my resume and to determine when an interview may be arranged. I look forward to speaking with you soon.

Cordially,

Katelyn Bieser
2001 Putt Drive
Cottage Grove, MN 55016
612-555-2728 or ktbieser@star.com

ENC: Resume

Box 18-8B	**Cover Letter: Internet Ad Response with No Contact Person Listed**

Please accept my resume as application for the Licensed Practical Nurse position advertised in Careerbuilder.com. I believe that my work experiences through the Rainy River Technical College nursing program and clinical rotation at St. Michael Hospital are a good match for the position.

As a recent graduate, I will be taking my NCLEX-PN® examination on September 27. My clinical work experiences include a focus on electronic patient documentation, care coordination under a multidisciplinary approach, follow-through on individualized patient/family care plans, working with a diverse population, patient advocacy, and participation in the evaluation process toward achievement of outcomes. Additionally, I have worked as a Certified Nursing Assistant, which honed a positive attitude when working with seniors.

I will contact your company on Tuesday, August 18, to confirm receipt of my resume and to determine when an interview may be arranged. I look forward to speaking with you soon.

Katelyn Bieser
612-555-2728 or ktbieser@star.com

ANSWERS TO APPLICATION QUESTIONS

You will be asked to fill out an application either before or after an interview. You must answer the questions truthfully. If you have had three or more jobs in the past 3 years, the employer will be concerned about this and expect you to supply good reasons for leaving the jobs. Reasons for leaving might include work interfered with school, a layoff, a relocation, career exploration and job stagnation. Employment gaps might be explained by responses such as laid off, job hunting, returned to school, travel, or family responsibilities.

If there are questions you wish to defer until the face-to-face interview, write "N/A" (for not applicable) or "Will discuss," or leave the space blank. However, do this sparingly. One such area might include expected wage and wages from former jobs. For current wage expected, write "Open" or "Prevailing wage"; do not specify a dollar amount. With wages in former employment, leave the spaces blank if you know you were underpaid, or tell the truth if the wage was fair.

Note that if applying via the Internet, several companies use software job application programs that are set to reject applicants if all the requested data are not provided. Some job experts recommend listing a mid-range salary in the box to position you to get the interview. Remember, lying on any application is typically grounds for termination. Be aware that you do not have to answer questions about age, religion, marital status, children, physical data (unless they are specific requirements for the job), or workers' compensation injuries. However, recognize the risk in refusing to answer questions either on the application or during an interview. An employer's eyes will naturally gravitate toward any blank spaces. Therefore answer every question, even if it does not apply to you (i.e., for military experience, write "N/A" in the space if you did not serve). Some employers view blanks or "Will explain" as an automatic screen for someone they do not want to employ. Should you choose to answer **illegal questions**, the examples in Box 18-9 will be helpful. Do not attempt to falsify information, because this will provide grounds for dismissal after hiring. Remember, the personnel department may contact your references, schools, former employers, licensing board, and others to verify the information on your job application and resume. The resume is your own painting, your own creation. The application is a legal document.

Box 18-9	Sample Answers to Illegal Questions

HAVE YOU BEEN HOSPITALIZED WITHIN THE PAST 5 YEARS?

Answer: I do not have any health problems that would interfere with fulfilling the described position.

HAVE YOU EVER BEEN ON WORKERS' COMPENSATION?

Answer: N/A (not applicable) [Or] I am able to perform all of the described job duties.

DO YOU HAVE A CRIMINAL RECORD?

Answer: I have received a speeding ticket, but I have never been convicted of crimes involving drugs, theft, or assault. [Or] I have paid for that error in judgment, taken special classes, and am now wise enough not to repeat it.

◎ Try This

Job Application

Using the suggestions in the text, fill out a practice job application for a nursing position.

PREPARING FOR THE INTERVIEW

During an interview, you should also be interviewing the potential employer. It is important to find a "great first fit" (Box 18-10). As Steve Jobs stated, "The only

Box 18-10	Sample Questions to Ask the Interviewer

Use four or five of the following questions:
- Can you explain the scheduling process?
- What types of patients will I work with?
- How big is the facility, and how many beds are in the unit?
- What is the nurse-to-patient ratio?
- Do you have 8-, 10-, or 12-hour shifts?
- Will I be routinely floated to other units?
- What type of electronic charting system is used?
- How long does orientation last, and what can I expect?
- Do you provide support or mentoring for new hires?
- What type of uniform is worn?
- How often is overtime available or mandated?
- Is there a weekend commitment?
- Is testing required before going to the floors?
- Is this a new position, or am I replacing someone? Why did they leave?
- Will I be required to do any on-call duty? If so, how often?
- Given my interests in the ___ unit, is it possible to move there if an opening occurs?
- Are there annual or review-based bonuses available?
- What can you tell me about the culture and environment here?
- What opportunities does the facility offer for career development?
- Tell me about your background and why you joined this organization.
- What were the results from the last survey? When is the next one scheduled?

way to do great work is to love what you do." Invest time in finding this great first fit! If you have prepared adequately, you will be able to evaluate whether your job skills, physical abilities, and interests match the objectives of the facility. Remember to bring a copy of your traditional resume, LPN/LVN license (if you have passed the NCLEX-PN® examination), current cardiopulmonary resuscitation (CPR) card, and medical records documenting tuberculosis skin tests, hepatitis B, tetanus vaccinations, and letters of recommendation and/or awards received.

If using the Internet via Skype, remember to look into the camera to simulate looking into the interviewer's eyes. For those who have difficulty looking into a camera, it is recommended you tape a picture of someone onto the computer monitor, at the same level as the camera, to look at. Then it will be as though you are speaking directly to the person and focused on what he or she is saying.

Interviews are stressful not only for you but also for employers. They have to fit interviews into their regular work duties, justify why one job candidate should be hired rather than another, and be on constant guard not to discriminate in matters of age, sex, race, and so on. Knowing that there are concerns on both sides (yours and the interviewer's) will help you be less defensive and answer in an honest and reassuring way.

Part of your responsibility is to help the interviewer become comfortable with who you are and why you should be selected for the job. There are ways to deal with cultural differences and age when encountered in an interview (Box 18-11).

Box 18-11	Tips for Handling Differences Between the Interviewer and You

Job seekers near or over the age of 50 may be vulnerable in interviews unless they adopt a vital, energetic, and positive approach. If the interviewer is younger than you and slights your age through a question, then a response like "I'm in excellent health, and as you can see by my resume, I have a solid work history and am not afraid to learn new things" would be appropriate. If the employer representative is older than you, an appropriate response is "I have always been surrounded by workers older than myself, which taught me to work hard and listen to what they had to say."

With respect to cultural background, when there are differences between you and the interviewer, you need to remember that different groups have different norms concerning eye contact, the loudness of your voice, personal distance, body language, joking/teasing, divulging too much information, and other subtle aspects of communication such as the use of metaphors, proverbs, and colloquialisms.

It is recommended you follow the interviewer's lead in the course of communication. Additionally, you can never go wrong by being polite, and if you are unclear about what was said, say, "Excuse me, I'm not quite following what you're asking. Could you ask it in another way?"

Also remember the need to be computer literate.

INTERVIEW QUESTIONS AND ANSWERS: A CHALLENGING OPPORTUNITY

Often the first interview question, "Tell me a little bit about yourself," is an icebreaker designed to make you comfortable and determine what is important to you. Take advantage of the question. Put both you and the interviewer on even ground. Do not use the first question as an opportunity to talk about their illegal job application questions, your dysfunctional family, the bad day you have had because of a fight with your significant other, or why nursing can be stressful.

Prepare for your interview by practicing sample responses to typical interview questions (Box 18-12). Do this as role-playing with another person in the role of the interviewer. For better preparation, ask the person

---

Box 18-12 Sample Interview Questions and Answers

TELL ME ABOUT YOURSELF.
Answer: Would you like to know about my work history or personal life? *If work history*, discuss your passion to help care for and treat people. Then provide a brief description of your schooling, past jobs, and goals to work as a staff/long-term care (or whatever) LPN. *For personal*, you might say, I have lived in this area all my life, (or) my plans are to make this area my home. I recently graduated from Rainey River Technical College and am looking for a career I can grow in.

HAVE YOU EVER DONE THIS TYPE OF WORK BEFORE?
Answer: Yes, in fact some of my experiences include direct patient care during clinical rotations, volunteer work as a hospital volunteer, experiences as a mother, and . . . .

WHY DO YOU WANT TO WORK HERE?
Answer: Your company has an excellent reputation in the community and has job opportunities that align with my training. Additionally, this company's mission statement of _____ reflects my views on _____.

WHAT MOTIVATES YOU?
As a nurse I am motivated by work and its challenge of my skills on a daily basis. I know with the right employer, I will continue to learn new skills as nursing changes.

WHY DID YOU LEAVE YOUR LAST JOB?
Answer: As you know, I am a recent graduate and am looking for employment in my field of study. *Note:* If you have worked as an LPN/LVN: I am looking for a new position to expand my work skills, keep the job interesting, and provide more opportunities for advancement.

TELL ME ABOUT YOUR LAST EMPLOYER.
Answer: I really enjoyed my work at _____, which has an excellent reputation for _____. But now it is time to move on to new opportunities.

WHAT HAVE YOU DONE TO KEEP YOUR CLINICAL SKILLS CURRENT?
Answer: Well, in addition to participating in several clinical rotations during school, I recently joined the _____ (LPN professional organization) to keep abreast of new developments in nursing.

HOW DO YOU COMPARE YOUR VERBAL SKILLS WITH YOUR WRITING SKILLS?
Answer: Organizations are more dependent than ever on their employees' communicating well both verbally and in writing. I am constantly taking advantage of opportunities to develop in both areas by asking for feedback and then putting the suggestions into practice.

WHY SHOULD I HIRE YOU INSTEAD OF SOMEONE ELSE?
Answer: I think my references can best answer that question. I am sure when you contact them, they will agree I am hardworking and dependable and get the job done correctly. In addition, I am flexible, adaptable and work well with a team.

WHEN ARE YOU AVAILABLE FOR WORK?
Answer: Right away. [Or] I would need to give my employer 2 weeks' notice. It will provide me time to tie up loose ends and give my employer time to find a replacement. *Note:* If the interviewer insists you terminate your job immediately, you are witnessing a power play. You need to ask yourself if you really want to work for this individual. This could be the tip of the iceberg for future power plays.

HOW IS YOUR HEALTH? ARE THERE ANY PARTS OF THE JOB YOU CAN'T PERFORM?
Answer: I have always been in good health. I see myself being able to perform all parts. I think the best approach to any job is to use common sense. If I need help, I am not afraid to ask for it.

WHAT ARE YOUR GREATEST STRENGTHS?
Answer: I would have to say that my strengths include (1) _____, (2) _____, (3) _____, (4) _____, and (5) _____. *Note:* Your responses should be consistent with what your references say about you.

WHAT IS YOUR GREATEST WEAKNESS?
Answer: As you know, everyone has weaknesses. My greatest weakness right now is my "driven" personality. It has certainly assisted me in getting the job done efficiently and effectively. However, at times, some colleagues will request that we slow down and have a break. I have learned to assess and carefully listen to the team to avoid "burnout."

WHAT ARE YOUR LONG-TERM GOALS?
Answer: Eventually, I would like to work as a Charge Nurse at this facility. My goal is to learn all I can. This will help me to develop skills to manage and lead a team, ultimately contributing to the mission of the institution, to advance the health of the residents.

HAS AN EMPLOYER EVER FIRED YOU?
Answer: Before going to nursing school and getting my priorities straight, an employer fired me for attendance problems. It was a valuable lesson that I learned from and will never repeat. My attendance was excellent in nursing school. I only missed one day due to illness. *Note:* Do not start your response with "Yes"; address the issue.

Continued

Box 18-12   Sample Interview Questions and Answers—cont'd

HOW DO YOU APPROACH DOING THINGS THAT YOU DON'T LIKE TO DO?

Answer: I tell myself, "Let's get it done, and done right." There is nothing worse than having to go back and redo work that was done incorrectly the first time.

CAN YOU WORK UNDER PRESSURE?

Answer: Yes, I have experienced working under pressure for many years. This has meant meeting deadlines, dealing with difficult people, and developing employer confidence that the job will be done right.

WILL CHILD CARE BE AN ISSUE?

Answer: No, I have found a good day care setting for my children. If they cannot go to day care, I have worked out a system of alternating days with another provider or relative to take care of them so that work is minimally affected. *Note:* Although some individuals believe this is an illegal question, it is important for the employer to anticipate any staffing issues. A stable staffing pattern is needed to maintain quality patient care.

WOULD YOU BE WILLING TO WORK OVERTIME?

Answer: Yes, if it will help the unit.

MAY WE CONTACT YOUR CURRENT EMPLOYER?

Answer: Yes, but only after a firm job offer has been made. I would appreciate it if before you contact my employer, you will allow me to talk with my supervisor first as a courtesy.

AREN'T YOU OVERQUALIFIED FOR THIS JOB?

Answer: I may be more qualified than other individuals you are considering, but this simply means that I will be able to make an immediate contribution. After learning your system, I hope to be eligible for advancement opportunities within the organization.

IS YOUR SPOUSE EMPLOYED? WILL THERE BE A CONFLICT?

Answer: Yes, my spouse has a job. No, I do not see that there would be a conflict. We are both looking forward to my working for you.

WHAT KIND OF SALARY OR WAGE DO YOU EXPECT?

Answer: What would a person with my background and qualifications typically earn in this position with your company? [Or] I am ready to consider your best offer. *Note:* If an employer insists you give a wage quote, give a range using your bottom dollar and a realistic top wage.

Answer: I would think we could agree on a salary between $00.00 per hour and $00.00 per hour. (Note that an hourly wage, not an annual salary, is stated.)

Salary resources include the Internet and labor market sites through your local Job Service/Workforce Centers. Right now, you can use the average median wage because you are new to the profession. Internet sources include www.salary.com; www1.salary.com/Licensed-Practical-Nurse-salary.html. Also check www.payscale.com/research/US/Job=Licensed_Practical_Nurse_(LPN)/Salary and www.glassdoor.com/Salaries/licensed-practical-nurse-salary-SRCH_KO0,24.htm. For an idea about the national average median wage, check www.bls.gov or your local state workforce web site. Additionally, if you are considering relocation to another city/state, you are encouraged to use http://swz.salary.com/CostOfLivingWizard/LayoutScripts/Coll_Start.aspx to determine how much salary you will need to maintain your current standard of living. For instance if, you are currently making $40,000/year in Miami, Florida, because the cost of living is 59.5% higher in New York City than Miami, you will need to earn $63,819 to maintain your current standard of living.

DO YOU HAVE ANY QUESTIONS?

Answer: (See Box 18-10 for questions to ask the interviewer.) After your questions, ask if it would be possible to take a tour of the facility.

HOW DO YOU DEAL WITH CRITICISM, AND DESCRIBE A TIME YOU WERE CRITICIZED FOR POOR PERFORMANCE.

Answer: A person who does not make mistakes will never grow. Most recently, in school, I had problems with time management. Because of this, I did not do very well on a couple of tests, and my teachers let me know they were disappointed because I had not done my best work. I agreed they were right and asked for assistance. One of my teachers then showed me how to improve my time management so the problem would not happen again. And it didn't.

HOW DO YOU VENT ANGER OR FRUSTRATION IF YOUR DAY HAS BEEN CHALLENGING OR STRESSFUL?

Answer: I am a walker and a talker. My first choice is to burn off the stress by walking/biking/going to the gym/whatever. I always feel better after exercising. If that is not available, I will go outside on my break alone or with one trusted peer and talk out the problem and associated emotion. It is amazing what talking for 10 minutes will do for getting perspective back. Of course, I would not violate HIPPA.

DO YOU HAVE A VALID DRIVER'S LICENSE?

Answer: I will use the city bus system to get to work. If the buses aren't running, there is always a taxicab available, plus I have a network of friends who can help me in a pinch. I have never been late to work.

IS THERE ANY TIME WHEN IT IS OKAY TO BREAK COMPANY RULES?

Answer: Yes, if someone's life is in danger or if there is a natural disaster. Even in these cases I would collaborate with the RN or physician, if possible, to confirm my decision making.

HOW DO YOU HANDLE CHANGE?

Answer: It is all about attitude! If you go in with the thought that the proposed change will help you do your job better and improve patient care, it is easy to embrace it. I also know that creating champions can work. I would try to identify a nurse aide who could be a champion for the proposed change.

ILLEGAL QUESTIONS/RESPONSES

You do not have to answer these questions.

Box 18-12 **Sample Interview Questions and Answers—cont'd**

WHAT RELIGIOUS FAITH ARE YOU?
Answer: Religion certainly is a part of this great country of ours, but I prefer to separate religion from work. (You can still choose to state your religion.)

THAT'S A NICE NAME. IS IT JEWISH/MUSLIM/IRISH/OTHER NATIONALITY?
Answer: America is a melting pot. That is why it is the greatest country on earth. I feel we are all Americans first and foremost, and that's the most important issue here. Don't you agree?

HAVE YOU EVER BEEN TESTED FOR HIV?
Answer: No, I have never had a reason to test for HIV, nor do I anticipate a reason to do so.

YOU LOOK GAY TO ME. ARE YOU GAY?
Answer: I've heard that employers will sometimes ask questions to see if they can make the applicant upset and observe their reaction. Personally I do not care if someone is gay as long as they are professional and do their job. I have always assumed this is important to employers, too.

[MALE NURSE] THE SUPERVISOR IS JANET SMITH, WHO, ALTHOUGH BEING VERY GOOD, IS ALSO VERY TOUGH AND CAN'T SEEM TO KEEP MALE STAFF ON HER UNIT. WHY DO YOU THINK YOU WOULD BE DIFFERENT?
Answer: First off, I work well with both male and female bosses. They, like me, have a job to do, want it done right, and want to go home at the end of the day feeling like something was accomplished. So if there is a better or faster way to accomplish job tasks and to communicate with everyone, it is her job to see that it is done that way.

YOU HAVE APPLIED FOR A PART-TIME JOB AND APPEAR TO BE IN YOUR FORTIES. WHY DO YOU WANT THIS JOB? (OLIVER, 2005)
Answer: Sometimes you have to take a step backward to move your career forward. Starting part-time will allow you to see what kind of employee I am and then think of me first when a full-time opportunity becomes available.

I SEE FROM YOUR RESUME THAT YOU CHANGED JOBS A LOT. DO YOU GET BORED IN A JOB QUICKLY AND FIND YOURSELF WANTING TO MOVE? (OLIVER, 2005)
Answer: I've enjoyed all my jobs and the challenges they presented. The reason I changed jobs was to bring my salary up to a living wage and to pay for school. My parents were not in a position to help me out financially, so each successive job helped to better pay expenses. I am now finished with school and am ready to build my career. I look forward to working here for several years.

PATIENTS AND THEIR FAMILIES CAN BE PRETTY MEAN. ARE YOU SENSITIVE ABOUT YOUR WEIGHT?
Answer: In my younger days, it was a problem, but now I like who I am and the profession I have chosen. Insults are like emptying bedpans. You flush them away and move on.

TELL ME A PERSONAL OR WORK STORY ABOUT SOMETHING THAT WENT WRONG AND WHAT YOU DID ABOUT IT.
Answer: Years ago, a friend of mine was celebrating her birthday on a weeknight at one of the local bars. There were folks there I had not seen in a long time, which meant staying longer to get caught up with them. The next thing I knew, it was 3:00 AM, and I had to be at work by 8:00 AM. Needless to say, I was pretty tired and useless that day at work. Never again did I stay out excessively late on a work night. It just was not worth it and can be unsafe.

IT'S YOUR LUNCH BREAK, AND YOU SEE A RESIDENT FALL. WHAT WOULD YOU DO?
Answer: I would stop eating, notify another staff member to let the charge nurse know, and then assist the resident as needed. Like CPR, we want help on the way in case the fall is more serious.

PLEASE DISCUSS HOW YOU HANDLED A SITUATION WHEN AN IRATE PHYSICIAN, COWORKER, PATIENT, OR PATIENT'S FAMILY MEMBER WAS INVOLVED.
Answer: There was a day at the nursing home when we were short-staffed, had a new resident moving in, and had to remove the belongings of one who had recently passed away. An out-of-town daughter of one resident turned on the call light and began yelling in the hallway that her father needed a drink of water. Upon entering the room, the daughter continued to yell about how her father was being neglected and that she would be making a complaint to the state.
The first thing I did was smile and thank her, in a quiet voice, for letting us know that her father needed assistance. I then went to her father, poured him a glass of water, and asked him how he was doing. When she began to yell again I asked her to lower her voice so I could hear what her father had to say. This was repeated twice more until her voice level dropped. After it was determined that her father was fine and in no distress, I smiled and asked the daughter her name and then introduced myself. Calling the daughter by name, I let her know that her father's care was very important to us, as were all the residents at the facility whose families expected the same. Also, at this point, I reminded her that in the future, if she needed assistance in a similar situation to come to the nurse's station and to ask for me rather than to yell down the hallway, which upsets the other residents. She agreed to this, and I then left, letting her know that I needed to care for some other residents and would be back in one hour to check on her father. Following this, I updated my supervisor about the incident.

IF YOU COULD BE DOING ANYTHING YOU WANTED TO RIGHT NOW, WHAT WOULD IT BE? (OLIVER, 2005)
Answer and smile: Celebrating with my friends at a restaurant after getting this job offer. The question now is "When can I make those reservations?"

to mix up the order of the questions. Have them include so-called illegal questions. This will prepare you to handle these questions effectively and make you appear confident when the actual interview occurs.

By being prepared, you will not fall victim to the interviewer's most powerful tool: **silence**. Candidates will usually try to fill the void of silence by providing more information (often revealing details beyond their prepared answers) than they should. If this should happen to you, smile at the interviewer and wait for the next question. An example of "too much information" is:

Question: Why did you leave your last job?

Answer: As you know, I am a recent graduate and am looking for employment in my field of study, *and I have never done anything before but work as a babysitter*. (The italicized portion constitutes "too much information.")

Also, never be afraid to ask the interviewer to repeat the question or clarify the question. This is a critical approach to ensure you understand the intent of the interviewer.

MAKING A LASTING IMPRESSION

◎ Try This

Impression Counts

The kind of person you are is an additional concern to the interviewer. The impression you make includes everything that has been previously discussed plus your appearance and habits during the interview.

PERSONAL HYGIENE

- Good hygiene is essential the day of the interview.
- Make sure your hair is arranged in a moderate style.
- Age can be a hidden bias. Consider removing the gray from your hair. To reduce the appearance of skin age, consider using a firming cream for your face and body and/or wear make-up.
- Men's hair, mustaches, and beards should be neatly trimmed.
- Keep nails short, clean, and nicely manicured, with clear nail polish (Research has identified long fingernails, fake nails, and nail polish as sites for infection, which subjected some health facilities to litigation.)
- If you are a smoker, remove yellow finger stains with bleach and water.
- Use an unscented or very lightly scented deodorant.
- Floss and brush your teeth, tongue, and palate. Do not consume any food, candy, or drink with a heavy, unpleasant odor or that will stain your teeth or tongue near the time of the interview. Also, carry and use two breath fresheners before you walk into the building. Do not chew gum.

- Go easy on the aftershave or perfume, and don't sprinkle any on your clothing. Limit yourself to light perfume (a "clean" look and smell go a long way).
- Smell your clothes; don't go into an interview smelling like you have come from a smoke-filled bar.

CLOTHING

Interview clothing should be conservative. You will always look your best in conservative clothes that are clean and ironed, with polished shoes. Go to thrift stores and consignment shops to find a suit that fits you well; they are resources waiting to be discovered. Additionally, check out www.dressforsuccess.org or Google "clothes closet" for possible sources. When looking for clothing, consider the following points:

Men: Wear a long-sleeved white dress shirt, a solid or pinstripe navy blue or gray suit, and a conservative tie that is 3 inches wide and length down to your belt. Wear dark-colored shoes, "long" dark socks, and a belt that matches the color of your shoes. A jacket may not be necessary but dress pants are essential. Cargo pants are not dress pants.

Women: Choose solid or conservative prints in navy, gray, or blue dresses, suits or a skirt and appropriate blouse. Look for simple, straight or pleated skirts that reach at least knee level and are comfortable to sit in. (Save the sexy, short skirts for other occasions.) If wearing a skirt or suit, consider wearing a white, off-white, or light blue cotton or silk blouse with a conservative neckline and buttons. For women with prominent cleavage, a camisole under the blouse is recommended to keep the focus on your face. No visible cleavage is acceptable for an interview. Wear dark, polished, low to moderate heeled shoes with primarily closed toes.

MAKEUP

Conservative makeup is always appropriate. Wearing too much makeup is a common mistake; try to keep it at a minimum. Remember: It is the confidence you display in the interview that makes you an attractive hire to the interviewer.

ACCESSORIES

Wear simple jewelry or none at all. Simple necklaces such as a single strand of pearls, colored beads, or a silver or gold chain work well. Avoid drop, dangle, or chandelier-type earrings and noisy charm bracelets that clank. Remove any piercings in the nose, tongue, or lips, and cover tattoos, particularly based on the culture of the institution. Also, limit yourself to a small portfolio that is large enough to hold any papers, resumes, and so on. If you have a coat or umbrella, leave it in the car or politely ask where you can hang or lay it. The main point is to avoid holding items or balancing them on your lap. The fewer distractions, the more calm and focused you will be on the interview.

EYEWEAR

Do not wear the latest craze in eyeglasses because they will only serve to distract the interviewer. Wear contact lenses or glasses that contrast the shape of your face and are seen as fashionable but not a "statement."

POSTURE

Walk tall and sit erect in the middle of the chair. Both feet should rest on the floor, and your head should be upright. Arms and hands should be in an open position and not crossed. (Remember, you have nothing to hide.) Keep your hands inactive, or if you habitually fidget, consider bringing a paper clip to hold in your hands during the interview. Some people may even need to slightly sit on their hands to prevent fidgeting.

MANNER

Your manner should be assured. Do not interrupt the interviewer or rush the interview. Pause to think as needed, and then answer without hesitating. Ask for an explanation or repetition of any questions you do not understand. Eye contact is essential, especially when answering questions. If you are uncomfortable with making eye contact, two techniques can be used to correct this: look at the person's nose or look at the space between the interviewer's eyebrows. Both techniques give the illusion of eye contact. Remember to look away periodically so you do not appear to be staring. Avoid making negative statements about your school, former bosses, jobs, current finances and personal problems. No one likes a whiner!

COURTESY

Arrive for the interview 5 minutes early, and remember to **shut off your cell phone** or leave it in the car; don't switch it to mute because the interviewer will still be able to hear it. When the employer enters the room, stand, smile, and extend your hand for a firm handshake. Do not use a limp, "dead fish" handshake or "bone-crusher" grip. To get the handshake right, find someone to practice with before the interview. Additionally, if your palms tend to sweat, slide your hands along the top of your thighs, towards your knees, when standing up. It will remove the moisture while appearing very natural.

With a handshake, say, "Hi, Mr. (Ms.) Smith, _____ (your name). I'm pleased to meet you." Wait until you are asked to be seated. If this does not occur, ask if you may be seated. When the interview is over, stand up, look the person in the eyes, and offer your hand for a firm handshake. Address the employer by surname: "Mr. (Ms.) Smith, thank you for the opportunity to interview with you. I am very interested in the job. Would it be all right if I call you next week to see if you have made a decision?" If you want the job, give the employer your work references or letters of recommendation. Last, ask the interviewer for his or her business card. The card will help you when sending your thank you letter (e.g., correct title, name, etc.).

HABITS

Make it a habit to go to bed early the night before so there are no dark circles under your eyes and you appear more energetic. Wear under eye cover if needed. Upon arriving at the interview location, do not chew gum while in the waiting room or during the interview. Also, do not smoke outside the building and then come in for the interview. Although the nicotine may make you feel calmer, you will be bringing in the fresh smell of smoke, which is often offensive to nonsmokers. Politely refuse an offer of a beverage. In addition, do not attempt to read any materials on the employer's desk or computer screen.

DISCUSSING PREGNANCY ISSUES

? Critical Thinking

Pregnancy

If you are pregnant, what do you need to consider before discussing it with an employer? When should you tell a new employer that you are pregnant? When should you discuss the pregnancy so it doesn't interfere with career advancement?

Even if the Pregnancy Discrimination Act and/or Family and Medical Leave Act will protect your job (FMLA applies if the company has 50 or more employees), pregnancy can lead to some tough questions. Consider disclosing your pregnancy when it is noticeable, before being asked.

Be prepared to discuss how long you plan to work, how long you intend to be on leave, and possibly how your work will be covered while you are away. Consider sharing your plan A and B for childcare. Although this is not necessary, this proactive approach can be viewed positively.

◎ Try This

Mock Interview

Enlist a peer to practice traditional and Skype webcam interviews (if planning to move). Take turns in the role of a nurse seeking a job and the employer. Practice asking and answering anticipated questions for an interview. Use the suggestions in this chapter, including appropriate dress and behavior, and stage a mock interview. Have a friend film the interview on their smartphone. Review the interview and ask your peers to evaluate your performance. Keep an open mind to any criticism given because the goal is to refine your techniques and get a job.

PREEMPLOYMENT PHYSICAL EXAMINATION, DRUG SCREENING, AND BACKGROUND CHECKS

More and more employers are requiring preemployment physical examinations as part of conditional job offers. A **conditional job offer** states that you have been offered the job contingent on your passing a physical examination, drug screening/urine analysis, and/or background check. If you fail, the job offer is withdrawn.

PHYSICAL EXAMINATION

Do not be surprised if you are required to meet with an employer-specified doctor who will perform an examination and can legally ask you about your past medical history. Think about any past surgeries, workers' compensation injuries, allergies, and family history, including cancer and heart trouble. Be prepared to provide the dates of these occurrences and the names of the physicians who provided treatment. If you have any personal concerns about the answers your physician might provide, call the doctor before the preemployment physical examination to discuss the prospective job and obtain their opinion.

DRUG SCREENING

If you are taking medications, be sure to notify the prospective employer before the screening, although they may state that the outside vendor performing the tests will be your point of contact. You will want to reaffirm in the employer's mind that your treating physician prescribed the medication and its effects will not interfere with your work. Be aware that you may need to provide a copy of your prescription to the employer testing vendor as verification. This is often called a medical officer review. Once the medical officer reviews your prescriptions and ensures that they are an exact match for the substance identified, your employer should receive a negative drug screening.

Also, although drug screening accuracy is improving, it is not 100% accurate. However, most drug screenings used by employers today are legally binding. Some false positive drug results may occur if medical conditions such as kidney infection/disease, liver disease, or diabetes exist. Common foods such as anything with poppy seeds, riboflavin in food (vitamin B_2 and hemp seed oil), or vitamin B_2 tablets may trigger false positive results. Additionally, false positive reactions can occur with some prescription medications and over-the-counter medications. If you are taking a prescribed or over-the-counter medication, **call your pharmacist** and ask if the medication could trigger a positive drug result.

Be careful not to drink excessive amounts of liquids before drug screening as this can trigger a "dilute" result. Some employers will view a second dilute as a positive drug test and will not hire you. Avoid this possibility by drinking normal volumes of fluid before your drug screening appointment. Do not overhydrate.

BACKGROUND CHECKS

Stories abound about individuals who have had successful job interviews, only to lose their opportunity when the employer saw what was on their personal web page or social network site. As such, discussions about partying, recreational drug use, religion, and views about certain classes of people or past employers should be avoided. Additionally, once you have a job, this is not the time to relax and feel you can post anything you'd like. Often teachers are highlighted in the news as they are fired for posting negative comments about their students and community members on social media (i.e., Facebook). Never forget that others, besides true friends, are reading and developing opinions about what you've written for the world to see. Always act as a professional! NCSBN provides guidance in their publication, *A Nurse's Guide to the Use of Social Media* (www.ncsbn.org).

In 2012, the Society for Human Resource Management (SHRM) surveyed its employers to see what was being done in the area of employment background checks. The survey showed that 69% conducted checks on all job candidates. In a health care setting, this number is higher and can prevent an otherwise strong candidate from obtaining a position. Following the issuing of your nursing license, you must notify the state board of nursing (SBON) if you are arrested or convicted of a crime. Visit your respective SBON website for details. With respect to employers requesting credit checks, only 13% report conducting credit checks on all job candidates and 34% on select candidates. Forty-five (45) percent indicated it was to reduce/prevent theft or other criminal activity, 22% to reduce legal liability, 19% to assess the trustworthiness of the candidate, and 7% to comply with applicable state laws. For more details, see https://www.shrm.org/research/documents/shrm-siop%20 background%20checks.pdf

There are many state and federal laws (i.e., SBON nursing assistant requirements and/or school law) that list prohibitive offenses for employment in health care. In most cases, these requirements were also necessary to participate in clinical assignments while enrolled in nursing school. Thus there are minimal surprises when beginning your job search unless the charge and/or conviction occurred while enrolled in the nursing program and you did not disclose it. This can be viewed as a violation of school policy and could result in dismissal. It will also cause issues as you seek licensure and employment. Honesty and integrity are integral to being a health care provider.

AFTER THE INTERVIEW

Follow up after a job interview is essential. It is a constant source of amazement to employers that 90% of the people who interview never follow up to see if they got the job. Recent graduates and even nurses who have been working in the field for some time are under the **follow-up illusion** that it is the employer's responsibility to contact *them*. If you are not interested enough to follow up after the interview, why did you bother to interview in the first place?

Write a handwritten or email thank you letter to the interviewer *the same day* you were interviewed. Write it while the information is fresh in your mind and before you become distracted by other projects. Remember, the more often the employer sees or hears your name, the better your chances are of being hired. Do not be the person left waiting for a telephone call. A thank you letter may be as simple as the one provided in

| Box 18-13 | Letter: Thank You for the Interview |

August 12, 2016

Ms. Irene Fedun, RN
Director of Nursing
St. Helen General Hospital
8354 177th Lane
St. Paul, MN 55084

Re: LPN Staff Nurse Position

Dear Ms. Fedun:

Thank you for meeting with me today to discuss the LPN staff position. After our conversation about the job duties and the tour of the hospital floor, I feel that my work experiences and education are a great match for the job. I am especially interested in working on the Memory Unit because this is a special interest of mine. Through our work together, the patients will receive timely, quality care.

I remain very interested in the position. I will contact you on Thursday, August 18, to see whether you have made a decision or whether a second interview will be arranged. I look forward to speaking with you soon.

Katelyn Bieser
2001 Putt Drive
Cottage Grove, MN 55016

612-555-2728 or ktbieser@star.com

Box 18-13. Be sure the letter is well written and free of grammatical and spelling errors.

Remember to follow up with the employer! Call the employer on the date stated in your letter. Make it a practice not to make follow-up contacts on Mondays, which are traditionally full because of staff meetings, weekend concerns, staff discipline, paperwork catch-up, and other duties. The best time to make follow-up calls is after 9:00 AM. The key to a successful follow-up call is to be courteous but firm with the assistant. Ask to speak with the person who interviewed you.

The following is a sample follow-up contact to an employer:

Assistant: Good morning, Human Resources (do not be surprised if no name is given).

You: Hi, I'm _____ (your name). Is Ms. George available? I am following up on our meeting.

Assistant: One minute, please. (Although the employer might be away from the office or on another line, the assistant will probably check whether he or she wants to take your call.)

Assistant: I am sorry. Ms. George is away from her desk/on another line/in a meeting. May I take a message, or would you like to leave a message on her voice mail?

You: Yes, thank you. Also, when is the best time to typically reach her?

You: (message if transferred to voice mail) Hi, Ms. George, this is _____ (your name), and I am

following up on our interview for the LPN staff position to see if you have made a decision. I remain very interested in the job and can be reached at _____ (telephone number). Again, that number is _____ (Say each number of the phone number slowly and clearly.)

You: (If the employer takes your call) Hi, Ms. George, this is _____ (your name), and I am following up on our interview for the LPN staff position. I was wondering if you have made a decision yet? Oh, you have not. Would it be okay to call you next Tuesday to see if you have made a decision? Great! I will call you then. [Or] Oh, you've decided on someone else? Is there any other position available that my qualifications meet? If the answer is no, add . . . can you please keep me in mind if any other positions become available, and I will continue to monitor your job postings. Thank you for your time. I hope our paths cross again soon.

Try This

Thank You Letter

Compose a thank you letter after an employment interview for a nursing position.

RESIGNATION WITH STYLE

Try This

Keep the Connections

Is there a difference between "burning bridges" and "untying the connection"? What is the value of recapping your accomplishments with a resignation letter?

In today's job market, employers continue to try to control their costs by limiting annual raises to 3% or less. However, in their desire to staff positions, some employers will offer job hoppers (i.e., frequent job changers) 10% to 20% over their current wages, offer sign-on bonuses, and/or provide higher shift differentials.

If you are contemplating a change, it is recommended that you work a minimum of 1 year to obtain experience and demonstrate stability. If you have made the decision to leave your employer, leave the job with a positive reputation. Perhaps the best expression is "Untie, don't sever, the connection." You never know who may call your former employer as a part of their follow-up. The nursing community, particularly a similar setting (i.e., nursing home), is like a small town. Everyone knows everyone. This can be helpful or harmful to your career. Continually take steps to ensure it is helpful. Always leave sharing a positive message.

It is strongly recommended that you have a position secured before leaving. Many employers today have what is called **"at will" employment**. Simply put, you or the employer can terminate your employment at any time for any reason without advance notice. As such, an employer may terminate your job the day you give notice.

Box 18-14   Sample Resignation Letter

September 24, 2016

Ms. Silvia Hinkkanen
Director of Nursing
George County Hospital
1515 Rodeo Lane

Minneapolis, MN 55401

Dear Ms. Hinkkanen:

Please accept my resignation as Charge Nurse on Unit 3, to be effective on October 1, 2016. My association with the George County Hospital has been rewarding professionally and personally. It is satisfying to have been able to contribute to the positive reputation of client care.

I am especially pleased to have been a member of the Quality Assurance Committee, which furthered my professional growth. In addition, I remain appreciative of having been honored as "Employee of the Month."

Please accept my thanks for the support you have provided me during the past one and a half years of employment. I wish the members of this hospital the very best.

Cordially,
Katelyn Bieser, LPN,
Alzheimer's Unit

That being said, we have found that several "at will" employers have personnel policies requiring that a 2-week notice be given when resigning. The policies typically indicate that if a 2-week notice is given, the employee will be eligible for future rehire and may be eligible for a reference.

It is **resignation courtesy** to give 2 weeks' notice whether or not a policy is in place. This is a courtesy to your coworkers and to the employer so a new person might be hired and orientated before you leave.

Use a business format and plain paper, and type the letter of resignation. Even if you are leaving because of unhappy circumstances on the job, do not vent these feelings in the letter. As mentioned before, you may need this employer as a work reference in the future. Additionally, your current supervisor may also leave in the future, and all there is to remind the employer about you is your personnel file.

Because resignation is part of your permanent record, it provides you with an opportunity to recap your accomplishments or special recognition. The employer may refer to the letter when employers with whom you are seeking employment contact him or her. See the sample resignation letter in Box 18-14.

⊚ Try This

Letter of Resignation

Compose a letter of resignation from a nursing position.

NATIONAL COUNCIL OF STATE BOARDS OF NURSING TRANSITION TO PRACTICE MODEL

In 2007, in an effort to help new RN and LPN/LVN graduates transition to the work environment from their nursing educational programs, increase retention in their employment, and improve patient outcomes, the NCSBN started to develop the **Transition to Practice** model. This model, similar to a **residency**, is a program in addition to orientation to a clinical area. The main parts of the model include:

- A trained nurse (**preceptor**) to assist the new graduate apply theory to practice, develop clinical reasoning, improve safety, and decrease practice errors in the care of patients.
- Five online modules of study: communication and teamwork, patient-centered care, evidence-based practice, quality improvement, and informatics.

In 2010, the IOM called for the implementation and evaluation of nursing residency programs. In collaboration with 35 nursing organizations, the evidence-based Transition to Practice Model was developed. Phase I took place in hospitals with RNs, whereas Phase II was conducted in public health, home health, and nursing home settings with RNs and LPNs. A full description of the model and study can be found at www.ncsbn.org/transition-to-practice.htm

⊚ Try This

Transitional Practice

Investigate if health care facilities in your area have a Transition to Practice model or Residency model for new employees.

STAYING SATISFIED AT YOUR JOB

You have landed your first job as an LPN/LVN. Orientation is great followed by a stressful first three months. You are proactive in asking for extended orientation as needed, have found a mentor and begin to love your job. It is now two years later and you feel that part of the spark is gone. You find yourself complaining more often about your job and joining others in finding continual fault with administration, patients, and families. Strong evidence exists supporting a relationship between nursing satisfaction, nursing retention, and patient outcomes. In fact, the average turnover rate is 49% for nurses in long-term care (Utley, Anderson, & Atwell, 2011). Knecht's (2014) qualitative study of LPNs working in six diverse long-term care settings found there are four critical job satisfaction attributes: value, growth, real connection, and empowerment. In addition, one dissatisfier was identified: working conditions. Working conditions were impacted by the availability of working equipment and the LPN's perception of an unrealistic workload fueled by staffing issues and regulatory demands (i.e., paperwork). It is critical for long-term care administrators and the LPN themselves to address these

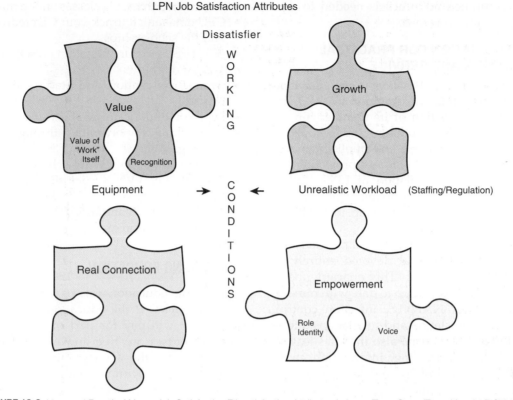

FIGURE 18-2 Licensed Practical Nurse Job Satisfaction/Dissatisfaction Attributes in Long-Term Care. (From Knecht P. [2014]. Demystifying job satisfaction in long-term care: The voices of licensed practical nurses [Doctoral dissertation]. Retrieved from http://gradworks.umi.com/35/83/3583372.html. The Pennsylvania State University, State College, Pennsylvania.)

attributes, thus improving their job satisfaction and decreasing their job dissatisfaction (Figure 18-2). Growth is an important attribute identified by the LPNs. A discussion follows describing professional organizations available to the LPN/LVN and nursing career pathways.

PROFESSIONAL ORGANIZATIONS

Becoming a part of and participating in at least one professional nursing organization is essential for career development. Becoming an active member permits you to have a voice in the future of nursing. It is an opportunity to meet nursing leaders, learn about current issues that affect your career, and take part in education opportunities, as well as serve on committees that influence nursing policy.

NATIONAL LEAGUE FOR NURSING

The **National League for Nursing (NLN)** membership is open to all levels of nurses and is focused on meeting the particular needs of the nursing educator, ultimately advancing the health of the nation. One of the goals of the NLN is to lead in setting standards that advance excellence and innovation in nursing education. The NLN's "Excellence in Education Model" has relevance for all levels of nursing education programs, from LP/LV nursing to doctoral level nursing.

Because of changes in health care, the NLN (2010) has developed a national model for nursing education that includes competencies that graduates of all levels of nursing programs should be able to do to meet workforce needs and the needs of an increasingly diverse population. The following are NLN competencies for graduates of LP/LV nursing programs:

- Promote the human dignity, integrity, self-determination, and personal growth of patients, oneself, and other members of the health care team.
- Provide a rationale for judgments used in the provision of safe, quality care and for decisions that promote the health of patients within a family context.
- Assess how one's personal strengths and values affect one's identity as a nurse and one's contributions as a member of the health care team.
- Question the basis for nursing actions, considering research, evidence, tradition, and patient preferences (National League for Nursing, 2010).

In 2014 the NLN supported the importance of the role of the LPN in their vision statement, *A Vision for Recognition of the Role of the Licensed Practical/Vocational Nurses in Advancing the Nation's Health.*

THE AMERICAN NURSES ASSOCIATION

The **American Nurses Association (ANA)** only represents registered nurses (RNs). Some state affiliates of the ANA allow LPNs/LVNs to join the association at the state level; however, because the LPN is not recognized at the national level they may not have a voice or vote in the organization. The ANA does not represent

LPNs/LVNs. Continued advocacy is needed to provide a unified nursing workforce.

NATIONAL ASSOCIATION FOR PRACTICAL NURSE EDUCATION AND SERVICE, INC

The **National Association for Practical Nurse Education and Service, Inc. (NAPNES)** was founded in 1941. The multidisciplinary composition of its membership includes LPNs/LVNs, RNs, students, and schools of practical nursing, organizations, and public members promoting the ideals of NAPNES and protecting the practice, education, and regulation of LPNs/LVNs, nursing educators, practical nursing schools, and practical nursing students. Membership in NAPNES provides the following benefits:

- A year's subscription to the *Journal of Practical Nursing* (*JPN*), the oldest journal devoted entirely to practical/vocational nursing. This quarterly, peer-reviewed journal keeps you up to date with nursing articles, news about NAPNES, infection control, nursing law, and legislation and regulations affecting LPNs/LVNs. The journal also includes feature articles about LP/LV nursing, information about certification in pharmacology and long-term care, and other educational opportunities. An *eJournal of Practical Nursing* is also a publication of NAPNES.
- The NAPNES website (www.napnes.org) includes information about certifications, regulation news and updates, clinical articles, continuing education units (CEUs), podcasts, webinars, blogs, and jobs.
- Networking with other LPNs/LVNs through the constituent state members throughout the United States.
- The NAPNES technology department has developed a tool for making nursing updates and education on line faster and easier.
- National representation and a voice for the future of nursing.
- NAPNES Standards of Practice for LPNs/LVNs (see www.napnes.org).

NATIONAL FEDERATION OF LICENSED PRACTICAL NURSES

The **National Federation of Licensed Practical Nurses (NFLPN)** was organized in 1949 (www.nflpn.org). It is the policy-making body for LPNs/LVNs. NFLPN is made up of LPNs/LVNs, SPNs/SVNs, and affiliate members. NFLPN was formed by LPNs/LVNs who wanted an organization to work for and speak on their behalf. It is the only nursing organization governed entirely by LPNs/LVNs. It is recognized by other national nursing organizations as the official voice of LPNs/LVNs. The NFLPN motto is "The Spirit of Care—The Heart of Nursing."

NFLPN membership includes the following benefits:

- National certification in The Spirit of Care—The Heart of Nursing therapy, gerontology

- Authorized free CEU classes online through NFLPN
- CEU databank to track your CE credits
- NFLPN scholarships
- Nurses Service Organization (NSO) insurance
- Vendor discounts
- Annual convention and trade show offering CE courses
- Legislative advocate on issues affecting LPNs/LVNs
- Networking opportunities through your chapter meetings
- Student Honor Society for achieving LPN students
- Annual LPN/LVN Recognition & Awareness Week (first week in October each year)

NFLPN Practice Standards for LPNs/LVNs can be found at www.nflpn.org.

CONTINUING EDUCATION

Continuing education classes are available through many agencies. If the education benefits the agency, they often will pay for part or the entire fee. Some agency courses are free and are part of continuing service within the agency. Initial licensure is being questioned as providing competency for life. Your continued study helps keep you up to date and ensures competency as an LPN/LVN. Some states require continuing education units (CEU) or continuing education (CE) to renew your practical nursing license. Continuing education includes the following options.

INSERVICE TRAINING

Inservice training is information chosen to meet specific needs in a facility. Attendance at some inservice programs, such as a yearly update on bloodborne pathogens, is required. Offer suggestions for content to your employer. Usually a specified amount of time is required for inservice programs, such as 1 hour per month or three times per year, according to the agency policy and accreditation standards. Depending on the credentials of the instructor and the content, continuing education credits may be available.

WORKSHOPS

Workshops present information and an opportunity to practice what is being taught. Workshops provide opportunities to learn new skills. Workshop length varies according to content. Some agencies pay the workshop fee or expenses if the topic is specific to, and enhances, your nursing skills. Workshops are also a major source of continuing education credits that are required by many states as a part of continued licensure in nursing. Workshops may be available through local or state Health Care Industry Partnerships at reduced costs, aimed at building a robust workforce.

CONTINUING EDUCATION UNITS

Classes are often taught involving complex nursing skills such as intravenous therapy, physical assessment,

LP/LV charge nurse (leadership/management), mental health concepts and the nursing process for LPNs/LVNs. Many vocational schools and community colleges will provide any course you request, if enough people are available to meet the required minimum enrollment. Many of these classes provide continuing education units (CEUs) as opposed to course credit. You receive a certificate if you complete course work satisfactorily.

One of the most valuable benefits of continuing education classes is the opportunity to get together with other working LPNs/LVNs. You discover similarities in challenges and satisfactions. Ideas are shared on how to deal with difficult situations in the work setting. You should keep a record of all inservice programs, seminars, and workshops taken (including dates, CEUs, and topics) for future reference. Ask for these records to be included in your file at your place of employment, and keep a copy for your own file. Some states require that you list the CEUs when you apply for license renewal. Other state boards of nursing want you to have the file available in case the board decides to check the accuracy of what you stated in your renewal application.

Continuing education contact hours are also available through your professional organizations.

INTERNET RESOURCES

Numerous sources are available online depending on what fits your needs:

- **Advance for Nurses** is available online with a free subscription (www.advanceweb.com). Current updates and nursing articles are available at the tip of your finger.
- **Podcasts.** A podcast is a digital recording of audio and visual information on the Internet that can be downloaded to a personal media player (for example, an iPod) or a computer. The term "pod" is derived from iPod of Apple Computer, Inc., but an iPod is not necessary to listen to a podcast. The term "cast" is derived from "broadcast," as many podcasts are radio-style shows. However, they are commercial-free, of interest to the listener, and can be listened to whenever convenient. Others include Google "Nursing Podcasts" for a wide selection of podcasts; and Google "iTunes Nursing Podcasts" for examples of free podcasts. Medscape also provides these programs by medical experts. Remember, anyone can upload anything to the Internet. Check podcasts for relevancy and accuracy, and check with your instructors for further suggestions and the accuracy of podcasts you discover. A good primer to understand podcasting is "How to Podcast" at http://howtopodcasttutorial.com.
- **Medscape** offers information on health care changes, new guidelines for care, emerging infectious diseases, sudden disasters, and more through daily summaries. Medscape offers partial CE hours through their Medscape Medical News service. Although the focus is primarily for RNs, there is useful information for all nurses on a daily basis. The subscription is free through www.Medscape.com.

CERTIFICATION OPPORTUNITIES

Take advantage of knowledge available during certification seminars and self-study courses. Knowledge is power! Knowledge is the basis for improved nursing skills and safety in patient care. In some agencies, certification is also the basis for salary increases and advancement. Enhancing your competence as a nurse increases both personal and professional satisfaction. Use the extended title you have earned and wear your pin(s) proudly. See specific certifications discussed earlier in this chapter.

NAPNES CERTIFICATION PROGRAMS

NAPNES offers **Long-Term Care Certification** (LPN CLTC or LVN CLTC), **Pharmacology Certification** (LPN NPC or LVN NPC), and IV Therapy (LPN IVT or LVN IVT), all of which are available online (www.napnes.org/certifications/index.htm). The website offers specific directions for each certification. After NAPNES notifies you of successful completion of the examinations, you may use the preceding title that applies in your signature/title.

NFLPN CERTIFICATION PROGRAMS

NFLPN offers **National Certification in Gerontology** (LPN GC or LVN GC) and **National Certification in IV Therapy** (LPN IVC or LVN IVC). Check out the website at www.nflpn.org/certification.html. Program details to complete the certification that you desire are explained. NFLPN notifies you after successful completion of the examination. You will be able to use the appropriate initials as part of your signature/title.

Recertification is required every 2 years to maintain a valid certificate. Do not assume that requirements are the same for all certifications. Visit www.nflpn.org for full details.

◎ Try This

Availability of Leadership Course

Almost half of the newly licensed practical/vocational nurses who participated in the 2012 NCSBN Job Analysis regularly assumed administrative responsibility, primarily in long-term care. Inquire whether a postgraduate LPN/LVN leadership/management course or certification is available. Ask for details about the course. This can increase your marketability as a LPN/LVN.

AMERICAN BOARD OF MANAGED CARE NURSING CERTIFICATION IN MANAGED CARE

American Board of Managed Care Nursing (ABMCN) **Certification in Managed Care Nursing (CMCN)** is available to LPNs/LVNs through a home study course. Order the course materials through ABMCN (www.abmcn.org).

The examination includes basic knowledge of managed care, health care economics, health care management, and patient issues. Upon successful completion of the examination, the nurse is certified and may use the title Certification in Managed Care in Nursing (CMCN). Certification is valid for 3 years.

REGISTERED NURSE CAREER PATHWAY

If you are an LPN/LVN who says, "I want to be an LPN/LVN, but I have no desire to be an RN," you have obviously given careful consideration to your personal goals. Being an LPN/LVN is an essential role on the health care team. Satisfaction in nursing, both for you and patients you care for, is closely related to defined goals. If you decided you want to be an LPN/LVN, chances are you will be satisfied with your choice and will provide high-quality care to your patients. If, however, someone else decided you should be a nurse, chances are you will never be entirely satisfied with the choice. This lack of satisfaction will be mirrored in the care you give to patients. The same process is true in regard to making a decision to become an RN. If you do not want to become an RN, avoid letting anyone push you into it. Only when a goal is truly your own will you be motivated to do your best both in the educational process and in the care of patients. Consider the following: If you want to enter an RN program, learn what programs of study are available. There are numerous reasons (beyond personal choice) for considering additional nursing education, including:

- You have investigated job opportunities in the area in which you plan to live and find that jobs for LPNs/LVNs are limited.
- The salary difference will be a good return on your investment.
- Your current place of employment will assist you in paying for additional schooling.
- You will enjoy the RN job role.

[?] Critical Thinking

What are some other reasons you can think of to pursue additional education and become an RN?

MOBILITY

A major problem in developing upward **mobility programs** for LPNs/LVNs is the belief held by some educators that a practical nursing course is terminal in nature; that some state boards of nursing will not permit upward mobility programs, nor will credit be given by some professional nursing programs. Although the same reasoning continues to be held in some parts of the country, other directors of nursing have successfully negotiated with state boards of nursing to develop progressive LPN/LVN-to-RN programs. Contact your state's board of nursing for a list of available accredited nursing programs in your state. Also, talk to your current school counselor about

accredited nursing programs available to you. Find out how to apply and if additional courses are needed for admission; the costs; the availability of grants, if local; and if transfer of credits is possible.

Distance learning nursing program

Excelsior College. Excelsior College (previously known as Regents College), of Albany, New York, is the first in the United States to have a distance learning nursing program (online). The associate degree in nursing program began in 1972 and has been continuously accredited by the National League for Nursing Accrediting Council (NLNAC), now the Accreditation Commission for Education in Nursing (ACEN). There are no or limited classes to attend, and the student can study when convenient and take examinations when ready. Interest-free financing may be available.

LPNs/LVNs must apply for admission and be accepted to the School of Nursing before enrolling. Requirements are found on their website at www.excelsior.edu. Licensed LPNs/LVNs are eligible to apply (except for California residents). The college is founded on the premise that what you know is more important than where you learned it. College faculty evaluate all previous credits you have earned. Possible credits include courses you have taken from other regionally accredited colleges and universities, military training, continuing education programs, and Internet-based programs. Generous learner support is made available to students from full-time advisors and nursing faculty. Students are able to study and prepare at their own pace while maintaining their jobs.

REGISTERED NURSE PROGRAMS; DO LPNS GET ADVANCED STANDING?

Turf issues continue to exist in all levels of nursing; certified nursing assistant (CNA) to LPN/LVN to Associate Degree in Nursing (and) to BSN to Master of Science in Nursing (MSN) to a Doctorate in Nursing. Plan to be a part of the solution, not the problem, when you are in a position to make a difference. This is an area where you, as a member of your professional nursing organization, can make your voice heard.

Some RN programs continue to ignore the value of practical/vocational education. These programs insist that LPNs/LVNs start from the beginning and repeat all previously covered theory and skills courses, including basic nursing skills. The bottom line is that a number of programs are available throughout the country that the LPN/LVN can use to become an RN, with credit given for being an LPN/LVN.

The state boards of nursing are an excellent source for locating approved nursing programs. Many of the programs have websites that make it possible to get information about a program before inquiring directly. Ask your board for a list of board-approved professional nursing programs preparing for registered nurse licensure that provide advanced standing for the LPN/LVN.

Box 18-15   Possible Response to Critical Thinking Scenario

From the day we are born until the day we die, we judge people and they judge us on how we look, act, talk, and respond to the environment. Based on this, decisions are made to like, dislike, or not care one way or the other about a person. For the Western culture there is a drive towards being youthful and fit, being a "man's man" or a "woman's woman," and having energy to burn. It is neither good nor bad; it just is! So play the game, get the job, and, afterwards, when you get the job, decide what to let go. Below is a checklist for Jeanne's consideration:

1. There are always many tasks to juggle. Are you getting a good night's rest before the interview?
2. Use all available resources, including make-up to avoid looking tired and improve youthful appearance.
3. Confirm you have a firm handshake and pleasant-sounding voice.
4. Practice quick responses to interview questions and project confidence. Use the power pose as described in Chapter 9 to build confidence prior to the interview.
5. Plan to highlight your ability to manage a household, school, and work effectively, emphasizing your time management skills.
5. Review key concepts in this chapter related to diverse job sources.
6. Check the health care business news and incorporate the information into a question for the employer to stand above the other candidates.

Lastly, it would benefit Jeanne to contact her references through LinkedIn, which will provide additional personal contacts within different companies. Those contacts will know if there are employment opportunities at their companies and may be used as a "name drop" to get an interview. The old adage is, "It is not what you know, but who you know," so use it.

Get Ready for the NCLEX-PN® Examination

Key Points

- LPN/LVNs are employed in a diverse array of settings providing many career options.
- Workforce trends include a decrease in LPNs working in hospitals, whereas LPNs working in long-term care and the community have increased.
- To be successful in your job search, begin your search with the first day of classes and continue from that day on.
- Opportunities present themselves to those who are willing to put forth a little effort and realize that the world does not owe them a living.
- The methods presented in this chapter have proved successful for graduates, people wishing to make career changes, or those wanting to institute a change in their work. Remember to treat your job search like a job.
- Make contacts by telephone or computer, forwarding resumes or cover letters, or by physically going to the employer to apply and schedule an interview.
- Explore the hidden job market via networking, the Internet, or using the telephone book and then calling employers, whether or not an ad has been placed.
- Dress for the job you want, not the job you have.
- Actively follow up on all interviews! Let the employer know you are interested. Remember, the more often the employer hears or sees your name, the better your chances of getting hired.
- If you are hired, send thank you notes to those who helped you. You may need them again someday. Remember, you are responsible for making your own luck.

Additional Learning Resources

evolve Go to your Evolve website (http://evolve.elsevier.com/Knecht/success) for the following FREE learning resources:

- Answers to Critical Thinking Scenarios
- Additional learning activities
- Additional Review Questions for the NCLEX-PN® exam
- Helpful phrases for communicating in Spanish and more!

Review Questions for the NCLEX-PN® Examination

1. What interpersonal style is representative of being easy-going, likes to blend in, has difficulty making decisions, and tends to be quiet and soft-spoken?
   a. Analytical type
   b. Driver type
   c. Amiable type
   d. Expressive type

2. Your employer has an employment policy of at-will employment. Which of the following reflects the meaning of this?
   a. The employer expects a 2-week notice before you leave their employment.
   b. The employer will determine the length or extension of probationary periods.
   c. The employer may terminate your job immediately without notice or reason.
   d. The employer will continue your job indefinitely, provided job requirements are met.

3. An interviewer asks you a question for which you do not have an answer. Which of the following would be an appropriate response?
    a. Ask the interviewer to please rephrase the question.
    b. Begin to answer and switch to a topic you know about.
    c. Smile pleasantly and say you don't know the answer.
    d. Take a key word from the question, and make up a response.

4. When creating a personal resume, the following statement is true:
    a. You are legally bound to include every employer (even if it was only for one month).
    b. It is critical to use special paper to print your resume.
    c. White space is beneficial.
    d. Most employers spend approximately 5 to 10 minutes reviewing a resume to determine the next step: an interview.

Alternate Format Item

1. Which of the following uses of the Internet are helpful in job hunting? *(Select all that apply.)*
    a. Identify salary range
    b. Complete job application
    c. Locate job opportunities
    d. Research facility information
    e. Professional and social networks

2. Which of the following should occur after an interview? *(Select all that apply.)*
    a. Write down, on paper, information learned and points stressed by the interviewer.
    b. Send a thank you letter to the interviewer noting some of the points discussed during the interview.
    c. Contact your references immediately after the interview and let them know that they may be contacted. Then discuss points about the job the employer stressed as being important.
    d. Follow up 4 weeks after the interview with the employer to see if there were additional questions to assist in making their hiring decision.
    e. Continue an active job search until a job offer is made.

Critical Thinking Scenarios

Scenario 1

Jeanne is in her late forties, with gray in her hair and recently divorced. She has three children at home, including a senior in high school who plans to go to college, a sophomore in high school, and a child in the eighth grade. Jeanne's ex-spouse was paying alimony until his manufacturing job went overseas. Wanting the best for her family, Jeanne returned to school and became a licensed practical nurse. Unfortunately, the interviews she has found through the newspaper have gone nowhere. Jeanne has the sense there is something more she can do to put her best foot forward. What would you recommend for a woman in her situation? See Box 18-15 for possible responses.

Scenario 2

Jack had been overweight for as long as he could remember, was a little nerdy, and had a slightly effeminate voice. During his clinical rotations, he was a star, and the staff said to let them know if he needed work references. Because Jack's true passion was helping people, his dream was within reach, but now he had to find a job. Unfortunately, when he went to interviews, he would catch strange looks from the interviewers. Jack saw his dream slowly slipping away, until a friend offered some ideas. What suggestions would you make to Jack after reading this chapter? See Box 18-15 for possible responses.

Licensure and Regulation: Becoming Licensed and Understanding Your State Nurse Practice Act

Objectives

On completing this chapter, you will be able to do the following:

1. Explain the purpose of the National Council Licensing Examination for Practical Nurses (NCLEX-PN®).
2. Explain the significance of the Authorization to Test (ATT).
3. Describe how Computerized Adaptive Testing (CAT) determines whether you pass or fail the NCLEX-PN®.
4. Discuss the proven way of preparing for the NCLEX-PN®.
5. Explain the legal implications of ignoring the NCLEX-PN® confidentiality agreement and sharing information about the NCLEX-PN® content with others.
6. Discuss the requirements of your state board of nursing for eligibility to take the NCLEX-PN®.
7. Explain the requirements of your state board of nursing for licensure renewal.
8. Explain the process of endorsement.
9. Differentiate between a temporary work permit and licensure.
10. Discuss how your state's nurse practice act speaks to the issue of assessment, supervision, and delegation.
11. Discuss how your state's nurse practice act regulates the LPN's role in the administration of intravenous therapy, including via a central line.
12. Explain why a state may be "silent" to a particular LPN job role, such as delegation, and how this impacts the LPN's practice.
13. Discuss why it is critical for the LPN to fully understand their state nurse practice act.

Key Terms

Authorization to Test (ATT) (ĂW-thŏr-ĭ-ZĀ-shŭn)
candidate (KĂN-dĭ-dāt)
computerized adaptive testing (CAT)
confidentiality agreement (kŏn-fĭ-dĕn-shē-ĂL-ĭ-tē ă-GRĒ-mĕnt)

endorsement (ĭn-DŌRS-mĕnt)
NCLEX-PN® examination
Nurse Practice Act (NPA)
state board of nursing (stāt bŏrd)

As graduation nears, it is natural for almost all practical nursing students to be focused on the National Council Licensing Examination for Practical Nurses (NCLEX-PN®) (often referred to as state boards). However, the reality is that NCLEX-PN® preparation begins the day you apply to a nursing program. Most licensed practical/licensed vocational (LP/LV) nursing programs, which consistently achieve NCLEX-PN® pass rates above the state and national norm, know that it is imperative to implement NCLEX-PN® preparation from the first day of the program. Unfortunately, sometimes it is difficult to convince students that this strategy is essential. Instead, students often feel burdened by the "computer work" and find "short cuts" to get the work done quickly, not realizing that this may haunt them in the near future. Trust in the program you have chosen. Accept the need to complete NCLEX-PN preparation computer work as assigned. This will enhance your ability to successfully pass the NCLEX-PN® the first time and improve your overall achievement of program outcomes. Once you have passed NCLEX-PN® and received your license, you want to keep it forever. A thorough understanding of your state **Nurse Practice Act (NPA)** is essential to being a safe and effective caregiver. Because each state has a unique NPA, you must be knowledgeable of the NPA for each state in which you are licensed.

WHAT IS THE STATE NURSE PRACTICE ACT?

The NPA exists to protect the public. Despite the intent of all nurses to provide competent, safe, and high-quality nursing care, assisting the patient and communities to regain, maintain, or advance their health, there is inherent harm that can occur as you perform your duties. The vast array of unique health care needs, complicated by constant technological advances taking place in a variety of health care settings, provides a constant challenge. The NPA provides a foundation to guide and govern nursing practice. It includes information regulating nursing education schools, the practice of nursing professionals, requirements for licensure, and grounds for disciplinary action and dismissal (National Council of State Boards of Nursing [NCSBN], 2015).

HOW DOES THE NURSE PRACTICE ACT GUIDE/GOVERN NURSING PRACTICE?

Each state has a specific NPA for all nurses, including LPNs/LVNs, which is enacted by the state legislature. Decades ago, State Boards of Nursing (SBON) were established to enact the NPA and give the authority to provide ongoing development of administrative rules and regulations to govern/guide nursing practice. This information is often referred to as the nurse's "scope of practice." The SBON is responsible to the public and as such any proposed changes to regulation go through a vigorous process where they are vetted by various stakeholders and accessible to the public for comment. As a licensed individual, it is the responsibility of LPNs/LVNs to know their NPA. Ignorance is not an excuse. Visit https://www.ncsbn.org/nurse-practice-act.htm to learn more details and find resources to access an NPA toolkit and a link to find your NPA.

VARIABILITY OF THE STATE'S NURSE PRACTICE ACT APPLICABLE TO LICENSED PRACTICAL NURSE/LICENSED VOCATIONAL NURSE PRACTICE

Corazzini et al. (2013) concluded that states varied considerably regarding their NPA. In addition, several states were silent regarding key aspects of nursing care, such as assessment or delegation (Corazzini et al., 2013). This variability and lack of clarity of the state NPAs can contribute to confusion and variability in LPN/LVN job roles. It is essential for the LPN/LVN to fully understand their NPA in any state in which they are licensed. Practice boundaries between the LPN and RN scope of practice can vary from facility to facility and state to state. A facility can limit the LPN scope of practice but can never expand the LPN job role beyond the scope as stated in the respective state's NPA. For example, it is possible as an LPN that you could be licensed and working in a facility in your home state where you are permitted to administer intravenous (IV) therapy via a central line device. However, you could travel across a state line to a neighboring state and work in a facility owned by the same corporation and this same act (IV therapy administration via a central line) could be prohibited.

You can see why this situation is complex and can be confusing to both the LPN, other members of the health care team, the public, and the employer. It is your responsibility as an LPN/LVN to know your NPA and educate your employer if a situation arises where you are being directed to perform a prohibited act. The issue becomes more confusing when the state NPA is silent regarding an LPN/LVN job duty such as delegation. When this occurs, carefully review your institutional policy and procedure and discuss the situation with your supervisor. Have your evidence (state NPA) available. This state NPA is easily found if you Google your state board of nursing and locate the NPA. The SBON staff can provide assistance; however, remember it is their role to regulate,

not advise. Thus they cannot advise regarding particular situations; however, their legal counsels can provide you with a recount of a similar situation and the outcome to guide you in your decision making. Most states have a decision-making guide that is located on their web site to assist nurses and employers.

> **? Critical Thinking: Nurse Practice Act**
>
> Locate your NPA for the state you anticipate obtaining a license. Review at least three other state sites and discuss the differences between each NPA related to the LPN's role in assessment, delegation, and IV therapy.

APPLYING FOR A PRACTICAL NURSING LICENSE OR A TEMPORARY PERMIT

Your practical nursing school will provide the information to assist you with an application for a practical nursing license or a temporary permit so you will be able to work as a graduate practical or vocational nurse (GPN or GVN) or an LPN/LVN. (See NCLEX-PN® discussion below for details regarding the application process for licensure and NCLEX-PN®.) All graduates must apply for a license to practice. However, some of you may wish to obtain a temporary permit. This is less of a necessity today as you can take your NCLEX-PN within a month or two following graduation. If you do decide to apply for a temporary permit, there can be restrictions to your practice. It is your responsibility to review the SBON web site and understand the restrictions as you seek employment with a temporary permit. For example, it may be required that a registered nurse (RN) is physically present on the unit where you work. In addition, once you have received results of the NCLEX-PN®, the temporary permit is automatically revoked if you did not successfully pass the examination. You will be required to surrender your temporary permit and no longer work as a GPN/GVN. Lastly, evidence exists showing a correlation between delayed first-time completion of the NCLEX-PN® more than three months following your program completion date and your predicted probability of passing the examination. Obtaining a temporary permit and beginning work may cause you to delay taking the exam. Thus scheduling the NCLEX-PN® as soon as possible, following execution of a well-developed study plan, is the best option. Passing the NCLEX-PN® means that you will work as a licensed practical or vocational nurse (LPN or LVN). Be sure to follow the guidelines carefully regarding the submission of the application for licensure. Your school will also need to submit the required documents indicating that you have successfully completed all the requirements of a state-approved practical nursing program. Be particularly attentive to the correct spelling of your name and use of a maiden, married, hyphenated, or middle name. This information must align exactly with the information submitted by your school or your application will be rejected, lengthening the time to receive your authorization to test and sit for the NCLEX-PN®.

🔆 Keep in Mind

Almost without exception, when student nurses are asked about their goal for the year, they respond by saying they want to pass the "boards," meaning pass the National Council Licensing Examination for Practical/Vocational Nursing (NCLEX-PN®) to become a licensed practical or vocational nurse (LPN/LVN). They should also always respond by saying they want to deliver competent, safe, high-quality care adhering to the guidelines of their state NPA. However, reality is that you will never be licensed unless you pass the NCLEX-PN®. As mentioned many times throughout this book, NCLEX-PN® preparation begins the first day you enter a nursing program.

WHAT IS THE NATIONAL COUNCIL LICENSING EXAMINATION FOR PRACTICAL NURSING?

The NCLEX-PN® is the National Council Licensing Examination for Practical/Vocational Nursing graduates. It is designed to test minimum knowledge, skills, and abilities needed to safely and effectively practice nursing as a new entry-level LPN/LVN. The NCLEX-PN® results provide the basis for licenses granted to LPNs/LVNs by **state boards of nursing**.

The NCSBN developed a secure method of examination. Since April 1994, practical/vocational nursing graduates (**candidates**) have taken the **NCLEX-PN®** by computer. This method is called **computerized adaptive testing (CAT)**. All candidates have different questions based on how they answer the previous question. Computer technology makes it possible to choose items from a large pool of questions classified by test category and difficulty to match the candidate's ability and fulfill NCLEX-PN® requirements.

All candidates answer a minimum of 85 items and up to a maximum of 205 items in the 5-hour period of time allotted for the examination. Twenty-five of the items are pretest items (possible future test questions) and are not scored. The time allotted includes the confidentiality agreement, tutorial instruction, and scheduled and unscheduled breaks. All breaks are optional. All answers are scored as right or wrong; no partial credit is given. The computer continues with questions until it determines that the candidate passes or fails the examination. If the candidate runs out of time, and the candidate has not answered the minimum number of questions, the candidate fails. If the candidate has answered the minimum number of questions, the computer evaluates the last 60 items, and if the answers were consistently above the passing standard, the candidate passes.

Computerized adaptive testing administers items with difficulty levels so that each candidate will answer about half correctly. These items provide the most information. All candidates answer about 50% correctly because the computer presents them with questions to match their ability. The next item should not be too easy or too difficult. The computer goes down a "pathway" or "branch," and no candidate has exactly the same test. Items that follow are based on the candidate's previous answer. This is why you *must* answer every item on the computer screen as they show up. You will not be able to go back and answer a previous question. The computer calculates each answer before it can choose the next item. Visit www.ncsbn.org for more details.

HOW THE NATIONAL COUNCIL LICENSING EXAMINATION FOR PRACTICAL NURSES IS KEPT UP TO DATE

The April 2014 NCLEX-PN® reflects the outcome of the *2012 LPN/LVN Practice Analysis: Linking the NCLEX-PN® Examination to Practice* (NCSBN, 2013). Currently, this survey is conducted every three years. Of the 12,000 surveys sent out, analyzable response rates were 14.4% for paper surveys and 16.4% for the web. The NCSBN (2013) explains the process as follows: The 2012 LPN/LVN Practice Analysis Survey used several methods to describe the practice of newly licensed LPN/LVNs in the U.S.: (1) document reviews; (2) daily logs of newly licensed LPN/LVNs; (3) subject matter expert's knowledge; and (4) a large scale survey. Based on evidence, the findings of this study can be used to evaluate and support an LPN/LVN test plan.

See Chapter 18 for some conclusions from the NCSBN LPN/LVN Practice Analysis. The entire study is available online at www.ncsbn.org.

CORE CONTENT

Four phases (steps) of the nursing process (see Chapter 12) are integrated into all areas of the NCLEX-PN®. The four phases are the basis for nursing care plans you developed for each patient assigned to you, before beginning nursing care on the clinical unit. The four steps (phases) are:
1. Data collection (assessment)
2. Planning
3. Implementation
4. Evaluation

TYPES OF TEST QUESTIONS

The NCLEX-PN® contains items (questions) in the cognitive level of knowledge, comprehension, application, and analysis. Most of the questions are at the application and analysis levels. These questions require prioritizing and decision-making. The two main types of test questions are multiple choice and alternate item format.

Multiple Choice

The majority of test questions are multiple choice. Each question describes a client or clinical situation. Four options are given from which to choose the correct response.

Alternate Item Format

The NCLEX-PN® also includes alternate item questions, including the following:

- *Fill-in-the-blank.* Medicine and IV rate calculations, intake, and output totals.
- *Multiple responses.* Select **all** responses that pertain to the question, with no partial credit given. For example: Which of the following drugs are antihypertensives?
- *Prioritizing* (ordered response). Options (nursing actions) are numbered as first, second, third, and so on, in order of priority, or the mouse is used to drag and drop options in the ordered priority. For example: When doing the Heimlich maneuver, which of the following actions would you do first, second, or third?
- *Figure or illustration* (hot spot). Questions are asked about a chart or figure. Either an answer is chosen from a list or the mouse is used to point and click a "hot spot" as the answer. For example: Click on the hypochondriac area.
- *Chart/exhibit questions.* A question is included with a chart or exhibit requiring use of the chart/exhibit to answer the question. For example: Which lab result is normal?
- An on-screen optional calculator is available for your use during the examination. Any format item, including standard multiple-choice items, might include charts, tables, or graphic images. A tutorial is provided on the computer screen regarding the operation of the computer and how to record answers. For general information questions about the NCLEX-PN®, use the FAQs at www.ncsbn.org as a resource. You can also email questions/comments to info@ncsbn.org.

◉ **Try This**

What Is an Alternate Item Question?

Write an example of an alternate item format using problem solving.

TEST FRAMEWORK: CLIENT NEEDS

The content of the NCLEX-PN® is divided into four client needs categories. Client needs provide an overall structure for defining nursing actions and competencies for a variety of patients in many settings and are in agreement with state laws and statutes. Two of the four categories are further subdivided. The percentage of test items assigned to each category and limited examples of content are included. Additional examples of content are found in the NCLEX-PN® Examination Test Bulletin and the 2016 NCLEX-PN® Examination Candidate Bulletin, available at https://www.ncsbn.org/089900_2016_Bulletin_Proof3.pdf. The categories and subcategories are as follows:

1. Safe, Effective Care Environment
   a. Coordinated Care: 16% to 22%
   Examples: Advance directives, client rights, concepts of management and supervision, confidentiality/ information security, establishing priorities, ethical practice, legal responsibilities
   b. Safety and Infection Control: 10% to 16%
   Examples: Accident/error/injury prevention, handling hazardous and infectious materials, standard precautions/transmission-based precautions/surgical asepsis, restraints, and safety devices
2. Health Promotion and Maintenance: 7% to 13%
   Examples: Aging process, ante/intra/postpartum and newborn care, data collection techniques, developmental stages and transitions, high-risk behaviors, lifestyle choices, and self-care
3. Psychosocial Integrity: 8% to 14%
   Examples: Abuse or neglect, behavioral management, crisis intervention, chemical and other dependencies, end-of-life concepts, mental health concepts, stress management, and therapeutic communication
4. Physiologic Integrity
   a. Basic Care and Comfort: 7% to 13%
   Examples: Assistive devices, elimination, nutrition and oral hydration, personal hygiene, and rest and sleep
   b. Pharmacologic Therapies: 11% to 17%
   Examples: Adverse effects/contraindications/side effects/interactions, medication administration, and pharmacologic pain management
   c. Reduction of Risk Potential: 10% to 16%
   Examples: Changes/abnormalities in vital signs, diagnostic tests, laboratory values, potential for complications from surgical procedures, and health alterations
   d. Physiologic Adaptation: 7% to 13%
   Examples: Basic pathophysiology, fluid and electrolyte imbalances, medical emergencies, radiation therapy, and unexpected response to therapies

In addition to the categories listed above, the following processes are integrated into all "Client Needs" categories of the *PN Test Plan:* Nursing Process, Caring, Communication and Documentation, and Teaching and Learning.

INTEGRATION OF NURSING CONCEPTS AND PROCESSES

Concepts and processes basic to the practice of LP/LV nursing are integrated into the four categories of patient needs.

- *Clinical problem-solving process* (nursing process): A scientific approach to patient care. It includes data collection, planning, implementation, and evaluation (four phases of nursing process that apply to the LPN/LVN).
- *Caring:* Interaction of the LPN/LVN and patient, in an atmosphere of mutual trust and respect.
- *Communication and documentation:* Verbal and nonverbal interaction between the practical/vocational nurse, patient, and others involved with care. Documentation (written or electronic) of all events and

activities associated with patient care reflect the standards of practice.

- *Teaching/learning:* Assist the patient to gain information, skills, and attitudes that lead to change in behavior.

[?] Critical Thinking

Client Need Categories

Provide a "real" example of a patient need for each of the categories and subcategories. Where in the scheduled studies of your program do you expect to learn what is needed for each subcategory? Relate information you give in preconference to the categories and subcategories.

[◎] Try This

Categories of Patient Care

Write a one-sentence example of how you might apply each of the four integrated processes in planning patient care.

OVERVIEW OF APPLICATION PROCESS

It is customary for an instructor to introduce you to the application process when it is time to apply to the state board of nursing (the Board) for a license as an LPN or LVN.

NATIONAL COUNCIL LICENSING EXAMINATION FOR PRACTICAL NURSES PROCESS OVERVIEW*

Submit an application for licensure/registration to the board of nursing/regulatory body (BON/RB) where you wish to be licensed/registered.

1. Meet all of the eligibility requirements of the BON/RB to take the NCLEX-PN®.
2. Register for the NCLEX-PN® with Pearson VUE.
3. Receive NCLEX-PN® Registration Acknowledgment email from Pearson VUE.
4. The BON/RB makes you eligible in the Pearson VUE system.
5. Receive Authorization to Test (ATT) email from Pearson VUE.
6. Schedule your exam with Pearson VUE.

Please note that all correspondence from Pearson VUE will arrive **only** by email.

If more than two weeks have passed since you have submitted a registration for the NCLEX-PN® and received acknowledgment from Pearson VUE, and you have not received an ATT email, please call Pearson VUE NCLEX-PN® Candidate Services (NCSBN, 2016).

---

*Excerpted from National Council of State Boards of Nursing. (2016). 2016 NCLEX-PN® Examination Candidate Bulletin, www.ncsbn.org/089900_2016_Bulletin_Proof3.pdf.

AUTHORIZATION TO TEST

You will receive an **Authorization to Test (ATT)** from Pearson VUE. The ATT letter has your authorization number, candidate identification number, and an expiration date. The ATT letter is valid for the time specified in the letter (determined by the board of nursing). The time period varies from 60 to 365 days. Once your board declares you eligible to test, you must test within that period of time. If you do not test within that period, you must reregister and repay to take the examination.

If you are not declared eligible within that time for taking the NCLEX-PN®, you forfeit the registration and the fee. To reapply, you must submit a new application and pay the fee. Do not send another registration form before calling about your status. Duplicate registration fees are not refunded.

- Schedule taking the NCLEX-PN® at a Pearson Center as soon as possible after receiving the ATT. Test centers may fill up quickly, and attempting to make a last-minute testing appointment may result in missing the ATT validity deadline. Most Pearson Centers are open Monday through Friday, except on holidays, and you may test at any Pearson Center. Some are busier than other sites. If you are flexible regarding time and site location, this author's experience has been that students can generally secure an appointment within two weeks.
- Take the NCLEX-PN® on the scheduled day. You must have the ATT and valid identification with you to be admitted to the Pearson Center.
- Validity dates for the ATT will not be extended for any reason. Once approved for testing, the candidate must take the NCLEX-PN® within the approved time frame.

[?] Critical Thinking

Authorization to Test

Explain the significance of attaining the ATT before scheduling your appointment to take the NCLEX-PN®.

FEES AND OTHER IMPORTANT INFORMATION

There is a fee for the NCLEX-PN® (https://www.ncsbn.org/089900_2016_Bulletin_Proof3.pdf). In addition, other fees are required by the nursing board where you are applying for licensure. Fees vary. There is no refund of a registration fee for any reason.

[◎] Try This

List any fees required by your state's board of nursing (or by the jurisdiction where you are applying).

HOW TO REGISTER (INTERNET OR TELEPHONE)

Internet or telephone can be used to register. Pearson VUE will confirm receipt of registration and send an

ATT to the candidate. Visit: www.ncsbn.org/089900_2016_Bulletin_Proof3.pdf for details.

NATIONAL COUNCIL LICENSING EXAMINATION FOR PRACTICAL NURSES ADMINISTRATION IN THE UNITED STATES AND ITS TERRITORIES

The NCLEX-PN® is given in the United States and territories including American Samoa, Guam, the Northern Mariana Islands, the Virgin Islands, and Canada. This makes it possible to provide licensure by endorsement from one board of nursing to another within the United States and its territories.

Endorsement means that an LPN/LVN may apply for licensure in a different state or territory without retesting. Taking the same examination in the United States and its territories facilitates endorsement from one nursing board to another.

⊚ Try This

Practicing in Other States

Research how to apply for licensure by endorsement in another state. Start by contacting the **state board of nursing** of a state in which you may be interested in applying for a job.

EXAMINATION SECURITY

The NCLEX-PN® ensures *minimal competency* to protect the public and, because of this, strict rules have been established for testing (Source: https://www.ncsbn.org/1219.htm):

- Arrive at the testing center 30 minutes before the scheduled time. If you arrive 30 minutes later than the appointed time, you may be required to forfeit your appointment.
- Avoid bringing children, family, or friends to the Pearson Center. They will not be permitted to wait at the testing center.
- *Name:* Use your name in *exactly* the same form you used when applying for the NCLEX-PN®. If your legal name has changed since you applied, the only legal documentation acceptable the day of the test is a marriage license, divorce decree, and/or court action legal name change documents.
- *Proper identification:* Your ATT and a valid form of picture identification in English and signed in English are required. The only proper identification is a valid (not expired) U.S. driver's license; U.S. state identification (issued by the Department of Motor Vehicles); a valid passport; U.S. Military Identification; or Permanent Residence Card.
- You will be asked to provide your signature. A digital fingerprint, palm vein scan, and photograph will be taken. No hats, scarves, or coats may be worn while the picture is taken. Hats, coats, or scarves may not be worn in the testing room. Your fingerprint, photograph, and signature accompany the examination results that are sent to the board and can be used to confirm your identity.
- Direct observation by staff, video, and audiorecording of the session occur at all times during the examination.
- Personal belongings are kept in secure storage outside of the classroom during the test. The storage space is small, so plan accordingly. A Pearson staff person escorts you to a secure area. A similar process is followed when you prepare to leave the Pearson Center. At no time does any candidate walk into the secure area without an escort. (Visualize a system similar to accessing a safe deposit box at the bank.) This can result in a failed test.
- All books, papers, unauthorized scratch paper, note boards, food, pens, purses, wallets, watches, beepers, cell phones, handheld computers, and personal digital devices are banned from the test room. The CAT includes both a calculator and a time device that tells you how much time remains to complete the NCLEX-PN®. (Refer to your candidate bulletin for a list of other items that are not permitted in the testing room.)
- Erasable note boards are provided for use during the test and collected before you leave the room during a break or at the end of testing. Note boards cannot be taken outside the room.
- Leaving the room is permitted with permission only. A palm vein scan is required each time you leave and return to the testing area after a break. A test administrator (TA) escorts the candidate to and from the room.
- Do not attempt to access any materials during a break without explicit permission from the test proctor.

Violation of center regulations such as attempting to take a test for someone else or inappropriate behavior such as attempting to tamper with the computer will result in dismissal from the testing center. It may also include test results being held or canceled, denial of a license, or denial of future registration for licensure.

⊚ Try This

Security Rules

Discuss why a student cannot access their cell phone (even for an urgent call) during a break.

Confidentiality Agreement (Source: https://www.ncsbn.org/1219.htm)

A confidentiality agreement will appear on the computer, which you must read and sign before you begin the examination. The **confidentiality agreement** includes not disclosing the contents of the examination items before, during, or after the examination. Disclosure includes, but is not limited to, discussing examination items with faculty, friends, family, and others. Please remember this and do not send information via email or discuss content verbally with anyone, including faculty. You may feel you are being helpful but this is a confidentiality breach. Any irregular behavior can result in criminal prosecution, civil liability, and/or disciplinary action by the nursing licensing board.

DURING THE TEST (Source: https://www.ncsbn.org/1219.htm)

You may ask for assistance with the computer at any time if needed or if the computer does not seem to be functioning properly. Raise your hand for assistance, or if you want to change note boards, or if you need a break. Remain in your seat, except when given permission to leave the room. Creating any disturbance can cause you to be dismissed from the room.

After you complete the exam, raise your hand. There will be a brief questionnaire on the computer for you to complete regarding the testing experience. You may also ask for a confidential comment sheet to write personal comments to the NCSBN. When all exam requirements are met, the test administrator will collect and inventory the note boards and dismiss you from the testing room.

REPORTING THE RESULTS OF THE EXAMINATION (Source: https://www.ncsbn.org/1219.htm)

The NCSBN Board of Directors reviewed evidence and voted to change the blueprint of the NCLEX-PN® and raised the passing standard for the NCLEX-PN® effective April 1, 2014.

Although the computer continuously computes the result of your answers, the Pearson Center does not release final results to you directly. The result is available only from the board approximately 1 month after testing. *Do not call the board, the NCLEX-PN® Candidate Services, the Pearson Centers, or the NCSBN for results.* The results will be sent to you by postal mail or email from the state board of nursing. In addition, you can check whether a license has been issued on our state's electronic website (by Googling "my license" and your state for possible links).

Your state's board of nursing (not Pearson Center) notifies you of the test results. Boards are the only agencies that can license a graduate of a practical/vocational program and release the test results to them. Do not contact Pearson VUE for test results; they will not release the results directly to you.

[?] Critical Thinking

Examination Results

Explain why the state board of nursing (rather than the Pearson Center) provides you with the results of the NCLEX-PN®.

[?] Critical Thinking

Computerized Adaptive Testing (CAT)

Explain why the CAT method of testing provides a clearer picture of the candidate's competency than does the usual paper/pencil test.

A WORD ABOUT NATIONAL COUNCIL LICENSING EXAMINATION FOR PRACTICAL NURSES REVIEW BOOKS AND NATIONAL COUNCIL LICENSING EXAMINATION FOR PRACTICAL NURSES PREPARATION PROGRAMS

The major nursing publishing companies have developed review books based on the NCLEX-PN® format. Each review book basically includes an outline of LP/LV nursing content, questions with explanations and rationale, and references for the answers. Questions are intended to simulate the NCLEX-PN® format. Realize that the test questions of the NCLEX-PN® itself are highly guarded and confidential. Actual NCLEX-PN® questions are not included in any review book. Some review books contain computer disks with test questions. These disks do not simulate CAT testing, but they do provide computer experience. Silvestri's (2016) book, *Comprehensive Review for NCLEX-PN® Examination* and its companion CD-ROM contains thousands of NCLEX-PN®-type questions and a comprehensive exam with multiple-choice, alternative item format, and audio questions. HESI's (2015) book, *Comprehensive Review for the NCLEX-PN® Examination* and companion CD-ROM include a study exam.

The best preparation is to study faithfully from the beginning of the program to its conclusion, on a regular basis until you take the NCLEX-PN®. Merely reading a review book at the end of the program without studying the nursing content throughout the program will rarely help you pass boards. The identified outcome of a nursing program is to learn, understand, and be able to apply basic nursing information in the safe, quality care of patients on clinical during your student year and when you graduate.

Countless other vendors provide NCLEX-PN® preparation and success products, including Comprehensive Practical Nurse Predictor Examinations, which can identify your weak areas and provide an in-depth remediation plan. Most importantly, follow your school's guidelines and/or the vendor's guidelines to maximize the positive impact of the product. Purchasing the product is only the first step, integrating the product throughout your program, focusing on remediation when indicated, and avoiding "short cuts" will prepare you well to excel on the NCLEX-PN® and graduate as a competent practitioner. In addition, some publishers provide adaptive testing as used by the NCLEX-PN® examination. If your school's pass rates are above the state and national mean, feel confident in the products assigned and use them effectively. If NCLEX-PN® pass rates at your school are below the state and national mean, question why this is so in a professional manner and discuss what other products or strategies that your school recommends to support your NCLEX-PN® preparation. Use these experiences as additional means of preparing for your nursing licensure examination. Good luck, and keep a positive mental attitude!

Get Ready for the NCLEX-PN® Examination

Key Points

- The Nurse Practice Act provides a foundation to guide and govern nursing practice. It exists to protect the public.
- The Nurse Practice Act varies from state to state, which can create some confusion regarding the LPN's job role boundaries.
- It is the LPN's responsibility to fully understand their state's NPA and educate others on the health care team if needed.
- Preparation for the NCLEX-PN® begins when the student enrolls in a practical nursing program.
- Graduate practical/vocational nurses (candidates) take the NCLEX-PN® to become licensed as LPNs/LVNs.
- The candidate applies to the board of nursing in the state or territory where he or she wishes to be licensed.
- The candidate also must apply to the vendor (e.g., Pearson) to complete the NCLEX-PN®.
- A computer administers the NCLEX-PN®, using the computerized adaptive testing (CAT) method of testing.
- Each candidate takes a different track (path) during the CAT method of testing. The zigzag track is based on the answer to the content area and difficulty level, not the item type.
- Neither pass nor fail is related to the number of items answered by the candidate.
- The NCLEX-PN® provides all candidates ample opportunity to demonstrate minimum competency in LP/LV nursing.
- The board of nursing to which you applied will provide results in approximately 1 month, although sometimes results will be available in less than 1 week.

Additional Learning Resources

evolve Go to your Evolve website (http://evolve.elsevier.com/Knecht/success) for the following FREE learning resources:
- Answers to Critical Thinking Review Scenarios
- Additional learning activities
- Additional Review Questions for the NCLEX-PN® exam
- Helpful phrases for communicating in Spanish and more!

Review Questions for the NCLEX-PN® Examination

1. The following statement best describes the Nurse Practice Act:
   a. The Nurse Practice Act provides a foundation to guide and govern nursing practice.
   b. The Nurse Practice Act provides a laundry list regarding all the tasks that an LPN is allowed to complete.
   c. The Nurse Practice Act is updated every three years.
   d. The Nurse Practice Act is the same in every state.
2. Which statement best describes how the CAT determines that a candidate has passed the NCLEX-PN®?
   a. The computer calculates accuracy or inaccuracy of a distracter chosen by a candidate.
   b. The computer subtracts the number of wrong answers from the number of right questions answers to determine the score.
   c. The computer makes a decision regarding minimum competency once the candidate has answered 100 questions.
   d. The computer continually reestimates the candidate's ability based on previous answers and difficulty level of the question until minimal competency is determined.

3. How is the NCLEX-PN® kept up to date with what LPNs/LVNs are really doing in nursing?
   a. Each nursing school surveys its students during the first year after graduation.
   b. The state board of nursing requires a work survey as a part of license renewal.
   c. The NCSBN sponsors a job analysis of newly licensed nurses throughout the United States.
   d. Each state board of nursing is required to do a work survey and submit questions.
4. A candidate attempts to access their cell phone while taking a break during the NCLEX-PN®. Which of the following is most likely to occur?
   a. The test center will confiscate the cell phone.
   b. The test administrator will ask to observe the text that was sent to ensure the candidate was not cheating.
   c. The test center will dismiss or cancel the testing result of the candidate.
   d. The candidate will return to the test area and resume testing.

Alternate Format Item

1. Which of the following are required as security during the NCLEX-PN®? *(Select all that apply.)*
   a. Fingerprint
   b. Palm vein technology
   c. Observation
   d. Identification
   e. Signature
2. Which of the following are examples of ignoring the confidentiality statement you signed before taking the examination? *(Select all that apply.)*
   a. Express relief to your family at passing the examination successfully.
   b. Make notes of questions you recall immediately after leaving the testing center.
   c. Contact your nursing program director to give her a list of questions you recall.
   d. Discuss the examination questions with a friend who has recently entered the PN program.
   e. Use of a white board while completing the NCLEX-PN®.

Critical Thinking Scenarios

Scenario 1
Kara, a friend of yours in another state, is also taking a practical nursing course. You both have completed about 25% of the program. Kara has expressed concern about being prepared for the NCLEX-PN®. Kara is an average student; however, she does not see the value in completing NCLEX type questions, as she will not be taking the NCLEX-PN for almost one year from now. What are you going to say to your friend?

Scenario 2
You are working for a staffing agency and they assign you to a facility in a neighboring state. You had obtained a license 6 months ago but have never worked in this state. Describe how you will prepare for this assignment.

National Association of Practical Nurse Education and Service Standards of Practice and Educational Competencies of Graduates of Practical/Vocational Nursing Programs*

These standards and competencies are intended to better define the range of capabilities, responsibilities, rights, and relationship to other health care providers for scope and content of licensed practical/licensed vocational nursing education programs. The guidelines will assist:

- Educators in development, implementation, and evaluation of licensed practical/licensed vocational nursing curricula
- Students in understanding expectations of their competencies upon completion of the educational program
- Prospective employers in appropriate use of the licensed practical/licensed vocational nurse
- Consumers in understanding the scope of practice and level of responsibility of the licensed practical/licensed vocational nurse

A. PROFESSIONAL BEHAVIORS

Professional behaviors, within the scope of nursing practice for a practical/vocational nurse, are characterized by adherence to standards of care, accountability for one's own actions and behaviors, and use of legal and ethical principles in nursing practice. Professionalism includes a commitment to nursing and a concern for others demonstrated by an attitude of caring. Professionalism also involves participation in life-long self-development activities to enhance and maintain current knowledge and skills for continuing competency in the practice of nursing for the LP/VN, as well as individual, group, community, and societal endeavors to improve health care.

Upon completion of the licensed practical/licensed vocational nursing program, the graduate will display the following program outcome:

Demonstrate professional behaviors of accountability and professionalism according to the legal and ethical standards for a competent, licensed practical/licensed vocational nurse.

*As approved and adopted by National Association of Practical Nurse Education and Service (NAPNES) Board of Directors May 6, 2007. Copyright © 2011 National Association for Practical Nurse Education and Service, Inc. All rights reserved.

Competencies which demonstrate this outcome has been attained:

1. Comply with the ethical, legal, and regulatory frameworks of nursing and the scope of practice as outlined in the LP/VN nurse practice act of the specific state in which licensed
2. Use educational opportunities for life-long learning and maintenance of competence
3. Identify personal capabilities and consider career mobility options
4. Identify own LP/VN strengths and limitations for the purpose of improving nursing performance
5. Demonstrate accountability for nursing care provided by self and/or directed to others
6. Function as an advocate for the health care consumer, maintaining confidentiality as required
7. Identify the impact of economic, political, social, cultural, spiritual, and demographic forces on the role of the licensed practical/vocational nurse in the delivery of health care
8. Serve as a positive role model within health care settings and the community
9. Participate as a member of a practical vocational nursing organization

B. COMMUNICATION

Communication is defined as the process by which information is exchanged between individuals verbally, non-verbally, and/or in writing or through information technology. Communication abilities are integral and essential to the nursing process. Those who are included in the nursing process are the licensed practical/licensed vocational nurse and other members of the nursing and health care team, client, and significant support person(s). Effective communication demonstrates caring, compassion, and cultural awareness and is directed toward promoting positive outcomes and establishing a trusting relationship.

Upon completion of the practical/vocational nursing program, the graduate will display the following program outcome:

Effectively communicate with patients, significant support person(s), and members of the interdisciplinary health care team, incorporating interpersonal and therapeutic communication skills.

Competencies which demonstrate this outcome has been attained:

1. Use effective communication skills when interacting with clients, significant others, and members of the interdisciplinary health care team
2. Communicate relevant, accurate, and complete information
3. Report to appropriate health care personnel and document assessments, interventions, and progress or impediments toward achieving client outcomes
4. Maintain organizational and client confidentiality
5. Use information technology to support and communicate the planning and provision of client care
6. Use appropriate channels of communication

C. ASSESSMENT

Assessment is the collection and processing of relevant data for the purposes of appraising the client's health status. Assessment provides a holistic view of the client which includes physical, developmental, emotional, psychosocial, cultural, spiritual, and functional status. Assessment involves the collection of information from multiple sources to provide the foundation for nursing care. Initial assessment provides the baseline for future comparisons to individualize client care. Ongoing assessment is required to meet the client's changing needs.

Upon completion of the licensed practical/licensed vocational nursing program, the graduate will display the following program outcome:

Collect holistic assessment data from multiple sources, communicate the data to appropriate health care providers, and evaluate client responses to interventions.

Competencies which demonstrate this outcome has been attained:

1. Assess data related to basic physical, developmental, spiritual, cultural, functional, and psychosocial needs of the client
2. Collect data within established protocols and guidelines from various sources, including client interviews, observations/measurements, health care team members, family, significant other(s), and review of health records
3. Assess data related to the client's health status, identify impediments to client progress, and evaluate response to interventions
4. Document data collection, assessment, and communicate findings to appropriate member(s) of the health care team

D. PLANNING

Planning encompasses the collection of health status information, the use of multiple methods to access information, and the analysis and integration of knowledge and information to formulate nursing care plans and care actions. The nursing care plan provides direction for individualized care and assures the delivery of accurate, safe care through a definitive pathway that promotes the clients and support persons' progress toward positive outcomes.

Upon completion of the licensed practical/licensed vocational nursing program, the graduate will display the following program outcome:

Collaborate with the registered nurse or other members of the health care team to organize and incorporate assessment data to plan/revise patient care and actions based on established nursing diagnoses, nursing protocols, and assessment and evaluation data.

Competencies which demonstrate this outcome has been attained:

1. Use knowledge of normal values to identify deviation in health status to plan care
2. Contribute to formulation of a nursing care plan for clients with non-complex conditions and in a stable state, in consultation with the registered nurse and as appropriate in collaboration with the client or support person(s), as well as members of the interdisciplinary health care team, using established nursing diagnoses and nursing protocols
3. Prioritize nursing care needs of clients
4. Assist in the review and revision of nursing care plans with the registered nurse to meet the changing needs of clients
5. Modify client care as indicated by the evaluation of stated outcomes
6. Provide information to client about aspects of the care plan within the LP/VN scope of practice
7. Refer client as appropriate to other members of the health care team about care outside the scope of practice of the LP/VN

E. CARING INTERVENTIONS

Caring interventions are those nursing behaviors and actions that assist clients and significant others in meeting their needs and the identified outcomes of the plan of care. These interventions are based on knowledge of the natural sciences, behavioral sciences, and past nursing experiences. Caring is the "being with" and "doing for" that assists clients to achieve the desired outcomes. Caring behaviors are nurturing, protective, compassionate, and person-centered. Caring creates an environment of hope and trust, where client choices related to cultural, religious, and spiritual values, beliefs, and lifestyles are respected.

Upon completion of the licensed practical/licensed vocational nursing program, the graduate will display the following program outcome:

Demonstrate a caring and empathic approach to the safe, therapeutic, and individualized care of each client.

Competencies which demonstrate this outcome has been attained:

1. Provide and promote the client's dignity
2. Identify and honor the emotional, cultural, religious, and spiritual influences on the client's health
3. Demonstrate caring behaviors toward the client and significant support person(s)
4. Provide competent, safe, therapeutic, and individualized nursing care in a variety of settings
5. Provide a safe physical and psychosocial environment for the client and significant other(s)
6. Implement the prescribed care regimen within the legal, ethical, and regulatory framework of licensed practical/licensed vocational nursing practice
7. Assist the client and significant support person(s) to cope with and adapt to stressful events and changes in health status
8. Assist the client and significant other(s) to achieve optimum comfort and functioning
9. Instruct client regarding individualized health needs in keeping with the licensed practical/licensed vocational nurse's knowledge, competence, and scope of practice
10. Recognize client's right to access information, and refer requests to appropriate person(s)
11. Act in an advocacy role to protect client rights

F. MANAGING

Managing care is the effective use of human, physical, financial, and technological resources to achieve the client-identified outcomes, while supporting organizational outcomes. The LP/VN manages care through the processes of planning, organizing, and directing.

Upon completion of the licensed practical/licensed vocational nursing program, the graduate will display the following program outcome:

Implement patient care, at the direction of a registered nurse, licensed physician, or dentist, through performance of nursing interventions or directing aspects of care, as appropriate, to unlicensed assistive personnel (UAP).

Competencies which demonstrate this outcome has been attained:

1. Assist in the coordination and implementation of an individualized plan of care for clients and significant support person(s)
2. Direct aspects of client care to qualified UAPs commensurate with abilities and level of preparation and consistent with the state's legal and regulatory framework for the scope of practice for the LP/VN
3. Supervise and evaluate the activities of UAPs and other personnel as appropriate within the state's legal and regulatory framework for the scope of practice for the LP/VN, as well as facility policy
4. Maintain accountability for outcomes of care directed to qualified UAPs
5. Organize nursing activities in a meaningful and cost-effective manner when providing nursing care for individuals or groups
6. Assist the client and significant support person(s) to access available resources and services
7. Demonstrate competence with current technologies
8. Function within the defined scope of practice for the LP/VN in the health care delivery system at the direction of a registered nurse, licensed physician, or dentist

National Federation Licensed Practical Nurses Association Nursing Practice Standards for the Licensed Practical/Vocational Nurse*

Nursing Practice Standards is one of the ways that the National Federation of Licensed Practical Nurses (NFLPN) meets the objective of its bylaws to address principles and ethics, and also to meet another Article II objective: "To interpret the standards of practical (vocational) nursing."

In recent years, licensed practical nurses (LPNs) and licensed vocational nurses (LVNs) have practiced in a changing environment. As LPNs and LVNs practice in expanding roles in the health care system, *Nursing Practice Standards* is essential reading for LPNs, LVNs, PN and VN students and their educators, and all who practice with LPNs and LVNs.

NURSING PRACTICE STANDARDS FOR THE LICENSED PRACTICAL NURSE/LICENSED VOCATIONAL NURSE

PREFACE

The Standards were developed and adopted by the NFLPN to provide a basic model whereby the quality of health service and nursing service and nursing care given by LP/VNs may be measured and evaluated.

These nursing practice standards are applicable in any practice setting. The degree to which individual standards are applied will vary according to the individual needs of the patient, the type of health care agency or services, and the community resources. The scope of licensed practical nursing has extended into specialized nursing services. Therefore, specialized fields of nursing are included in this document.

THE CODE FOR LICENSED PRACTICAL NURSE/ LICENSED VOCATIONAL NURSES

The Code, adopted by the NFLPN in 1961 and revised in 1979, provides a motivation for establishing, maintaining, and elevating professional standards. Each LP/VN, upon entering the profession, inherits the responsibility to adhere to the standards of ethical practice and conduct as set forth in this Code:

1. Know the scope of maximum use of the LP/VN as specified by the nurse practice act and function within this scope.

2. Safeguard the confidential information acquired from any source about the patient.
3. Provide health care to all patients regardless of race, creed, cultural background, disease, or lifestyle.
4. Uphold the highest standards in personal appearance, language, dress, and demeanor.
5. Stay informed about issues affecting the practice of nursing and delivery of health care and, when appropriate, participate in government and policy decisions.
6. Accept the responsibility for safe nursing by keeping oneself mentally and physically fit and educationally prepared to practice.
7. Accept responsibility for membership in the NFLPN, and participate in its efforts to maintain the established standards of nursing practice and employment policies that lead to quality patient care.

INTRODUCTORY STATEMENT

Definition

Practical/Vocational nursing means the performance for compensation of authorized acts of nursing that use specialized knowledge and skills and that meet the health needs of people in a variety of settings under the direction of qualified health professionals.

Scope

Licensed practical/licensed vocational nurses represent the established entry into the nursing profession and include specialized fields of nursing practice. Opportunities exist for practicing in a milieu where different professions unite their particular skills in a team effort to preserve or improve an individual patient's functioning and to protect health and safety of patients.

Opportunities also exist for career advancement in the profession through academic education and for lateral expansion of knowledge and expertise through both academic/continuing education and certification.

STANDARDS

Education

The licensed practical/licensed vocational nurse:
1. Shall complete a formal education program in practical nursing approved by the appropriate nursing authority in a state

2. Shall successfully pass the National Council Licensure Examination for Practical Nurses
3. Shall participate in initial orientation within the employing institution

Legal/Ethical Status

The licensed practical/licensed vocational nurse:
1. Shall hold a current license to practice nursing as an LP/VN in accordance with the law of the state wherein employed
2. Shall know the scope of nursing practice authorized by the nurse practice act in the state wherein employed
3. Shall have a personal commitment to fulfill the legal responsibilities inherent in good nursing practice
4. Shall take responsible actions in situations wherein there is unprofessional conduct by a peer or other health care provider
5. Shall recognize and have a commitment to meet the ethical and moral obligations of the practice of nursing
6. Shall not accept or perform professional responsibilities that the individual knows he or she is not competent to perform

Practice

The licensed practical/licensed vocational nurse:
1. Shall accept assigned responsibilities as an accountable member of the health care team
2. Shall function within the limits of educational preparation and experience as related to the assigned duties
3. Shall function with other members of the health care team in promoting and maintaining health, preventing disease and disability, caring for and rehabilitating individuals who are experiencing an altered health state, and contributing to the ultimate quality of life until death
4. Shall know and use the nursing process in planning, implementing, and evaluating health services and nursing care for the individual patient or group
   a. Planning: The planning of nursing includes:
      - Assessing and collecting data on the health status of the individual patient, the family, and community groups
      - Reporting information gained from the assessment/data collection
      - Identifying health goals
   b. Implementing: The plan for nursing care is put into practice to achieve the stated goals and includes:
      - Observing, recording, and reporting significant changes that require intervention or different goals
      - Applying nursing knowledge and skills to promote and maintain health, to prevent disease and disability, and to optimize functional capabilities of an individual patient

- Assisting the patient and family with activities of daily living and encouraging self-care as appropriate
- Carrying out therapeutic regimens and protocols prescribed by personnel pursuant to authorized state law
   c. Evaluating: The plan for nursing care and its implementations are evaluated to measure the progress toward the stated goals and will include appropriate persons and/or groups to determine:
      - The relevancy of current goals in relation to the progress of the individual patient
      - The involvement of the recipients of care in the evaluation process
      - The quality of the nursing action in the implementation of the plan
      - A reordering of priorities or new goal setting in the care plan
5. Shall participate in peer review and other evaluation processes
6. Shall participate in the development of policies concerning the health and nursing needs of society and in the roles and functions of the LP/VN

Continuing Education

The licensed practical/licensed vocational nurse:
1. Shall be responsible for maintaining the highest possible level of professional competence at all times
2. Shall periodically reassess career goals and select continuing education activities that will help achieve these goals
3. Shall take advantage of continuing education and certification opportunities that will lead to personal growth and professional development
4. Shall seek and participate in continued education activities that are approved for credit by appropriate organizations, such as the NFLPN

Specialized Nursing Practice

The licensed practical/licensed vocational nurse:
1. Shall have had at least 1 year's experience in nursing at the staff level
2. Shall present personal qualifications that are indicative of potential abilities for practice in the chosen specialized nursing area
3. Shall present evidence of completion of a program or course that is approved by an appropriate agency to provide the knowledge and skills necessary for effective nursing services in the specialized field
4. Shall meet all of the standards of practice as set forth in this document

GLOSSARY

Authorized (acts of nursing) Those nursing activities made legal through State Nurse Practice Acts.

Lateral expansion of knowledge An extension of the basic core of information learned in the school of practical nursing.

Peer review A formal evaluation of performance on the job by other LP/VNS.

Special nursing practice A restricted field of nursing in which a person is particularly skilled and has specific knowledge.

Therapeutic regimens Regulated plans designed to bring about effective treatment of disease.

Career advancement A change of career goal.

LP/LV A combined abbreviation for licensed practical nurse and licensed vocational nurse; LVN is the title used in California and Texas for the nurses who are called LPNs in other states.

Milieu One's environment and surroundings.

Protocols Courses of treatment that include specific steps to be performed in a stated order.

Review Questions for the National Council Licensure Examination for Licensed Practical/Licensed Vocational Nurses (NCLEX-PN®) Answer Key

Chapter 1
1. a
2. c
3. a
4. d

Alternate Format Item
1. a, d
2. a, e

Chapter 2
1. d
2. b
3. a
4. a
5. d
6. b

Alternate Format Item
1. a, b, c, d, e
2. a, b
3. a, d

Chapter 3
1. a
2. b
3. a

Alternate Format Item
1. a, b, c
2. a, b, c, d, e

Chapter 4
1. d
2. c

Alternate Format Item
1. a, b, c, d
2. b, c, d

Chapter 5
1. c
2. d
3. d
4. b

Alternate Format Item
1. a, b, d, e
2. b, c, d, e

Chapter 6
1. c
2. a
3. a
4. b

Alternate Format Item
1. a, b, d
2. b, c, d, e

Chapter 7
1. b
2. d
3. c
4. d

Alternate Format Item
1. a, b, c, e
2. c, d, e

Chapter 8
1. d
2. c
3. c
4. b

Alternate Format Item
1. c, d
2. a, d

Chapter 9
1. d
2. b
3. c
4. a

Alternate Format Item
1. a, b, c
2. a, b, c

Chapter 10
1. a
2. a
3. d
4. c

Alternate Format Item
1. a, d

Chapter 11
1. c
2. b
3. d
4. a

Alternate Format Item
1. d
2. a, b, c, d, e

Chapter 12
1. d
2. b
3. d
4. a

Alternate Format Item
1. a, c, e
2. a, b, c, d, e

Chapter 13
1. d
2. c
3. d
4. a

Alternate Format Item
1. a, b, d, c
2. a, b, c, d, e

Chapter 14
1. d
2. b
3. a

Alternate Format Item
1. a, b, d
2. b
3. a, b, c, d

Chapter 15
1. b
2. c
3. c

Alternate Format Item
1. a, b, c, d
2. c, d, e
3. a, b, c, d

Chapter 16
1. a
2. c
3. d
4. d

Alternate Format Item
1. a, b, c

Chapter 17
1. a
2. b
3. d
4. a
5. a

Alternate Format Item
1. a
2. b, c, d
3. a, c, d

Chapter 18
1. c
2. c
3. a
4. c

Alternate Format Item
1. a, b, c, d, e
2. a, b, c, e

Chapter 19
1. a
2. d
3. c
4. c

Alternate Format Item
1. a, b, c, d, e
2. b, c, d

Glossary

A

Accountability: Obligation to answer for personal actions.

Active learning: Taking charge of own education.

Active listener: Listener who is open minded and curious and is always asking questions about content.

Active listening: Hearing sounds and searching for information relevant to those sounds so the sounds may be understood.

Acute care: Higher level of care required for seriously ill patients.

Adult day care center: A service that provides mental stimulation, socialization, assistance with some activities of daily living (ADLs), and basic observation. Services often include transportation, meals, therapeutic activities, nursing interventions, and rehabilitation activities. The service is hospital-based or freestanding.

Advance directives: Written documents to state personal wishes regarding future health care.

Affective communication: Sending or receiving information through feeling tone.

Aggressive: An attacking type of behavior that occurs in response to frustration and hostile feelings.

Agnostic: A person who holds the belief that the existence of God can neither be proved nor disproved.

Allah: Muslim name of the one supreme being; God of Islam.

Alliances: New partnerships among hospitals, clinics, laboratories, health care systems, and physicians. They coordinate the delivery of care, contain costs, and attempt to provide a seamless system.

Ambulatory care facilities: Primary health care services for walk-in patients. Also known as Urgent Care, Express Care, and Quick Care.

Ambulatory surgery centers: One-day surgery centers that perform surgery at a scheduled date and time. Patient discharged home when recovered from surgery and is stable.

Analysis: Break down complex information into its basic parts and relate it to the whole picture.

Application: Use learned information in new situations.

Apps: Abbreviation for applications; programs that can be stored on an electronic device.

Assault: An unjustified attempt or threat to touch someone.

Assertiveness: A way of accepting responsibility for oneself by expressing thoughts and feelings directly and honestly, without blaming oneself or others.

Assigning (assignment): Allotting tasks that are in the job description of workers. Assigned tasks are the ones that workers are hired and paid to perform.

Assimilation: Giving up parts of your own culture and adopting parts of the culture of the dominant group.

Assisted care: Residences that provide "a home with services."

Assisting: Licensed practical nurse/licensed vocational nurse (LPN/LVN) role in 4 phases (steps) of nursing process.

Associate degree nursing: A 2-year community college or technical school program. The title registered nurse (RN) is used after passing the National Council Licensure Examination-Registered Nurse (NCLEX-RN®).

Atheist: A person who does not believe the supernatural exists and therefore does not believe in God.

Attitude: Nonverbal expression of the way a person thinks or feels.

Auditory learner: Talks to himself or herself or hears sounds when thinking. Learns best by hearing.

Authorization to test (ATT): Denotes that the graduate practical/vocational nurse has met the requirements for eligibility to take the National Council Licensure Examination-Registered Nurse (NCLEX-RN®). ATT applied for and obtained from the testing center.

Authorized consent: Parents cannot give informed consent for medical care of a child but can give authorized consent instead.

Autocratic leadership: A purely task-centered leadership style that thrives on power.

Automatic responses: Both passive and aggressive responses result from being caught by an emotional hook. These responses are not based on choice.

Autonomy: Control over personal decisions.

B

Barton, Clara: Founder of the American Red Cross.

Basic patient situation: Patient's clinical condition is predictable. Medical and nursing orders are not changing continuously. No complex modifications of nursing care are needed.

Battery: Causing acute physical harm to someone.

Belittling: Mimicking or making fun of a person in some way.

Beneficence: Doing good.

Beneficent paternalism: Health care provider making decisions for the patient based on "I know what's best for you." Discounts patient autonomy.

Biomedicine: Belief that abnormalities in structure and function of body organs are caused by pathogens, biochemical alterations, and/or environmental factors.

Blended course: A course that combines face-to-face instruction with online learning.

Board and care homes: Offer housing and custodial care. Also known as adult care homes or group homes.

Bodily/kinesthetic learner: Learns best by touching, moving, and processing knowledge through bodily sensations.

Breach of duty: One of the elements needed to prove negligence; means that the nurse did not adhere to standards of care.

Bucket theory: Suggests that merely by lecturing, the teacher can transfer knowledge from the teacher's mind to the student's mind.

Buddha: The enlightened one; Siddhartha Gautama, founder of Buddhism.

Bullying: Negative acts perpetrated by one at a higher level.

C

Cadet Nurse Corps: 1943 Bolton Act was the basis of the government subsidizing schools to teach nursing skills in 2 1/2 years. More than 150,000 nurses graduated from these programs. Discontinued in 1948.

Call number: Series of letters and numbers used to identify library materials and assist in locating materials.

Candidate: Graduate practical/vocational nurse who will take (or is taking) the National Council Licensure Examination-Registered Nurse (NCLEX-RN®).

Capability: Ability or capacity.

Capitation: Set fee for health care, paid annually regardless of the number of health services provided.

Case management method: Focus is on quality, service, and cost.

Case method: A method of patient care in which one nurse is assigned to give total care to one patient.

Case scenarios: A printed or computer patient story that brings reality to theory in the form of a clinical situation.

Centers for Medicare and Medicaid Services (CMS): Formerly Health Care Financing Administration (HCFA). Federal agency of Department of Health and Human Services. Certifies nursing homes for Medicare and Medicaid reimbursement.

Certification: Certificate awarded to a registered nurse (RN) or licensed practical nurse/licensed vocational nurse (LPN/LVN) after passing a comprehensive examination in a select area of practice.

Certification in Long-Term Care (CLTC): Postgraduate course offered by the National Association of Practical Nurse Education and Service (NAPNES). Replaces previous gerontology certification. Recertification is every 5 years.

Certification in Managed Care Nursing: Postgraduate course including basic knowledge of managed care, health care economics, health care management, and patient issues.

Certification in Pharmacology (NCP): Postgraduate course offered by the National Association of Practical Nurse Education and Service (NAPNES. Recertification is every 5 years.

Change-of-shift report: Report on patient condition at beginning and end of shift.

Choice: Act of choosing. For example, to speak assertively is to speak out of choice.

Civil action (related to individual rights): Involves the relationships between individuals and the violation of those rights.

Clark, Mildred L: Chief of Army Nurse Corps from 1963 to 1967.

Clerk receptionist: Assumes responsibility for many clerical duties in the patient care area.

Clinical pathway: Blueprint for patient care. Includes time frame of significant events that are expected to occur each day a patient with a specific diagnosis is in the hospital.

Closed-ended questions: Questions that require specific answers from a patient.

Clustering: A form of mapping is a method of note making.

Cognitive level: Intellectual level of functioning.

Coinsurance: Percentage of total bill paid for by insurance company once deductible is paid.

Commitment: Pledge to do one's best.

Common law: Judge-made law, which has its origins in the courts.

Communication blocks: Stops meaningful conversation. Examples include chiding, belittling, probing, giving advice, and providing pat answers.

Community health nursing: Nursing that focuses on improving the health status of communities or groups of people through public education, screening for early detection of disease, and providing services for people who need care outside the acute care setting.

Community resources: Include a diverse group of people, organizations, and facilities (in-person and virtual) that assist community members in achieving their personal and professional goals. This includes social service, educational, health, workforce, and professional-related services.

Compensation: Coping mechanism used to cover for real or imagined inadequacy by developing or exaggerating a desirable trait.

Complementary and alternative medicine (CAM): Focus is on assisting the body's own healing powers and restoring body balance.

Complex nursing situation: Patient's clinical condition is not predictable. Medical and nursing orders are likely to involve continuous changes or complex modifications.

Comprehension: Basically understand information, recall it, and identify examples of that information.

Computer-aided instruction: An increasingly used teaching strategy in nursing education.

Computerized adaptive testing (CAT): Method by which the National Council Licensure Examination for Licensed Practical Nurses (NCLEX-PN®) examination is administered to the candidate (a nursing graduate who has fulfilled requirements for testing).

Computer simulation: Learning activities on a CD-ROM or floppy disc that use an imaginary patient situation. The student uses the nursing process as he or she would in an actual clinical situation.

Conditional job offer: Job offer contingent on passing physical, drug screening, and/or background check.

Confidentiality: Avoid sharing patient information with anyone not directly involved in care without the patient's permission.

Confidentiality agreement: Before taking the National Council Licensure Examination for Licensed Practical Nurses (NCLEX-PN®) examination, read and sign agreement not to disclose contents of examination.

Conflict resolution: A method of resolving differences in a peaceful way.

Constructive evaluation: Critique directed toward performance and behavior; has no bearing on one's value as a person.

Continuous care retirement community: Provides a continuum living option from independent living, assisted living, and skilled nursing home, all on one campus.

Continuous quality improvements (CQIs): Search for new ways to improve patient care, prevent errors, and identify and fix problems.

Continuum: A way to look at two extremes (from least complex to most complex).

Cooperative learning: Emphasis on individual accountability for learning a specific academic task while working in small groups.

Copayment: Percentage of the bill that is paid by a person (subscriber) who is enrolled in a health insurance plan.

Copyright laws: These laws permit a single copy of an article for personal use. Instructors may not make copies of articles, chapters, or books for distribution to each student.

Cost containment: Holding costs within fixed limits.

Course outlines: Up-to-date listings of what is covered in a course. Provided by the instructor.

Criminal action: Involves persons and society as a whole, for example, murder.

Critical thinking: Used to resolve problems and find ways to make improvements, even when no problem exists.

Cultural bias: Unquestioned, unproved way of thinking.

Cultural competence: The continuous attempt of licensed practical nurses/licensed vocational nurses to gain the knowledge and skills that will allow them to effectively provide care for patients of different cultures.

Cultural diversity: Differences in elements of culture in groups of people.

Cultural sensitivity: Learning about other cultures and being respectful of their customs, rites, and beliefs.

Culture: The total of all the ideas, beliefs, values, attitudes, communication, customs, traditions, and objects that a group of people possess. Culture includes ways of doing things.

Customs: Ways of doing things that are common to a group of people of the same culture.

D

Damages: One of four elements needed to prove negligence. Patient must be able to show the nurse's negligent act injured the patient in some way.

Data collection: Phase 1 of nursing process for practical/vocational nurses. Involves systematic gathering and reviewing of information about the patient.

Deductibles: Amount the subscriber must pay before health insurance begins to cover costs.

Defamation: Damage to someone's reputation through false communication or communication without permission.

Delano, Jane: Of the American Red Cross and who began to recruit and train nurses for overseas duty in World War I.

Delegated medical act: Physician's orders given to a registered nurse (RN), licensed practical nurse (LPN), or licensed vocational nurse (LVN) by a physician, dentist, or podiatrist.

Delegating (delegation): Generally, duties within the licensed practical nurse/licensed vocational nurse (LPN/LVN) job description that can be given to another worker to perform.

Denial: Coping mechanism that includes rejection of events as they really are. Eliminates need for anxiety.

Department of Health and Human Services (HHS): A federal agency funded by taxes. Advises President on national health matters.

Dependent role: The licensed practical nurse/licensed vocational nurse (LPN/LVN) functions with supervision in a dependent role to the registered nurse (RN), physician, or dentist.

Depositions: Gathering information under oath. One of the steps in bringing legal action.

Desired patient outcome: Observable result. Focuses directly on what the patient will accomplish (not what the nurse will do).

Diagnosis-related group (DRG): Prospective payment system. Specifies number of days for which Medicare will pay, based on illness category.

Diploma program: A 3-year nursing educational program conducted by a hospital-based school of nursing.

Direct supervision: Supervisor is continuously present to coordinate, direct, or inspect nursing care. Supervisor is in building.

Directed (or focused) thinking: Purposeful and outcome-oriented thinking. Focuses on particular problem to find solution.

Discrimination: Rights and privileges are withheld from those of another cultural group.

Discussion buddy: Another student with whom you discuss a topic to comprehend the information.

Distance learning: A course in which the teacher and student are separated by physical distance, using such tools as two-way television, videotapes, audiotapes, and the Internet.

Distracters: Incorrect options for multiple-choice items.

Dix, Dorothea Lynde: Appointed Superintendent of Nurses during the American Civil War to organize a corps of nurses to tend to wounded soldiers.

Do-not-resuscitate (DNR): Order written by physician. Patient will not recover. Patient may have signed an advance directive regarding end-of-life care that states personal wishes.

Durable medical power of attorney: Identifies who will make decisions regarding future care, extent of treatment, and kinds of treatment if the person is unable to make his or her own decisions. Written while the person is mentally competent.

Duty: One of four elements needed to prove negligence. Refers to nurse's responsibility to provide care in an acceptable way. As used in the text, responsibilities directly related to nursing licensure and scope of practice. Usually not delegated to someone with less education and nursing skill.

E

Electronic device: Smartphone (BlackBerry, Android, iPhone), notebook, tablet, laptop, computer.

Electronic simulation: Uses mannequins that are high-tech, more costly simulation models that can be programmed to set up different patient situations and allow practice of nursing procedures and data collection (assessment).

Emotional needs: How people respond and deal with feelings of joy, anger, sadness, guilt, remorse, sorrow, love, etc.

Empathy: Respectful, detached concern.

Enculturation: Process of learning your culture: the way your group does things, resulting in a worldview.

End-of-life principles: Support core principles for end-of-life care.

Endorsement: Agreement among states that nurses licensed in one state may become licensed in another if they meet the state nursing board criteria.

Entitlement program: Those eligible because of age, disability, or economic status are entitled by law to benefits of certain programs, namely, Social Security, Medicare, and Medicaid.

Ethics: Rules or principles that govern correct conduct.

Ethnic groups: Cultural groups composed of people who are members of the same race, religion, or nation, or who speak the same language.

Ethnocentrism: The belief that one's own culture is best; the belief that one's way of doing things is superior/right/best.

Euthanasia: Physician or other person administering lethal dose of medication to end life; illegal in the United States and Canada.

Evaluation: Phase 4 of nursing process for licensed practical nurses/licensed vocational nurses (LPNs/LVNs). Compares actual patient outcomes to expected outcomes.

Evidence-based practice: Nursing procedures/interventions that have been proven to be effective.

External distractions: Interruptions in concentration from outside oneself, such as background sounds, lighting, peers, and so forth.

F

Facilitator: Instructor who creates a learning environment by arranging for a variety of activities and experiences.

False reassurance: Promising patient something you cannot deliver, such as saying, "You'll be just fine."

Feedback: Response to sender's message as a part of meaningful conversation.

Fee-for-service: Patient pays the physician a fee for each service provided.

Felony: Serious offense, with a penalty that ranges from 1 year in prison to death.

Fidelity: In nursing, to be faithful to the charge of acting in the patient's best interest when the capacity to make free choice is no longer available.

First Amendment: Guarantees freedom of expression as long as it is not at the expense of harming others.

Focused questions: Questions that require definitive, precise information from a patient.

Follow-up illusion: Irrational belief that it is the employer's responsibility to contact applicants after an interview.

Formal education: Planned, organized learning, such as the nursing course of study.

Free clinic: Used by persons who cannot afford traditional health care. May have an age and income range. The clinic charges a minimal fee.

Freestanding: Health facility not attached to a hospital.

Functional method: A method of patient care that is task-oriented and involves dividing the tasks to be done among staff members according to their abilities.

G

General hospitals: Set up to treat a variety of medical/surgical problems.

General (implied) consent: By entering a health facility voluntarily, a patient gives permission for treatment with noninvasive procedures. However, a patient may revoke this consent verbally and refuse to be treated.

General supervision: Supervisor regularly coordinates, directs, or inspects nursing care and is within reach either in the building or by phone.

Generalization: Broad, sweeping statements made about a group.

Generational personality: Personality of people born around the same period of time and shaped by a common history of cultural events, images, and experiences.

Giving advice: Telling someone what to do.

Goals (outcomes): Realistic, measurable, time-limited statements of resolution of a problem or need.

Good Samaritan Act: Stipulates that a person who provides emergency care at the scene of an accident is immune from civil liability for actions done in good faith. There is some variation of the law within states.

Goodacres, Glenna: Designed and sculpted Vietnam Women's Memorial. Located on the National Mall in Washington, D.C.

Goodrich, Anna: Helped form the National Emergency Committee on Nursing during World War I.

Green House: Designed to deinstitutionalize long-term care by eliminating large nursing facilities. These are homes with 6 to 12 elders in a residential setting.

Gretter, Lystra: Modified the Hippocratic Oath in 1893 and named it The Nightingale Pledge.

Guest speakers: Nurses or other health professionals invited to present up-to-date information on areas of expertise.

H

Hays, Colonel Anna Mae: Led Army Nurse Corps during the Vietnam War. First woman to become a brigadier general and first woman in American military to attain general officer rank.

Health care provider: A licensed health care person, such as a physician, dentist, or nurse practitioner, whose health care services are covered by a health insurance plan.

Health Insurance Portability and Accountability Act (HIPAA) 2003: Federal law commonly called the Privacy Act.

Health maintenance organization (HMO): A comprehensive care system of medical services based on a set, prepaid fee.

Hidden job market: Unadvertised jobs.

Higbee, Lenah S.: World War I Navy nurse. Received the Navy Cross. Was the first nurse to have a destroyer named in her honor.

Home health nursing: Provides health services supervised by a licensed professional in a patient's home. Examples include visiting nurse associations, health departments, home health agencies, etc.

Honesty: To not deliberately deceive to present oneself in a better light.

Hospice care: End-of-life care for the terminally ill. The philosophy is to maintain comfort as death approaches.

Howlett hierarchy: Hierarchy of work motivators. Adapted from Maslow's hierarchy of needs.

Humor: Communication characteristic to help "lighten up" a situation.

I

Idea sketches: Representing a verbal concept with a picture.

Illegal questions: Interview questions that do not have to be answered, such as age, marital status, number of children, and health problems, unless directly related to job.

Implementation: Phase 3 of the nursing process for licensed practical nurses/licensed vocational nurses (LPNs/LVNs). Provides required nursing care to accomplish established patient goals.

Independent: Function without supervision, for example, the registered nurse (RN) role in the nursing process.

Informational interview: By appointment, meet with an administrator to learn about a facility. This is not a job interview, although it is treated with the same courtesy.

Informed consent: Obtained by physician for invasive procedures after physician has provided patient with facts about effects, side effects, alternative treatments, prognosis, and so on. May be revoked verbally at any time up to time of procedure.

Institute of Medicine (IOM): An independent, nonprofit organization that advises the public and decision makers with ways to improve health.

Institutional liability: Form of vicarious liability. Health setting sued for negligence of employee.

Intentional tort: Intent to do a wrongful act.

Interdependent: Both registered nurses (RNs) and licensed practical nurses/licensed vocational nurses (LPNs/LVNs) collaboratively carry out orders for treatments and medications written by a physician.

Interlibrary loan services: Allow libraries to borrow materials from other libraries that are not a part of their holdings.

Internal distractions: Interruptions in concentration from inside oneself, such as daydreaming and boredom.

Internet: Physical infrastructure that allows the electronic circulation of vast amounts of information to computer users. This information is unregulated and cannot always be taken at face value.

Interpersonal learner: Learns best by sharing, comparing, cooperating, and interviewing.

Interpersonal styles: Four major styles: analytical type, driver type, amicable type, and expressive type.

Interstate endorsement: Agreement among states that licensed nurses do not have to repeat the National Council Licensure Examination for Licensed Practical Nurses (NCLEX-PN®) examination if they meet criteria for working in the state.

Intervention: Action taken to reach a patient outcome.

Intrapersonal learner: Learns best by working alone, self-paced instruction, and having own space.

Intravenous Therapy Certification (IVC): Postgraduate education on intravenous therapy, offered through National Federation of Licensed Professional Nurses (NFLPN) and National Association for Practical Nurse Education and Service (NAPNES).

Irrational thinking: Based on Ellis (1994). Self-talk is often irrational thinking: Judgments are subjective and have no bearing on facts. Leads to negative emotions and stress.

J

Jesus Christ: Founder of Christian religion.

Judging: Arriving at an opinion based on some evidence. Can be a communication block, particularly if judging is perceived as "thinking less" of the person.

Justice: Giving patients their due and treating them fairly.

K

Key: Correct option(s) for a multiple choice or alternate item format question.

Kinesthetic/tactual learner: Have two sub-channels: movement and touch.

Kinkela-Keil, Captain Lillian: Member of the Air Force Nurse Corps. Flew over 200 air evacuation missions during World War II, as well as 25 trans-Atlantic crossings. Went back to civilian flying until the Korean War. Flew several hundred more missions as a flight nurse in Korea. Numerous decorations. Inspiration for the movie *Flight Nurse*.

Knowledge: Repeat information exactly as read or told. Does not imply an understanding of the information.

L

Lateral violence: Between nursing colleagues. Includes both overt and covert physical, verbal, and emotional abuse by one nurse against another.

Law: Nursing law is based on each state's Nurse Practice Act.

Leadership: Manner in which the leader gets along with co-workers, with the goal of producing workplace changes to meet the goals of the employing agency.

Learner: One who acquires knowledge and skills.

Learning Management System (LMS): Electronic platform such as Moodle, Blackboard, and Angel where resources are housed.

Learning resource center (LRC): The library.

Lecture-discussion strategy: A strategy in which the instructor shares several ideas with the class and then stops to let the class discuss the ideas.

Left-brain dominant: A person who is more orderly, is logical, reads and writes well, and excels at analytical thinking. Also called *linear thinkers.*

Leininger's Culture Care Theory: Recognition of the link between a person's cultural background and his or her response to nursing care.

Libel: Damage to someone's reputation through written communication or pictures.

Linguistic learner: Learns best by saying, hearing, and seeing words.

Living will: Written directive stating personal wishes regarding future health care. Not recognized as a legal document in every state or other countries.

Logical learner: Learns best by using an organized method of study.

Long-term care: Range of medical care to assist persons with disability or chronic care needs.

M

Malpractice (professional negligence): A part of negligence that relates to lack of skill or misconduct by professional persons.

Managed care: A system of controlling cost of health care by arranging health care at predetermined rates. A health maintenance organization (HMO) is an example of managed care.

Management: Organizing all care required for patients in a health care setting for a specific period.

Manipulation: An indirect way of dealing with issues that may be positive or negative. Negative (maladaptive) manipulation occurs if the feelings of others are disregarded or other people are treated as objects.

Mapping: A form of note making in which information and its relationships are put in a visual pattern.

Maslow's human needs theory: A way to look at identifying patient care priorities and responding to the patient's needs according to the patient's level of functioning.

Medicaid: Financial assistance provided by the federal government for states and counties to pay for medical services for eligible poor.

Medicare: Federally sponsored and supervised health insurance plan for persons 65 years of age and older and persons under 65 years who are totally and permanently disabled.

Medicare Quality Improvement Organizations (QIOs): Formerly known as peer review organizations. Under the direction of Centers for Medicare and Medicaid Services.

Melting pot: The United States became known as the "melting pot" in the nineteenth century, when immigrants would assimilate into the dominant culture.

Mental imagery: Uses the right side of the brain to generate pictures of an idea; the left side supplies the script.

Message: The idea being conveyed or the question being asked.

Misdemeanor: Least serious infraction of the law, except for a summary offense. Can result in a fine or up to 1 year in jail.

Mission statement: A statement that defines the purpose and goals of a health care organization.

Mnemonic devices: Memory aids such as rhymes or acronyms.

Mobile device: PDA, smartphone (iPhone, BlackBerry), iPod Touch, e-book reader, and tablet.

Mobility program: Seamless program of study from certified nursing assistant (CNA) to licensed practical nurse/licensed vocational nurse (LPN/LVN) to associate degree registered nurse (RN) to Bachelor of Science in Nursing (BSN) to Master of Science in Nursing (MSN) to Doctorate Degree in Nursing.

Morals: Dealing with right and wrong behavior.

Multistate licensure (Nursing Licensure Compact): Legislation in some states that renders a nursing license obtained in that state valid for practice in other states with multistate legislation. Each state's individual regulations must still be followed.

Musical learner: Learns best by humming, singing, or playing an instrument.

N

NANDA-I: North American Nursing Diagnosis Association.

NAPNES: National Association for Practical Nurse Education and Service, Inc.

National Certification in Intravenous Therapy: Postgraduate course through National Association for Practical Nurse Education and Service (NAPNES).

National Certification in Gerontology: Postgraduate NFLPN program leading to certification in gerontology.

National Patient Safety Foundation (NPSF): An organization that aims to improve safety in health care.

Naturalistic system: Beliefs developed from the traditional medical practices of the ancient civilizations of China, India, and Greece.

NCLEX-PN® examination: National Council Licensing Examination for Practical Nursing.

Negligence: Conduct that falls below the standard of care established by law for the protection of others.

Networking: Building relationships with instructors, employers, and peers for the purposes of finding new jobs, better pay, faster promotions, and greater job satisfaction.

NFLPN: National Federation of Licensed Practical Nurses.

NIC: Nursing Interventions Classification.

Nightingale, Florence: Founder of modern nursing who is known as "The Lady with the Lamp" because of her after-hours rounds with her lamp during the Crimean War.

NLN: National League for Nursing.

NOC: Nursing Outcomes Classification

Nonassertive (passive): Fear-based, emotionally dishonest, self-defeating type of behavior. Gives message of "I don't count, but you count."

Nonjudgmental: Taking at face value. Accepting people as they are.

Nonmaleficence: First, do no harm.

Nonprofit community hospital: Nonprofit hospital operated by community association or religious organization.

Nonverbal communication: Sending or receiving information by facial expressions or body language.

Notes on Nursing: Written by Florence Nightingale.

Nursing manager: A registered nurse (RN) who has graduated from a baccalaureate nursing program (4-year) and is enrolled in a Master of Science in Nursing (MSN) program.

Nurse Practice Act: Governs the practice of nursing.

Nursing assistant: Minimum 75-hour course prepares nursing assistant to give bedside care. Successful completion makes Certified Nursing Assistant (CNA) eligible for state registry.

Nursing research: An organized way of finding information that supports existing knowledge and develops new knowledge for clinical practice, nursing education, and nursing services.

Nursing diagnosis: Second step of the nursing process for registered nurses (RNs): Actual and high-risk problems that nurses can respond to. Exclusive responsibility of RN in nursing process.

Nursing ethics: System of principles governing conduct of nurses.

Nursing organizations: Groups for nurses focused on nursing issues of importance.

Nursing process: An orderly way of developing a plan of care for the individual patient. The registered nurse (RN) is responsible for developing the nursing diagnosis.

Nursing skills lab: Resource that allows student nurses to practice and develop nursing skills.

Nursing standard of care: Guideline for good nursing care. Standards are based on what an ordinary, prudent nurse with similar education and nursing experience would do in a similar situation.

Nursing theories: Often used as a basis for developing nursing curricula.

Nutting, Adelaide: Helped form the National Emergency Committee on Nursing during World War I.

O

Objective information: Data that can be observed and verified. Data obtained by seeing, hearing, touching, smelling, tasting, measuring, counting, and so on. Does not include subjective judgment.

Official (government) health care agencies: Local, state, and federal health agencies supported by tax dollars.

Omnibus Reconciliation Act of 1987 (OBRA): Major federal legislation that addresses the quality of life, health, and safety of residents.

One-way communication: When the sender controls a situation and offers no opportunity for feedback from the receiver; used to give a command.

Online catalog: Computerized card catalog in the library.

Open-ended questions: Questions that permit the patient to respond in a way most meaningful to him or her. These type of questions often begin with what, where, when.

Options: Choices; for example, choices for an answer in a multiple-choice item.

Oregon Death with Dignity Act: Allows terminally ill Oregonians to end their lives through voluntary self-administration of lethal medication.

Orem's Self-Care Deficit Theory: This nursing theory has three subtheories: self-care, self-care deficit, and the nursing system. Nursing data collection can be used to identify the particular deficit to choose interventions that will have the desired outcomes for the patient.

Outcome: Identifies the degree of progress made (or not made) by the patient toward reaching a goal.

Outpatient clinic: Provides health care outside of the hospital setting. Staffed by physicians and nurses.

P

Palliative care: According to the World Health Organization (WHO; www.who.int/cancer/palliative/definition/en/), an approach that improves the quality of life of patients and their families facing the problem associated with life-threatening illness, through the prevention and relief of suffering by means of early identification and impeccable assessment and treatment of pain and other problems, physical, psychosocial, and spiritual.

Paradigm: A way of thinking.

Parish nurse: Works in various church settings in a health ministry.

Passive listener: A person who receives sounds with little recognition or personal involvement.

Pastoral care team: Members of the health team who assist nurses in meeting the spiritual needs of the patients.

Patience: Willingness to put up with waiting and being okay about doing so.

Patient competency: Relates to ability to understand and make decisions. Has both legal and clinical meaning.

Patient outcomes: Focus on whether patient has accomplished what was desired during treatment. Does not focus on what the nurse did.

Patient Self-Determination Act (PSDA): Basis for advanced directives. Federal law mandates that Medicare and Medicaid patients must be told of their right to formulate advance directives.

Peer-reviewed: Information reviewed by others in a subject for accuracy, quality, and appropriateness.

Peplau's Interpersonal Relations Theory: Basis for developing a therapeutic relationship with a patient (especially useful for working with adult or child psychiatric patients). The relationship has certain parameters that are a major part of the treatment. The overlapping phases are orientation, identification, exploitation, and resolution.

Perceptual learning style: Refers to learning by three main sensory receivers: visual, auditory, and kinesthetic.

Performance evaluation: Evaluation of clinical performance that involves input from the instructor and the student.

Periodical indexes: List of periodicals by author, title, and subject.

Periodicals: Magazines published weekly, monthly, and quarterly.

Personal ethics: Provide personal guidelines for living.

Personal liability: Holds person (nurse) responsible for own actions.

Personalistic system: Belief that a deity, ghost, god, evil spirit, witch, or angry ancestor is punishing the sick person.

Physician-assisted suicide: Name tagged onto "Oregon Death with Dignity Law." Physician writes prescription for medication to end life but does not administer it. Patient self-administers lethal medication.

Planning: Phase 2 of the nursing process for licensed practical nurses/licensed vocational nurses (LPNs/LVNs). Involves collaborating with the registered nurse (RN) in development of the nursing diagnosis, goals, and interventions for the patient's plan of care and maintaining patient safety.

Podcast: A digital audio/visual recording of information on the Internet that can be downloaded to a personal media player or a computer.

Positive mental attitude: Expectation to succeed combined with hard work.

Practical/vocational nurse: A person who performs, for compensation, any basic acts in the care of convalescent, subacutely, or chronically ill, injured, or infirm persons, or any act or procedure in the care of the acutely ill, injured, or infirm under the specific direction of a registered nurse, physician, podiatrist, or dentist.

Preceptor: An experienced nurse who guides a newly licensed nurse or senior nursing student to adjust/learn how to "tie it all together" in the first job.

Preferred provider organizations (PPOs): Similar to health maintenance organizations (HMOs), except that physicians maintain their own practice and continue to be part of their own physician group. Part of the day is spent treating patients enrolled in a PPO.

Prejudice: The opinion that a person has about something, even though facts dispute the opinion.

Premium: Monthly fee a subscriber must pay for health care insurance coverage.

Preponderance: Evidence that is beyond a reasonable doubt.

Primary care: The point at which a person enters the health care system.

Privacy: Both a legal and ethical issue. Patient's right to choose what is done to his or her body, based on personal beliefs, feelings, and attitude.

Private health care agencies: Agencies that are generally proprietary (for profit) and that charge a fee for service. The primary focus is curing illness.

Private pay: The patient pays out of pocket for services received.

Probing: Pushing for information beyond what is medically necessary to know.

Problem solving: A series of steps used to solve problems long before the nursing process was developed.

Problem-oriented thinking: Focus on a particular problem to find a solution (e.g., planning your school, work, and home schedule).

Projection: A coping or mental mechanism in which an individual attributes his or her own weaknesses to others.

Proprietary hospitals (for profit): For-profit hospitals.

Prospective payment system (PPS): A system in which the federal government announces to a hospital in advance what it will pay for health care costs.

Proximate cause: One of four elements needed to prove negligence. Refers to reasonable cause-and-effect relationship between omission and commission of nursing act and harm to patient.

Public health care agencies: Made up of official and voluntary health care agencies.

Purpose: Reason.

Q

Qualitative research study: Subjective study that gathers data as a narrative description of the "lived experience" of individuals.

Quantitative research study: Objective study that collects numerical data that are measured using statistics. Establishes a cause-effect relationship.

R

Rationalization: A coping or mental mechanism in which the individual offers a logical but untrue reason as an excuse for his or her behavior.

Receiver: Person receiving the message, idea, or question.

Reference hierarchy: Ranking of references from best to least by employers: current and former supervisors from work and volunteer experiences, unit managers, and teachers; workers who have seen your work; and personal references or friends.

Reference materials: Includes medical and nursing dictionaries, almanacs, yearbooks, atlases, encyclopedias, handbooks, and so on. Generally cannot be checked out, but needed material can be copied.

Referral: Send or direct for help.

Reflective thinking: Thinking about what you are thinking about.

Registered nurse (RN): A member of the nursing team who has gone to nursing school for two, three, or four years and has passed the National Council Licensure Examination-Registered Nurse (NCLEX-RN®) to be registered. The person on the nursing team who functions independently in decision making regarding the nursing care of patients.

Rehabilitation: After acute care is completed, treatment may continue to bring person up to maximum functioning.

Reincarnation: Belief in rebirth of the soul in many bodies as many times as necessary to achieve enlightenment.

Religion: Attempts to give form to spiritual beliefs by adopting specific beliefs and rituals.

Religious denomination: An organized group of persons with a philosophy that supports their particular concept of God.

Residency: Further "training" in nursing after initial schooling and licensure.

Residential care: Broadly defined as 24-hour supervision of persons, for reasons of age or impairments. Falls between skilled care and intermediate care facilities.

Resignation courtesy: A two-week notice of ending employment is considered courteous even if not part of the contract.

Respect: Consideration, regard.

Restructuring: Changing something that is not working out as planned.

Resume: Summary of what you have accomplished; work, skills, education, experience, and sometimes personal achievements. Used to persuade an employer that you are the right person for the job. Limit to one or two pages.

Returning adult learner: A learner in the age bracket of the mid-twenties or older who has entered an educational program and has not experienced formal education for a period of time.

Right-brain dominant: This person shows more advanced spatial relationships, recognizes negative emotions more quickly, is less verbal, adds tone and inflection to voice, and sees the total picture. Also called *global thinkers*.

Rituals: Religious practices that affirm believers' connection to a higher power.

Rosenstock's health belief theory: Attempts to explain why a person will or will not seek help to prevent or detect illness.

S

SBAR: A method of clear communication between nurses and physicians. S, situation; B, background; A, assessment; and R, recommendation.

Scope of practice: What the nurse is able to do legally.

Seacole, Mary: Black nurse from Jamaica, West Indies. Helped Florence Nightingale during the Crimean War. Used knowledge of tropical medicine, herbs, and natural plant medicines to treat soldiers with cholera, yellow fever, malaria, and diarrhea.

"Seamless" nursing systems: Provide progressive nursing programs without the need to repeat courses as the person goes from certified nursing assistant (CNA), to licensed practical nurse/licensed vocational nurse (LPN/LVN) to associate degree registered nurse (RN) to Bachelor of Science in Nursing (BSN) to Master of Science in Nursing (MSN) to Doctorate Degree in Nursing degrees; provide ease of movement from one nursing education program to another.

Self-directed learner: Takes responsibility for own learning and performance.

Self-esteem: Special sense that it is okay to receive credit for something you did well.

Self-evaluation: Objective look at personal performance with a plan for improvement.

Sender: Person conveying an idea or asking a question.

Sensitivity: Awareness of what others are feeling. Tunes in on affective and nonverbal communication.

Sexual harassment: A form of assault. Abuse of power. Not about sex or passion.

Silence: Avoid filling the interviewer's void of silence by providing information beyond what is needed.

Simple answer: General responses. Can be a communication block and discount the patient as a person.

Simulation: A learning activity that uses imaginary patient situations and mimics the reality of the clinical environment.

Sister Callista Roy's adaptation model: Describes the patient as a holistic adaptive system influenced by both internal and external stimuli.

Situational leadership: Varying the leadership style to meet the demands of the situation in the work environment.

Skill mix: Health care staff made up of workers with different levels of education and training.

Skilled nursing facility (SNF): Patients with more serious problems need a higher level of care by skilled and well-trained staff.

Slander: Damage to someone's reputation by verbalizing untrue or confidential information.

Social media: Ways of using the Internet for interactive dialogue, such as Facebook, Twitter, and LinkedIn.

Social networking: Gathering of individuals to share information; specifically used in this book as online communities.

Spatial learner: Learns best by studying diagrams, boxes, and special lists.

Specialized hospital: Offer services related to a particular disease or condition.

Spirit: Life force that penetrates the person's entire body. Gives meaning to life.

Spirit of inquiry: Trait of licensed practical nurses/licensed vocational nurses (LPNs/LVNs) that challenges traditional and existing practices and seeks creative approaches to problems.

Spiritual caring: Recognize and support spiritual need of the patient in the health care setting.

Spiritual dimension: That which gives insight into the person's meaning of life, suffering, and death.

Spiritual distress: Observed in patients who are unable to practice their rituals or seen in those who experience conflict between their religious or spiritual beliefs and prescribed medical regimen.

Spiritual needs: Requirements that arise out of the desire of human beings to find meaning in life, suffering, and death.

Spirituality: Pertaining to the soul, one's life force.

Stacks: Place in library where material that can be checked out is located.

Standards of care: What a prudent nurse is expected to do.

State board of nursing: Develops and enforces nurse practice act, which is the basis for nursing law. There is some variation among states.

Static simulation: Simulation that uses full-size body models or models of specific parts of the body made to be realistic.

Statutory law: Law developed by the legislative branch of state and federal governments.

Stem: First line of a multiple-choice item.

Stereotype: Casting all people in a culture as being the same in regard to thinking, feeling, and acting.

Stress management: Maintenance of stress at a moderate level. The reaction to both high and low levels of stress may be overwhelming.

Student nurse: Person involved in a course of study to become a nurse.

Study group: Peers who are actively involved in understanding information by discussing it in a small group.

Study skills lab: A place where schools provide services to assist a student with academic problems.

Subjective information: Information based on a patient's opinion.

Syllabus: Up-to-date course document distributed at the beginning of a course. This document usually includes a course description, course objectives, course requirements, required text, grading scale, and instructor information.

T

Taxonomy: Standardized, orderly, systematic language (example, NANDA-I).

Teaching: Originally thought of as lecturing to students. All responsibility was on the instructor. Current method equalizes responsibility between student and instructor and encourages a wide range of learning/teaching methods.

Teaching and research hospital: Private or public hospitals that focus on treating patients; training physicians, nurses, and other health professionals; and research and development.

Team method: A method of patient care in which small teams of nursing personnel are assigned to give total care to groups of patients.

The Joint Commission (TJC): Sets the standards of care for hospitals and long-term care agencies. Agencies receive accreditation if they elect to be reviewed and meet standards.

Therapeutic communication: Between the patient and the nurse. The focus is on the patient.

Third-party coverage: Health insurance.

Time management: The effective use of time to meet goals.

Total patient care: The registered nurse (RN) is responsible for all aspects of patient care: assessing, planning, organizing, and delivering patient care. This model is often used in critical care and specialty health care settings. This model generally does not use licensed practical nurses (LPNs) to provide nursing care.

Traditional adult learner: A learner who comes to an educational program directly from high school or from another program of study, usually in his or her late teens or early twenties.

Transitional practice model: Helps new graduate nurses transition from their educational program to the work environment.

Trust: Rely on, depend on.

Tutoring: Select study group. Student arranges for special help through instructor referral or self-referral.

Two-way communication: When there is feedback or discussion between the sender and receiver; the usual form of conversation.

U

Understanding: Comprehension. Able to recall and provide examples.

Unintentional torts: Nurse did not intend to injure patient. Negligence and malpractice are examples.

Unit manager: Has supervisor and management functions for patient units.

United Nations (UN): International organization that deals with world issues. Has representatives of many countries.

Unlicensed assistive personnel (UAP): Trained by health care organizations to function in an assistive role to registered nurses (RNs) and licensed practical nurses/licensed vocational nurses (LPNs/LVNs). Also known as patient care technicians, patient care associates, nurse extenders, and multiskilled workers.

U.S. Public Health Service (USPHS): Division of Department of Health and Human Services. Made up of six agencies.

V

Validate information: Verify data.

Values: Assigned to an idea or action. Freely chosen and affected by age, experience, and maturity.

Verbal communication: Sending or receiving communication through the spoken or written word.

Vertical violence: Occurs between persons of unequal power, for example, an instructor and a student.

Vicarious liability: Responsible for actions of another because of a special relationship with the other person.

Virtual clinical excursion: A real clinical experience simulated on a computer, including changing physician orders.

Visual learner: Generates visual images, that is, thinks primarily in pictures. Learns best by watching a demonstration first.

Visual/linguistic learner: Learns best through reading and writing.

Visual/spatial learner: Learns best through charts, demonstrations, videos, and other visual materials.

Voice control: Be aware of how your voice sounds. A well-modulated voice makes a better impression.

Voluntary health care agencies: Not-for-profit, nonofficial health care agencies that complement official health agencies and meet the needs of persons with a specific disease.

W

Wald, Lillian: Began Henry Street Settlement visiting nurse service in New York in 1893 to care for indigent persons.

Watson's theory of human care: Health is a harmony among body, mind, and spirit. It involves self-perception and how the self is experienced. Illness is a lack of harmony within the self and the soul.

Wellness and illness: Relative terms. Have different meanings for different cultures.

Wellness center: Promotes wellness. Includes nutritional counseling, exercise programs, stress reduction, and weight control programs.

World Health Organization (WHO): International health agency of the United Nations, located in Geneva.

Worldview: Shared by persons with same cultural background.

Reference List

CHAPTER 1

Billings, D., Halstead, J. (2009). *Teaching in nursing: A guide for faculty*. St. Louis: Elsevier/Saunders.

Halfer, D., Saver, C. (2008). Bridging the generation gaps. *Nursing Spectrum/Nurse Week*. <http://ce.nurse.com/course/ce478/bridging-the-generation-gaps/>.

Hartner, K. (2007). Generational diversity. *ADVANCE News magazines for LPNs*. <http://nursing.advanceweb.com/Article/Generational-Diversity.aspx>.

Mehallow, C. *Generational conflict in nursing: How to relate to colleagues across generations*. <http://career-advice.monster.com/in-the-office/workplace-issues/generational-conflict-in-nursing/article.aspx>. Accessed June 13, 2016.

Olson, M. (2009). The millennials: First year in practice. *Nursing Outlook*, 57(1), 10–17.

Riggs, C. (2013). Multiple generations in the nursing workplace: Part I. *The Journal of Continuing Education in Nursing*, 44(3), 105–106.

U.S. Department of Health and Human Services Health Resources and Services Administration. (2014). *The future of the nursing workforce: National and state level projections 2012-2025*. <http://bhpr.hrsa.gov/healthworkforce/supplydemand/nursing/workforceprojections/index.html>.

CHAPTER 2

Barsch Learning Style Inventory. (2015). <http://valenciacollege.edu/east/academicsuccess/spa/BarschLearningStyles.cfm>

Bixler, B. *Penn State Learning Style Inventory*. <www.personal.psu.edu/bxb11/LSI/LSI.htm>.

Brightman, H. (2015). *GSU master teacher program: on learning styles*. <www2.gsu.edu/~dschjb/wwwmbti.html>.

Chall, J. S. (1958). *Readability: An appraisal of research and application*. Columbus, OH: The Bureau of Educational Research, Ohio State University.

Gardner, H., Hatch, T. (1990). *Multiple intelligences go to school: Educational implications of the theory of multiple intelligences*. (Technical Report No. 4). New York: Center for Technology in Education.

Gardner, H. (1999). *Intelligence reframed: Multiple intelligences for the 21st century*. New York: Basic Books: Perseus Books Group.

Giles, E., Pitre, S., Womack, S. (2013). Multiple intelligences and learning styles. In: M. Orey (ed.), *Emerging perspectives on learning, teaching, and technology*. <http://epltt.coe.uga.edu/>.

Jensen, E. (1998). *The learning brain. Teaching with the brain in mind*. Alexandria, VA: Association for Supervision and Curriculum Development.

National Council of State Board of Nursing (NCSBN). (2014). *NCLEX PN Test Plan-Basic*. <www.ncsbn.org/3793.htm>. (need to update in chapter submitted).

Web Site Resources Cited

www.lucidchart.com
http://help4adhd.org

CHAPTER 3

Duffy, M. (2011). Facebook, Twitter, and LinkedIn, oh my! *American Journal of Nursing*, 111(4), 56–59.

National Council of State Board of Nursing (NCSBN). (2011). *A nurse's guide to the use of social media*. <www.ncsbn.org/3739.htm>

Web Site Resources Cited

allnurses.com
www.napnes.org
www.nflpn.org
nursegroups.com
http://ajnoffthecharts.com
www.practicalclinicalskills.com
http://www.nursingworld.org/socialnetworkingtoolkit.aspx

CHAPTER 4

Bolvin, J. *War on the mind, part 1: Nurses deployed in Iraq and Afghanistan struggle with PTSD*. <https://news.nurse.com/2010/10/04/war-on-the-mind-part-1-nurses-deployed-to-iraq-and-afghanistan-struggle-with-ptsd/>.

Carlson, M. *Women, the Unknown soldiers*. <www.deanza.edu/faculty/swensson/bestresearch_womensoldiers.html>.

Cherry, B., Jacob, S. (2011). *Contemporary nursing: Issues, trends, and management*. St. Louis: Elsevier.

Desch, E., Doherty, M. E. (2010). Experiences of U.S. military nurses in Iraq and Afghanistan wars, 2003-2009. *Nursing Scholarship*, 42(1), 3–12.

Halfer, D., Saver, C. (2008). Bridging the generation gaps. *Nursing Spectrum/Nurse Week*. <http://ce.nurse.com/course/ce478/bridging-the-generation-gaps/>

Hartner, K. (2007). Generational diversity. *ADVANCE Newsmagazines for LPNs*, <http://nursing.advanceweb.com/Article/Generational-Diversity.aspx>.

Institute of Medicine (IOM). (2010). *Future of nursing: Leading change, advancing health*. Washington, DC: The National Academies Press, <www.iom.edu/Reports/2010/The-future-of-nursing-leading-change-advancing-health.aspx>.

Kalish, P., Kalish, B. (1995). *The advance of American nursing* (3rd ed.). Boston: Little, Brown.

LeVasseur, J. (1998). Plato, Nightingale, and contemporary nursing. *IMAGE: Journal of Nursing Scholarship*, 30(3), 281–285.

Martinez, O. L. (2010). *The Honor Society of Vietnam War Nurses*. <www.experienceproject.com/stories/Am-A-Registered-Nurse/1005174>.

Mehallow, C. *Generational conflict in nursing: how to relate to colleagues across generations*. <http://career-advice.monster.com/in-the-office/Workplace-Issues/Generational-Conflict-in-Nursing/article.aspx>. Accessed June 13, 2016.

National Black Nurse's Association (NBNA) Mission. (2015). <www.nbna.org/mission>.

National League for Nursing. (2014). *A vision for recognition of the role of the Licensed Practical/Licensed Vocational Nurses in advancing the nation's health*. <www.nln.org/about/position-statements/nln-living-documents>.

Olson, M. (2009). The millennials: First year in practice. *Nursing Outlook*, 57(1), 10–17.

Riggs, C. (2013). Multiple generations in the nursing workplace: Part I. *The Journal of Continuing Education in Nursing*, 44(3), 105–106.

Romanoff, B. (2006). Facts about Flo you may not know. *Nurse Week*, 7(3), 32–33.

U.S. Department of Health and Human Services Health Resources and Services Administration. (2013). *The U.S. nursing workforce: Trends in supply and education*. <http://bhpr.hrsa.gov/healthworkforce/supplydemand/nursing/nursing-workforce/nursingworkforcefullreport.pdf>.

Wilson, B. (2011). *Women in the Korean conflict. Women in war.* <http://userpages.aug.com/captbarb/femvets6.html>.

CHAPTER 5

Alfaro-LeFevre, R. (2006). *Critical thinking indicators.* <www.AlfaroTeachSmart.com>.

Alfaro-Lefevre, R. (2009). *Critical thinking and clinical judgement: A practical approach* (4th ed.). Philadelphia: WB Saunders.

Alfaro-Lefevre, R. (2013). *Critical thinking and clinical judgement: A practical approach* (5th ed.). Philadelphia: WB Saunders.

Bureau of Labor Statistics, U.S. Department of Labor, U.S. (2014). *Women in the labor force: A databook.* <www.bls.gov/opub/reports/cps/womenlaborforce_2013.pdf>.

Ignatavicius, D, Workman, M. L. (2013). *Medical surgical nursing* (7th ed.). Philadelphia: WB Saunders.

National Council of State Boards of Nursing. (2014). *NCLEX-PN examination test plan for the National Council Licensure Examination for licensed practical/vocational nurse.* Chicago: NCSBN. <www.ncsbn.org/3778.htm>.

Project Implicit. (2015). <https://implicit.harvard.edu/implicit/>.

Silvestri, L. A. (2012). *Saunders Q and A Review for NCLEX-PN® Examination.* Philadelphia: WB Saunders.

Web Site Resources Cited

www.ncsbn.org

CHAPTER 6

Bureau of Labor Statistics, U.S. (2014). Department of Labor. *Highlights of women's earnings in 2013.* <www.bls.gov/opub/reports/cps/highlights-of-womens-earnings-in-2013.pdf>.

Mosby. (2012). *Mosby Dictionary of Medicine, Nursing & Health Professions.* St. Louis: Elsevier.

Rumbold, G. (2002). *Ethics in nursing practice.* Edinburgh: Elsevier Science Ltd.

Ulrich, B. (1992). *Leadership and management according to Florence Nightingale.* Norwalk, CT: Appleton and Lange.

World Health Organization. (2015). *Baby-friendly hospital initiative.* <www.who.int/nutrition/topics/bfhi/en/>.

CHAPTER 7

American Association of Retired Persons (AARP). (2015). *FAQ about estate planning.* <www.aarp.org/money/estate-planning/info-03-2009/faq_power_of_attorney.html>.

American Cancer Society (ACS). (2015). *Patient self determination act.* <www.cancer.org/treatment/findingandpayingfortreatment/understandingfinancialandlegalmatters/advancedirectives/advance-directives-patient-self-determination-act>.

American Hospital Association. (2003). *The patient care partnership.* <www.aha.org/advocacy-issues/communicatingpts/pt-care-partnership.shtml>.

American Nurses Association. (2005). *Joint ANA and National Council of State Boards of nursing position statement.* <www.nursingworld.org/MainMenuCategories/Policy-Advocacy/Positions-and-Resolutions/ANAPositionStatements/Position-Statements-Alphabetically/Joint-Statement-on-Delegation-American-Nurses-Association-ANA-and-National-Council-of-State-Boards.html>.

American Nurses Association. (2013). *Euthanasia, assisted suicide, and aid in dying.* <www.nursingworld.org/euthanasiaanddying>.

Brent, N. J. (2001). *Nurses and the law: A guide to principles and applications* (2nd ed.). Philadelphia: Saunders. 58–59.

California Health Care Foundation. (2012). *Conversation project.* <http://theconversationproject.org>.

Christensen, E, Kokrow, B. (2011). *Foundations of adult health nursing* (6th ed.) St. Louis: Mosby.

Death with Dignity National Center. (2015). *Death with dignity around the US.* <www.deathwithdignity.org/advocates/national>.

Institute of Medicine (IOM) (2008). *Report Brief. Retooling for an aging America: Building the health care workforce.* National Academy of Sciences http://www.nationalacademies.org/hmd/~/media/Files/Report%20Files/2008/Retooling-for-an-Aging-America-Building-the-Health-Care-Workforce/ReportBriefRetoolingforanAgingAmericaBuildingtheHealthCareWorkforce.pdf

Institute of Medicine (IOM). (2010). *Future of nursing: Leading change, advancing health.* Washington, DC: The National Academies Press. <www.iom.edu/Reports/2010/The-future-of-nursing-leading-change-advancing health.aspx>.

National Association for Practical Nurse Education and Service. (2003). *NAPNES Standards of practice for Licensed Practical/Vocational Nurses.* Silver Spring, MD: author.

National Council of State Boards of Nursing. (2010). *Boards of nursing complaint process.* <www.ncsbn.org/transcript_BON_Complaint_Process.pdf>.

National Council of State Board of Nursing (NCSBN). (2011). *A Nurse's Guide to the Use of Social Media.* <www.ncsbn.org/3739.htm>.

National Council of State Boards of Nursing. (2015). *Nurse licensure compact.* <www.ncsbn.org/nurse-licensure-compact.htm>.

National Institutes of Health. (2014). Med Line Plus. *Advanced directives.* <www.nlm.nih.gov/medlineplus/advancedirectives.html>.

National League for Nursing. (2014). *A vision for recognition of the role of the Licensed Practical/Licensed Vocational Nurses in advancing the nation's health.* <www.nln.org/about/position-statements/nln-living-documents>.

Oregon Health Authority. (2014). *Death with dignity act.* <http://public.health.oregon.gov/ProviderPartnerResources/EvaluationResearch/DeathwithDignityAct/Pages/index.aspx>.

Pennsylvania Department of State. (2015). *Title 4, Chapter 2.* <www.pacode.com/secure/data/049/chapter21/s21.141.html>.

Starks, H., Dudzinski, D., White, N. (2013). (Original text written by Braddock, C., & Tonelli, M. [1998]) *Physician aid in dying.* <http://depts.washington.edu/bioethx/topics/pas.html>.

Society for Human Resource Management. (2014). *Good Samaritan laws.* <www.shrm.org/legalissues/stateandlocalresources/stateandlocalstatutesandregulations/documents/goodsamaritanlaws.pdf>.

The Joint Commission. (2015). *National patient safety goals.* <www.jointcommission.org/standards_information/npsgs.aspx>.

The National Association for Home Care and Hospice. (2015). *Hospice Association of America.* <www.nahc.org/haa/consumer-information/>.

Watson, E. (2014). Nursing malpractice: Costs, trends, and issues. *Journal of Legal Nurse Consulting*, 25(1), 26–33.

Weydt, A. (2010). Developing delegation skills. *The Online Journal of Issues in Nursing*, 15(2), Manuscript 1.

CHAPTER 8

Arnold, E., Boggs, K. U. (2003). *Interpersonal relationships: professional communication skills for nurses* (4th ed.). Philadelphia: WB Saunders.

Cherry, B., Jacob, S. (2014). *Contemporary nursing: Issues, trends, and management.* St. Louis: Mosby.

Cuddy, A. (2012). *TED Talk.* <www.ted.com/talks/amy_cuddy_your_body_language_shapes_who_you_are?language=en>.

National Council State Board of Nursing. (2015). *Transition to practice (TTP) toolkit.* <www.ncsbn.org/687.htm>.

National Council State Board of Nursing. (2015). *Communication and teamwork module (TEAMSTEPPS).* <www.ncsbn.org>.

National League for Nursing. (2015). *ACE.S.* <www.nln.org/professional-development-programs/teaching-resources/aging>.

Pagana, K. (2008). *The nurse's etiquette advantage.* Indianapolis, IN: Sigma.

CHAPTER 9

Belanger, D. (2000). Nurses and suicide: The risk is real. *RN,* 63(10), 61–64.

Cuddy, A. (2012). *TED Talk.* <www.ted.com/talks/amy_cuddy_your_body_language_shapes_who_you_are?language=en>.

Jahner, J. (2011). *Building bridges: An inquiry into horizontal hostility in nursing culture and the use of contemplative practices to facilitate cultural change.* <www.upaya.org/uploads/pdfs/Jahnersthesis.pdf>.

Knecht, P. (2014). *Demystifying job satisfaction in long-term care: The voices of licensed practical nurses. ProQuest Digital Dissertations.* The Pennsylvania State University. <http://gradworks.umi.com/35/83/3583372.html>.

Kurz, J. (2002). Combating sexual harassment. *RN,* 65(7), 65–68.

Occupational Safety and Health Administration. (2015). *Guidelines for preventing workforce violence for health care and social service workers.* <www.osha.gov/Publications/osha3148.pdf>.

PACERS. (2015). *Stop bullying tool kit.* <http://stopbullyingtoolkit.org>. Retrieved June 13, 2016.

Romano, S. J, Levi-Minzi, M. E, Rugala, E. A., et al. (2011). Workplace violence prevention: Readiness and response. *FBI Law Enforcement Bulletin,* 80(1), 1–10.

Spector, P. E, Zhou, Z. E, Xin Xuan, C. (2014). Nurse exposure to physical and nonphysical violence, bullying, and sexual harassment: A quantitative review. *International Journal of Nursing Studies,* 51(1), 72–84.

Speroni, K. G, Fitch, T., Dawson, E., et al. (2014). Incidence and cost of nurse workplace violence perpetrated by hospital patients or patient visitors. *Journal of Emergency Nursing,* 40(3), 218–228.

CHAPTER 10

Cherry, B., Jacob, S. (2014). *Contemporary nursing: Issues, trends, and management.* St. Louis: Mosby.

D'Avanzo, C., Geissler, E. (2008). *Pocket guide to cultural assessment.* St. Louis: Mosby.

Douglas, M. K, Pierce, J. U., Rosenkoetter, M., et al. (2011). Standards of practice for culturally competent nursing care: 2011 update. *Journal of Transcultural Nursing,* 22(4), 317–333.

Giger, J., Davidhizar, R. (1990). Transcultural nursing assessment: A method for advancing practice. *International Nursing Review,* 37(1), 199–203.

Giger, J., Davidhizar, R. (2008). The Giger and Davidhizar Transcultural Assessment Model. *Journal of Transcultural Nursing,* 13, 185–188.

Giger, J. (2013). *Transcultural nursing, assessment & intervention.* St. Louis: Elsevier.

Jackson, L. (1993). Understanding, eliciting and negotiating patients' multicultural health beliefs. *Nurse Pract,* 18(4), 30–32, 37–43.

Kutner, M., Greenberg, E., Jin, Y., Paulsen, C. (2006). *The health literacy of America's adults: Results from the 2003 National Assessment of Health Literacy.* Washington, DC: National Center for Education Statistics. <https://nces.ed.gov/pubs2006/2006483.pdf>.

Lipson, J., Dibble, S. (2006). *Culture and nursing care: A pocket guide.* San Francisco: The Regents of the University of California.

Project Implicit. (2011). <https://implicit.harvard.edu/implicit/>. Accessed June 13, 2016.

Reinhardt, E. (1995). *Through the eyes of others—Intercultural resource directory for health care professionals.* Minneapolis: Hennepin County Medical Society, United Way Intercultural Awareness.

U.S. Department of Health and Human Services. (2013). *Enhanced National CLAS Standards.* <www.thinkculturalhealth.hhs.gov/Content/clas.asp>.

U.S. Census Bureau. (2010). *US Census bureau predicts that minorities will make up 55% of the US population by 2025.*

World Bank. (2015). *Population growth rate.* <www.worldbank.org/depweb/english/modules/social/pgr/chart1a.html>.

Yen, H. (2011). New York: *Census estimates show big gains for U.S. minorities.* Associated Press. <http://www.wcpo.com/news/national/census-estimates-show-big-gains-for-us-minorities>. Accessed June13, 2016.

Web Site Resources Cited

www.nccam.nih.gov.

www.dimensionsofculture.com.

www.thinkculturalhealth.hhs.gov/Content/clas.asp.

www.jointcommission.org/Advancing_Effective_Communication/.

www.dimensionsofculture.com/2010/10/traditional-asian-health-beliefs-healing practices/.

www.dimensionsofculture.com/2010/10/folk-illnesses-and-remedies-in-latino-communities/.

www.cancer.org/treatment/treatmentsandsideeffects/complementaryandalternativemedicine/mindbodyandspirit/curanderismo.

www.minoritynurse.com/about/index.html.

CHAPTER 11

Carson, V. (1989). *Spiritual dimensions of nursing practice.* Philadelphia: WB Saunders.

Delgado, D. A., Ness, S., Ferguson, K., et al. (2013). Cultural competence training for clinical staff: Measuring the effect of a one-hour class on cultural competence. *Journal of Transcultural Nursing,* 24(2), 204–213.

Esposito, J. (1998). *Islam: The straight path.* New York: Oxford University Press.

Friends. (2011). Religious Society of *The Columbia Electronic Encyclopedia* (6th ed.). Columbia University Press. <www.infoplease.com/ce6/society/A0819726.html>.

Gellman, M., Hartman, T. (2002). *Religion for dummies.* New York: Wiley.

Giger, J. (2013). *Transcultural nursing, assessment & intervention.* St. Louis: Elsevier.

Gritsch, E. (2002). *A history of Lutheranism.* Minneapolis: Augsburg Fortress.

International Council of Nurses. (2013). *Vision for the future of nurses.* <www.icn.ch/who-we-are/icns-vision-for-the-future-of-nursing/>.

The Joint Commission. (2008). *Standards FAQ – Spiritual assessment.* <www.jointcommission.org/standards_information/jcfaqdetails.aspx?StandardsFaqId=290&ProgramId=47>.

Kosmin, B., Keysar, A. (2009). *American Religious Identification Survey.* <http://commons.trincoll.edu/aris/files/2011/08/ARIS_Report_2008.pdf>.

Lipson, J., Dibble, S. (2006). *Culture and nursing care: a pocket guide.* San Francisco: The Regents of the University of California.

North American Nursing Diagnosis Association (NANDA). (2015). *Nursing diagnoses: 2015–2017.* <www.nanda.org>.

Web Site Resources Cited

www.beliefnet.com

CHAPTER 12

Corazzini, K. N., Anderson, R. A., Mueller, C., et al. (2013). Licensed practical nurse scope of practice and quality of nursing home care. *Nursing Research*, 62(5), 315–324.

Johnson, M., Bulechek, G., Dochterman, J., et al. (2006). *Nursing diagnoses, outcomes, and interventions: NANDA, NOC and NIC Linkages* (2nd ed.). St. Louis: Mosby.

Johnson, M., Maas, M., Moorhead, S. (2000). *Nursing outcomes classification (NOC)* (2nd ed.). St. Louis: Mosby.

National Council of State Boards of Nursing. (2014). *2014 NCLEX-PN examination test plan for the National Council Licensure Examination for licensed practical/vocational nurse*. Chicago: NCSBN. <www.ncsbn.org>.

Nightingale, F. (1860). *Notes on nursing: What it is and what it is not*. New York: D. Appleton and Company.

North American Nursing Diagnosis Association (NANDA). (2008). *International Journal of Nursing Terminologies and Classifications*. <www.nanda.org>.

Peseit, D. J., Herman, J. (1998). OPT: Transformation of nursing process for contemporary practice. *Nursing Outlook*, 46(1), 29–36.

CHAPTER 13

Ackley, B. J., Ladwig, G. B., Swan, B. A., Tucker, S. J. (2008). *Evidence-based nursing care guidelines*. St. Louis: Elsevier/Mosby.

Cherry, B., Jacob, S. (2011). *Contemporary nursing: Issues, trends, and management*. St. Louis: Mosby, Inc.

Institute of Medicine (IOM). (2001). *Report brief: Crossing the quality chasm: A new health system for the 21st century*. <www.iom.edu/Reports/2001/Crossing-the-Quality-Chasm-A-New-Health-System-for-the-21st-Century.aspx>.

Institute of Medicine (IOM). (1999). *Report brief: To err is human: Building a safer health care system*. <http://iom.edu/Reports/1999/To-Err-is-Human-Building-A-Safer-Health-System.aspx>.

Koh, H., Sebelius, K. (2010). Promoting prevention through the Affordable Care Act. *New England Journal of Medicine*, 363, 1296–1299.

National League for Nursing. (2015). *Practical/Vocational nursing program outcomes*. <www.nln.org/professional-development-programs/teaching-resources/practical-nursing>.

CHAPTER 14

Aiken. L. H., Clarke, S. P., Sloane, D. M., et al. (2008). Effects of hospital care environment on patient mortality and nurse outcomes. *Journal of Nursing Administration*, 38(5), 223–229.

Buerhaus, P., Auerbach, D. (2011). The recession's effect on hospital registered nurse employment growth. *Nursing Economics*, 29(4), 163–167.

Bureau of Labor Statistics, U.S. Department of Labor. (2013). *Occupations with the most job growth, 2012 and projected 2022*. <www.bls.gov/news.release/ecopro.t05.htm>.

Bureau of Labor Statistics, U.S. Department of Labor. (2016). *Occupational outlook handbook, Licensed Practical and Licensed Vocational Nurses, 2016–2017 edition*. <http://www.bls.gov/ooh/healthcare/licensed-practical-and-licensed-vocational-nurses.htm>.

Henderson, V. (1966). *The nature of nursing: a definition and its implications for practice, research and education*. New York: MacMillan.

National League for Nursing. (2013). *A vision for doctoral education for nurse educators*. <www.nln.org/docs/default-source/about/nln-vision-series-(position-statements)/nlnvision_6.pdf>.

National League for Nursing. (2014). *A vision for recognition of the role of the Licensed Practical/Licensed Vocational Nurses in advancing the nation's health*. <www.nln.org/about/position-statements/nln-living-documents>.

Tri-Council for Nursing. (2010). *Educational advancement of registered nurses: A consensus position*. <www.aacn.nche.edu/education-resources/TricouncilEdStatement.pdf>.

U.S. Department of Health and Human Services Health Resources and Services Administration. (2014). *The future of the nursing workforce: National and state level projections 2012 -2025*. <http://bhpr.hrsa.gov/healthworkforce/supplydemand/nursing/workforceprojections/nursingprojections.pdf>.

U.S. Department of Health and Human Services Health Resources and Services Administration. (2013). *The US nursing workforce: Trends in supply and education*. <http://bhpr.hrsa.gov/healthworkforce/supplydemand/nursing/nursingworkforce/nursingworkforcefullreport.pdf>.

Web Site Resources Cited

www.iom.edu/About-IOM.aspx.
www.aacn.org
www.nursingworld.org/EspeciallyForYou/What-is-Nursing
www.icn.ch/who-we-are/icn-definition-of-nursing/

CHAPTER 15

Christensen, E., Kokrow, B. (2011). *Foundations of adult health nursing* (6th ed.). St. Louis: Mosby.

Health Forum. (2015). *American Hospital Association 2013 annual survey*. <www.aha.org/research/rc/stat-studies/fast-facts.shtml>.

Web Site Resources Cited

aarp.org
www.hhs.gov
www.hrsa.gov
www.longtermcarelink.net/eldercare/long_term_care.htm
www.medicare.gov/coverage/skilled-nursing-facility-care.html
www.longtermcarelink.net/eldercare/long_term_care.htm

CHAPTER 16

Cherry, B., Jacob, S. (2014). *Contemporary nursing: Issues, trends, and management*. St. Louis: Mosby.

Institute of Medicine (IOM). (2010). *Future of nursing: Leading change, advancing health*. Washington, DC: The National Academies Press. <www.iom.edu/Reports/2010/The-future-of-nursing-leading-change-advancing health.aspx>.

Institute of Medicine (IOM). (2008). *Report Brief Retooling for an aging America: Building the health care workforce*. Washington, DC: National Academy of Aciences http://www.nationalacademies.org/hmd/~/media/Files/Report%20Files/2008/Retooling-for-an-Aging-America-Building-the-Health-Care-Workforce/ReportBriefRetoolingforanAgingAmericaBuildingtheHealthCareWorkforce.pdf.

Institute of Medicine (IOM). (2001). *Report brief: Crossing the quality chasm: A new health system for the 21st century*. <www.iom.edu/Reports/2001/Crossing-the-Quality-Chasm-A-New-Health-System-for-the-21st-Century.aspx>.

Institute of Medicine (IOM). (1999). *Report brief: To err is human: Building a safer health care system*. <http://iom.edu/Reports/1999/To-Err-is-Human-Building-A-Safer-Health-System.aspx>.

The Joint Commission. (2011). *National patient safety goals*. <www.jointcommission.org/assets/1/6/2015_NPSG_LT2.pdf>.

The Kaiser Family Foundation. (2015). *Health reform quiz*. <http://kff.org/quiz/health-reform-quiz/>.

The Kaiser Family Foundation. (2015). *Medicare beneficiaries*.

Knecht, P. (2014). *Demystifying job satisfaction in long-term care: The voices of licensed practical nurses*. ProQuest Digital Dissertations. The Pennsylvania State University. <http://gradworks.umi.com/35/83/3583372.html>.

Knecht, P., Sosik, J. J. (2012). *Institute of Business and Management Conference (IBAM) Transformational leadership of nurses in long-term care: Propositions and implications for practice.*

Kovner, C., Spetz, J. (2011). The future of nursing: An interview with Susan B. Hassmiller. *Medscape.* <www.medscape.com?viewarticle/739963_print>.

Medicare and You 2012. (2012). *(CMS Publication Product Number 10050-24).* Baltimore, MD: U.S. Department of Health and Human Services. <http://healthreform.kff.org/faq/how-does-law-change-the-medicare-part-d-donut-hole.aspx>.

Smith, J., Medalia, C. (2014). *U.S. Census Bureau, Current Population Reports, P60-250, Health insurance coverage in the United States.* Washington, DC: U.S. Government Printing Office.

Websites Resources Cited

www.medicare.gov
www.medicaid.gov
www.healthcare.gov
http://www.ahrq.gov
www.cms.gov
www.jointcommission.org/PatientSafety Goals
www.npsf.org
www.ncsbn.org/6889
www.va.gov

CHAPTER 17

American Nurses Association. (2015). *Joint ANA and National Council of State Boards of Nursing position statement.* <www.nursingworld.org/MainMenuCategories/Policy-Advocacy/Positions-and-Resolutions/ANAPositionStatements/Position-Statements-Alphabetically/Joint-Statement-on-Delegation-American-Nurses-Association-ANA-and-National-Council-of-State-Boards.html>.

Bass, B. M. (1985). *Leadership and performance beyond expectations.* New York: Free Press.

Bass, B. M. (2008). *The Bass handbook of leadership – Theory, research and managerial applications.* New York: Free Press.

Blanchard, K., Zigarmi, P., Zigarmi, D. (1994). *Leadership and the one-minute manager.* UK: Clays Ltd.

Ellis, A. (1994). *Reason and emotion in psychotherapy.* New York: Carol Publishing Group.

Grumet, J. (June 12, 2005). Effective delegation. *Nursing Management,* 50–60.

Frantz, A. (1998). Nursing pride: Clara Barton in the Spanish-American War. *American Journal of Nursing,* 98(10), 39–41.

Herzberg, F., Mausner, B., Snyderman, B. (1959). *The motivation to work.* New York: John Wiley.

National Council State Board of Nursing. (2013). *2012 LPN/VN practice analysis: Linking the NCLEX-PN examination to practice.* <www.ncsbn.org/4313.htm?iframe=true&width=500&height=270>.

National Association for Practical Nurse Education and Service. (2007). Standards of practice and educational competencies of graduates of practical/vocational nursing programs. *Journal of Practical Nursing,* 57(2), 20–22.

National Council of State Boards of Nursing. (1998). *Implementation of the 1999 NCLEX-PN® test plan.* In *Issues.* Chicago: NCSBN. (pp. 4–5)

National Council of State Boards of Nursing. (2007). *NCLEX-PN® test plan for the National Council Licensure Examination for Practical Nurses.* Chicago: NCSBN.

National Council of State Boards of Nursing. (2010). *NCLEX-PN® test plan for the National Council Licensure Examination for Practical/Vocational Nurses.* Chicago: NCSBN.

National Council of State Boards of Nursing. (2005). *ANA and NCSBN joint statement on delegation.* Chicago: IL.

National Federation of Licensed Practical Nurses. (2003). *Nursing practice standards for the Licensed Practical/Vocational Nurse.* <www.nflpn.org>.

Nightingale, F. (2009). *Notes on nursing.* New York: Fall River Press.

Residents Bill of Rights. <www.forltc.org/nhrbillrights.html>.

Sosik, J. J, Jung, D. I. (2010). *Full range leadership development: Pathways for people, profit and planet.* New York: Routledge.

Wong, C, Cummings, G. (2007). The relationship between nursing leadership and patient outcomes: A systematic review. *Journal of Nursing Management,* 15(5), 508–521.

Web Site Resources Cited

www.jointcommission.org.
www.cms.gov
www.napnes.org
www.nflpn.org

CHAPTER 18

American Health Care Association. (2011). *LTC stats: Nursing facility operationalcharacteristics report, December 2011 update.* Washington DC: author.

Barry, D. (2011). *A milestone for baby boomers, 65 years in the making.* New York: New York Times. <http://www.nytimes.com/2011/01/01/us/01boomers.html?_r=0>.

Beshara, T. (2008). *Acing the Interview: How to Ask and Answer the Questions That Will Get You the Job.* New York: AMACON.

Bureau of Labor Statistics, U.S. Department of Labor. (2016). *Occupational outlook handbook, Licensed Practical and Licensed Vocational Nurses, 2016–2017 edition.* <http://www.bls.gov/ooh/healthcare/licensed-practical-and-licensed-vocational-nurses.htm>.

Institute of Medicine (IOM). Committee on the Future Health Care Workforce for Older Americans. (2005). *Retooling for an aging America: Building the health care workforce.* Washington, DC: The National Academies Press. <www.nap.edu/catalog.php?record_id=12089>.

Institute of Medicine (IOM). (2010). *Future of nursing: Leading change, advancing health.* Washington, DC: The National Academies Press. <www.iom.edu/Reports/2010/The-future-of-nursing-leading-change advancing health.aspx>.

National Council State Board of Nursing (NCSBN). (2013). *2012 LPN/VN practice analysis: Linking the NCLEX-PN examination to practice.* <www.ncsbn.org/4313.htm?iframe=true&width=500&height=270>.

National Council of State Boards of Nursing (NCSBN). (1998). *Implementation of the 1999 NCLEX-PN test plan. Issues.* Chicago: NCSBN.

National Council of State Boards of Nursing (NCSBN). (2007). *NCLEX-PN® test plan for the National Council Licensure Examination for Practical/Vocational Nurses.* Chicago: NCSBN.

National Council of State Boards of Nursing (NCSBN). (2010). *NCLEX-PN® test plan for the National Council Licensure Examination for Practical/Vocational Nurses.* Chicago: NCSBN.

National Council of State Board of Nursing (NCSBN). (2011). *A nurse's guide to the use of social media.* <www.ncsb.org>.

National League for Nursing. (2014). *A vision for recognition of the role of the Licensed Practical/Licensed Vocational Nurses in advancing the nation's health.* <www.nln.org/about/position-statements/nln-living-documents>.

Pyrtle, B. (2014). Tips to recognize scam job ads. Minneapolis: *Star Tribune.* Section W., WI.

U.S. Department of Health and Human Services Health Resources and Services Administration. (2013). *The US nursing workforce: Trends in supply and education.* <http://bhpr.hrsa.gov/healthworkforce/supplydemand/nursing/nursingworkforce/nursingworkforcefullreport.pdf>.

Web Site Resources Cited

www.napnes.org
www.nflpn.org
www.abmcn.org
www.mycareeratva.va.gov/careers/career/062000
www.paworkstats.state.pa.us.
www.linkedin.com

www.simplyhired.com

www.indeed.com

www.jobvite.co

twitter.com

www.facebook.com

www.careerbuilder.com

www.healthcarefinancenews.com

www.abyznewslinks.com

www.employmentguide.com/job-fairs/browse

www.resumehelp.com/home-1?utm_source=bing%
20&utm_medium=cpc&utm_keyword=%2Bresume%
20%2Btemplates

www.resumetemplates.org/

owl.english.purdue.edu/owl/resource/719/1/

www.ncsbn.org

www.shrm.org

www.ncsbn.org/transition-to-practice.htm

http://howtopodcasttutorial.com

www.Medscape.com.

www.napnes.org/certifications/index.htm

www.nflpn.org/certification.html.

www.abmcn.org

www.excelsior.edu.

www.bls.gov/oes/current/oessrcst.htm

www.careerowl.com

www.salary.com;   www1.salary.com/Licensed-Practical-Nurse-
salary.html. www.payscale.com/research/US/Job=Licensed_
Practical_Nurse_(LPN)/Salary www.glassdoor.com/Salaries/
licensed-practical-nurse-salary-SRCH_KO0,24.htm. www.bls.gov.
http://swz.salary.com/CostOfLivingWizard/LayoutScripts/
Coll_Start.aspx to

CHAPTER 19

Corazzini, K. N., Anderson, R. A., Mueller, C., et al. (2013). Licensed practical nurse scope of practice and quality of nursing home care. *Nursing Research, 62*(5), 315–324.

National Council of State Boards of Nursing (NCSBN). (2016). *2016 NCLEX-PN® Examination Candidate Bulletin.* <www.ncsbn.org/089900_2016_Bulletin_Proof3.pdf>.

National Council of State Boards of Nursing (NCSBN). (2014). *2014 NCLEX-PN® examination test plan for the National Council Licensure Examination for licensed practical/vocational nurse.* Chicago: NCSBN. <www.ncsbn.org>.

National Council of State Boards of Nursing (NCSBN). (2014). *Report of findings from the 2014 LPN/LVN practice analysis: Linking the NCLEX-PN® examination to practice.* <www.ncsbn.org>.

National Council of State Boards of Nursing (NCSBN). (2015). *Nurse practice act rules and regulations.* <www.ncsbn.org/nurse-practice-act.htm>.

Web Site Resources Cited

https://portal.ncsbn.org

Suggested Readings

CHAPTER 1

American Council on Exercise. (2007). <www.acefitness.org/acefit/exercise-library-main/>.

Aleccia, J. (2008). *Hey, doc, wash your hands: Patients shouldn't be shy about asking providers to hit the sink, experts say.* <www.msnbc.com/id/22827499/print1./displaymode/1098/>.

Cohen, E. (2011). *The chart.* <http://thechart.blogs.cnn.com/2011/04/14/the-gruesome-math-of-hospital-infections/>.

Center for Advancing Heath. (2014). *Obese employers cost employers thousands in extra medical costs.* <www.cfah.org/hbns/2014/obese-employees-cost-employers-thousands-in-extra-medical-costs>.

Baxley, S, Ibitayo, K. (2009). *De-stress for success!* <www.reflectionsonnursingleadership.org/Pages/Vol35_1_Baxley_Ibitayo.aspx>.

Beattie, M. (1992). *Codependent no more: How to stop controlling others and start caring for yourself.* Center City, MN: Hazelton.

Billings, D, Halstead, J. (2009). *Teaching in nursing: A guide for faculty.* St. Louis: Elsevier/Saunders.

Borrello, S. (2011). Nursing as a second career. *Nursing Made Incredibly Easy,* 9(1), 6–7.

(2015). *Burnout: Signs, symptoms, and burnout recovery.* <http://proactivechange.com/stress/burnout.htm>.

Calfee, D. (2009). *Emergence of carbapenem-resistant* Klebsiella pneumoniae *as a significant healthcare-associated pathogen.* Presented at Jacksonville, FL.

Centers for Disease Control and Prevention (CDC). (2009). *General information on hand hygiene.* <www.cdc.gov/nceh/vsp/cruiselines/hand_hygiene_general.htm>.

Centers for Disease Control and Prevention (CDC). (2016). *Handwashing: Clean hands save lives.* <www.cdc.gov/handwashing/>.

Chenevert, M. (2011). *Mosby's tour guide to nursing school: A student's road survival kit.* St Louis: Mosby.

Cohen, M. (2008). The next best thing. *Real Simple,* 173–178.

Converso, A, Murphy, C. (2004). Winning the battle against back injuries. *RN,* 67(2), 52–57.

Delahanty, K, Myers, F. (2010). 3 bad bugs. *Nursing,* 40(3), 24–30.

DeNoon, D. (2010). *Healthy aging center hospital infections kill 48,000 each year.*

DeNoon, D. (2010). *USDA ditches Food Pyramid for a Healthy Plate.* <www.medscape.com/viewarticle/743889>.

deWit, S. (2015). *Saunders student nurse planner: A guide to success in nursing school.* Philadelphia: Elsevier Saunders.

Dietary Guidelines for Americans 2010. USDA and HHS.

Dunbar, D. (2006). Infection squads. *Nurs Spectr.*

Dunbar, S, Levitt, S. (Sept 24, 2006). Freakonomics: Selling soap. *The New York Times.* <www.nytimes.com/2006/09/24/magazine/24wwln_freak.html>

Edmunds, M, Scudder, L. (2009). *Do nurses practice what they preach?* <www.medscape.com/viewarticle/712966>.

Emery, C. (2006). *Simple measures to reduce infections: Hopkins study finds catheter rules, clean hands aid hospitals.* <http://articles.baltimoresun.com/2006-12-28/news/0612280018_1_infections-johns-hopkins-patient-safety>.

Galbraith, M. (2003). *Adult learning methods: A guide for effective instruction.* Melbourne, FL: Krieger Publishing.

Gerber, S. (2009). *Public health and long-term care: A cautionary tale.* Chicago: Cook County Department of Public Health.

Goldman, D. (2006). System failure versus personal accountability: The case for clean hands. *N Engl J Med,* 355(2), 121–123.

Haas, J, Larson, E. (2008). Compliance with hand hygiene. *American Journal of Nursing,* 108(8), 40–44.

Hislop, J. (2010). Paper chart nurse. *American Journal of Nursing,* 110(10), 72.

Keepnews, D. M, Brewer, C. S, Kovner, C. T, Shin, J. H. (2010). Generational differences among newly licensed registered nurses. *Nursing Outlook,* 58(3), 155–163.

Knowles, M, Holton, E, Swanson, R. (2005). *The adult learner: The definitive classic in adult education and human resource development* (6th ed.). New York: Butterworth-Heinemann.

Lakein, A. (1973). *How to get control of your time and your life.* New York: New American Library-Dutton.

Landsberger, J. (2011). Time management. *Study Guides Strategies.* <www.studygs.net/timman.htm>.

Leung-Chen, P. (2008). Everybody's crying MRSA. *American Journal of Nursing,* 108(8), 29–31.

Lieberman, S, Berardo, K. (2008). Closing age gaps. *ADVANCE for Nurses,* <http://nursing.advanceweb.com/Article/Closing-Age-Gaps.aspx>.

Maxworthy, J. (2008). *The dirty hands of health care: What would Florence think?* <www.reflectionsonnursingleadership.org/pages/SplashAuthors.aspx?_stht=Juli%20C.%20Maxworthy>.

Nelson, A, Fragala, G, Menzel, N. (2003). Myths and facts about back injuries in nursing. *American Journal of Nursing,* 103(2), 32–41.

National Institute on Alcohol Abuse and Alcoholism (NIAAA). (2009). *A snapshot of annual high-risk college drinking consequences.* <www.collegedrinkingprevention.gov/StatsSummaries/snapshot.aspx>.

Olson, M. (2009). The millennials: First year in practice. *Nursing Outlook,* (1), 10–17.

Palfrey, J, Gasser, U. (2008). *Born digital: Understanding the first generation of digital natives.* NY: Basic Books: A Member of the Perseus Books Group.

Rettner, R. (2011). *Deadly drug-resistant bacteria found in L.A.* <www.livescience.com/35570-drug-resistant-bacteria-los-angeles.html>.

Rothrock, J. C. (2006). What are the current guidelines about wearing artificial nails and nail polish in the healthcare setting? *Medscape,* <www.medscape.com/viewarticle/547793>.

Sack, D. (2013). *5 myths about addiction that undermine recovery.* <www.psychologytoday.com/blog/where-science-meets-the-steps/201305/5-myths-about-addiction-undermine-recovery>.

Sagon, C. (2014). Ebola's here, should you be worried? *AARP Bulletin Today,* <http://blog.aarp.org/2014/10/01/ebolas-here-should-you-be-worried/>.

Sagon, C. (2014). Hopsital infections kill 200 patients per day. *AARP Health Talk,* <http://blog.aarp.org/2014/03/27/hospital-infections-kill-200-patients-a-day/>.

Skiba, D, Barton, A. (2006). Adapting your teaching to accommodate the next generation of learners. *OJIN: The Online Journal of Issues in Nursing,* 11(2), Manuscript 4.

Study Guides and Strategies. (1996). *How to deal with stress.* <www.studygs.net/stress.htm>.

Tierro, P. (2007). *Germ-fighting secrets: A leading microbiologist tells how to stay healthy*. Boulder, CO: Bottom Line.

Townsend, A. (2014). *Hospital's hand washing strategies effective in reducing patient infection rates*. <www.cleveland.com/healthfit/index.ssf/2014/08/hospitals_hand_washing_strategies_effective_in_reducing_patient_infection_rates.html>.

United States Department of Agriculture (USDA) Press Release. (2011). *USDA and HHS announces new dietary guidelines to help Americans make healthier food choices and confront obesity epidemic*. USDA. <www.choosemyplate.gov>.

United States Department of Agriculture (USDA). (2011). *First Lady and agriculture secretary Vilsack to launch new food icon as a reminder to help consumers make healthier food choices*. <www.usda.gov/wps/portal/usda/usdamediafb?contentid=2011/06/0225.xml&printable=true&contentidonly=true>.

United States Department of Agriculture (USDA). (2015). *Dietary Guidelines.gov. Guidelines for Americans*. <www.cnpp.usda.gov/DietaryGuidelines>.

U.S. Department of Agriculture and U.S. Department of Health and Human Services. (2010). Dietary Guidelines for Americans, 2010. 7th Edition, Washington, DC: U.S. Government Printing Office. <http://health.gov/dietaryguidelines/2010/>

University of Maryland Medical Center. (2007). *What are some specific stress reduction methods?* <www.umm.edu/patended/articles/>.

WebMD. <www.webmd.com>.

Weiss, B. (2005). Winning the battle with addiction. *RN*, 68(7), 63–66.

Wu, D, Cal, J, Liu, J. (2011). Risk factors for the acquisition of nosocomial infection with carbapenem-resistant *Klebsiella pneumoniae*. *South Med Journal*, 104(2), 106–110.

Yamamoto, L, Marten, M. (2007). Listen up, MRSA. The bug stops here. *Nursing*, 37(12), 55–56.

CHAPTER 2

Baron-Cohen, S. (2003). *They just can't help it*. <www.theguardian.com/education/2003/apr/17/research.highereducation>.

Barsch, J. (1999). *Understanding your learning preference*. Ventura, CA: Ventura College Learning Disability Clinic.

Billings, D, Halstead, J. (2009). *Teaching in nursing*. St. Louis: Elsevier/Saunders.

Burke, M, Harper, J. (2010). I've arrived in cyberspace: Have you seen my lecture? *Nurse Educator*, 35(3), 101–102.

Byrne, M. (2001). Uncovering racial bias in nursing fundamentals textbooks. *Nurse Health Care Perspect*, 22(6), 299–303.

Carey, B. (2010). Forget what you know about good study habits. *The New York Times*, <www.nytimes.com/2010/09/07/health/views/07mind.html?pagewanted=all>.

Chatterbean. (2007). *Are you a right-brain thinker?* <www.chatterbean.com/newsroom/Thinking_Style.php>.

Chenevert, M. (2011). *Mosby's tour guide to nursing school: A student's road survival kit*. St. Louis: Mosby.

Clinton, P. (2000). The crisis you don't know about. In Book 4th anniversary issue. (pp. L4–L11).

Craig, E. (2009). *Personal digital assistants and smart phones: Clinical tools for nurses*. From Medscape Multispecialty. <www.medscape.com/viewarticle/709144>.

Cunningham, D. (2010). Incorporating medium fidelity simulation in a practical nurse education program. *Journal of Practical Nursing*, 60(1), 2–5.

Delpier, T. (2006). Cases 101: Learning to teach with cases. *Nurs Educ Perspect*, 27(4), 204–209.

deWitt, S. (2014). *Virtual clinical excursions—General hospital*.

deWitt, S., Williams, P. Fundamental concepts and skills for nursing (4th ed.). St. Louis: Elsevier.

Dryden, G, Vos, J. (2010). *Check your personal thinking style. Based on research from Gregoric*. <www.thelearningweb.net/personalthink.html>.

Dryden, G, Vos, J. (2010). *Learning styles: Learning methods to identify and build on your strengths*. <www.thelearningweb.net>.

Duffy, M. (2011). Facebook, Twitter, and LinkedIn, oh my! *American Journal of Nursing*, 111(4), 56–59, 2011.

Eagleman, D. (2007). 10 unsolved mysteries of the brain. *Discover*. <http://discovermagazine.com/2007/aug/unsolved-brain-mysteries>.

Felder, R, Soloman, B. (April 11, 2007). *Learning styles and strategies*. <www4.ncsu.edu/unity/lockers/users/f/felder/public/ILSdir/styles.htm>.

Felder-Silverman Model. (April 11, 2007). *Learning styles*. <www4.ncsu.edu/unity/lockers/users/f/felder/public/Learning_Styles.html>.

Filer, D. (2010). Using technology to increase classroom participation. *Nursing Education Perspectives*, 31(4): 247–250.

Gardner, H, Hatch, T. (1990). *Multiple intelligences go to school: Educational implications of the theory of multiple intelligences*. (Technical Report No. 4). New York: Center for Technology in Education.

Gardner, H. (1999). *Intelligence reframed: Multiple intelligences for the 21st century*. New York: Basic Books: a member of the Perseus Books Group.

Gurian, M. (1997). *The wonder of boys*. New York: Jeremy P. Tarcher/Putnum.

Hallowell, E, Ratey, J. (2010). *Adult ADHD: 50 tips on management*. <www.addresources.org/>.

Hallowell, E, Ratey, J. (2010). *50 tips on the management of adult deficit disorder*. <www.faslink.org/adhdtips.htm>.

Houghton Mifflin College. (2010). Thinking and Learning Styles. Retrieved from ISD-Development. *Learning styles or, how we go from the unknown to the known*. <www.itu.dk/~metteott/ITU_stud/Speciale/L%E6ring/learningStyles/Learning%20styles1.doc>.

Jensen, E. (1998). *The learning brain. Teaching with the brain in mind*. Alexandria, VA: Association for Supervision and Curriculum Development.

Kelly, K, Ramundo, P. (1993). *You mean I'm not lazy, stupid or crazy?!* New York: Scribner.

Kett, A.R. Social Networking for Student Nurses. *Nursing Times.net*. <www.nursingtimes.net/social-networking-for-student-nurses/5018573.fullarticle>.

King, V. (2010). *Learning & thinking styles*. <www.hoagiesgifted.org/>.

Levine, J, Young, M. (2010). *The Internet for dummies*. Indianapolis, IN: Wiley.

Lim, F. (2010). I simulate. Therefore I am nursed. *American Journal of Nursing*, 110(9), 72, 2010.

Mastersportal. (2014). What type of learner are you? (2010). <http://www.mastersportal.eu/articles/905/what-kind-of-learner-are-you-identifying-your-preferred-learning-styles-and-methods.html>.

National League for Nursing Board of Governors (Position Statement). (2008). *Preparing the next generation of nurses to practice in a technology-rich environment: An informatics agenda*. NLN. <http://www.nln.org/docs/default-source/professional-development-programs/preparing-the-next-generation-of-nurses.pdf?sfvrsn=6>.

Patillo, R.E. (2011). How private is your Facebook? *Nurse Educator*, 36(3), 102.

Paul, R, Elder, L. (2002). *Critical thinking: Tools for taking charge of your personal and professional life*. Upper Saddle River, NJ: Financial Times Prentice Hall.

Pauk, W, Owens, J. (2010). *How to study in college* (10th ed.). Independence, KY: Wadsworth Publishing.

Reis, R. (2005). *Learning styles. Tomorrow's professor listserv*. <www.fresnostate.edu/academics/csalt/documents/DisplayingaPersonalInterestinStudentsandTheirLearning.pdf>.

Staton, T. (1959). *How to study*. Circle Pines, MN: American Guidance Service, Inc.

Springer, S, Deuttsch, G. (2001). Attempts at applying asymmetry. Hemisphericity, education, and culture. *Left brain right brain: A perspective on cognitive neuroscience* (5th ed.). New York: W.H. Freeman & Co.

Springer, S, Deutsch, G. *Left brain right brain: A perspective on cognitive neuroscience* (5th ed.). New York: W.H. Freeman & Co.

Williams, M, Dittmer, A. (2009). Textbooks on tap: Using electronic books housed in electronic devices in nursing clinical courses. *Nursing Education Perspectives*, 30(4), 220–225.

Wink, D. (2010). Online lectures. *Nurse Educator*, 35(3), 95–97.

Wink, D. (2010). Social networking sites. *Nurse Educator*, 35(2), 49–51.

Wink, D. (2010). Teaching with technology: Automatically receiving information from the Internet and web. *Nurse Educator*, 35(4), 141–143, 2010.

Wink, D, Killingsworth, E. (2010). Organizing use of library technology. *Nurse Educator*, 36(2), 48–51, 2010.

CHAPTER 3

Disability.gov. <www.disability.gov>.

Office of Vocational Rehab. <www.portal.state.pa.us/portal/server.pt/community/vocational_rehabilitation/10356>.

Workforce Development Board. <www.chesco.org/159/Workforce-Development-Board>.

CHAPTER 4

ANA Report. (1944). Trained attendants and practical nurses. *American Journal of Nursing*, 44(1), 7–8.

Backer, B. (1993). The Nightingale pledge: A commitment that survives the passage of time. *Nurs Health Care*, 14, 3.

Brown, E. (1948). *Nursing for the future*. New York: Russell Sage Foundation.

D'Antonio, P. (1997). Nineteenth century nursing: Science, and the values of duty, will and power. *Reflections*, 23(3), 16–17.

Deloughery, G. (1998). *Issues and trends in nursing* (3rd ed.). St. Louis: Mosby.

Deming, D. (1994). Practical nurses—A professional responsibility. *American Journal of Nursing*, 44, 36–43.

Desch, E, Doherty, M. E. (2010). Experiences of U. S. military nurses in Iraq and Afghanistan Wars, 2003–2009. *Nursing Scholarship*, 42(1), 3–12.

Donahue, M. P. (1985). *Nursing, the finest art*. St. Louis: C.V. Mosby.

Donley, R., Flaherty, M. (2002). Revisiting the American Nurses Association's first position on education for nurses. *Online J Issues Nursing*. <www.nursingworld.org/MainMenuCategories/ANAMarketplace/ANAPeriodicals/OJIN/TableofContents/vol132008/No2May08/ArticlePreviousTopic/EntryIntoPracticeUpdate.html>.

Dryden, P. (2002). *Afghanistan: Nursing in a war zone*. <www.medscape.com/viewarticle/433919>.

Dryden, P. (2004). *Nursing in Iraq: Starting from scratch*. <www.medscape.com/viewarticle/470849>.

Fahy, E. (1993). Covering the history of nursing. *Nurs Health Care*, 14(3), 115.

Frantz, A. (1998). Nursing pride: Clara Barton in the Spanish-American War. *American Journal of Nursing*, 98(10), 39–41.

Go, P. (2009). *Role of Canadian Nurses in World War One*. <http://ezinearticles.com/?Role-of-Canadian-Nurses-in-World-War-One&id=2631265>.

Goldsmith, J. (1942). New York's practical nurse program. *American Journal of Nursing*, 42, 1026–1031.

Goldstein, J. (2001). *War and gender*. <http://catdir.loc.gov/catdir/samples/cam031/2001277554.pdf>.

Gosnell, D. (2002). Overview and summary: The 1965 entry into practice proposal—Is it relevant today? *Online J Issues Nurs*, 7(2). <www.nursingworld.org/MainMenuCategories/ANAMarketplace/ANAPeriodicals/OJIN/TableofContents/Volume72002/No2May2002/EntryIntoPracticeOverview.html>.

James, E. (2003). *Legacy lives on in advance for nurses*. 5(12), 11. <http://nursing.advanceweb.com/Article/Legacy-Lives-On.aspx>.

Joel, L. (2002). Education for entry into nursing practice: Revisited for the 21st century. *Online J Issues Nurs*, 7(2), <www.nursingworld.org/MainMenuCategories/ANA-Marketplace/ANAPeriodicals/OJIN/TableofContents/Volume72002/No2May2002/EntryintoNursingPractice.aspx>.

Kalish, P, Kalish, B. (1995). *The advance of American nursing* (3rd ed.). Boston: Little, Brown.

Kinder, J. (1986). President NLN. *Letter*.

LeVasseur, J. (1998). Plato, Nightingale, and contemporary nursing. *IMAGE: Journal of Nursing Scholarship*, 30(3), 281–285.

Longfellow, H. W. (1975). *The political works of Longfellow*. Cambridge ed. Boston: Houghton-Mifflin.

Martinez, O. L. (2010). *The Honor Society of Vietnam War Nurses*, (posted April 24, 2010). <www.experienceproject.com/stories/Am-A-Registered-Nu>.

McGuane, E, Bullough, B. (1992). Proud history, promising future. *Pract Nurs*, 42(4), 40–42.

Metules, T. (1998). Pins and pinning—The traditions continue. *RN*, 61(12), 49–50.

National Archives and Records Administration. (2012). *Records of Nurse Casualties in the Korean War*.<www.archives.gov/research/military/korean-war/nurses.html>.

Nightingale, F. (2009). *Notes on nursing*. Reprinted New York: Fall River Press.

NLN Research and Policy. (1994). Practical nursing's role in a community-based health care system. *Prism: NLN*, 2, 1–8.

Philips, E. C. (1944). Practical nurses in a public health agency. *American Journal of Nursing*, 44(10), 974–975.

Pillitteri, A. (1994). One nursing curriculum 100 years ago: A retrospective view as a prospective necessity. *J Nurs Ed*, 33(6), 286–287.

Romanoff, B. (2006). Facts about Flo you may not know. *Nurse Week*, 7(3), 32–33.

Russel, L. (1987). *Women in Vietnam*. <www.tourofdutyinfo.com/Notebook.htm>.

Server, S. (1998). The story of the lamp. *Am J Pract Nurs*, 5(1).

Seymour, M. (2004). Nightingale's nurses aides. *The New York Times*, <www.nytimes.com/2004/10/24/books/review/24SEYMOUR.html?_r=0>.

Sigma Theta Tau International. (2006). *Helping nurses help others*. Indianapolis: Nursing Knowledge International. Sigma Theta Tau, 3rd/4th Quarter, 3, 3.

Thompson, M. (1955). *The cry and the covenant*. New York: Signet Books.

U.S. Army Center of Military History. (2003). *The Army Nurse Corps in World War II*. <www.history.army.mil/books/wwii/72–14/72–14HTM>.

Vanfosson, C. (2011). Letters from Afghanistan: Daily Life and "Dirty" Work. *AJN*, 111(2), 52–57.

West, I. J. The women of the Army Nurse Corps during the Vietnam War. *U.S. Army Center of Military History*. <www.vietnamwomensmemorial.org/pdf/iwest.pdf>

Widerquist, J. (1992). The spirituality of Florence Nightingale. *Nurs Res*, 41(1), 49–55.

Wilde, R. *Women in World War I*. <http://europeanhistory.about.com/od/worldwar1/a/ww1women.htm>. Accessed December 30, 2010.

Wilson, B. (2011). Women in the Korean Conflict. *Women in War*, <http://userpages.aug.com/captbarb/femvets6.html>.

Wilson, B. (2011). WWI thirty thousand women were there. *Women in War*, <http://userpages.aug.com/captbarb/femvets4.html>.

Yourk, D. (2008). *American Nurse Today. Nursing in Afghanistan: A cultural perspective*. <www.americannursetoday.com/nursing-in-afghanistan-a-cultural-perspective/>.

CHAPTER 5

Alfaro-LeFevre, R. (2000). *Applying nursing process: Promoting collaborative care* (5th ed.). Philadelphia: Lippincott.

Alfaro-LeFevre, R. (2003). Improving your ability to think critically. *Healthcare Traveler*, 11(1), 72–76.

Austhink Software Pty Ltd., Australia. (2015). *Augment mapping and critical thinking.* <www.austhink.com/critical/>.

Bauer, B, Hill, S. (2000). *Mental health nursing: An introductory text* (2nd ed.). Philadelphia: WB Saunders.

Foundation of Critical Thinking. (2009). *Nursing and health care.* <www.criticalthinking.org/pages/nursing-and-health-care/801>.

Heaslip, P. (2008). *Critical thinking: To think like a nurse.* <www.criticalthinking.org/pages/critical-thinking-and-nursing/834>.

Ignatavicius, D, Workman, M. L. (2011). *Medical surgical nursing* (6th ed.) Philadelphia: WB Saunders.

Khosravani, S, Manoochehri, H, Memarian, R. (2004). Developing critical thinking skills in nursing students by group dynamics. *The Internet Journal of Advanced Practice Nursing*, 7(2).

Martin, C. (2002). The theory of critical thinking of nursing. *Nursing Education Perspective*, 23(5), 243–247.

CHAPTER 6

Armstrong, R. M. (2003). *Turning to Islam: African-American conversion stories.* Chicago: Christian Century.

Carpenter, A. (2007). Ethical suspicion and Katrina's nurses. *AJN*, 107(3), 15.

Christensen, B, Parker-Feliciano, K. (2011). Legal and ethical aspects of nursing. *Christenson & Kockrow's foundations and adult health nursing* (6th ed.). St. Louis: Mosby/Elsevier.

deWit, S. (2009). *Fundamental concepts and skills for nursing* (3rd ed.). Philadelphia: Saunders/Elsevier.

Haddad, A. (2005). Ethics in action. *RN*, 68(3), 31–32

Ham, K. (2000). Legal/ethical components of nursing. *From LPN to RN role transitions.* Philadelphia: WB Saunders.

Health workers can refuse to participate in procedures. (2003). *Midwest/Heartland NurseWeek.* 4, 3.

Rumbold, G. (2002). *Ethics in nursing practice.* Edinburgh: Elsevier Science Ltd.

Shannon, J. (2003). *Legal and ethical issues in counseling: A primer for mental health and substance abuse professionals.* Duluth, MN: Workshop.

Soglin, B. (2005). *Teaching medical students to examine ethics.* Iowa City: Spectator, University of Iowa.

Tyson, S. (2002). Ethical issues with age. *Gerontological nursing care.* Philadelphia: WB Saunders.

Venes, D. (Ed.) (2005). *Taber cyclopedic medical dictionary* (20th ed.). Philadelphia: FA Davis.

Ulrick, B. (1992). *Florence Nightingale leadership and management.* Norwalk, CT: Appleton and Lange.

CHAPTER 7

Alfaro-LeFevre, R. (2009). *Critical thinking and clinical judgment: A practical approach* (4th ed.). Philadelphia: WB Saunders.

American Hospital Association. (2003). *The patient care partnership: Understanding expectations, rights and responsibilities.*

Anderson, F. (2007). Finding HIPPA in your soup. *American Journal of Nursing*, 107(2), 66–71.

Brekken, S. (2014). *MN Board of Nursing.* <www.nursingboard.state.mn.us/>.

Charting Checkup. (2006). Making it clear with an incident report. *LPN*, 2(3), 17–19.

Christensen, E, Kockrow, E. (2011). *Foundations and adult health nursing* (6th ed.). St. Louis: Elsevier Mosby.

Cleveland Clinic Department of Bioethics. (2005). *Policy on do not resuscitate.* <www.clevelandclinic.org/bioethics/policies/dnr.html>.

Daly, B. J, Berry, D, Fitzpatrick J. J, et al. (1997). Assisted suicide: Implications for nurses and nursing. *Nurs Outlook*, 45: 209–214.

Dempski, K. (2000). If you have to give a deposition. *RN*, 63(1), 59–60.

deWit, S. (2009). *Fundamental concepts and skills for nursing* (2nd ed.). Philadelphia: Elsevier Saunders.

Gelfand, J. (2010). *The living will and durable power of attorney for health care.* <www.webmd.com/a-to-z-guides/frequently-asked-questions-about-advance-directives>.

Glazer, G. (1999). *Legislative and policy issues related to interstate practice.* <www.nursingworld.org/MainMenuCategories/ANAMarketplace/ANAPeriodicals/OJIN/TableofContents/Volume41999/No1May1999/InterstatePracticeStateBill.html>.

Glazer, G. (1999). *Multistate licensure: Overview and summary.* <www.nursingworld.org/MainMenuCategories/ANAMarketplace/ANAPeriodicals/OJIN/TableofContents/Volume41999/No1May1999/Overview.html>.

Hanawalt, A. (2001). End of life issues advanced directives—A health professional's guide to their use. *NFLPN*, 1(1), 8–11.

Helm, A, Kihm, N. (2006). Liability insurance: Is it for you? *LPN*, 2(3), 14–15.

Main, A, Todd, F. (2005). *Depositions 101.* Louisville, KY: American Bar Association Young Lawyers Division.

McNeil, D. (2003). *First study on patients who fast to end their lives.* <www.nytimes.com/2003/07/31/us/first-study-on-patients-who-fast-to-end-lives.html>.

Medline Plus. *Advance directives.* (2014). <https://www.nlm.nih.gov/medlineplus/advancedirectives.html>.

NAPNES. (2004). *Standards of practice for licensed practical/vocational nurses.* Silver Spring, MD: NAPNES.

National Council of State Boards of Nursing. (2011). *Filing a complaint.* <www.ncsbn.org/filing-a-complaint.htm>.

NiCastro, D. (2010). *HIPAA proposed rule—A breakdown.* <http://blogs.hcpro.com/hipaa/2010/07/hipaa-proposed-rule-a-breakdown/>.

O'Keefe M. (2001). *Nursing practice and the law: Avoiding malpractice and other legal risks.* Philadelphia: FA Davis.

Ryan, B, Sullivan, G, Mackay, T, et al. (2007). *RN*, 70(1), 26–31.

Starks, H, Dudzinski, D, White, W. (2013). Ethics in medicine. *Physician-aided suicide.* <http://depts.washington.edu/bioethx/topics/pad.html>.

U.S. Department of Health and Human Services. (2012). *The HIPAA privacy rule.* <www.hhs.gov/ocr/privacy/hipaa/administrative/privacyrule/>.

Ventura, M. J. (1999). Report tracks impact of Oregon's assisted suicide law. *RN*, 62(5), 16.

Ventura, M. J. (1999). When information must be revealed. *RN*, 62(2), 61–64.

(2007). You're on trial: How to protect yourself. *LPN*, 3(2), 16–18.

Zittel B. (2007). Profession update in teaching techniques. *ADVANCE for LPNs*, 7(5), New York Tri-State Area.

CHAPTER 8

Alessandra, T. (2005). Sixteen common-sense listening tips. *ADVANCE for LPNs.* <http://www.alessandra.com/freeresources/16CommonSenseListeningTips.asp>.

Arnold, E, Boggs, K. U. (2003). *Interpersonal relationships: professional communication skills for nurses* (4th ed.). Philadelphia: WB Saunders.

Banotai, A. (2007). Simplified strategies. *Advance Healthcare Network for Speech and Hearing.* <http://speech-language-pathology-audiology.advanceweb.com/Article/Simplified-Strategies.aspx>.

Carey, B. (2005). *In the hospital, a degrading shift from person to patient.* New York: The New York Times. <www.nytimes.com/2005/08/16/health/in-the-hospital-a-degrading-shift-from-person-to-patient.html>.

Carson, V. B. (2000). The vehicle for healing: Communication as part of a therapeutic relationship.

Carson, V. B., ed. *Mental health nursing, the nurse-patient journey* (2nd ed.). Philadelphia: WB Saunders.

Christenson, B, Kockrow, E. (2011). *Foundations and adult health nursing* (6th ed.). St. Louis: Elsevier.

Gurian, M. (1997). *The wonder of boys*. New York: Jeremy P. Tacher/Putnam.

Mascioli, S, Laskowski-Jones, L, Urban, S, Moran, S. (2009). Improving handoff communication. February. *Nursing*, 39(2), 52–55.

Newsroom. (2015). Medical errors drop with improved communication during hospital shift changes. Washington University in St. Louis. <http://news.wustl.edu/news/Pages/27628.aspx>.

Pagana, K. (2008). *The nurse's etiquette advantage*. Indianapolis: Sigma Theta Tau.

Pope, B. B, Rodzen, L, Spross, G. (2008). Raising the SBAR. *Nursing*, 38(3), 41–43.

Ustun, B. (2008). Communication skills training as part of a problem-based learning curriculum. *J Nurs Educ*, 45(10), 421–424.

CHAPTER 9

Belanger, D. (2000). Nurses and suicide: The risk is real. *RN*, 63(10), 61–64.

Carrol, V. (1997). Health and safety in workplace violence. *Sm J Nurs*, 99(3).

Center for American Nurses (2008). *Lateral violence and bullying in the work place*. <www.mc.vanderbilt.edu/root/pdfs/nursing/center_lateral_violence_and_bullying_position_statement_from_center_for_american_nurses.pdf>.

Demers, J. (2015). *10 Signs you are headed for burnout*. </www.inc.com/jayson-demers/10-signs-you-re-headed-for-burnout.html>.

Jahner, J. (2011). *Building bridges: An inquiry into horizontal hostility in nursing culture and the use of contemplative practices to facilitate cultural change*. <www.upaya.org/uploads/pdfs/Jahnersthesis.pdf>.

Kurz, J. (2002). Combating sexual harassment. *RN*, 65(7), 65–68.

Levine, P, Hewitt, J, Misner, S. (1998). Insights of nurses about assault in hospital-based emergency rooms. *Image J Nurs Schol*, 30(3), 9–10.

Lipson, J, Dibble, S. (2006). *Culture and clinical care*. San Francisco: Nursing Press.

McKay, D. (2011). *Job burnout: Causes, symptoms and cures.* <http://careerplanning.about.com>.

National Council State Boards of Nursing (NCSBN). (2012). The Nurse Licensure Compact. <www.ncsbn.org/nlc.htm>.

Needleman, J. Buerhaus, P. (2003). Nurse staffing and patient safety: Current knowledge and implications for safety. *Int J Quality Health Care*, 15:275–277. <http://intqhc.oxfordjournals.org/content/15/4/275>.

New York State Nurse Association. (2011). *Position statement. Workplace violence.* <http://www.nysna.org/position-statement-workplace-violence#.V2oXPldzrdk>.

Pagana, K. (2008). *The nurse's etiquette advantage*. Indianapolis, IN: Sigma Theta Tau.

Patients Rights Council. (2013). *Frequently Asked Questions/Patient Rights Council.* <http://www.patientsrightscouncil.org/site/frequently-asked-questions/>.

Patients Rights Council. (2013). *Montana.* <http://www.patientsrightscouncil.org/site/montana/>.

U.S. Department of Labor. (2004). *OSHA guidelines for preventing workplace violence for health care and social service workers.* <www.osha.gov>.

CHAPTER 10

Carroll, R. (March 1, 2011). The evil eye. *The skeptic's dictionary.* <http://skepdic.com/evileye.html>.

Cook, L. (2010). Convicted: The job description doesn't say you get to choose your patients. *American Journal of Nursing*, 110(3), 72.

Culver, V. (1974). *Modern bedside care* (8th ed.). Philadelphia: WB Saunders.

D'Avanzo, C, Geissler, E. (2008). *Pocket guide to cultural assessment*. St. Louis: Mosby.

deWit, S. (2007). Medical-surgical nursing: Concepts and practice. Philadelphia: WB Saunders.

Darrah, J. (2009). Expanding the diversity definition: LTC facilities are learning how to better accommodate the LGBT population. *Advance for LPNs*, 9(2), 9.

Dibble, S, Robertson, P. (2010). *Lesbian health 101: A clinician's guide*. San Francisco: UCSF Nursing Press.

Eliason, M, Dibble, S, DeJoseph, J, Chinn, P. (2012). LGBTQ issues in nursing. *Nursing Made Incredibly Easy*, 10(2), 4.

Fadiman. A. (1997). *The spirit catches you and you fall down*. New York: Farrar, Strauss, and Giroux.

Foster, G. (1978). *Medical anthropology*. New York: John Wiley and Sons.

Goulette, C. (2010). Cultural competence and kids: Sensitivity to patients' needs is a must for pediatric nurses. *Advance for Nurses*. <http://nursing.advanceweb.com/Regional-Articles/Features/Cultural-Competence-Kids-2.aspx>.

Hall, E. (1973). *The silent language*. Westport, CT: Greenwood Press.

Hall, E. (1966). *The hidden dimension*. New York: Doubleday.

Honer, D, Hoppie, P. (2004). The enigma of the Gypsy patient. *RN*, 67(8), 33–36.

Jackson, L. (1993), Understanding, eliciting and negotiating patients' multicultural health beliefs. *Nurse Pract*, 18(4), 30–32, 37–43.

Jacobs, J. (2015). Workplace initiatives that promote diversity and inclusion. *Minority Nurse*, 44–45. <http://minoritynurse.com/workplace-initiatives-that-promote-diversity-and-inclusion/>.

Joyce, E, deGonzalez, M. (2004). *Say it in Spanish*. Philadelphia: WB Saunders.

Kutner, M, Greenberg, E, Jin, Y, Paulsen, C. (2006). *The health literacy of America's adults: Results from the 2003 National Assessment of Health Literacy*. National Center for Education Statistics. <https://nces.ed.gov/pubs2006/2006483.pdf>.

Leininger, M, McFarland, M. (2002). *Transcultural nursing: Concepts, theory, research, and practice*. New York: McGraw-Hill.

Lipson, J, Dibble, S. (2006). *Culture and clinical care*. San Francisco: UCSF Nursing Press.

Murphy, K. (2011). The importance of cultural competence. *Nursing Made Incredibly Easy*, 9(2), 5.

Narayan, M. (2010). Culture's effects on pain assessment and management: Cultural patterns influence nurses' and their patients' responses to pain. *American Journal of Nursing*, 110(4), 38–45.

Pagana, K. (2008). *The nurse's etiquette advantage*. Indianapolis: Sigma Theta Tau International.

Randall-David, E. (1992). *Strategies for working with culturally diverse patients*. Bethesda, MD: Association for the Care of Children's Health.

Roberts, S. (2009). Projections put whites in minority by 2050. New York: New York Times, <www.nytimes.com/2009/12/18/us/18census.html?_r=0>.

Rodriguez, B. (1995). *Understanding and integrating cultural awareness and related issues into specialized health curricula*. Green Bay, WI: Seminar at Northeast Wisconsin Technical College.

Spector, R. (2003). *Cultural diversity in health and illness*. Englewood Cliffs, NJ: Prentice Hall.

Srivastava, R. (Ed.). (2007). *The healthcare professional's guide to clinical cultural competence*. Canada: Elsevier.

U.S. Census 2010. *Explore the form*. (2010). <http://www.census.gov/2010census/about/interactive-form.php>.

Varcarolis, E, Shoemaker, N. (2006). *Foundations of psychiatric-mental health nursing* (5th ed.). Philadelphia: Elsevier/Saunders.

Yen, H. (2011). Census estimates show big gains for U.S. minorities. New York: Associated Press. <http://www.wcpo.com/news/national/census-estimates-show-big-gains-for-us-minorities>.

Yoder-Wise, P. (2011). *Leading and managing in nursing*. St. Louis: Mosby.

CHAPTER 11

Anonymous. (2007). Om. *ReligionFacts*. <www.religionfacts.com/hinduism/symbols/aum.htm>.

Anonymous. (2010). Christian crosses. *Religion Facts*. <www.religionfacts.com/christianity/symbols/cross.htm>.

Anonymous. (2010). Islamic symbols. *Religion Facts*. <www.religionfacts.com/islam/symbols.htm>.

Atwood, D, Mead, F, Hill, S. (2010). *Handbook of denominations in the United States*. Nashville, TN: Abingdon Press.

Armstrong, K. (2001). *Buddha*. New York: Penguin Group Penguin Putnam.

Armstrong, K. (2000). *Islam*. New York: Random House.

Baha'ism. (2007). *The Columbia electronic encyclopedia* (6th ed.). New York: Columbia University Press.

Bauer, B, Hill, S. (2000). *Mental health nursing: An introductory text*. Philadelphia: WB Saunders.

Bowker, J. (Ed.). (2007). *The Oxford dictionary of world religions*. Cambridge, MA: Oxford University Press.

Carson, V. (1989). *Spiritual dimensions of nursing practice*. Philadelphia: WB Saunders.

Christian Science. (2011). *The Columbia electronic encyclopedia* (6th ed.). New York: Columbia University Press. <www.infoplease.com/ce6/society/A0812103.html>.

D'Avanzo, C, Geissler, E. (2003). *Pocket guide to cultural assessment*. St. Louis: Mosby.

Episcopal Church. (2011). *The Columbia Electronic Encyclopedia* (6th ed.). New York: Columbia University Press. <www.infoplease.com/ce6/society/A0817503.html>.

Esposito, J. (1998). *Islam: The straight path*. New York: Oxford University Press.

Gellman, M, Hartman, T. (2002). *Religion for dummies*. New York: Wiley.

General Conference of Seventh-day Adventists. (2016). *Beliefs*. <www.adventist.org/beliefs/index.html>.

Gerardi, R. (1989). Western spirituality and health care. In V. Carson (Ed.), *Spiritual dimensions of nursing practice*. Philadelphia: WB Saunders.

Gritsch, E. (2002). *A history of Lutheranism*. Minneapolis: Augsburg Fortress.

Grossman, C. (2011). Number of U.S. Muslims to double. *USA Today*. <http://usatoday30.usatoday.com/news/religion/2011-01-27-1Amuslim27_ST_N.htm>.

Grossman, C. (2015). *The future map of religion reveals a world of change for Christians, Muslims and Jews*. <www.religionnews.com/2015/04/02/future-map-religions-reveals-world-change-christians-muslims-jews/>

Harderwijk, R. (2011). *A view on Buddhism*. <http://viewonbuddhism.org/4_noble_truths.html>.

Islamic Food and Nutrition Council. (2015). *What is Halal?* <http://www.ifanca.org/Pages/Faq.aspx>.

Leininger, M, McFarland, M. (2002). *Transcultural nursing: Concepts, theory, research, and practice*. New York: Hill.

Lewis, B. (2003). *The crisis of Islam*. New York: Modern Library.

Lindner, E. W. (2010). *Yearbook of American and Canadian churches 2010*. Nashville: Abingdon Press.

Lipson, J, Dibble, S. (2006). *Culture and nursing care: A pocket guide*. San Francisco: The Regents of the University of California.

McCurdy, D. (2008). Ethical spiritual care at the end of life. *American Journal of Nursing*, 108(5), 11.

Mennonite Church. (2015). *Who we are—A quick visual guide*. <http://mennoniteusa.org/who-we-are/>.

More Good Foundation. (1998). *Mormon underwear*. <www.ldschurchtemples.com/mormon/underwear/>.

National Council of Churches. (2011). Yearbook of American and Canadian Churches. Nashville: Abingdon Press.

Nomani, A. (2005). *Standing alone in Mecca*. New York: Harper Collins Publishers, Inc.

Ontario Consultants on Religious Tolerance. (2010). *Hinduism: The world's third largest religion*. <www.religioustolerance.org/hinduism.htm>.

Pennington, R. (2009). *Do Muslims observe the Sabbath?* <http://muslimvoices.org/do-muslims-observe-the-sabbath/>.

Pentecostalism. (2011). *The Columbia electronic encyclopedia* (6th ed.). New York: University Press. <www.infoplease.com/ce6/society/A0838204.html>.

Religious Society of Friends. (2011). *The Columbia Electronic Encyclopedia* (6th ed.). New York: Columbia University Press. <www.infoplease.com/ce6/society/A0819726.html>.

Rich, T. (2012). *Star of David*. <www.jewishvirtuallibrary.org/jsource/Judaism/star.html>.

Rocca, F. (2011). Vatican: Number of Catholics is up, still behind Muslims. *USA Today*. <www.usatoday.com/news/religion/2011-02-23-catholic_vatican_22_ST_N.htm?csp=34&utm_source=feedburner&utm_medium=email&utm_campaign=Feed%3Aþ Religion-TopStoriesþ%28Newsþ-þ Religionþ-þTopþStories%29>.

Schoenbeck, S. (1994). Called to care: Addressing the spiritual needs of patients. *J Pract Nurs*, 44, 19–23.

Sheskin, I, Dashefsky, A. (2006). Jewish population of the United States. *American Jewish Year Book*, 106, 133–193.

Society of St. Pius X. (2011). *What is the Society of St. Pius X?* <http://sspx.org>.

Sumner, C. (1998). Recognizing and responding to spiritual distress. *American Journal of Nursing*, 98(1), 26–30.

United Church of Christ. (2011). *Testimonies, not tests of the faith*. <www.ucc.org/beliefs/>.

United Methodist Church. (2012). *The Columbia Electronic Encyclopedia* (6th ed.). New York: Columbia University Press. <http://www.infoplease.com/encyclopedia/society/united-methodist-church.html>.

United States Conference of Catholic Bishops. (2006). *Compendium of the catechism of the Catholic Church*. Washington, D.C.: USCCB Publishing.

Wendt, K. (2010). *Report on findings from the 2009 LPN/LVN practice analysis: Linking the NCLEX-PN examination to practice*. Chicago: National Council of State Boards of Nursing, Inc.

Wisegeek. (2011). *Why do Some Muslim women wear head scarves?* <www.wisegeek.org/why-do-some-muslim-women-wear-head-scarves.htm>.

Yearbook of American and Canadian Churches. (2011). *National Council of Churches in the USA*: Abingdon Press.

CHAPTER 12

Alfaro-LeFevre, R. (2002). *Applying nursing process: Promoting collaborative care* (5th ed.). Philadelphia: Lippincott.

Christensen, B, Kockrow, E. (2011). *Foundations and adult health nursing* (6th ed.). St. Louis: Mosby.

Frederick, J, Scherb, C A, Smith-Foreman, K, et al. (2002). Speaking a common language. *American Journal of Nursing*, 101(3), 2400.

Gordon, M. (1998). Nursing nomenclature and classification system development. *Online Journal of Issues in Nursing*, 3(2).

Ham, K. (2002). *From LPN to RN: Role transitions* (Ch. 7). Philadelphia: WB Saunders.

Herdman, T. H. (2008). Nursing diagnosis: Is it time for a new definition? *Int J Nurs Terminol Classif*, 19(1), 2–13.

Johnson, M, Bulechek, G, Dochterman, J, et al. (2006). *Nursing diagnoses, outcomes, and interventions: NANDA, NOC and NIC Linkages* (2nd ed.). St. Louis: Mosby.

Johnson, M, Bulechek, G, Doterman, J, et al. (2006). *NANDA, NOC, and NIC LINKAGES* (2nd ed.). St. Louis: Mosby-Elsevier.

Maslow, A. (1943). A theory of human motivation. *Psych Rev*, 50, 370.

McCloskey, J. C, Bulechek, G. M. (2000). *Nursing interventions classification* (3rd ed.). St. Louis: Mosby.

Nursing Degrees. (1999). *Study tips from former nursing students.* <www.nursingdegrees.com/study-tips.htm>.

National Association for Practical Nurse Education and Service (NAPNES). (2007). Standards of practice and educational competencies of graduates of practical/vocational nursing programs. *JPN*, 57(2), 20–22.

National Council of State Boards of Nursing (NCSBN). (1998). Implementation of the 1999 NCLEX-PN test plan. *Issues.* Chicago: NCSBN. (pp. 4–5).

National Council of State Boards of Nursing (NCSBN). (2007). *NCLEX-PN® test plan for the National Council Licensure Examination for Practical Nurses.* Chicago: NCSBN.

National Council of State Boards of Nursing (NCSBN). (2010). *NCLEX-PN® test plan for the National Council Licensure Examination for Practical/Vocational Nurses.* Chicago: NCSBN.

CHAPTER 13

Ackley, B. J, Ladwig, G. B, Swan, B. A, Tucker, S. J. (2008). *Evidence-based nursing care guidelines.* St. Louis: Elsevier/Mosby.

Alligood, M. (2010). *Nursing theory: Utilization and application* (4th ed.). Mosby: Elsevier.

Burns, N, Grove, S. (2011). *Understanding nursing research: Building an evidence-based practice.* St. Louis: Elsevier/ Saunders.

Cherry, B, Jacob, S. (2011). *Contemporary nursing: Issues and trends, and management.* St. Louis: Elsevier/Mosby.

Chinn, P, Kramer, M. (2011). *Integrated theory and knowledge development in nursing* (8th ed.). Philadelphia: Elsevier.

deWit, S. (2009). *Fundamental concepts and skills for nursing* (3rd ed.). Philadelphia: Saunders/Elsevier.

Massey, V. (1998). Theories and models in nursing practice. In J. Leahy & P. Kizilay (Eds.), *Foundations of nursing practice.* Philadelphia: WB Saunders.

Mazurek, B, Fineout-Overholt, E. (2011). *Evidence-based practice in nursing and healthcare: A guide to best practice.* Philadelphia: Wolters Kluwer Health/Lippincott Williams and Wilkins.

Motacki, K, & Burke, K. (2011). *Nursing delegation and management of patient care.* St. Louis: Elsevier.

Nightingale, F. (1860). *Notes on nursing: What it is, and what it is not.* New York: D. Appleton and Company.

The Cochrane Collaboration. (June 12, 2011). *Working together to provide the best evidence in health care.* <www.cochrane.org/about-us>.

CHAPTER 14

American Nurses Credentialing Center (AANC). (2015). *AANC Nurse Certification.* <www.nursecredentialing.org/Certification.aspx#>.

Aiken, L. (2011). News for the future. *New England Journal of Medicine*, 364(3), 280–281.

American Nurses Association. (2015). *Nursing World.* <www.nursingworld.org>.

Clark, A. (2009). Advanced practice nursing. *American Journal of Nursing Career Guide*, 109(1), 17–18.

Cherry, B, Jacob, S. (2011). *Contemporary nursing: Issues, trends, and management.* St. Louis: Elsevier.

Doheny, K. (2009). How old is too old to work? Economic woes add a twist to the age-old question. <https://consumer.healthday.com/senior-citizen-information-31/misc-aging-news-10/how-old-is-too-old-to-work-623882.html>.

Gibson, S. (2009). Intergenerational communication in the classroom: Recommendations for successful teacher-student relationships. *Nursing Education Perspectives*, 30(1), 37–39.

Hader, R. (2009). Is being a chief nursing officer in your future? *NSNA imprint.* <www.nsna.org/Portals/0/Skins/NSNA/pdf/Imprint_Jan09_Feat_Hader.pdf>.

Kennedy, M. (2010). Don't call us, we'll call you: But will new nurses be available when we need them? *American Journal of Nursing*, 110(6), 7.

Mahaffey, E. (2002). The relevance of associate degree nursing education: Past, present, future. *Online Journal of Issues in Nursing*, 7(2), 11.

Mitchell, PH. (2008). Patient-centered care—a new focus on a time-honored concept. *Nursing Outlook*, 56(5), 197–198.

National Academies of Sciences, Engineering and Medicine. (2016). *About the Health and Medicine Division (formerly the IOM).* <http://www.nationalacademies.org/hmd/About-HMD.aspx>.

National League for Nursing. (2010). *Outcomes and competencies for graduates of practical/vocational, diploma, associate degree, baccalaureate, master's, practice doctorate, and research doctorate programs in nursing.* New York: NLN.

Nelson, R. (2010). The clinical nurse leader. *American Journal of Nursing*, 110(1), 22–23.

Northam, S. (2009). Conflict in the workplace (Part 1): Sex, age, hierarchy, and culture influence the nursing environment. *American Journal of Nursing*, 109(6), 70–73.

Nurse.com. (2015). *Nurses shortage not as severe, but more nurses needed.* <https://news.nurse.com/2015/10/15/nursing-shortage-not-as-severe-but-more-nurses-still-needed/>.

Seago, J, Spetz, J, Chapman, S, et al. (2004). *Supply, demand, and use of licensed practical nurses. Health Resources and Services Administration, Bureau of Health Professions.* Washington, DC: National Center for Health Workforce Analysis.

Sorrentino, S. (2011). *Mosby's textbook for long-term care nursing assistants.* St. Louis: Elsevier/Mosby.

Stokowski, L. (2008). Old, but not out: The aging nurse in today's workplace. *Medscape Multispeciality.* <www.medscape.com/viewarticle/585454>.

Willard, K, Haley-Moyer, C, Arbour, R. (2008). *Synergy model, role of clinical nurse.*

CHAPTER 15

Bauer, J. (2009). *Green house concept combines best new thinking for elderly.* Grand Rapids, MI: The Grand Rapids Press. <www.globalaging.org/elderrights/us/2009/green.htm>.

Brandeisky, K. (2015). Here's how much an average American worker has to pay for health care. Money. <http://time.com/money/4044394/average-health-deductible-premium/>.

Callantine, P, Sheridan, W. Y. (2011). *Green House Board, Task Force, and Chair of Operations Committee.*

Christensen, E, Kokrow, B. (2011). *Foundations of adult health nursing* (6th ed.). St. Louis: Mosby.

Day, T. (May 7, 2011). *What is long-term care?* <www.long-termcarelink.net/eldercare/long_term_care.htm>.

CHAPTER 16

Bihari, M. (2015). Patient rights—Health reform and patient's rights. *About Health.* <http://healthinsurance.about.com/od/reform/a/Health-Reform-And-Patients-Rights.htm>.

Brandeisky, K. (2015). Here's how much an average American worker has to pay for health care. Money. <http://time.com/money/4044394/average-health-deductible-premium/>.

Center for Medicare and Medicaid. (2013). *National Health Expenditure (NHE) Fact Sheet.* <www.cms.gov/research-statistics-data-and-systems/statistics-trends-and-reports/nationalhealthexpenddata/nhe-fact-sheet.html>.

Cherry, B, Jacob, S. (2011). *Contemporary nursing: Issues, trends, and management.* St. Louis: Elsevier.

Chester, H. (2011). What does health care reform mean for you. *Nursing Made Incredibly Easy!* 9(2), 6–9.

DeParle, N. (2011). The facts about the Independent Advisory Board. *The White House Blog*. <www.whitehouse.gov/blog/2011/04/20/facts-about-independent-payment-advisory-board>.

Federal officials try again to bolster plans for people with medical conditions. (2011). *Kaiser Health News*. <www.kaiserhealthnews.org/Features/Insuring-Your-Health/Michelle-Andrews-on-high-risk- plans.aspx>. Retrieved July 6, 2011.

Gawande, A. (2009). *The checklist manifesto: How to get things right*. NY: Metropolitan Books.

Health Reform Quiz. (2011). *The Henry J. Kaiser Family Foundation*. <http://healthreform.kff.org/quizzes/health-reform-quiz.aspx>.

Highlights from the National Healthcare Quality and Disparities Reports. (2012). *Agency for Healthcare Research and Quality*. <http://archive.ahrq.gov/research/findings/nhqrdr/nhdr12/>.

Hoadley, J. (2015). *Medicare Part D at ten years: The 2015 marketplace and key trends, 2006–2015*. <http://kff.org/medicare/report/medicare-part-d-at-ten-years-the-2015-marketplace-and-key-trends-2006-2015/>.

Holly, C. (2011). What does healthcare reform mean to you? *Nursing Made Incredibly Easy*, 9(2), 6–9.

Ip, G. (2010). *The little book of economics*. Hoboken: John Wiley and Sons.

Kaiser Health Foundation. (2015). *Costs for Medicare Advantage plans*. Kaiser Health News. <http://khn.org/news/michelle-andrews-on-high-risk-plans/>

Levitt, L, Pollitz, K, Claxton, G, Damico, A. (2013). How buying insurance will change under Obama care. <http://kff.org/health-reform/perspective/how-buying-insurance-will-change-under-obamacare/>.

Masson, D. (2011). What future for the affordable care act? *The American Journal of Nursing*, 111(1), 23–24.

Medicaid. (2011). *Annual report on the quality of care for children in Medicaid and CHIP*. <www.medicaid.gov/Medicaid-CHIP-Program-Information/By-Topics/Quality-of-Care/Downloads/2011_StateReporttoCongress.pdf>.

Prater, C. (2008). *15 tips for paying high medical bills: Negotiate before using credit cards to finance medical expenses*. <credit cards.com. www.creditcards.com/credit-card-news/medical-bill-payment-tips-1266.php>.

Schorn, D. (2009). FAQs on hospital bills. *Sixty Minutes*. <www.cbsnews.com/stories/2006/03/03/60minutes/main1369185.shtml>.

CHAPTER 17

Akrani, G. (2010). Frederic Herzberg's two factor theory—Motivation hygiene. <http://kalyan-city.blogspot.com/2010/06/frederick-herzberg-two-factor-theory.html>.

Bauer, B, Hill, S. (2000). *Mental health nursing: An introductory text*. Philadelphia: Elsevier.

Bennis, W. (2003). *On becoming a leader: The leadership classic—Updated and expanded*. Boulder, CO: Perseus Publishing.

Blanchard, K, Zigarmi, P, Zigarmi, D. (1994). *Leadership and the one minute manager*. UK: Clays Ltd.

Blanchard, K, Parisi-Carew, E. (2009). *The one minute manager builds high performance teams*. New York: Morrow.

Blanchard, K, Fowler, S, Hawkins, L. (2005). *Self leadership and the one minute manager: Increasing Effectiveness through Situational Self-Leadership*. NY: William Morrow/Harper Collins Publishers, Inc.

Blanchard, K, Johnson, S. (2000). *The one minute manager*. New York: Berkeley Publishing.

Blanchard, K, Oncken, W, Burrows, H. (1991). *The one minute manager meets the monkey*. New York: William Morrow and Co.

Chapman, A. (2016). *Frederick Herzberg's motivation and hygiene factors*. <www.businessballs.com/herzberg.htm>.

Cherry, B, Jacob, S. (2011). *Contemporary nursing: Issues, trends, and management*. St. Louis: Mosby, Inc.

Covey, S. (2004). *The 7 habits of highly effective people*. New York: Free Press.

Ellis, A. (1994). *Reason and emotion in psychotherapy*. New York: Carol Publishing Group.

Fisher, R, Ury, W, Patton, B. (1991). *Getting to yes: Negotiating agreement without giving in*. New York: Random House Business Books.

Hansten, R, Jackson, M. (2008). *Clinical delegation skills: A handbook for professional practice*. Boston: James and Bartlett.

Hansten, R, Washburn, M. (2001). Delegating to UAPs—Making it work. *Nurse Week*, 2(3), 21–22.

Hearthfield, S. (2011). *What people want from work: Motivation*. <http://humanresources.about.com/od/rewardrecognition/a/needs_work.htm>

Herzberg, F. (1993). *The motivation to work*. New Brunswick, NJ: Transaction Pubs.

Huber, D. (2010). *Leadership and nursing care management*. St. Louis: Elsevier.

Huston, C. (2009). 10 tips for successful delegation. *Nursing*, 39(3), 54–56.

Javitch, D. (2009). *5 employee motivation myths debunked*. <www.entrepreneur.com/humanresources/employeemanagement-columnistdavi djavitch/article202352.html>.

LaCharity, L, Kumagai, C, Bartz, B. (2006). *Prioritization, delegation, assignment*. St. Louis: Elsevier.

Linton, A. (2007). *Introduction to medical-surgical nursing*. St. Louis: Elsevier.

Maslow, A. (1998). *Maslow on management*. New York: John Wiley and Sons.

Motacki, K, Burke, K. (2011). *Nursing delegation and management of patient care*. St. Louis: Elsevier/Mosby.

National Council of State Boards of Nursing. (2005). *Working with others: A position paper*. (2005). <https://www.ncsbn.org/3945.htm>.

Pink, D. (2009). *Drive: The surprising truth about what motivates us*. New York: Riverhead Books.

Quality Improvement Organizations. U.S. (2015). *Department of Health and Human Services, Centers for Medicare & Medicaid Services*. <www.cms.gov/QualityImprovementOrgs/>.

Safer Healthcare Partners. (2010). *SBAR: A communication technique for today's healthcare professional*. <www.saferhealthcare.com/cat-shc/sbar-a-communication-technique>.

Sorrentino, S. (2011). *Mosby's textbook for long-term care assistants*. St. Louis: Mosby.

Ulrich, B. (1992). *Leadership and management according to Florence Nightingale*. Norwalk, CT: Appleton and Lange.

Ury, W. (1993). *Getting past no: Negotiating your way from confrontation to cooperation*. New York: Bantam Books.

Wywialowski, E. (2004). *Managing patient care*. St. Louis: Mosby.

Yoder-Wise, P. (2011). *Leading and managing in nursing*. St. Louis: Mosby.

Yoder-Wise, P, Hansten, R, Jackson, M. (2011). *Leading and managing in nursing*. St. Louis: Mosby.

CHAPTER 18

Ahl, ME. In, C. Lemburg, (Ed.), (1975). *Open learning and career mobility in nursing*. St. Louis: Mosby.

American Board of Managed Care Nursing (ABMCN). (1998). *What is the American Board of Managed Care Nursing?* <http://www.abmcn.org>.

Beshara, T. (2008). *Acing the interview: How to ask and answer the questions that will get you the job*. New York: AMACON.

Department of Veterans Affairs. (2016). *Licensed practical nursing*. <www.mycareeratva.va.gov/careers/career/062000>.

Fox News. (2010). *Teacher fired over Facebook post, 2010*. <http://video.foxnews.com/v/4316834/teacher-fired-over-facebook-post>.

Levinson, J, Perry, D. E. (2009). *Guerilla marketing for job hunters 2.0: 1001 unconventional tips, tricks, and tactics for landing your dream job.* Hoboken: John Wiley & Son, Inc.

National League for Nursing. (2013). *A vision for doctoral preparation for nurse educators.*<http://www.nln.org/docs/default-source/about/nln-vision-series-(position-statements)/nln-vision_6.pdf>.

Oliver, V. (2005). *301 smart answers to tough interview questions.* Naperville, IL: Source Books, Inc.

Pyrtle, B. (2009). Tips to recognize scam job ads. Minneapolis: *Star Tribune Newspaper*, Section W., WI.

Schepp, B, Schepp, D. (2010). *How to find a job on Linkedin, Facebook, Twitter, MySpace and other social networks.* New York, NY: McGraw-Hill.

Society for Human Resource Management. (2010). *Background checking: The implications of credit background checks on the decision to hire SHRM poll.* <https://www.shrm.org/research/surveyfindings/articles/pages/backgroundcheckingimplications.aspx>.

CHAPTER 19

Heisel, J. (2012). *Comprehensive review for NCLEX-PN examination.* St. Louis: Elsevier Saunders.

National Council State Boards of Nursing (NCSBN). (2011). *Dispelling NCLEX myths.* <http://mail.google.com/mail/?ui=2&ik=9621232bde&view=pt&se>.

National Council State Boards of Nursing (NCSBN). (2015). *Transitions to Practice toolkit.* <www.ncsbn.org/687.htr>.

Index